THE ENC

PHARMAC
DRUGS

THE ENCYCLOPEDIA OF

PHARMACEUTICAL DRUGS

THE ENCYCLOPEDIA OF

PHARMACEUTICAL DRUGS

Dana K. Cassell

and

Cynthia A. Sanoski, Pharm. D.

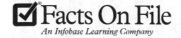

☑ Facts On File
An Infobase Learning Company

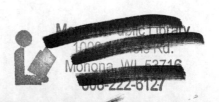

The Encyclopedia of Pharmaceutical Drugs

Facts On File
An imprint of Infobase Learning, Inc.
132 West 31st Street
New York NY 10001

Library of Congress Cataloging-in-Publication
Cassell, Dana K.
The encyclopedia of pharmaceutical drugs / Dana K. Cassell and Cynthia A. Sanoski.
p. cm.—(Library of health and living)
Includes bibliographical references and index.
ISBN-13: 978-0-8160-6287-4 (hardcover : alk. paper)
ISBN-10: 0-8160-6287-0 (hardcover : alk. paper) 1. Drugs—Encyclopedias, Juvenile.
I. Sanoski, Cynthia A. II. Title.
RM301.17.C37 2012
615'.103—dc22   2011005637

Facts On File books are available at special discounts when purchased in bulk quantities for businesses, associations, institutions, or sales promotions. Please call our Special Sales Department in New York at (212) 967-8800 or (800) 322-8755.

You can find Facts On File on the World Wide Web at http://www.factsonfile.com

Text design by Cathy Rincon
Composition by Hermitage Publishing Services
Cover printed by Yurchak Printing, Landisville, Pa.
Book printed and bound by Yurchak Printing, Landisville, Pa.
Date printed: March 2012

Printed in the United States of America

10 9 8 7 6 5 4 3 2 1

This book is printed on acid-free paper.

In memory of my parents, Bob and Mayadell Amacher,
both of whom our family lost during
the writing of this book.
—dkc

CONTENTS

ACKNOWLEDGMENTS

Over the years of putting this work together, we have turned to several experts in particular branches of pharmacy for their input, clarifications, and suggestions. Among those who have been especially helpful are AstraZenica, a global research-based biopharmaceutical company, for their explanation of how drugs work. A number of industry and scientific experts have answered questions, reviewed manuscript sections, or supplied quotes, including Mario Ehlers, M.D., Ph.D., Pacific Biometrics, Seattle, Washington; John D. Rhodes, U.S. & Global Managing Partner, Life Sciences, Deloitte & Touche USA, New York; William K. Sietsema, Ph.D., Vice President, Regulatory Consulting and Submissions, Kendle International, Cincinnati, Ohio; Albert I. Wertheimer, Ph.D., M.B.A., Director, Center for Pharmaceutical Health Services Research, Temple University School of Pharmacy; Charisse Johnson, Pharm.D., Professional Affairs Manager, National Association of Boards of Pharmacy; Jon Hess, Research Team Leader, Cutting Edge Information, Durham, North Carolina; and Linda McCoy, Pharm.D., Assistant Director of Pharmacy, Yavapai Regional Medical Center, Prescott, Arizona.

One always risks leaving out contributors when attempting to recall all who have helped make a project of this size a more valuable book. Our apologies to any others we have failed to mention; the slight is unintentional, and their contributions have been equally valuable.

A special appreciation goes to our long-suffering editor, James Chambers, whose patience and invaluable suggestions have been a godsend. He is an exceptional editor to work with.

And last, but never least, Christine Adamec and Mary Harwell Sayler, who are also Facts On File authors as well as friends, have been there throughout, always ready to offer empathy and encouragement and ever ready to take time out of their busy days to answer questions related to their own areas of expertise. They are forever appreciated.

FOREWORD

The Encyclopedia of Pharmaceutical Drugs is an introduction to drugs as a major component of the disease prevention, treatment, and healing process. From infants to the geriatric population, drugs are used for the prevention and treatment of disease states in every age group. In fact, the most recent statistics have shown that nearly half of all Americans take at least one prescription drug each month, and about 20% take more than two prescription drugs on a monthly basis. Approximately 60% of Americans have also taken at least one over-the-counter medication in the past six months. Even though these prescription and over-the-counter drugs have become so commonplace in our lives, we often give little thought to why they were developed, how they work, or what are the potential benefits and hazards associated with their use.

The importance of this book is that it helps us better understand drugs – both generally as a medical option and specifically as a particular group or class. It is designed to enhance our overall appreciation for the history of drugs, the development of the pharmaceutical industry, and the issues we all face relative to pharmaceutical drugs – whether from the viewpoint of a pharmacy professional, caregiver, or patient.

One of the issues that pharmacists have had to face over the years has been their changing role in healthcare. Historically, pharmacists primarily served in the role of compounding, preparing, and dispensing medications. However, over time, the roles of pharmacists have evolved from being once product-focused to being much more patient-focused. Currently, while the pharmacist still commonly plays a role in dispensing medications, they have also become vital members of the healthcare team in providing patient care because of their skill in providing services such as medication therapy management, patient counseling, and immunizations. The involvement of pharmacists in providing direct patient care in a variety of inpatient and outpatient settings has been associated with an improvement in patient outcomes, including a reduction in hospitalizations and an improvement in survival. As the "drug expert," pharmacists need to remain current on the medications being used to treat the numerous disease states that affect their patients. Therefore, pharmacists need to keep up-to-date on the mechanisms of action, side effects, drug interactions, and dosing regimens of current as well as newly approved medications. This book will serve as an excellent resource for pharmacists as it provides a useful overview of the most commonly used drug classes, including how they work, approved and off-label uses, routes of administration, contraindications, warnings, and cautions associated with their use, side effects, and drug interactions. Additionally, interesting information regarding sales numbers, the impact of using the drugs in specific racial/ethnic groups, and how the drugs were developed within the pharmaceutical industry is included in each of the drug-specific chapters.

One of the biggest issues that both patients and pharmacists face is the impact of poor compliance with prescribed medications. The term "compliance" may include both medication adherence and medication persistence. Medication adherence refers to the appropriate use of therapy as recommended by a healthcare provider. Medication persistence refers to the continued use of therapy. The statistics are quite staggering regarding the impact that medication non-adherence has on patient outcomes. According to recent reports, only about half of all patients with chronic diseases are compliant with their medications. This rather high rate of medication non-adherence has had a significant impact on mortality as well as economic outcomes. In fact, medication non-adherence is the fourth leading cause of death, just behind stroke, accounting for an estimated 125,000 deaths annually in the United States. Medication non-adherence also accounts for an estimated $290 billion in avoidable medical spending per year in the United States. While there are a number of factors that can influence medication adherence and persistence, educating patients regarding their disease states and the drug therapies being used to treat these conditions has been associated with an improvement in adherence rates. This book will serve as a helpful resource for caregivers and patients to learn more about the medications they may be taking. By becoming more informed about their drug therapies, these individuals can become better equipped to ask the appropriate questions to their healthcare providers regarding why certain drugs are being used, the side effects or drug interactions that may occur, or the instructions for use. As a result, these individuals can assume more control over their disease state management process, which may make them more likely to be adherent to their medications.

While one can certainly obtain information on individual drugs from any number of sources, both in print and on the Internet, this encyclopedia enhances that information by providing background on where drugs have come from and how they work. Even though a large portion of this book is about specific drugs, it is not meant to be a complete A-Z listing of all drugs available. Rather, the most commonly used drug classes and drugs have been included in this book so that both health care practitioners and patients would find the information to be useful.

While this book contains a plethora of information regarding numerous drugs and drug classes, it is important to realize that the pharmaceutical industry is continually evolving as new research and ongoing clinical experience discover new problems and new treatments. The drug information included in this book is current as of the time it was included in the text. Since that time, new drugs may have been approved, existing drugs may have been removed from the market, or new drug safety concerns may have been issued. Because of the constantly fluctuating dynamics of the pharmaceutical industry and their drug products, coupled with the time involved in writing and producing a work such as this, not every recent drug or drug labeling change can be included in this resource. Please remember that it is always a good idea to check with your doctor and pharmacist before taking any new drug or if you are concerned with a warning that you heard about for a medication that you are currently taking.

I sincerely hope that pharmacists and patients will find this drug encyclopedia to be a useful reference for their various medication needs.

—Cynthia A. Sanoski, Pharm.D.
Chair, Department of Pharmacy Practice,
Jefferson School of Pharmacy,
Jefferson College of Health Professions,
Thomas Jefferson University

INTRODUCTION

The Encyclopedia of Pharmaceutical Drugs provides a comprehensive overview of the development of pharmacy as an art and science and outlines the risks and benefits of the drugs readers are most likely to encounter. The book is divided into two major sections: an introduction that addresses the history and scope of pharmaceutical drugs, and A-to-Z listings of major drug therapeutic groups. In addition, appendixes offer reference material of special interest.

This introduction recounts the story of how drugs have evolved from medicinal plants to today's complex chemical products. It also addresses how drugs work in the body, the effects of drugs on different population groups, the evolution of the pharmaceutical industry, governmental oversight of drugs, drug discovery and development, prescription drug types and classification, marketing of drugs and related issues, prescription drug abuse and misuse, and the future of pharmaceutical drugs.

In their Career Guide to Industries, 2010–11 Edition, the Bureau of Labor Statistics, U.S. Department of Labor, notes that "thousands of medications are available today for diagnostic, preventive, and therapeutic uses." Other references targeting the pharmacological community list all those thousands of individual drugs. Our purpose was not to repeat those listings. Rather, in the A–Z section, you will find major drug groups, defined by the conditions they are primarily used to prevent or treat. Each drug group lists drug classes within that group; how the drugs within the group work; approved uses for each drug, off-label uses, where applicable; companion drugs, when a drug is frequently used in addition to another specific drug for optimal results; how the drugs are administered; any cautions and concerns about drugs within the group; any warnings issued by the Food and Drug Administration (FDA); and any contraindications, potential side effects, and potential interactions between drugs within the group and other drugs or foods. Most entries on drug groups will also provide statistics for the top-selling drugs; demographics and cultural groups, where pertinent; development history of the group; and drugs in the pipeline for that group.

History of Making and Dispensing Drugs

The word drug has been traced back to the Middle English drogge, which came from the Old French drogue, which may have derived from the Dutch/Low German word droog, which means "dry"—believed to have been used because originally most drugs were dried plant parts.

Under the Federal Food, Drug, and Cosmetic Act, a "drug" is any of the following: (A) articles recognized in the official United States Pharmacopoeia, official Homeopathic Pharmacopoeia of the United States, or official national formulary, or any supplement to any of them; (B) articles intended for use in the diagnosis, cure, mitigation, treatment, or prevention of disease in humans or animals; (C) articles (other than food) intended to affect the structure or any function of the body of humans or animals; and (D) articles intended for use as a component of any article specified above.

Although today we typically think of drugs as being manufactured in pristine pharmaceutical plants, usually in pill, powder, or liquid form, for most of history, drugs were directly derived from plants, minerals, and animal parts.

Prehistoric drugs

Stone Age cave dwellers are believed to have dug for medicinal plants, although Burger notes that wall paintings and carvings on rocks from earliest prehistory "give us little insight into any healing arts those forebears may have invented. Probably accidental discovery of the healing powers of roots, barks, leaves, and berries and of nutritional sources of proteins and starch occurred even during those earliest stages." Medicinal plants were found in a Neanderthal grave more than 60,000 years old.

As the nomadic wanderers began settling down, planting seeds, and developing actual societies, certain individuals emerged as leaders. Burger explains, "Part of the influence of these commanding individuals came from the personal help they could give to sick, wounded, and otherwise afflicted members of their groups. The medicine man, witch doctor, or shaman was the first person to turn to in distress." The medicine man turned to healing herbs taken from trees, shrubs, and other plants for most of his medicines. "It must have been hard for a medicine man to decide which plant to give a patient. Trial and error was the order of the day. Even after a healing effect was found in a certain plant, it was probably used for a variety of illnesses, whether identical in symptoms or only vaguely similar."

South and Central American Indians made many prehistoric discoveries of drug-bearing plants, according to Burger. "Mexican Aztecs even recorded their properties in hieroglyphics on rocks, but our knowledge of their studies comes mainly from manuscripts of Spanish monks and medical men attached to the forces of the conquistador Hernan Cortes (1485–1547)." Among the plants in their "drug cabinets" were tobacco and mind-altering plants such as hallucinatory sacred mushrooms and the small cactus peyote.

Early Indians in the Andes mountains discovered several drug-bearing plants, including the coca shrub, the dried leaves of which contain alkaloids that became cocaine, and cinchona bark, which yields the alkaloid quinine.

Sumerian drugs, 2500 to 2300 B.C.

Sumer, believed by some historians to have been the first civilization in the world, was a collection of city-states around the lower Tigris and Euphrates Rivers in what is now southern Iraq. The Sumerians may have migrated from ancient India or Iran—their language was unrelated to the various groups speaking Semitic languages in the ancient Near East. Begun as a collection of farming villages 5,000 years ago, the Sumerians developed a religion and a society that influenced both their neighbors and their conquerors. Sumerian cuneiform—the earliest written language—described well-established medicinal uses for such plants as laurel, caraway, and thyme. A 4,000-year-old Sumerian clay tablet is the earliest known recorded medical document.

Ancient Egyptian drugs, 2000 B.C.

Because Egyptian doctors were often priests, they believed that the gods were responsible for the general health and healing of individuals. Believing that evil spirits or poisons in the body caused disease and most illnesses, physicians would offer prayers to the gods, who could cure the disease. Thus, medicines were not used for healing as much as they were for reducing pain.

The Egyptians are believed to have been the first to use opium as an anesthetic at around 1500 B.C. Their preparations also included cannabis, linseed oil, and senna. The Egyptians were among the first to allocate different physicians to specialize in treating particular body parts, and certain physicians became early pharmacists, responsible for processing plant materials to prepare ointments, inhalers, and pills for various ailments. Many modern drugs have originated from the study and isolation of active ingredients from plants with healing properties.

Egyptian physicians prescribed figs, dates, and castor oil as laxatives and used tannic acid to treat burns. Other potent drugs used by the Egyptians that continue in use today included colchicine (a poisonous alkaloid from the autumn crocus used to treat gout) and mercury. Some of the natural remedies described in Egyptian medical texts included: colocynth (bitter apple—a strong laxative), henbane (source of the drug hyoscyamine), manna (used as a laxative), aloe, and numerous other plants and herbs.

Ancient Chinese drugs, 3000 B.C.

Chinese medicine evolved during the same centuries as Egypt, Greece, and Rome, but in relative isolation from other cultures. Around 2750 B.C., the legendary Chinese emperor Shen Nung first documented the use of the Indian hemp plant *Cannabis sativa* for pharmacological purposes in his *Shen-Nung Pen Ts'ao Ching* (Divine husbandman's materia medica), the earliest Chinese pharmacopoeia still in existence. Venerated as the Father of Chinese Medicine, Shen Nung is said to have tasted hundreds of herbs to test their medicinal value, and his text includes 365 medicines derived from minerals, plants, and animals, which became the basis for Chinese medicine.

Burger writes, "He found that the drug *Ch'ang Shan* was helpful in treating fevers. Such fevers were, and still are, caused by malaria parasites. The drug consists of the powdered roots of a plant in the breakstone family (Saxifragaceae, now identified as *Dichroa febrifuga, Lour.*). Almost 4700 years later, a group of Chinese chemists isolated two compounds (the dichroines) from the plants, one of which later proved to control bird malaria. The leaves of this plant—called *Shun Chi* or chuine in present-day China—also contain antimalarial chemicals (the febrifugines), one

of which is identical with one of the dichroines. These alkaloids (organic bases) were studied and synthesized during World War II in an effort to protect Americans from malaria in the Pacific and other tropical campaigns."

Other drugs listed as being in use at this time included opium (to relieve pain and aid sleep), rhubarb, croton oil (for purging), arsenic, sulphur, and ma huang. Now known as ephedra, ma huang has stems and roots yielding ephedrine and other alkaloids. Ephedrine was first isolated by the Japanese chemist Nagai in 1887 and later used as a bronchial dilator and decongestant. In April 2004, the FDA banned the use of ephedra since it presented an unreasonable risk of illness or injury. Ephedra had been linked to significant adverse health effects, including heart attack and stroke.

According to the National Library of Medicine, "Chinese medicine seems to have reached its peak during the Ming dynasty (1368–1644) when Li Shih-Chen wrote his *Pen Ts'ao Kang Mu* (The Great Herbal). This great pharmacopoeia, which summarizes what was known of herbal medicine up to the late 16th century, describes in detail more than 1,800 plants, animal substances, minerals, and metals, along with their medicinal properties and applications. Li Shih-Chen was 35 years old when he began to compile his *Pen Ts'ao Kang Mu*. He took 27 years to finish it." Iversen adds, "Li was one of the first to study drugs scientifically; he personally studied the actions of many traditional remedies. As a result he discarded a lot of useless information and eliminated some toxic preparations."

Collectively, the Chinese pharmacopoeia was the most extensive of all the older civilizations. Carr writes, "The extensive Chinese pharmacopoeia was classified by function: Different classes of drugs were held to be specific to induce perspiration, to reduce excessive heat inside the body, to counteract rheumatism, to reduce cold sensation in the body, to reduce dampness in the body, to lubricate dry symptoms, to induce vomiting, to induce bowel movements, to promote digestion, to suppress cough and sputum, to regulate energy, to regulate blood, to regain consciousness, to constrict and obstruct movements, to expel or destroy parasites, for ulcers and tumors, for external applications."

Ancient Indian medicine, 3000 B.C.

The ayurvedic texts of ancient India, written 5,000 years ago, referenced botanical drugs to treat hardening of the arteries. Hindus used the cannabis and henbane plants as anesthetics and the root of the plant *Rauwolfia serpentina*, which contains reserpine, as a tranquilizer. Ayurvedic medicine is still a popular form of health care in India, and it has gained acceptance in the West as a form of alternative medicine. According to Iversen, "Unlike the relatively benign and nontoxic effects of most Chinese medicines, however, the ayurvedic approach seems often to be more aggressive—with drug-induced vomiting, purging of the gut with laxatives and enemas, and bleeding as common remedies."

Drugs and the Greeks and Romans, 400 B.C. to A.D. 300

The origin of the word *pharmacy* is generally traced to the Greek *pharmakon* (remedy or drug).

The Greeks used acetylsalicylic acid (known today as aspirin), derived from salicin, the active ingredient in the bark of the willow tree, to reduce fever and pain.

Hippocrates (460–377 B.C.), the father of modern day medicine and medical ethics, broke away from the traditional search for plant-based drugs and instead pursued inorganic salts as medications. Burger writes, "Hippocrates' authority lasted throughout the Middle Ages and reminded alchemists and medical experimenters of the potential of inorganic drugs. In fact, a distant descendant of Hippocrates' prescriptions was the use of antimony salts in elixirs (alcoholic solutions) advocated by Basilius Valentius in the middle of the 15th century and later by the medical alchemist Paracelsus. We still use magnesium sulfate (named Epsom salts for the British town of Epsom), both internally and externally; aluminum salt astringents; sodium

and potassium chlorides and calcium salts for various deficiencies; barium sulfate as an X-ray contrast agent; and sodium iodide to prevent thyroid disorders, as well as stannous fluoride to prevent tooth decay."

Following Hippocrates, the Greek physician and teacher Claudius Galenus, or Galen (around A.D. 129–199) introduced drug delivery by soaking (infusion) or boiling (decoction) plants. Burger writes, "Galen insisted on carefully identifying the type and age of botanical materials and thus foreshadowed the value of controlling the purity of drugs. Among his favorite potent drugs were hyoscyamus (which contains atropine), opium (the source of morphine), and squill (which contains heart stimulants)" such as cardiac glycosides, which include digitalis.

Dioscorides of Anazarbus, a Greek physician born in southeast Asia Minor in the Roman Empire in the first few decades A.D., traveled extensively seeking medicinal substances from all over the Roman and Greek world. About A.D. 50–70, he wrote his fundamental work, known in Latin as *De materia medica*. This five-book study focused upon "the preparation, properties, and testing of drugs" and became the most central pharmacological work in Europe and the Middle East for the next 16 centuries.

Drugs during the Middle Ages, 500–1400 A.D.

Following the fall of the Roman Empire, medicine returned to the purview of priests and religious scholars, with illness believed to be a punishment from God. Prayers for forgiveness usually replaced drugs, with patients given food and comfort by nursing staff, but little else. Traditional cures, using herbal remedies and potions, were seen as witchcraft and outlawed by the church.

Although surgery was a crude practice during the Middle Ages, amputations, setting broken bones, replacing dislocations, and binding wounds were relatively common. Opium was sometimes used as an anesthetic, and wounds were cleaned with wine in an attempt to prevent infections. Most drugs were more likely used for the euphoric effect to relieve pain rather than to heal the patient.

As time went on, schools and universities began to educate wealthy individuals in religion, the arts, law, and medicine. Men and even a few women were trained and allowed to become physicians. As more universities developed, more and more were not religious-based, and eventually it was not necessary to be a cleric to practice medicine.

Burger writes, "The little that was known about healing plants, minerals, and tissues was called materia medica, a term still used for drug information at the turn of this century. Latin was used throughout the collective accounts of this subject because it was the professional language of the monks and also because it kept the common people in ignorance. The late Middle Ages coincided with the upsurge of alchemy, a primitive chemistry dealing mostly with inorganic substances. The renewed interest in inorganic materials pushed botanical sources of medicines into second place temporarily."

Islamic medicines, 700–1500

For many centuries after the fall of the Roman Empire, the Arabic world was the center of scientific and medical knowledge. Texts from Greece and Rome were translated into Arabic and studied by Islamic scholars. They developed and refined Hippocrates' theories, and Islamic physicians began to use the regulation of diet and exercise and the prescription of medicinal herbs in the treatment of their patients. Arabic pharmacists became skilled in the formulation of medicines from plants and minerals. Even though they did not know about microbes, they used alcohol to clean wounds, allowing them to heal better and not become infected.

A school of pharmacy established in Arabia from 750 to 1258 discovered many substances effective against illness, such as burned sponge (which contains iodine) for the treatment of goiters—a noncancerous enlargement of the thyroid gland, visible as a swelling at the front of the neck.

Hospitals treated rich and poor alike. Early in the ninth century, Islamic hospitals around Baghdad had medical and surgical wards, operating theaters, and pharmacies for the dispensing of medicines—the first specialization in pharmacy in the civilized world. By A.D. 931, large hospitals were involved in the training and licensing of doctors and pharmacists. Officials tested medicines to certify that they were safe and visited pharmacists to make sure that prescriptions were being made correctly. All of these events took place at a time when medicine in Europe was still governed by religion and superstition.

Records show that Arabic doctors performed many different surgical operations including the removal of varicose veins and kidney stones and the replacement of dislocated limbs. They used sponges soaked in narcotic drugs which were placed over the patient's nose as early anesthetics.

One of the most important medical books of its time was written by the physician Ali al-Husayn Abd Allah Ibn Sina (also known as Avicenna). His massive manuscript, called the *Laws of Medicine,* was completed about A.D. 1030 and translated into Latin in the 12th century. This encyclopedia of medicine contained five books detailing the formulation of medicines, diagnosis of disorders, general medicine, and detailed therapies. It continued to be a great influence in the development of medicine in medieval Europe for hundreds of years.

The Renaissance and medicines, 1400–1700

During the Renaissance, as studies about science and medicine expanded, physicians began to learn more about the human body. Burger writes, "When pamphlets could no longer hold the accumulating knowledge of materia medica, larger, more formal collections were gathered in national pharmacopoeias. The first of these books appeared in Florence in 1498, six years after Christopher Columbus landed in Dominica, followed by others in Nuremberg (1535), Basel (1561), Augsburg (1564), and London (1618). Standards of purity and methods of preparing various drug products accompanied the descriptions of botanical and mineralogical specimens. One item tells how to make a sort of candy of red rose petals for pale tired people and of using white roses for those with too ruddy complexions."

In the 16th century, a German-Swiss physician named Paracelsus (born Theophrastus Bombast von Hohenheim, in Switzerland, 1493–1541) identified the characteristics of numerous diseases such as syphilis, a chronic infectious disease usually transmitted in sexual intercourse. By preparing and using new chemical remedies, including those containing mercury, sulfur, iron, and copper sulfate, to counter various diseases, Paracelsus was among the first to unite medicine with chemistry.

About 1530, Paracelsus experimented with the medical value of opium, a narcotic drug obtained from the unripe seedpods of the opium poppy. Unaware of its addictive properties, he determined that its analgesic value was of such magnitude that he called it Laudanum, from the Latin *laudare*, to praise, or from *labdanum*, the term for a plant extract. Laudanum was prescribed for many disorders and remained in use up until Victorian times.

By the mid-16th century, Dioscorides' message that investigation and experimentation were crucial to pharmacology began to emerge, and modern research into medicines began. In 1546, the first list of drugs with instructions for preparation, called a pharmacopoeia, appeared in Nuremberg, Germany.

Physicians now read books translated from Arabic medical texts and began to study anatomy in a scientific and systematic way. As the understanding of the body increased, so did the development of new medicines. Building on knowledge of herbs and minerals taken from Arabic writings, Renaissance pharmacists (or apothecaries) experimented with new plants brought from distant lands by explorers like Christopher Columbus. The bark of the cinchona tree (called quina quina by the indigenous Peruvians), found in the rain forests along the Amazon river in the Andes of South America, contained an ingredient called quinine, which is still used in the treatment of malaria, a disease transmitted by the bite of an infected mosquito and one of the oldest plagues of mankind. Although cinchona bark was introduced in Europe around 1640 and first sold in England in 1658, it would be nearly 200 years before the alkaloid quinine would be isolated as its potent ingredient.

Although knowledge of drugs was expanding, progress was slow, and many medicines remained little more than superstitious potions containing ingredients like worms' livers and tongue of newt.

Medicines during the eighteenth and nineteenth centuries

During the 18th century, heart failure was treated with the leaves of the foxglove plant (which contains digitalis); scurvy, a disease caused by vitamin C deficiency, was treated with citrus fruit (which contains vitamin C); and smallpox was prevented using inoculations of cells infected with a similar viral disease known as cowpox. The therapy developed for smallpox stimulated the body's immune system, which defends against disease-causing agents, to produce cowpox- and smallpox-specific antibodies.

Pharmacy began to develop as a profession separate from medicine in the 18th century, with pharmacists becoming the compounders of medications while physicians were the therapists.

Medicine made great advances during the 18th and 19th centuries as Edward Jenner pioneered the earliest vaccinations, and discoveries by Louis Pasteur and Robert Koch led to the understanding that infections were caused by certain bacteria or germs. The study of microbes, or microbiology, was born. Increased knowledge of pathogenic microbes led to the development of new medicines to tackle infectious diseases and to the birth of the pharmaceutical industry.

In 1821, the first school of pharmacy in North America was established—the Philadelphia College of Pharmacy.

Nineteenth-century scientists continued to discover new drugs including ether, morphine, and a vaccine for rabies, an infectious, often fatal, viral disease of mammals that attacks the central nervous system and is transmitted by the bite of infected animals. These drugs, however, were limited to those occurring naturally in plants, minerals, and animals. A growing understanding of chemistry soon changed the way drugs were developed. Heroin and aspirin, two of the first synthetic drugs created from other elements or compounds using chemical reactions, were produced in the late 1800s.

In 1853, the French chemist Charles Gerhardt first synthesized the acetyl derivative from salicylic acid, developing the first synthetic aspirin. However, Felix Hoffman, a German chemist and employee of Fredrich Bayer & Co., was the first to realize its medical value in 1897.

Heroin was first synthesized in 1874 by C. R. A. Wright, a British chemist working at St. Mary's Hospital Medical School, London. While combining morphine with various acids during experimentation, he boiled anhydrous morphine alkaloid with acetic anhydride over a stove for several hours and produced a more potent, acetylated form of morphine. We now call it diacetylmorphine. Heinrich Dreser of Bayer noticed that diacetylmorphine was more potent than morphine; thus Bayer registered Heroin (meaning "heroic treatment" from the German word *heroisch*) as a trademark. From 1898 through 1910, it was marketed as a nonaddictive morphine substitute and cough medicine for children. As with Aspirin, Bayer lost some of its trademark rights to Heroin following World War I. In 1914, the Harrison Narcotics Tax Act made it illegal to manufacture or possess heroin in the United States.

These developments, combined with the establishment of a new discipline called pharmacology, the study of drugs (or chemicals) and their actions on the body, signaled the birth of the modern drug industry.

But it was in 19th-century Germany that the modern era of drug development began, according to Iversen. "Germany was a leader in the scientific approach to medicine, and students flocked to German medical schools from all over the world. German chemists were the first to isolate pure drug chemicals from herbal medicines, beginning with the isolation of morphine in 1803 and quinine in 1820."

Paul Ehrlich (1854–1915), a German bacteriologist, determined that certain tissues have a selective affinity for certain chemicals. Davis explains, "Although Ehrlich's original idea seems perfectly obvious now, it was considered very strange at the time. He proposed that every disease should be treated with a chemical specific for that disease, and that the pharmacologist's task was to find these treatments by systematically testing potential drugs."

Iversen adds, "This led in turn to the modern concept that drugs are recognized by specific receptors in the body, and indeed Ehrlich was one of the first to use the term 'receptor.'"

Ehrlich's greatest triumph was his discovery of salvarsan, the first effective treatment for the sexually transmitted disease syphilis. Ehrlich discovered salvarsan after screening 605 different arsenic-containing compounds. Iversen writes, "It inaugurated the era of 'chemotherapy,' which was to revolutionize the treatment and control of infectious diseases, which had hitherto been largely untreatable."

Later, researchers around the world had great success in developing new drugs by following Ehrlich's methods. For example, testing of sulfur-containing dyes led to the 20th century's first "miracle drugs"—the sulfa drugs, used to treat bacterial infections.

Pharmaceuticals during the twentieth century

Between 1901 and 2000, the average life expectancy rose from 47 years to 77 years. New medicines, improved air quality, and better public hygiene contributed to this 64-percent increase in life expectancy.

At the turn of the century, only a few medically effective substances were widely used scientifically, among them ether, morphine, digitalis, diphtheria antitoxin, smallpox vaccine, iron, quinine, iodine, alcohol, and mercury. Then in the 20th century, biology and chemistry came into their own and medicine was transformed. For the first time, the crude plants and mineral materials that act on living tissues could be analyzed, separated, and used as medicine. With the introduction of anesthetics, screams were no longer heard in the operating room.

Since 1900, and particularly since World War II, many important new drugs have been developed. Among the major advances in pharmacy during the 20th century were the work of Banting and Best (1921) to show that insulin can be used to treat diabetes, the development of penicillin by Fleming (1928), and the development of antibiotics by Domagk, Florey, and Chain (1935–45). Pharmaceutical laboratories around the world began to constantly produce new treatments for diseases.

Mass vaccination programs were undertaken to prevent deaths from diseases such as yellow fever, poliomyelitis, measles, mumps, and rubella. In 1980, the World Health Organization announced that the deadly smallpox virus had been completely eradicated.

Iversen writes, "The last half of the twentieth century saw an unprecedented flourishing of basic medical research and a remarkable increase in the kinds and numbers of drugs available for clinical use. The list of disease conditions that could be treated expanded enormously, and the discovery and production of new drugs for sale became a major industry. Annual sales of medical drugs in the USA, for example, increased from $149 million in 1939 to $130 billion in 1999—an increase of nearly a thousandfold."

During the past several decades, further progress in drug treatment has been characterized by the rise of chemotherapy, the use of new antibiotics, increased understanding of the mechanisms of the immune system, and the increased use of vaccination to prevent disease and insulin to treat diabetes.

The pharmacy field itself has undergone great changes during the past several decades. Prior to 1950, approximately 60 percent of all medications were compounded (mixed by the pharmacist) to meet the requests of the prescribing physicians and needs of the individual patients. With the growth of commercial drug manufacturers, compounding declined. Spencer and Mathews explained, "Until the 1950s, pharmacists whipped up nearly all prescriptions with a mortar and pestle behind the drugstore counter. Pharmacists were often called 'doc' and they worked in close consultations with physicians to make personalized treatments for each patient. The earliest pharmaceutical companies, such as today's Merck & Co., supplied raw ingredients to pharmacists, instead of finished products. But as the commercial pharmaceutical industry expanded in the 1960s and 1970s, pharmacists found themselves counting out pills rather than mixing powders." Today, an estimated 43,000 prescriptions are compounded daily, which represents 1 percent of the total prescriptions dispensed.

Burger, Alfred. *Understanding Medications: What the Label Doesn't Tell You*. Washington, D.C.: American Chemical Society, 1995.

Carr, Ian. "Folk Healing, Alternative, and Parallel Medicines." Hippocrates on the Web. Faculty of Medicine, University of Manitoba. Available online. URL: http://www.umanitoba.ca/faculties/medicine/history/histories/folk.html. Accessed May 30, 2005.

David, Allison. *Medicines By Design*, NIH Publication No. 03-474. Bethesda, Md.: National Institutes of Health, revised June 2003.

Iversen, Leslie. *Drugs: A Very Short Introduction*. Oxford: Oxford University Press, 2001.

Spencer, Jane, and Anna Wilde Mathews. "As Druggists Mix Customized Brews, FDA Raises Alarm." *Wall Street Journal*, February 27, 2004, A1.

Pharmacology: How Drugs Work in the Body

The word *pharmacology*, derived from the Greek *pharmacon* (drug) and *logos* (study), is the study of how drugs (chemical substances) act on or interfere with the body and, conversely, how the body affects the drugs themselves.

When these chemical substances have medicinal properties, they are referred to as pharmaceuticals or therapeutic drugs. The field of pharmacology encompasses drug composition, drug sources, drug appearance, drug properties, drug interactions, toxicology, undesirable effects (also called adverse or side effects), and desirable effects that can be used in therapy of diseases.

The major challenge in pharmacology is that no drug produces a single effect. Medicines work in many different ways on many different organs of the body. As medicines find their way to their "targets" or "job sites" in the body, hundreds of things happen along the way, with each action triggering another. Complicating this process, different bodies can respond differently to the same drugs.

Many factors can lead to one person reacting differently to a particular drug compared to a neighbor or a person in another state, including eating different foods, lifestyles, living and working environments, amount of exercise each one gets, presence of other medications, and different health status and medical histories. But a key factor that can lead to these different responses is a person's DNA, which contains one's genes and makes that person unique.

As the National Institute of General Medical Sciences booklet, *Medicines by Design*, explains, a gene is a unit of heredity—a segment of a DNA molecule containing the code for making a protein which can affect how one responds to medicines. According to this booklet, "Your genetic code instructs your body how to make hundreds of thousands of different molecules called proteins. Some proteins determine hair color, and some of them are enzymes that pro-cess or metabolize food or medicines. Slightly different, but normal, variations in the human genetic code can yield proteins that work better or worse when they are metabolizing many different types of drugs and other substances. Scientists use the term *pharmacogenetics* to describe research on the link between genes and drug response." Specifically, it is the study of inherited differences in drug metabolism and response.

As scientists work to figure out how the makeup of DNA can contribute to a body's response to medicines, their findings will help guide doctors in prescribing the precisely correct amount of the correct medicine—maximizing drug efficacy and safety.

Another term often used interchangeably with pharmacogenetics is *pharmacogenomics*. However, there is a difference between them. Dingle explains, "Pharmacogenomics differs from classical pharmacogenetics in that it encompasses a broader subject matter, including variability in toxicity of medications, in response to medications and in the risk of developing disease following drug or xenobiotic (foreign to the body) exposure. Nevertheless, the differences between these two subjects are ill-defined and vary from author to author."

Joly explains further, "Pharmacogenetics was first coined in 1959 when it was observed that individuals differ in the way they respond to medicines due to individual genetic profiles. In the 1980s, with the identification of the molecular bases of hereditary traits and then later the completion of the human genome draft, pharmacogenomics became possible. Compared to pharmacogenetics, pharmacogenomics goes even further by identifying genes or whole genomes responsible for modifying an organism's response to drugs. Pharmacogenomics also includes the use of genomics in the search for new therapeutic targets." The role of pharmacogenomics is discussed further in the section on "Future of Prescription Drugs" (p. lxxxvi).

ADME

A drug goes through four basic stages as it progresses through the body: absorption, distribution, metabolism, and excretion (or elimination). The entire process is commonly referred to by its acronym of ADME.

Absorption   This first stage includes getting the drug into the body's circulation (bloodstream). Medicines can enter the body in many different ways, and they are absorbed when they travel from the site of administration into the body's circulation.

Drugs are introduced or administered into the body in a number of ways. Among these:

- buccal—placing the drug in the mouth between the gums and cheek, without swallowing it
- inhalation—inhaling the drug
- intramuscular—getting an injection in an arm muscle
- intravenous (parenteral)—receiving a drug through a vein
- ocular—administering the drug into the eye
- oral—swallowing the drug
- rectal—inserting a suppository into the rectum
- subcutaneous—injecting the drug just under the skin
- sublingual—placing the drug under the tongue
- topical or cutaneous—applying the drug to the skin surface
- transdermal—wearing a skin patch
- vaginal—inserting the drug into the vagina

In addition to the method of administration, a drug's physical and chemical properties, design, and dosage impact its absorption. How much of and how quickly a drug is absorbed into the blood are of particular importance and concern. If a drug's active ingredients do not get into the blood, it will not achieve its desired effect. When developing drugs, scientists may add other chemicals to the drug to help the body absorb it or, on the other side, to prevent it from being broken down and excreted too soon. Also, various physiologic characteristics of the person taking the drug can affect absorption of a drug into the body, including the person's age, weight, stomach acidity and time to empty (for drugs taken by mouth), and kidney and liver function.

A drug faces significant hurdles during absorption. Medicines taken by mouth are shuttled via a blood vessel leading from the digestive tract to the liver, the place where the body processes chemicals and where a large amount may be destroyed by metabolic enzymes in the so-called first pass effect. Drugs taken in other ways— such as getting an injection, using an inhaler, or applying a skin patch—bypass the liver and enter the bloodstream directly or through the skin or lungs.

Distribution   Once a drug gets absorbed, the next stage is distribution. Most often, the bloodstream carries medicines throughout the body, where they can interact with many organs in the body. During this step, side effects can occur when a drug has an effect in an organ other than its target organ. For a pain reliever, the target organ might be a sore muscle in the leg; however, irritation of the stomach could be a side effect. Many factors influence distribution, such as the presence of protein and fat molecules in the blood that can put drug molecules out of commission by grabbing on to them.

Drugs destined for the central nervous system (the brain and spinal cord) face an enormous hurdle: a nearly impenetrable barricade called the blood-brain barrier. This blockade is built from a tightly woven mesh of capillaries cemented together to protect the brain from potentially dangerous substances such as poisons or viruses, yet pharmacologists have devised various ways to sneak some drugs past this barrier.

Metabolism   In their journey through the body, medicines interact with many different molecules called proteins. Some of these proteins work to get rid of medicines, while others help medicines do their jobs. Some proteins actually "turn on" certain medicines, by switching them from an inactive form to an active one. For example, the painkiller codeine is a medicine that is switched on in this way by proteins. This "turning on" or "switch" is not sudden like a light switch, but rather a process. Genes provide the manufacturing instructions for all of the proteins in the body. Small differences between one's genes and those of a relative or neighbor can affect how one reacts—or does not react—to a drug. In addition, some drugs work to mask a symptom, like a stuffy nose; others work to fix a problem, like a bacterial infection.

After a medicine has been distributed throughout the body and has done its job, the drug is broken down, or metabolized. The breaking down of a drug molecule usually involves two steps that take place mostly in the body's chemical processing plant, the liver. The liver is a site of continuous and frenzied, yet carefully controlled, activity. Everything that enters the bloodstream—whether swallowed, injected, inhaled, absorbed through the skin, or produced by the body itself—is carried to this largest internal organ. In the liver, substances are chemically broken down and transformed.

The biotransformations that take place in the liver are performed by the body's busiest proteins, its enzymes. Every cell in the body has a variety of enzymes. Each enzyme specializes in a particular job. Some break molecules apart, while others link small molecules into long chains. With drugs, the first step is usually to make the substance easier to get rid of in urine.

Many of the products of enzymatic breakdown, which are called metabolites, are less chemically active than the original molecule. For this reason, scientists refer to the liver as a detoxifying organ. Occasionally, however, drug metabolites can have chemical activities of their own—sometimes as powerful as those of the original drug. Because of this, the liver can be prone to damage caused by too much medicine

in the body. Thus, when prescribing certain drugs, doctors must take into account these added effects.

Excretion (elimination)   Once liver enzymes are finished working on a medicine, the now inactive drug and any of its active metabolites enter the excretion stage and exit the body in the urine or feces. Age-related changes in kidney function can have significant effects on how fast a drug is eliminated from the body. Age-related changes in liver function can also affect the rate of elimination ultimately by slowing down metabolism.

The study of how the body absorbs, distributes, metabolizes (breaks down), and eliminates (or excretes) a drug—or how the body affects the drug—is called pharmacokinetics. And opposite to that, pharmacodynamics is the study of the effects of drugs on living organisms—what a drug does to the body or how it acts at target sites of action.

How drugs achieve what they set out to do

Generally, drugs are formulated to do one of three things:

- replace substances that are deficient or missing in the body

- alter the activity of cells

- destroy infectious microorganisms or abnormal cells

AstraZeneca, an international pharmaceutical company that spends more than $15 million every working day on the research and development of new medicines, explains how medicines work:

Replacing substances that are deficient or missing in the body   The body needs certain levels of proteins (or amino acids), vitamins, and minerals in order to work normally. If these important substances are insufficient or lacking, this can lead to medical disorders. These are called deficiency disorders. Examples include iron deficiency (anemia) and vitamin C deficiency (scurvy).

Deficiency disorders can also occur as a result of a lack of hormones in the body (hormone deficiencies). Common examples include Type I diabetes mellitus and hypothyroidism (thyroid hormone deficiency).

Deficiency disorders can be treated with medicines or hormones that replace or restore the levels of the missing substances, for example insulin injections for diabetics.

Altering the activity of cells   Cells are the basic "building blocks" of the body. All human tissue is made up of groups of cells. Many medicines work by altering the activity of cells. For example, anti-inflammatories such as ibuprofen and diclofenac block the action or stop the production of chemical substances (mediators) that are released by cells in response to tissue damage and which cause inflammation and pain.

Medicines that interfere with the way cells work are used to treat a variety of conditions, such as blood-clotting disorders (e.g., ANTICOAGULANTS) and heart diseases (e.g., calcium channel blockers).

Some medicines work by attaching themselves (binding) to sites found on the surface of cells (receptors) and either increase or decrease the activity of the cell (e.g., medicines used in the treatment of epilepsy and Parkinson's disease).

Destroying infectious microorganisms or abnormal cells   Infectious diseases occur when viruses, bacteria, protozoa, or fungi invade the body. Antibiotics (e.g., penicillin) can destroy bacteria by killing them directly or by preventing them from multiplying. ANTIFUNGALS commonly used for infections of the skin and mouth (e.g., clotrimazole and miconazole) work by disrupting infected cells. (Other antifungals can also be used for infections in the bloodstream or urine.) Still other medicines work by killing abnormal cells; for example, some anticancer drugs directly target and kill harmful cancer cells.

Other ramifications of pharmaceutical drug use

In a perfect world, the precise dosage of a drug would reach its target site, do its job, and leave the body with no complications. Of course, such an ideal scenario does not always occur. The combination of chemical drugs and the human body can lead to challenges. Among these:

Drug tolerance   When certain drugs are taken regularly for a length of time, the body does not respond to them as well as it once did, and the drugs at a fixed dose become less effective. Larger or more frequent doses must be taken to obtain the effect that was achieved with the original dose. For example, people who take narcotics (e.g., morphine) for pain control sometimes find that over time they will need to take larger doses. This may be due to either an increase in the pain or the development of drug tolerance. Increasing the doses of narcotics to relieve increasing pain or to overcome drug tolerance is not addiction. When the body gets used to a medicine so that more medicine is needed than is safe, the physician may prescribe a different drug. Tachyphylaxis is the rapid development of drug tolerance.

Drug dependence   Most controlled drugs (narcotics, central nervous system depressants or stimulants, hallucinogens, and anabolic steroids) are capable of producing dependence, either physical or psychological. Physical dependence refers to the changes that have occurred in the body after repeated use of a drug that necessitate the continued administration of the drug to prevent a withdrawal syndrome. This withdrawal syndrome can range from mildly unpleasant to life-threatening effects and is dependent on a number of factors. The type of withdrawal experienced is related to the drug being used; the dose and route of administration; concurrent use of other drugs; frequency and duration of drug use; and the age, gender, health, and genetic makeup of the user. Psychological dependence refers to the perceived "need" or "craving" for a drug.

Individuals who are psychologically dependent on a particular substance often feel that they cannot function without continued use of that substance. While physical dependence disappears within days or weeks after drug use stops, psychological dependence can last much longer and is one of the primary reasons for relapse/initiation of drug use after a period of abstinence.

Contrary to common belief, physical dependence is not addiction. While addicts are usually physically dependent on the drug they are abusing, physical dependence can exist without addiction (e.g., patients who take narcotics for chronic pain management or benzodiazepines to treat anxiety).

Prescription drug addiction Addiction rarely occurs among those who use pain relievers, central nervous system depressants (useful in the treatment of anxiety and sleep disorders), or stimulants as prescribed; the risk for addiction exists when these medications are used in ways other than as prescribed. Addiction is often described as compulsive drug-seeking behavior where acquiring and using a drug becomes the most important activity in the user's life. This definition implies a loss of control regarding drug use, and the addict will continue to use a drug despite serious medical and/or social consequences. The National Institute on Drug Abuse (NIDA) estimates that about 5 million Americans suffer from drug addiction.

Overdose All medicines can be dangerous if they are not taken properly. Too large a dose of a narcotic may cause breathing to slow down or stop (respiratory depression). Typically, doses required for good pain relief are rarely, if ever, large enough to cause death. Doctors carefully adjust the doses of narcotic pain relievers so that pain is relieved with little effect on breathing.

Drug interactions In the National Institutes of Health (NIH) *Pharmacy Update Special Edition*, a drug interaction is defined as "the pharmacologic or clinical response to the administration of a drug combination different from that anticipated from the known effects of the two agents when given alone. The incidence of drug interactions varies widely in the literature ranging from 2.2 to 70.3 percent." The report notes that although the term *drug interaction* usually has a negative connotation, and while drug interactions may lead to a loss of therapeutic effect or toxicity, they may also benefit the patient. The use of certain drugs in combination can lead to improved outcomes or improve a drug regimen's convenience, reduce costs, or improve the side effect profile. For example, the prescribing of probenecid and ampicillin together has been used to achieve high and prolonged concentrations of the antibiotic. However, this synergy approach is rarely used in clinical practice, because these interactions may also lead to an increase in the drug's therapeutic effect or toxicity, which may also be harmful. It is only in less common situations that clinicians purposely employ a drug interaction to increase a drug's therapeutic effects.

In addition to drug-drug interactions, a variety of other substances can alter the pharmacokinetics and/or effect of drugs. These include foods, nutritional supplements, formulation excipients (substances used to dilute a drug), and environmental factors (e.g., cigarette smoke). In the A-to-Z section of this encyclopedia, each drug group lists potential drug interactions where applicable.

The potential for drug interactions is especially important to consider in elderly patients, who often have various chronic diseases for which they receive multiple medications. Patients who receive their care from more than one provider and their medications from more than one pharmacy are also prone to drug interactions. In addition, drug interactions are common in disease states for which multidrug therapy is the standard of care, such as tuberculosis, HIV infection, organ transplantation, and cancer.

Combinations of narcotics, alcohol, and tranquilizers can be particularly dangerous. Patients drinking alcohol or taking tranquilizers, sleeping aids, antidepressants, antihistamines, or any other drugs that make them sleepy need to tell their doctors how much and how often they are taking these substances. Even small doses might cause problems. The use of alcohol or any of these drugs with narcotics can lead to overdose symptoms such as weakness, difficulty in breathing, confusion, anxiety, or more severe drowsiness or dizziness. These drug interactions may result in unconsciousness and death.

The United States Food and Drug Administration (FDA) has removed several drugs, including mibefradil, terfenadine, astemizole, and cisapride, from the U.S. market solely because of the life-threatening potential of interactions with these drugs.

Taking more than one antidepressant at the same time can result in serotonin syndrome, which is potentially fatal. Serotonin syndrome is rare and is due to excessive serotonergic activity that is usually associated with the use of multiple serotonergic agents, such as selective serotonin reuptake inhibitors (SSRIs) together with monoamine oxidase inhibitors (MAOIs), but can occur with SSRIs alone. The syndrome can include abdominal pain, diarrhea, flushing, sweating, hyperthermia, lethargy, mental status changes, tremor, myoclonus, rhabdomyolysis, renal failure, cardiovascular shock, and possible death.

Drug hypersensitivity   A reaction to a therapeutic drug can occasionally occur after the patient has been exposed to the drug one or more times without incident. The body produces antibodies to the drug, and subsequent exposure to the same drug causes an allergic reaction in the body. Hypersensitivity reactions can include skin rash, itching, hives, flushed skin, unexpected fever, anxiety, wheezing and breathing difficulty (anaphylaxis), and anemia. In rare cases, blood vessel inflammation (vasculitis) may develop after repeated exposure to a drug.

Drug intolerance   Drug intolerance means that side effects occur, making it difficult or impossible to take particular drugs as directed. The adverse reaction may occur the very first time

the drug is administered. When this occurs, the physician may replace one or more of the drugs being taken with different ones.

Drug eruptions   Some medications cause skin reactions, which are also referred to as adverse cutaneous lesions or drug eruptions, after they have been administered. Drug eruptions are relatively common; studies have shown they affect 2 to 3 percent of hospitalized patients, with an estimated one in 1,000 hospitalized patients having a serious cutaneous drug reaction. Drug eruptions may be caused by either hypersensitivity or allergy to a medication.

Symptoms vary according to the drug and the sensitivity of the patient, ranging from a mild rash to hives (urticaria), serum sickness, and, rarely, life-threatening anaphylaxis. A "fixed" drug eruption has been described as single or multiple, round, sharply demarcated, dusky red plaques appearing soon after drug exposure and reappearing in exactly the same spot (hence, fixed) each time that drug is taken. Generally, itching and burning accompany these eruptions. In addition to prescription drugs, over-the-counter (OTC) medicines such as Sudafed can cause a fixed drug eruption.

Some drugs, such as digitalis, rarely provoke allergies, while others, such as penicillin, frequently cause drug eruptions. (Penicillin can also cause anaphylaxis from breathing difficulties.) Sulfa drugs and antiseizure medications may also cause drug eruptions. Once a person is found to be susceptible to skin reactions from any drug, he or she must avoid taking that medication; thus, doctors and pharmacists need to always be alerted. If a person has these allergic tendencies, skin tests may be performed prior to prescribing new medications to help determine the new drugs' safety for that person.

Special concerns when taking prescription drugs

Drugs can also cause harm when taken incorrectly. While patients may be aware of the more widely discussed issues of drug abuse and side effects, less obvious harmful practices and effect can also lead to drug-related problems.

Mixing with OTC medications Because OTC medications do not require a prescription, many people erroneously think they are safe for any circumstance. However, many OTC medicines contain the same ingredients as prescription drugs, so patients, physicians, and pharmacists need to be consulted before taking OTCs along with prescribed drugs.

Splitting pills Because double-strength pills often do not cost much more than a pill with single strength, many patients would rather buy pills that are double the strength of what they really should be taking, so that they can cut them in half to obtain the strength they need. And it is not only individuals who are splitting pills to save money; various health organizations have also been splitting pills to cut prescription drug costs. Researchers at Stanford University Medical Center confirmed that pill-splitting could mean lower costs for health maintenance organizations without losing any drug effectiveness or safety. They stressed that pill-splitting must begin with a doctor-patient or pharmacist-patient conversation so that the patient can be informed about its potential limitations.

In order to guarantee patient safety, pill-splitting must be used only with specific drugs and by specific patients. Certain types of medications are unsuitable for pill-splitting, including time release medications and those with special coatings. Some pills have a softer texture, making them crumble easily when cut, which results in loss of some of the drug. Capsules cannot be split. Time-release pills have a protective coating that plays a role in the drug's gradual release. Destroying that coating can impact proper delivery of the drug. Stacy noted that pills with hard, enteric coating to prevent stomach irritation should not be split. "Cutting such pills can cause crumbling, and ruin the stomach protection." Also, certain patients may be unable to split tablets consistently and accurately. These patients may include those with poor eyesight, loss of limbs, tremors, advanced arthritis, dementia, or psychosis. The researchers noted that results are best when the patient used a pill-splitting device; these are available at pharmacies for around $5.

Pharmacists can tell if a tablet is one that can be split. Pill-splitting may save money, but this approach can be dangerous and lead to overdosage or underdosage. In addition, pill-splitting can be difficult to do properly. Some pharmacies may do the pill-splitting for their patients.

Researchers from the Rutgers University Ernest Mario School of Pharmacy found that patients who had split the generic version of the muscle relaxant Flexeril (cyclobenzaprine HCl 10-milligram), using a tablet splitter or kitchen knife, into two 5-mg portions, were receiving anywhere from half the recommended dose to one and a half times more. The generic pills were not scored to make splitting easier.

Acknowledging that people will split pills regardless of the possible dangers, experts advise that for those pills approved for splitting by physicians or pharmacists, one tablet at a time be divided, with the two halves then taken on consecutive days. This will help compensate for any over- or underdosage.

Drug-resistant bacteria Antibiotic drugs kill bacteria, which cause most ear infections, some sinus infections, strep throat, and urinary tract infections. Sometimes bacteria may be resistant or become resistant. Resistant bacteria do not respond to antibiotics and continue to cause infection. Studies have shown that this increase in antibiotic resistance parallels the increase in antibiotic use in humans.

Some of the blame for this increased antibiotic use has been placed on consumers who insist that their doctors prescribe antibiotics for their colds and flu, which are often caused by viruses and not by bacteria. Each unnecessary or improper use of an antibiotic increases the chance of developing drug-resistant bacteria. Therefore, it is very important to take antibiotics only when necessary. Because of these resistant bacteria, some diseases that used to be easy to treat are now becoming very difficult to treat with the antibiotics that are currently available.

Therapeutic drug levels   Certain drugs have a narrow therapeutic dose window for effectiveness. Below this therapeutic window, the drug is ineffective; above it, the drug is toxic. According to the NIH, therapeutic drug level testing is especially important in people taking procainamide or digoxin (used to treat abnormal beating of the heart), phenytoin, carbamazepine, or valproic acid (used to treat seizures), and gentamicin, tobramycin, or amikacin (antibiotics used to treat infections). Therapeutic drug levels are monitored via a blood test.

Self-medicating   The classical definition of self-medication is "the taking of drugs, herbs or home remedies on one's own initiative, or on the advice of another person, without consulting a doctor." With some 700 prescription drugs cleared over the past two dozen years to be sold OTC, self-medication has escalated to be an issue of concern. Treating oneself or altering the treatment plan of a doctor without that doctor's knowledge can lead to negative consequences. Some people overmedicate on the mistaken assumption that more is better. When people combine drugs without consulting a pharmacist or doctor, serious harm can be done. Also, should the person misdiagnose his or her condition or complications, then later seek professional medical attention when self-medicating proves ineffective, it can take the professionally prescribed treatment longer to work.

Calis, Karim Anton, ed. "Drug Interactions: A Guide for Clinicians." *Pharmacy Update Special Issue*. Bethesda, Md.: National Institutes of Health, November–December 2001.

Dingle, Brian. "Pharmacogenomics in Oncology." *Oncology Exchange* 3, no. 5 (December 2004): 8–11.

Joly, Y., B. M. Knoppers, and M. T. Nguyen. "Stored Tissue Samples: Through the Confidentiality Maze." *Pharmacogenomics Journal* 5, no. 1 (2005): 2–5.

National Institute of General Medical Sciences. *Medicines by Design*. Bethesda, Md.: National Institutes of Health, revised October 2003.

Stacy, Kelli Miller. "Split Decisions." *Arthritis Today* May/June 2005, p. 44.

Stafford, Randall S., and D. C. Radley. "The Potential of Pill Splitting to Achieve Cost Savings." *American Journal of Managed Care* 8, no. 8 (August 2002): 706–712.

Walch, J. M., et al. "The Effect of Sunlight on Postoperative Analgesic Medication Use: A Prospective Study of Patients Undergoing Spinal Surgery." *Psychosomatic Medicine* 67, no. 1 (January–February 2005): 156–163.

Prescription Drug Issues with Different Population Groups

Certain groups of people may need to be particularly careful when taking prescription drugs.

Children, the elderly, and pregnant and nursing women, for example, have special concerns and needs with regard to taking certain drugs. As the National Institute of Mental Health cautions, "Some effects of medications on the growing body, the aging body, and the childbearing body are known, but much remains to be learned. Research in these areas is ongoing." In addition, some drugs affect different ethnic groups differently.

Pediatrics and medicines

Developing drug formulations appropriate for growing children is a challenge for scientists. Nunn and Williams explain, "Childhood is a period of maturation requiring knowledge of developmental pharmacology to establish dose, but the ability of the child to manage different dosage forms and devices also changes. Pediatric formulations must allow accurate administration of the dose to children of widely varying age and weight." While tablet forms of medications may be the only formulation available for a particular drug, not all young children can safely take tablets. Even when liquid formulations are available, unpleasant or bitter tastes have to be masked to assure appropriate compliance. Nunn and Williams caution that many gaps exist in the knowledge of pediatric formulations.

Many of the prescription drugs that are given to children have undergone testing in adults, but not in infants or children. Although pediatricians have called for testing in children in order to provide information vital for proper dosing, greater safety, and enhanced effectiveness, the drug industry has generally argued that such testing could be unethical because those being tested are not old enough to give consent. While parents may be enthusiastic about a study, the seven-year-olds who learn what is involved often say, "No way!" Meadows also noted that technical procedures seemingly simple for adults, such as drawing blood or getting a urine sample, can be difficult with children.

Some in the medical community counter that it is a matter of money—that extending drug trials to children would add to the already high research and development costs for drugs. Meadows explained further, "Pharmaceutical companies generally have viewed children as a market that would only bring small financial benefits. The drugs that have been adequately studied in children—vaccines, some antibiotics, and some cough and cold medicines—have a large market."

According to the Pediatric Pharmacology Research Unit Network established by the National Institute of Child Health and Human Development, which is part of the National Institutes of Health (NIH), only five in 80 drugs most frequently used in newborns and infants are labeled for pediatric use, and fewer than one-quarter of all medications currently on the market have been approved by the FDA for use in children. Thus, three-quarters do not carry FDA labeling for use in newborns, infants, children, and adolescents.

Fortescue et al. noted problems in giving medications to children. "Medication errors in pediatric inpatients occur at similar rates as in adults but have three times the potential to cause harm. Children pose special challenges in the drug ordering and delivery process; for example, drug dosages often must be calculated individu-

ally, leading to increased opportunities for error with a relatively high risk of 10-fold errors over time, especially in small infants, requiring frequent dosing recalculations. Medicine dispensing in children is complicated by the fact that stock solutions of medicines are often available only at adult concentrations and must be diluted for use in children. Children, particularly those who are young and critically ill, may be more prone to adverse drug events than adults because they have less physiologic reserve with which to buffer errors such as overdoses." In their study of 1,020 pediatric patients admitted to two academic medical centers during a six-week period, 616 of 10,778 medication orders contained errors. Most errors occurred at the ordering stage (74 percent) and involved errors in dosing (28 percent), route (18 percent), or frequency (9 percent).

Although neonates (birth to one month) are reported to be at greater risk of medication error than infants and older children, little is known about the causes and characteristics of error in this patient group, according to Kunac and Reith. In their study to identify and prioritize potential failures in the neonatal intensive care unit, the researchers found "common potential failures related to errors in the dose, timing of administration, infusion pump settings and route of administration."

Spending on prescription drugs for infants, children, adolescents, and young adults increased by 85 percent between 1997 and 2002, with spending in some categories of pediatric prescriptions soaring by more than 600 percent, according to research reported in the *Medco Health Solutions 2002 Drug Trend Report*. In 2001, young patients surpassed senior citizens and baby boomers in representing the fastest-growing segment of prescription drug consumers, the report said. According to the research, more pediatric patients are taking more—and more costly—medications for longer periods of time. The three primary drivers of drug spending in the under-19 age group were asthma, allergy, and anti-infectives, followed by neurological/psychological treatments and dermatologics. Other findings in the report:

- More than half of the increase in drug spending for children was due to an increase in the cost of drugs, including price inflation, and the introduction of new and more effective therapies.

- Spending on proton pump inhibitors to treat heartburn and other gastrointestinal disorders in children, a class of drugs whose use was virtually nonexistent in that age group five years prior, increased by 660 percent, as pediatricians broadly embraced use of these medications.

- An increase in pediatric asthma diagnosis and treatment and the introduction of new allergy medications contributed to a 211 percent rise in spending.

- Spending on drug therapies prescribed for attention-deficit/hyperactivity disorder (ADHD) increased by 122 percent over the previous four years.

- Spending on antibiotics increased by 42 percent; however, recent studies have shown that physician prescribing in this category is on the decline.

Higgins reported that children and adolescents are taking more mood-altering drugs that treat disorders such as ADHD, anxiety attacks, and depression. "The use of antidepressants jumped about 10 percent annually from 1998 to 2002 among children and adolescents, according to an April 2004 survey by Express Scripts Inc., a St. Louis pharmacy-benefit management company." According to the report, the fastest-growing segment of users was among infants to five-year-olds. Medication use among preschool girls more than doubled, while use by boys rose 64 percent. This was followed in 2005 with data released by pharmacy-benefit manager Medco Health Solutions Inc., which revealed that antidepressant prescriptions for patients younger than 18 years old fell 10 percent in 2004. The decreased use was attributed to the FDA's requirement that pharmaceutical companies strengthen warning labels on the drugs to alert parents and physicians that the drugs increase the risk of suicidal thoughts and behaviors in children and adolescents.

Drugs commonly prescribed for children and adolescents that carry black-box warnings include

- *all ANTIDEPRESSANTS:* treat depression and anxiety. Warnings are for suicidal thoughts and behaviors.

- *fluvoxamine:* treats obsessive-compulsive disorder. May need to be prescribed in lower than recommended doses for girls ages eight to 11.

- *lamotrigine:* treats epilepsy. Warning is for serious skin rashes that require hospitalization.

- *gabapentin:* treats seizures. Warning is for new adverse effects not seen in adults, such as hostility and aggressive behavior.

- *isotretinoin:* treats severe acne. Warnings are for birth defects, depression, and suicidal thoughts.

- *propofol:* an anesthesia drug. A research study showed an increase in deaths when the drug was used for pediatric ICU sedation in comparison with standard sedative agents. Administration of propofol with the pain medication fentanyl may result in serious slowing of the heart rate.

- *salmeterol xinafoate:* treats asthma. Warnings are for respiratory arrest and seizures.

- *buspirone:* treats generalized anxiety disorder. Safety and effectiveness were not established in patients ages six to 17 at doses recommended for use in adults.

- *midazolam:* used as a sedative. Warning is for respiratory problems.

- *etodolac:* treats the signs and symptoms of juvenile rheumatoid arthritis. Research shows that higher doses are needed in younger children. Warning is for the potential for increased risk of cardiovascular events (including heart attack and stroke) and serious and potentially life-threatening gastrointestinal (GI) bleeding associated with its use.

In June 2004, the Pharmaceutical Research and Manufacturers of America (PhRMA) announced that 158 new medicines for children were then being tested in clinical trials or awaiting review by the FDA. These medicines included:

- a new generation of inhaled corticosteroid, with novel release and distribution properties, for the treatment of asthma. The medicine is activated only when it enters the lungs, reducing potential side effects in the mouth and throat. Asthma is the leading cause of school absenteeism, affecting an estimated 6.3 million American children under the age of 18.

- a medicine that addresses relapsed pediatric malignancies. It is comprised of a widely used anticancer drug encapsulated in a unique drug-delivery system. Cancer, while rare in children, is the chief cause of death by disease in children between ages one and 14.

- a potential gene treatment to deliver a functional copy of the mutated gene that plays a role in cystic fibrosis. Cystic fibrosis is a genetic disease affecting approximately 30,000 American children and adults. Each year about 3,200 babies are born with this lung disease.

The elderly and medicines

Older adults are prescribed the greatest number of medications, use the greatest number of non-prescription medications, and are more likely to be administered several medications at once for longer periods of time. Although they constitute only 13 percent of the U.S. population, they receive 32 percent of all prescription drugs dispensed. Although elderly persons use prescription medications approximately three times as frequently as the general population, they have been found to have the poorest rates of compliance with directions for taking a medication. The most cited reasons for older adults not taking medications appropriately include forgetting to take them, forgetting that they have already taken a dose, not understanding or remembering the verbal instructions, being unable to afford the drugs, not wanting to deal with the side effects, having difficulty with swallowing larger capsules and tablets, and difficulty with opening the medicine containers (especially those with arthritis).

Curry et al. elaborated, "Because their medication regimens often are complicated by many medications and different doses, times, and administration methods, older adults are at high risk for medication mismanagement. The most common errors associated with medication mismanagement include mixing OTC and prescription medications, discontinuing prescriptions, taking wrong dosages, using incorrect techniques, and consuming inappropriate foods with specific medications."

Wooten and Galavis note that although absorption of medicines in the elderly is generally slower, "[a]bsorption through the skin after topical administration may actually increase in the elderly as the aging skin becomes thin and frail." They add that distribution of drugs throughout the body also changes with age. "A medication gets distributed into either fat or water, depending on its chemical characteristics. As a patient ages, his percentage of body fat increases, so a drug that's lipid-soluble, such as diazepam (Valium), may stay in the body longer because there are more fat stores into which it can be distributed. And, because older patients have proportionately less body water than younger ones, blood levels of a drug that is water-soluble may be higher than expected. It's difficult, though, to anticipate the effect that changes in fat stores or body water will have on drug distribution because other body functions, such as protein binding, can also complicate drug distribution." In addition, liver and kidney function also affect how the elderly respond to a particular drug. Typically, elderly patients have reduced hepatic and renal function compared to younger individuals. Therefore, drugs that are eliminated hepatically or renally may stay in the body longer and have the potential to cause an increased risk of side effects.

Because older people tend to have a larger number of concurrent chronic health problems than younger people, they are more apt to be multiple medication users, so are at increased risk for drug-drug interactions.

Curtis et al. of Duke University found that over the course of a year one in five elderly Americans in their large study filled a prescription for at least one drug classified as a "drug of concern," according to the Beers Criteria. This list of criteria for determining the appropriate use of medication in elderly living in nursing homes was developed in 1991 by a team led by Mark Beers at the University of California, Los Angeles. In 1997, Beers updated the original list, initially intended primarily for institutional use, for use in any setting. The list named 28 medications or classes of medications considered inappropriate for use in elderly patients. Then in 2003, a U.S. consensus panel of experts led by Fick et al. expanded the Beers Criteria by identifying 48 individual medications or classes of medications to avoid in older adults and their potential concerns, and 20 diseases/conditions and medications to be avoided in older adults with these conditions. Of these potentially inappropriate drugs, 66 were considered by the panel to have adverse outcomes of high severity.

The Duke University study population included 765,423 people from all 50 states, the District of Columbia, Puerto Rico, and two U.S. territories. More than 20 percent filled a prescription for one or more drugs—including the antidepressant amitriptyline and antianxiety drug diazepam—with potential for severe adverse effects in older people. Nearly 16 percent filled prescriptions for two risky drugs and 4 percent for three or more Beers list drugs within the same year. The authors noted that many drugs present increasing risk for people as they age due to changes in metabolism and excretion. In addition, the effects of drugs are complicated by the number of prescription drugs taken. (See Polypharmacy in "Other Drug Industry and Prescription Drug–Related Issues," p. lxix.)

Data from the Veterans Affairs Hospital System suggest that elderly patients may be prescribed inappropriately high doses of medications such as benzodiazepines and may be prescribed these medications for longer periods than younger adults. In general, older people should be prescribed lower doses of medications, because the body's ability to metabolize many medications decreases with age. In addition, the doses of medication should be increased at more extended intervals. This approach has been termed "Start low, go slow." An association between age-related morbidity and misuse of prescription medications probably exists. For example, elderly persons who take benzodiazepines are at increased risk for falls that cause hip and thigh fractures, as well as for vehicle accidents. Cognitive impairment also is associated with benzodiazepine use, although memory impairment may be reversible when the drug is discontinued. Finally, use of benzodiazepines for longer than four months is not recommended for elderly patients because of the possibility of physical dependence.

In September 2004, PhRMA announced that more than 800 medicines were in development for diseases of aging, including 123 for heart disease and stroke, 395 for cancer, and 329 for such debilitating diseases as Alzheimer's, diabetes, and osteoporosis. The medicines in development for diseases of aging included:

- 22 for Alzheimer's disease, which could afflict 16 million people by the middle of the 21st century unless a cure or prevention is found
- 11 for depression, which affects an estimated 6.5 million Americans 65 and older
- 53 for diabetes, which affects 7 million Americans 65 and older, or 20.1 percent of all people in this age group
- 18 for osteoporosis, which affects more than half of all women over the age of 65, although it is usually not diagnosed until a fracture or break occurs
- 14 for Parkinson's disease, which affects about one in 100 people age 65 and older

Other medicines in development target bladder and kidney diseases, eye disorders, gastrointestinal disorders, osteoarthritis, pain, prostate disease, respiratory and lung disorders, rheumatoid arthritis, skin conditions, and other conditions of aging. All of the medicines are either in clinical trials or awaiting approval by the FDA. Many of the medicines use cutting edge knowledge and technology to attack diseases in different ways. These include a potential medicine that blocks the new blood vessel growth that causes one form of macular degeneration, the leading cause of blindness in Americans over 65, and a medicine for Alzheimer's that both inhibits plaque formation and blocks the degradation of the neurotransmitter acetylcholine.

Women and medications

Gender differences in drug pharmacokinetics and pharmacodynamics have been recognized for some time, according to Sica et al. "This issue has generally been ignored in clinical practice, despite there being ample evidence to suggest that gender can influence multiple aspects of pharmacokinetics. Gastric acid secretion, gastrointestinal blood flow, proportions of muscular and adipose tissue, the amount of drug-binding proteins, gender-specific changes in the available amount of P450 isozymes, physiologic and hormonal changes during the menstrual cycle, and differences in renal blood flow are several factors that may have some bearing on gender-related differences in pharmacokinetics. Furthermore, female-specific issues such as pregnancy, menopause, oral contraceptive use, and menstruation may independently influence drug metabolism and serve as confounders to the interpretation of gender differences in drug handling or effect."

Kaiser notes that studies of how women's and men's bodies process drugs have turned up mostly minor differences. "But some drugs may be less or more effective in women or cause more side effects, and other variations may await discovery." Because women are smaller on average than men are, Kaiser explains that "they may absorb drugs more slowly, and their kidneys may filter excreted drugs out more slowly. Because women tend to have more body fat, fat-soluble drugs stay in their bodies longer. All this means a woman who swallows the same number of pills as a man may end up with a larger or smaller

level in her blood." While some experts remain skeptical that gender makes a difference in drug efficacy, others argue that drug researchers have barely scratched the surface in this area.

Pregnant women Certain medications taken during pregnancy may cause serious birth defects in the baby. Therefore, these medications should be avoided by all pregnant women. In 1979, the FDA introduced a classification of fetal risks due to pharmaceuticals based on a similar system that had been introduced in Sweden one year earlier. The Pregnancy Risk Categories are assigned to all drugs, and range from A (safest drugs) to X (least-safe drugs) as defined on the following chart:

PREGNANCY RISK CATEGORIES	
Pregnancy Category A	Adequate and well-controlled studies have failed to demonstrate a risk to the fetus in the first trimester of pregnancy (and there is no evidence of risk in later trimesters).
Pregnancy Category B	Animal reproduction studies have failed to demonstrate a risk to the fetus, and there are no adequate and well-controlled studies in pregnant women OR Animal studies have shown an adverse effect, but adequate and well-controlled studies in pregnant women have failed to demonstrate a risk to the fetus in any trimester.
Pregnancy Category C	Animal reproduction studies have shown an adverse effect on the fetus and there are no adequate and well-controlled studies in humans, but potential benefits may warrant use of the drug in pregnant women despite potential risks.
Pregnancy Category D	There is positive evidence of human fetal risk based on adverse reaction data from investigational or marketing experience or studies in humans, but potential benefits may warrant use of the drug in pregnant women despite potential risks.
Pregnancy Category X	Studies in animals or humans have demonstrated fetal abnormalities and/or there is positive evidence of human fetal risk based on adverse reaction data from investigational or marketing experience, and the risks involved in use of the drug in pregnant women clearly outweigh potential benefits.

However, according to the Centers for Disease Control and Prevention (CDC), not enough is known about the safety of many other drugs when they are taken by pregnant women. The CDC notes that although women are often told not to use any medications while pregnant, this is not always possible. Some pregnant women must take medications to treat health conditions such as asthma, epilepsy, high blood pressure, and depression. Not treating these conditions could harm the mother or the child. Also, many women take medications before they even know they are pregnant.

Although drugs are tested in pregnant animals to see if there are problems, human clinical trials do not usually include pregnant women because of possible risks to the unborn children. While animal testing can help to identify potential problems, these tests do not always predict how medications will affect pregnant women, who can have effects that pregnant animals do not have.

Drug companies sometimes conduct special studies called pregnancy registries. They enroll pregnant women who have taken certain medications. Then after birth, their babies are compared to the babies of women who did not take the medication. For a list of current pregnancy registries and how to enroll, see http://www.fda.gov/womens/registries.

The Organization of Teratology Information Services (OTIS) gives information to health care providers and pregnant women about the risks and safety of taking medications during pregnancy and while breastfeeding. They also conduct studies of pregnant women who contact them after taking certain medications. Their Web site is at http://www.otispregnancy.org.

Nursing women   Many prescription and over-the-counter drugs, herbals, and dietary supplements can reach a nursing baby through breast milk. Fortunately, according to the CDC, most medications enter breast milk in small amounts that will not affect a nursing baby very much. However, more information is needed about the actual effects of most medications on nursing babies to be certain they are safe to use while breastfeeding.

In March 2004, PhRMA announced that pharmaceutical researchers were developing 371 medicines for diseases that disproportionately affect American women. The medicines in development were either in clinical trials or awaiting FDA review. The potential medicines included 41 for breast cancer, 33 for ovarian cancer, 41 for diabetes, 36 for arthritis, 23 for depression, 21 for Alzheimer's disease, 20 for osteoporosis, and 13 for multiple sclerosis.

Other medicines in development targeted systemic lupus erythematosus, psoriasis, scleroderma, cervical cancer, glaucoma, incontinence, urinary tract infections, asthma, chronic bronchitis, migraine, obstetrical and gynecological disorders, anxiety, irritable bowel syndrome, sepsis, and other diseases.

Ethnic groups and medications

Racial and ethnic groups make up important populations whose special needs and drug responses traditionally have been undervalued or ignored, according to Burroughs et al.: "Research in the last 35 years has uncovered significant differences among these groups in their rates of drug metabolism, in clinical responses to drugs, and in drug side effects due to genetic variations, suggesting that those treating these patients need to take special care when prescribing drug therapies."

Blacks   Racial differences may play a significant role in determining a patient's response to asthma medications, according to one study. Federico et al. found that asthmatic and non-asthmatic blacks required higher doses of glucocorticoids to suppress lymphocytes, which play an important role in airway inflammation. As a result, the researchers speculate that blacks may have a predisposition to a diminished medication response, which can contribute to more difficult asthma control.

Blacks have been found to metabolize antidepressants more slowly than whites and may experience serious side effects from inappropriate dosages.

In a continuing drive to close the health gap between blacks and the majority population, pharmaceutical and biotechnology companies are developing 249 new medicines for disease that disproportionately afflict blacks or diseases that are among the top 10 causes of death among blacks, according to a survey released by PhRMA in 2002.

The 249 medicines in the pipeline represented a more than 50 percent increase in research on drugs for diseases disproportionately affecting blacks since a 1999 survey, which found 156 medicines in development. The potential medicines were either in clinical trials or awaiting approval by the FDA.

Ninety of the new medicines targeted cancer, the second leading killer of all Americans. Overall, blacks are more likely to develop cancer than whites and are about 30 percent more likely to die of cancer than whites. They have disproportionately higher rates of multiple myeloma and cancers of the esophagus, cervix, uterus, larynx, stomach, mouth, pancreas, and prostate. In fact, black men may have the highest incidence of prostate cancer in the world, and the death rate among African-American men is twice as high as that of white American men. The medicines in the pipeline target cancers of the cervix, colon/rectum, esophagus, larynx, liver, lung, pancreas, prostate, stomach, and uterus, as well as multiple myeloma and non-Hodgkin's lymphoma.

Fifty-three potential medicines focus on respiratory disorders, including asthma, which kills blacks at three times the rate of the majority population, and chronic obstructive pulmonary disease, which takes more than 5,000 black lives each year. Forty-eight of the medicines in development are for diabetes, whose incidence in the black community is on the rise. The number of blacks with diabetes has tripled since the 1960s, and black Americans experience higher rates of the disease's most serious complications—blindness, amputation, and kidney failure—than do white Americans with diabetes.

Fifty-eight medicines targeted HIV/AIDS. AIDS death rates for blacks are nearly 10 times higher than for whites, and blacks are experiencing less dramatic decline in AIDS deaths than the majority population.

Nineteen medicines are designed to treat cardiovascular disease, including coronary artery disease, heart attack, heart failure, stroke, and hypertension. The death rate from cardiovascular disease is nearly 50 percent higher for black men than for white men and 67 percent higher for black women than for white women. Other medicines in development tackled kidney failure, eye disorders, obesity, and sickle-cell disease.

On June 23, 2005, the FDA approved BiDil (combination of hydralazine and isosorbide dinitrate), a drug for the treatment of heart failure in self-identified black patients, which represented a step toward the promise of personalized medicine. The approval of BiDil was based in part on the results of the African-American Heart Failure Trial (A-HeFT) involving 1,050 self-identified black patients with severe heart failure who had already been treated with the best available therapy. This follow-up trial of blacks only was conducted when two previous trials of the drug had found no benefit in the general population of severe heart failure patients, but had suggested a benefit in black patients. In the A-HeFT study, black patients on BiDil experienced a 43 percent reduction in death and a 39 percent decrease in hospitalization for heart failure compared to placebo, and a decrease of their symptoms of heart failure.

Asian Americans In another step toward personalized medicine, University of Washington researchers found that people of Asian descent were more sensitive to the blood-thinning drug warfarin, while African Americans were more resistant. People of European descent were about evenly split among low, medium, and high sensitivity. If further testing validates these findings, genetic testing could lead to better and more effective treatment.

Following the FDA's findings about the risk of rhabdomyolysis (serious muscle damage) in patients taking rosuvastatin (Crestor), Astra-Zeneca Pharmaceuticals (Crestor's manufacturer) revised the package insert for Crestor to reemphasize recommendations made in the original label about the need for physicians to consider using lower starting doses of the drug in some individuals as a means of reducing the risk of rhabdomyolysis. The revised labeling notes that this may be particularly important for treating Asian-American patients, since clinical trial data suggest that they (along with patients on cyclosporine or patients with severe renal insufficiency) may have higher drug levels and therefore be at greater risk for muscle injury due to Crestor than the general population.

Hispanic Americans/Mexican Americans In addition to searching for possible differences in drug effectiveness among various ethnic groups, experts have looked into disparities in prescription drug use among groups. A University of Maryland School of Pharmacy study compared drug coverage and prescription drug use by race and Hispanic ethnicity for Medicare beneficiaries with three chronic conditions: diabetes, hypertension, or heart disease. "We found that among beneficiaries without any drug coverage black persons and Hispanics used 10 to 40 percent fewer medications, on average, than white persons with the same illness, and spent up to 60 percent less in total drug costs. Having drug coverage somewhat lessened these differences although the effect was consistent with only M + C (Medicare+Choice) prescription benefits. Substantially lower medication use remained for dually eligible black beneficiaries and Hispanics with employer-sponsored drug benefits."

Marin noted that despite the fact of Hispanics being the largest minority group in the United States, no truly reliable data about treating mentally ill Hispanic Americans with psychotropic medications exists. "Most of the comparative clinical trials with Hispanics have been performed for antidepressants. Because

of design shortcomings and sample size, their significance is limited, but several studies point toward a better response, higher attrition and higher side-effect reporting in Hispanics given antidepressants."

Pharmaceutical and biotechnology companies are developing 258 new medicines for diseases that disproportionately affect the nation's 35.3 million Hispanic Americans, according to a 2004 survey by PhRMA. Among the key findings of the survey:

- Although Hispanic Americans make up only 14 percent of the U.S. population, they account for nearly 20 percent of new AIDS cases. Pharmaceutical companies were developing 58 new medicines to fight HIV and AIDS.

- Hispanic Americans have high rates of cervical cancer, colorectal cancer, and lung cancer. Pharmaceutical researchers were working on 71 potential medicines for these types of cancer.

- Hispanic Americans are twice as likely to develop Type 2 diabetes as do non-Hispanic whites. There were 48 medicines in the pipeline for this disease.

Note: The number of drugs being developed, as described by PhRMA, are for the overall population, and not for a particular disease in a particular patient population. However, they may have potential benefit for some patient populations more so than others because of the higher disease incidence rates in these particular groups.

Briesacher, B., R. Limcangco, and D. Gaskin. "Racial and Ethnic Disparities in Prescription Coverage and Medication Use." *Health Care Financing Review* 25, no. 2 (Winter 2003): 63–76.

Burroughs, Valentine J., Randall W. Maxey, and Richard A. Levy. "Racial and Ethnic Differences in Response to Medicines: Towards Individualized Treatment." *Journal of the National Medical Association* 94, no. 10 Suppl (October 2002): 1–26.

Curry, L. C., et al. "Teaching Older Adults to Self-manage Medications: Preventing Adverse Drug Reactions." *Journal of Gerontological Nursing* 31, no. 4 (April 2005): 32–42.

Curtis, Lesley H., et al. "Inappropriate Prescribing for Elderly Americans in a Large Outpatient Population." *Archives of Internal Medicine* 164, no. 15 (August 9–23): 1,621–1,625.

Federico, M. J., et al. "Racial Differences in T-lymphocyte Response to Glucocorticoids." *Chest* 127, no. 2 (February 2005): 571–578.

Fick, Donna M., et al. "Updating the Beers Criteria for Potentially Inappropriate Medication Use in Older Adults." *Archives of Internal Medicine* 163, no. 22 (December 8, 2003): 2,716–2,724.

Fortescue, E. B., et al. "Prioritizing Strategies for Preventing Medication Errors and Adverse Drug Events in Pediatric Inpatients." *Pediatrics* 111, no. 4 pt. 1 (April 2003): 722–729.

Higgins, Marguerite. "Aging America Fuels Drug Industry." *Washington Times,* March 27, 2005, A01.

James, Frank. "Pediatricians Want Medications Tested on Children; Drug Industry Disagrees." *Chicago Tribune,* February 5, 2003, 8.

Kaiser, Jocelyn. "Gender in the Pharmacy: Does It Matter?" *Science* 308, no. 5,728 (June 10, 2005): 1,572.

Kunac, D. L., and D. M. Reith. "Identification of Priorities for Medication Safety in Neonatal Intensive Care." *Drug Safety* 28, no. 3 (March 2005): 251–261.

Marin, Humberto. "Hispanics and Psychiatric Medications: An Overview." *Psychiatric Times* 20, no. 10 (October 2003). Available online. URL: http://www.psychiatrictimes.com/p031080.html. Accessed February 4, 2011.

Meadows, Michelle. "Drug Research and Children." *FDA Consumer* 37, no. 1 (January–February 2003): 12–17.

National Institute on Drug Abuse. *Prescription Drugs: Abuse and Addiction.* NIDA Research Report Series, NIH Publication 01-4881, July 2001.

Nunn, T., and J. Williams. "Formulation of Medicines for Children." *British Journal of Clinical Pharmacology* 59, no. 6 (June 2005): 674–676.

Rieder, M. J., et al. "Effect of VKORC1 Haplotypes on Transcriptional Regulation and Warfarin Dose." *New England Journal of Medicine* 352, no. 22 (June 2, 2005): 2,285–2,293.

Sica, D. A., M. Wood, and M. Hess. "Gender and Its Effect in Cardiovascular Pharmacotherapeutics: Recent Considerations." *Congestive Heart Failure* 11, no. 3 (May–June 2005): 163–166.

Wooten, James, and Julie Galavis. "Polypharmacy: Keeping the Elderly Safe." *RN* 68, no. 8 (August 2005): 44–50.

Pharmaceutical Industry—Beginnings through Today

Prior to the Revolutionary War, American apothecaries adopted some native herbs and plants that were used by Native Americans for their medical needs, but "the vast majority of drugs needed in this country before the 19th century were imported from Europe, either as raw material or as finished pharmaceutical products," according to Allen. Pharmaceutical manufacturing as an industry separate from retail pharmacy had its beginnings about 1600 but did not really begin to mature until the middle 1700s. Once the Revolutionary War began, Allen writes, "It became more difficult to import drugs, and the American pharmacist was motivated to acquire the scientific and technologic expertise of his European contemporary. From this period until the Civil War, pharmaceutical manufacturing was in its infancy in this country. A few of the pharmaceutical firms established during the early 1800s were the forerunners of some of the large pharmaceutical companies of today." Among those, Philadelphia druggist John K. Smith founded in 1830 what was to eventually become Smith, Kline and French Laboratories. Also, Cowen writes, "The firm established by pharmacist William R. Warner in Philadelphia became one of the constituents of Warner-Lambert in 1856."

The pharmaceutical industry as we know it today developed first in Germany, then in England and in France. In America, it was "the child of wars," as described by the Fort Carson Medical Department Activity (MEDDAC) of the U.S. Army Medical Command Department of Pharmacy on their Web site, which explains that the industry was "born in the Revolution; grew rapidly during and following the Civil War; became independent of Europe during World War I; came of age during and following World War II."

The Civil War was "the spark" that ignited the industry's phenomenal expansion in the late 1800s and into the 20th century, according to

Flannery. "The Civil War permanently changed American pharmacy, and the roots of that transformation lie in the four years of conflict that created unprecedented demand for mass-produced drugs. Statistics partly tell the tale. In 1860 there were 84 chemical manufacturers (including pharmaceutical firms) in the United States; the vast majority of which, as with other industrial concerns, were in the North; by 1870 the number had grown to nearly 300. The product value of drugs rose from $3.4 million in 1860 to $16.2 million in 1870—then to nearly $118 million fifty years later."

Haynes noted that although hundreds of opportunists responded to the "war-born influences" of shortages, skyrocketing prices, and improvisation to increase output, few survived beyond the war. "But the able managements of established companies greatly strengthened their positions." One effect of the war, according to Haynes, was the migration of the industry. "Philadelphia remained for years the largest single producer of fine chemicals, but it was no longer undisputed national headquarters. . . . St. Louis, Cincinnati, Indianapolis, and especially Detroit developing as pharmaceutical centers were outgrowths of this decentralization which logically flowed westward." Among those was Eli Lilly, who trained as a pharmacist prior to founding the Eli Lilly Company in Indianapolis in 1876.

If the Civil War was its spark, then the industrialization of America following the war fanned the pharmaceutical industry's flames. Allen explained,

The second half of the 19th century brought great and far-reaching changes. The United States was now under the full impact of the industrial revolution. The steam engine, which used water power to turn mills that powdered crude botanic drugs, was replaced by the gas, diesel or electric motor. New machinery was substituted for the old whenever possible, and often machinery from other industries was adapted to the special needs of pharmaceutical manufacturing. Mixers from the baking industry, centrifugal machines from the laundry industry, and sugarcoating pans from the candy industry were a few examples of the type of improvisations made. Production increased rapidly, but the new industry had to wait for the scientific revolution before it could claim newer and better drugs for mankind. A synergism was needed between science and the advancing technology.

By 1880, the industrial manufacture of chemicals and pharmaceutical products had become well established in this country, and the pharmacist was relying heavily on commercial sources for drug supply. Synthetic organic chemistry began to have its influence on drug therapy. The isolation of some active constituents of plant drugs had led to knowledge of their chemical structure. From this arose methods of synthetically duplicating the same structures, as well as manipulating molecular structure to produce organic chemicals yet undiscovered in nature. This new source of drugs—synthetic organic chemistry—welcomed the turn into the 20th century.

Tansey explains further the confluence of science and industry and its effect on the pharmaceutical industry:

During the late nineteenth and early twentieth centuries, there was an extraordinarily rapid increase in new ways of treating and preventing many bacterial diseases with antitoxins and vaccines. These therapies were of biological origin, derived from animals, and were the practical outcome of cell theory and germ theory. They continued to be used and refined well into the twentieth century and provided a major stimulus to the development of the pharmaceutical industry. At the same time, the demand for "wonder drugs" encouraged the production of new chemical agents, and these two lines of research, into biological and chemical therapies, continued hand in hand.

There was already, especially in Germany, a well-established chemical industry that developed and exploited these new therapies. This industrial development had resulted from the growth of the coal-tar and associated dye-stuff industries, and from synergistic advances in both organic and inorganic chemistry. The first synthetic dye, "mauve," had actually been developed in Britain, but it was German, and to a lesser extent Swiss, industrial machinery that extended the technical know-how into producing synthetic chemical therapeutic agents.

Many large pharmaceutical companies such as Hoechst, Bayer, Ciba, and Sandoz originated from the dye-stuff industry. Commercial companies and some academic institutes, such as Pasteur Institute in Paris, attempted to produce Roux's therapeutic serum on a large scale. In Britain, the London-based pharmaceutical firm of Burroughs, Wellcome & Co. and the Brown Animal Sanatory Institution, a small research laboratory associated with the University of London, first produced diphtheria antitoxins towards the end of 1894.

The search for new synthetic chemicals for treating disease accelerated towards the end of the nineteenth century. The potions, pills, and nostrums of the quack began to give way to rational, mass-produced, and mass-marketed therapies.

During these early industry years, the individual pharmacists continued to compound their own medications for the most part, but some were expanding their reach. Flannery explains, "Many pharmacists who had success running their drugstores were trying their hand at small-scale manufacturing and billing themselves as wholesalers. In Philadelphia, the nation's pharmaceutical capital, small manufacturers such as the Charles Ellis Company and Dulles, Earl, and Cope were producing a few select items for the wholesale trade."

But the pharmacist acting as a small manufacturer could not last long. As Cowen and Helfand explain, "Phytochemistry and synthetic chemistry created new derivatives of old drugs and new chemical entities of medicinal value that strained the capacity of the individual pharmacy. Large scale drug manufacturing had its strong hold on society with the advent of machines and patents. The progress made by this new industry is demonstrated by the catalogue of the American firm G. D. Searle, which by the late 1880s listed 400 fluid extracts, 150 elixirs, 100 syrups, 75 powdered extracts, and 25 tinctures and other drug forms."

The pharmacy as the manufacturer, rather than the local compounder of herbs and other raw materials, utilized the latest technical advances from every branch of science to economically develop and produce the latest and greatest in drugs in immense quantities—allowing physicians everywhere to prescribe and pharmacists to dispense them under controlled quality assurance.

Following World War II, the pharmaceutical industry expanded greatly, as Weatherall explains. "By the 1980s, around ten companies were usually among the top fifty major corporations in the USA, and there was similar growth in Britain and elsewhere in Europe. Research laboratories grew even faster than the companies; typically, the old-fashioned American firm of Smith, Kline & French had a research staff of eight in 1936, which grew to hundreds in the 1950s and now is enlarged by amalgamations with other enterprises into Smith Kline Beecham."

Allen, Loyd V., Jr. "A History of Pharmaceutical Compounding." *Secundum Artem* 11, no. 3 (2003): 1–6.

Cowen, David L. "Industrial Origins and Pharmacy." *Apothecary's Cabinet* no. 5 (Fall 2002): 10.

Cowen, David L., and William H. Helfand. *Pharmacy: An Illustrated History.* New York: Harry N. Abrams, 1990.

Flannery, Michael A. *Civil War Pharmacy: A History of Drugs, Drug Supply and Provisions, and Therapeutics for the Union and Confederacy.* Binghamton, N.Y.: Haworth Press, 2004.

Haynes, Williams. *American Chemical Industry. Vol. 1, Background and Beginnings: 1609–1911.* New York: Van Nostrand, 1945.

Tansey, E. M. "From the Germ Theory to 1945." Chap. 7 in *Western Medicine: An Illustrated History,* edited by Irvine Loudon. New York: Oxford University Press, 1997.

Modern Pharmacy Industry and Its Players

From research to manufacturing to dispensing, getting the proper drugs to the patients who need them can involve any number of companies and specialists. Generally, according to the

American Association of Pharmaceutical Scientists, those involved directly with pharmaceutical drugs fall into two camps:

Pharmaceutical scientists are typically involved in the development of new drugs: discovery, drug delivery systems, drug absorption, distribution, metabolism, and elimination characteristics. They spend most of their time doing research in a laboratory or office setting.

Pharmacists work with existing drugs, patients, and other health-care practitioners to optimize patient care and drug use. They often work face-to-face with physicians (drug selection and use) and patients (best use of medications).

Thus, those involved in beginning stages of drug development—at the research or manufacturing front end—do not necessarily interact directly with those at end stages of drug application—in the patient-care pharmacy arena. Among the various players between the beginning and end stages of the modern pharmacy industry:

Drug companies

Drug companies develop, produce, and market drugs licensed for use as medications, which relieve millions of people from various diseases and permit many suffering from illness to recover and lead productive lives. According to the Bureau of Labor Statistics, U.S. Department of Labor, *Career Guide to Industries, 2010–11 Edition,* Pharmaceutical and Medicine Manufacturing (on the Internet at http://www.bls.gov/oco/cg/cgs009.htm—accessed May 30, 2011), the pharmaceutical and medicine manufacturing industry consists of more than 2,500 places of employment, located throughout the country. The industry is composed of several different types of drug companies.

Brand-name drug companies   These companies concentrate on developing and marketing drugs with proprietary, trademark-protected names

(also called patented drugs). These major companies are also referred to as "Pharma" or "Big Pharma." According to their trade organization, the Pharmaceutical Research and Manufacturers of America (PhRMA), total U.S. drug sales from members reached nearly $163.3 billion in 2004, which was a 20 percent increase over 2003. During that same time period, their global sales reached $243.8 billion, a 13.8 percent increase. IMS Health Inc., a provider of business intelligence for the pharmaceutical and health-care industries, reported U.S. brand pharmaceutical sales for 2004 to be $217.4 billion.

Pioneer drug companies   Brand-name companies that develop the first versions of drugs, which are marketed under their brand names. For example, Valium is the brand name for the first marketed version of the antianxiety drug diazepam.

Generic drug companies   Companies that develop versions of drugs that are equivalent to the pioneer or brand-name drugs and are not marketed until the pioneer drugs' patent exclusivity has expired. These "copies" are often marketed under just the generic name of the drug—for example, diazepam. IMS Health Inc. reported U.S. generic pharmaceutical sales for 2004 to be $18.1 billion. According to the industry trade group Generic Pharmaceutical Association (GphA), generic drugs account for 53 percent of all prescriptions dispensed in the United States.

Specialty pharmaceutical companies   Specialty pharmaceutical companies focus on specific stages and aspects of drug development and marketing or on certain therapeutic areas. For example, PediaMed—The Pediatrics Company specializes in providing medicine to pediatric patients. Pollack explained, "Specialty pharmaceutical companies, like Forest Laboratories and King Pharmaceuticals, have long licensed drugs from pharmaceutical giants that had decided not to develop them. As big pharmaceutical companies have become even larger, they have concentrated on drugs with blockbuster potential rather than devote time to drugs with smaller markets. But for a small company, a crumb from a pharmaceutical giant can look like a feast. Moreover, as big companies have merged, overlapping projects have been cut. Some companies have decided it is better to get a return on these redundant or minor drugs by letting someone else sell them in exchange for a payment or royalties." In the area of research and development, brand name drug companies reportedly outsource a little more than a quarter of all their clinical trials and other drug development work to pharmaceutical specialty labs—amounting to an estimated $10.5 billion in 2005.

Drug delivery companies Companies that take existing drugs and develop systems to release those drugs into the body in new ways. For example, drug delivery technologies can make injectable drugs available in an oral form or make oral drugs available in a skin patch. With new delivery systems, patients may need less frequent dosing or may have less discomfort (such as patch delivery instead of injections) and may even enjoy better health outcomes. Drug delivery companies usually draw royalty streams for the products they improve for other companies. Their customers are most often large pharmaceutical companies that want to improve upon already marketed products.

Biopharmaceutical companies Pharmaceutical companies that have adopted a number of new technologies, allowing for broader and more efficient screening of chemical compounds. The PhRMA explains,

> One type of technological advance, the advent of biotechnology, has been particularly applicable to pharmaceutical chemistry. Biotechnology is a collection of technologies that capitalize on the attributes of cells, such as their manufacturing capabilities, and put biological molecules, such as DNA and proteins, to work for medicine development and other uses. This discipline uses new techniques such as bioprocessing (using living cells to manufacture products such as human insulin); monoclonal antibody technology (using immune system cells that make proteins called antibodies to target treatments to specific cells); molecular cloning (creating genetically identical DNA molecules); and recombinant DNA technology (combining and modifying genes to create new therapies). The convergence of traditional pharmaceutical chemistry and biotechnology has led the pharmaceutical and biotechnology industries, once thought of as being distinct and independent, to become more similar than dissimilar.

Pharmacists

Pharmacists are most often the direct link between drug and patient. Although a physician will usually prescribe the medication, and in a hospital setting, the nursing staff will likely do the administering of the drugs, for the vast majority of prescription drug–taking, the pharmacist will distribute the drug to the patient and educate the patient on usage. But today, pharmacists have much greater influence on the use of drugs than a few decades ago. They advise physicians and other health care practitioners on the selection, dosages, interactions, and side effects of medications. Pharmacists also monitor the patients' response to drug therapy to ensure safe and effective use of medication. Pharmacists must understand the use, clinical effects, and composition of drugs, including their chemical, biological, and physical properties. Among the roles they play are:

Community/retail pharmacists Pharmacists working behind the drug counter in chain and independent drug stores present the picture most people see when thinking about pharmacists. Community pharmacists counsel patients and answer questions about prescription drugs, including questions regarding possible side effects or interactions among various drugs. They provide information about over-the-counter drugs and make recommendations after talking with the patient. Some community pharmacists provide specialized services to help patients manage conditions such as diabetes, asthma, smoking cessation, or high blood pressure. Some community pharmacists are also certified to administer vaccinations. In addition to "counting out the pills," a few community pharmacists practice compounding—the actual mixing of ingredients to form powders, tablets, capsules, ointments, and solutions.

Health-care facilities pharmacists   Many pharmacists work in hospitals, nursing homes, mental health institutions, or neighborhood health clinics. Medical treatments in clinical settings rely more and more on drugs; therefore, pharmacists are increasingly seen as an integral part of the medical team. Pharmacists in health-care facilities dispense medications and advise the medical staff on the selection and effects of drugs. They also assess, plan, and monitor drug therapies and play a pivotal role in the facility's adherence to drug safety regulations. They counsel patients on the use of drugs while in the hospital and on their use at home when the patients are discharged. Pharmacists also may evaluate drug use patterns and outcomes for patients in hospitals.

Home health care and drugs   Pharmacists who work in home health care monitor drug therapy and prepare infusions—solutions that are injected into patients—and other medications for use in the home.

Consultant pharmacists   According to the American Society of Consultant Pharmacists, a consultant pharmacist is "paid to provide expert advice on the use of medications by individuals or within institutions, or on the provision of pharmacy services to institutions. The phrase 'consultant pharmacist,' coined by George F. Archambault who is referred to as the founding father of consultant pharmacy, originated in the nursing home environment when a group of innovative pharmacists focused on improving the use of medications in these facilities. However, consultant pharmacists are found today in a wide variety of other settings, including subacute care and assisted living facilities, psychiatric hospitals, hospice programs, and in home and community-based care."

Drug therapy specialists   Some pharmacists specialize in specific drug therapy areas, such as intravenous nutrition support, cardiovascular disease, infectious disease, oncology (cancer), nuclear pharmacy (used for chemotherapy), geriatric pharmacy, and psychopharmacotherapy (the treatment of mental disorders with drugs). In some states, specially trained pharmacists are developing collaborative practices—working alongside physicians to provide disease management services, especially for patients with diabetes, asthma, and heart disease.

Most pharmacists keep confidential computerized records of patients' drug therapies to ensure that harmful drug interactions do not occur. Pharmacists are responsible for the accuracy of every prescription that is filled, but they often rely upon pharmacy technicians to assist them in the dispensing process. Thus, the pharmacist may delegate prescription-filling and administrative tasks and supervise their completion. They also frequently oversee pharmacy students serving as interns in preparation for graduation and licensure.

Increasingly, pharmacists pursue work outside the pharmacy itself. Some are involved in research for pharmaceutical manufacturers, developing new drugs and therapies and testing their effects on people. Others work in marketing or sales, providing expertise to clients on a drug's use, effectiveness, and possible side effects. Some also work in industry as medical science liaisons outside the sales and marketing area. Some pharmacists also work for managed care organizations, developing pharmacy benefit packages and carrying out cost-benefit analyses on certain drugs. There are also pharmacists who work for medical education companies that provide educational programs (in a variety of formats) for health-care providers. Other pharmacists work for the government and pharmacy associations. Finally, some pharmacists are employed as college faculty, teaching classes and performing research in a wide range of areas.

American Association of Colleges of Pharmacy. "Is a Career in the Pharmaceutical Sciences Right for Me?" Available online. URL: http://www.aacp.org. Accessed May 30, 2011.

Pharmaceutical Research and Manufacturers of America. *Pharmaceutical Industry Profile 2005*. Washington, D.C.: PhRMA, March 2005.

Pollack, Andrew. "Is Biotechnology Losing Its Nerve?" *New York Times*, February 29, 2004. Sec. 3, 1.

Governmental Oversight of Drugs

Prior to the 20th century, little regulation of drugs existed—and then only at the local or state level. Drugs were considered consumer goods, not much different from foods or dry goods. Also, with most drugs compounded by individual pharmacists, uniformity in the final product could not easily be regulated. However, as scientific research led to more powerful drugs, which could do harm when used inappropriately or produced incorrectly, it became apparent that some government regulation on a national scale was warranted. Also, improvements in medical technology made it more likely that drugs could be manufactured and tested for uniformity.

Over-the-counter and prescription drugs, including generic drugs, are regulated by the FDA's Center for Drug Evaluation and Research (CDER). The center is a consumer watchdog whose best-known job is to evaluate new drugs before they can be sold. The center's review of new drug applications not only prevents quackery but provides doctors and patients with the information they need to use medicines wisely. The CDER ensures that drugs work correctly and that their health benefits outweigh known risks.

Drug manufacturers submit full reports of drug studies so that the center can evaluate the data. The studies answer the question: "Does this drug work for the proposed use?" By analyzing the data, the CDER reviewers assess the benefit-to-risk relationship and determine if the drug will be approved. In addition, the FDA makes sure the labeling (package insert) outlines the benefits and risks reported in the tested population.

Once a drug gets CDER approval, the drug is on the market as soon as the firm gets its production and distribution systems going.

Chronology of drug regulation in the United States

1820 Physicians met in Washington, D.C., to establish the U.S. Pharmacopeia (USP), the first compendium of standard drugs for the United States. Although all state societies of medicine were invited to send delegates, only 11 attended. According to the United States Pharmacopeial Convention Inc., "USP created a system of standards, a system of quality control (formulae), and a national formulary. Only 217 drugs that met the criteria of 'most fully established and best understood' were admitted. The original USP practitioners recognized that by setting public standards for drug products, they would help ensure the consistency and quality of drugs."

1846 Publication of Lewis Caleb Beck's *Adulteration of Various Substances Used in Medicine and the Arts* (New York: S. S. and W. Wood) helped document problems in the various substances used in medicine, addressing specifically impurities in the U.S. drug supply and the means of detecting them. Intended as a manual for the physician, the apothecary, and the artisan, it led to federal legislation two years later.

1848 Drug Importation Act passed by Congress, requiring U.S. Customs Service inspection to stop entry of adulterated drugs from overseas. This was the first national law pertaining to drugs.

1903 Lyman Frederic Kebler, M.D., Ph.C. (Pharmaceutical Chemist), assumed duties as director of the Drug Laboratory, Bureau of Chemistry. This new position had been established by Harvey Wiley, the chief chemist of the Bureau of Chemistry, who intended the laboratory to assist with standardizing pharmaceuticals and unifying analytical results. Dr. Kebler had been the chief chemist at Smith Kline and French and was a recognized expert in the detection of drug adulteration. Hamilton wrote, "Initially, the Drug Laboratory worked on a variety of projects. One of the first was an investigation of the reagents used by the Bureau, which Kebler soon learned were not completely pure. The Laboratory spent much of its time in search of methods to improve pharmaceutical analyses. Kebler also alerted the public to problems with the drug supply in general."

1905 Investigative journalist (called a muckraker at the time) Samuel Hopkins Adams's 10-part exposé of the patent medicine industry, "The Great American Fraud," began appearing in the October 7 issue of *Collier's, The National Weekly*. In the series, Adams exposed many of the false claims made about patent medicines, pointing out that in some cases these medicines were damaging the health of the people using them. The series had a huge impact and led to the passage of the 1906 Federal Food and Drugs Act.

Also in 1905, the American Medical Association, through its Council on Pharmacy and Chemistry, initiated a voluntary program of drug approval that would last until 1955. To earn the right to advertise in AMA and related journals, companies submitted evidence, for review by the council and outside experts, to support their therapeutic claims for drugs.

1906 The original Federal Food and Drugs Act (also called the Pure Food and Drug Act) was passed by Congress on June 30 and signed by President Theodore Roosevelt. It prohibited interstate commerce of misbranded and adulterated foods and drugs. The complete Federal Food and Drugs Act of 1906

(the Wiley Act) and its later amendments can be viewed at http://www.fda.gov/opacom/laws/wileyact.htm. This act, which the Bureau of Chemistry was charged to administer, prohibited the interstate transport of unlawful food and drugs under penalty of seizure of the questionable products and/or prosecution of the responsible parties. According to Food and Drug Administration (FDA) historian John P. Swann, "The basis of the law rested on the regulation of product labeling rather than pre-market approval. Drugs, defined in accordance with the standards of strength, quality, and purity in the USP and the National Formulary, could not be sold in any other condition unless the specific variations from the applicable standards were plainly stated on the label."

1911 In *U.S. v. Johnson*, the Supreme Court ruled that the 1906 Food and Drugs Act did not prohibit false therapeutic claims but only false and misleading statements about the ingredients or identity of a drug.

1912 Congress enacted the Sherley Amendment to overcome the ruling in *U.S. v. Johnson*. It prohibited labeling medicines with false therapeutic claims intended to defraud the purchaser. Although the amendment attempted to correct the language of the law, Swann explains, "It put the bureau in the difficult position of attempting to prove in court that manufacturers of drugs labeled with false therapeutic claims intended to defraud consumers. The Bureau lost several cases against egregious products, but seizures of misbranded and adulterated drugs nevertheless increased in the 1920s and 1930s."

1914 The Harrison Narcotic Act imposed upper limits on the amount of opium, opium-derived products, and cocaine allowed in products available to the public. It required prescriptions for products exceeding the allowable limit of narcotics and mandated increased record-keeping for physicians and pharmacists that dispensed narcotics. A separate law dealing with marijuana would be enacted in 1937.

1933 The FDA recommended a complete revision of the obsolete 1906 Food and Drugs Act, introducing the first bill into the Senate, and launching a five-year legislative battle.

1937 An untested liquid form of the new sulfa wonder drug that was raspberry-flavored to appeal to pediatric patients, Elixir Sulfanilamide, marketed by a Tennessee drug company, contained the poisonous solvent diethylene glycol. It killed 107 persons, many of whom were children. This event dramatized the need to establish drug safety before marketing. According to Swann, "The public outcry not only reshaped the drug provisions of the new law to prevent such an event from happening again, it propelled the bill itself (Federal Food, Drug, and Cosmetic Act) through Congress."

1938 The Federal Food, Drug, and Cosmetic (FDC) Act of 1938, which was passed by Congress and signed by President Franklin D. Roosevelt on June 25, contained new provisions:

- requiring new drugs to be shown safe before marketing, with the results to be submitted to the FDA in a New Drug Application (NDA)—starting a new system of drug regulation. Hamilton notes, "Within the first year of this requirement, the FDA issued over 1200 NDAs."

- eliminating the Sherley Amendment requirement to prove intent to defraud in drug misbranding cases

- regulating cosmetics and therapeutic devices for the first time

- prohibiting addition of poisonous substances to foods except where unavoidable or required in production. Safe tolerances were authorized for residues of such substances, for example, pesticides.

- authorizing standards of identity, quality, and fill-of-container for foods

- authorizing factory inspections

- adding the remedy of court injunctions to the previous penalties of seizures and prosecutions

The Wheeler-Lea Act of 1938 gave the Federal Trade Commission specific authority to prevent false and misleading advertising of products, including pharmaceuticals, otherwise regulated by the FDA.

In August 1938, the FDA announced a new policy that sulfanilamide and selected other dangerous drugs must be administered under the direction of a qualified expert, thus launching the requirement for prescription only (nonnarcotic) drugs.

1941 The Insulin Amendment required the FDA to test and certify purity, quality, strength, and potency of this life-saving drug for diabetes before marketing.

Also in 1941, after nearly 300 deaths and injuries resulted from distribution of sulfathiazole tablets tainted with the sedative phenobarbital, the FDA revised manufacturing and quality controls drastically, the beginning of what would later be called good manufacturing practices (GMPs). Swann elaborated, "FDA's investigation into Winthrop's [Winthrop Chemical Company of New York] sulfathiazole production and the agency's efforts to retrieve the Winthrop drug remaining on the market revealed numerous control deficiencies in the plant and serious irregularities in the firm's attempt to recall the tainted tablets. The incident prompted the FDA to require detailed controls in sulfathiazole production at Winthrop and throughout the industry, an approach that became the basis for production control standards for all pharmaceuticals."

1945 The Penicillin Amendment required FDA testing and certification of safety and effectiveness of all penicillin products. Later amendments would extend this requirement to all antibiotics. In 1983, after all drugs had been "approved" or removed, and new laws requiring drug testing and FDA approval were in place, such control would no longer be needed and would be subsequently abolished.

1948 The Supreme Court ruled in *U.S. v. Sullivan* that the FDA's jurisdiction extends to retail distribution, thereby permitting the FDA to interdict pharmacies' illegal sales of drugs—the most problematical being barbiturates and amphetamines.

1951 The Durham-Humphrey Amendment defined the kinds of drugs that cannot be used safely without medical supervision and restricted their sale to prescription by a licensed practitioner. As a result of this amendment, two classes of drugs came into existence: prescription and over-the-counter. Also from this amendment came the prescription legend: "Caution: Federal law prohibits dispensing without prescription."

1952 In *U.S. v. Cardiff*, the Supreme Court ruled that the factory inspection provision of the 1938 FDC Act is too vague to be enforced as criminal law. The ruling stated that it was not an offense for the president of a corporation operating a factory engaged in packing and preparing food or drugs for interstate distribution to refuse to grant permission for inspectors of the Food and Drug Administration to enter and inspect the factory at reasonable times. (See 1953.)

Also in 1952, a nationwide investigation by the FDA revealed that chloramphenicol, a broad-spectrum antibiotic, had caused nearly 180 cases of deadly aplastic anemia. Two years later, the FDA enlisted the aid of the American Society of Hospital Pharmacists, the American Association of Medical Record Librarians, and later the American Medical Association in a voluntary program of drug reaction reporting. The chloram-

phenicol investigation resulted in mandated revised drug labeling.

1953 The Factory Inspection Amendment clarified previous law and required the FDA to give manufacturers written reports of conditions observed during inspections and analyses of factory samples.

1960 Senate hearings, held in June and chaired by Senator Estes Kefauver of the Subcommittee on Antitrust and Monopoly of the Committee on the Judiciary, resulted in the Factory Inspection and Drug Amendment, sec. 3(a)(1960) S.3815. This bill aimed to protect the public by instituting certain manufacturing practices, in particular requiring manufacturers to establish the safety of color additives in foods, drugs, and cosmetics.

1962 Thalidomide, a new sleeping pill and pill to treat morning sickness in pregnancy, was found to have caused birth defects in thousands of babies born in western Europe. Prior to this revelation, the FDA had received an NDA for Kevadon, the brand of thalidomide that the William Merrell Company hoped to market in the United States. However, FDA medical officer Dr. Frances Kelsey refused to allow Kevadon to be approved because of insufficient safety data. However, Hamilton writes, "Even though Kevadon was never approved for marketing, Merrell had distributed over two million tablets for investigational use, use which the law and regulations left mostly unchecked. Once thalidomide's deleterious effects became known, the agency moved quickly to recover the supply from physicians, pharmacists, and patients." News reports on the role of Dr. Kelsey in keeping the drug off the U.S. market stirred public support for stronger drug regulation.

As a result, the Kefauver-Harris Drug Amendments passed unanimously to ensure drug efficacy and greater drug safety. For the first time, drug manufacturers were required to prove to the FDA that their products were both safe and effective before they could market them. In addition, the FDA was given closer control over investigational drug studies, FDA inspectors were granted access to additional company records, drug firms were required to send adverse reaction reports to the FDA, and all antibiotics now had to be certified. In addition, manufacturers had to demonstraté the efficacy of products approved prior to 1962. Also, the FDA now had control over prescription drug advertising; ads in medical journals now had to provide complete information to the doctor—the risks as well as the benefits. Hamilton adds, "The Drug Amendments also addressed the use of drugs in clinical trials, including a requirement of informed consent by subjects. FDA had to be provided with full details of the clinical investigations, including drug distribution, and the clinical studies had to be based on previous animal investigations to assure safety."

1963 The Advisory Committee on Investigational Drugs met; it was the first meeting of a committee to advise the FDA on product approval and policy on an ongoing basis.

1965 Drug Abuse Control Amendments were enacted to deal with problems caused by abuse of depressants, stimulants, and hallucinogens.

1966 The FDA contracted with the National Academy of Sciences/National Research Council to evaluate the effectiveness of 4,000 drugs that had been approved on the basis of safety alone between 1938 and 1962, in order to comply with the 1962 amendments.

1968 The FDA Bureau of Drug Abuse Control and the Treasury Department's Bureau of Narcotics were transferred to the Department of Justice to form the Bureau of Narcotics and Dangerous Drugs (BNDD), thereby consolidating efforts to police traffic of abused drugs.

Also in 1968, the FDA formed the Drug Efficacy Study Implementation (DESI) on the recommendation of the 1966 National Academy of Sciences investigation. According to Hamilton, one of the early effects of the DESI was "the development of the Abbreviated New Drug Application (ANDA). ANDAs were accepted for reviewed products that required changes in existing labeling to be in compliance."

Also in 1968, Animal Drug Amendments placed regulation of new animal drugs under one section of the FDC Act—Section 512—making approval of animal drugs and medicated feeds more efficient.

1970 In *Upjohn v. Finch,* the Court of Appeals upheld enforcement of the 1962 drug effectiveness amendments by ruling that commercial success alone does not constitute substantial evidence of drug safety and efficacy.

Also in 1970, the FDA required the first patient package insert for oral contraceptives, which had to contain information for the patient about specific risks and benefits.

Also in 1970, the Comprehensive Drug Abuse Prevention and Control Act—which established the Controlled Substances Act (CSA) under Title II and Title III of the bill—replaced previous laws and categorized drugs based on abuse and addiction potential in relation to therapeutic value. The CSA placed all substances that were regulated under existing federal law into one of five schedules. This placement is based upon the substance's medicinal value, harmfulness, and potential for abuse or addiction. Schedule I is reserved for the most dangerous drugs that have no recognized medical use, while Schedule V is the classification used for the least dangerous drugs. The act also provided a mechanism for substances to be controlled, added to a schedule, decontrolled, removed from control, rescheduled, or transferred from one schedule to another. CSA was the legal foundation of the U.S. government's fight against the abuse of drugs and other substances.

1972   The Over-the-Counter Drug Review was initiated to enhance the safety, effectiveness, and appropriate labeling of drugs sold without a prescription.

Also in 1972, the Drug Listing Act Amendment was established to provide the FDA with a current list of all drugs manufactured, prepared, propagated, compounded, or processed by a drug establishment that were registered under the Federal FDC Act. Until this amendment took effect in 1973, the FDA had no means of obtaining this information except by periodic inspection of registered establishments. The current drug list is called the National Drug Code Directory and is available on the Internet at http://www.fda.gov/cder/ndc/database/default.htm.

1973   The U.S. Supreme Court upheld the 1962 drug effectiveness law and endorsed FDA action to control entire classes of products by regulations rather than to rely only on time-consuming litigation. A reorganization of BNDD formed the Drug Enforcement Administration (DEA).

Also in 1973, the Indian Health Service developed the Pharmacist Practitioner Program, in which specially trained pharmacists provided drug therapy management services in collaboration with physicians. Hammond et al. noted that later reviews of the program found that quality of care, as judged by physicians, was satisfactory, patient acceptance was excellent, and the patient monitoring provided by pharmacists between physician visits extended the interval needed between physician visits. The program remains in existence today.

Also in 1973, the National Association of Boards of Pharmacy (NABP) published the first NABP Model State Pharmacy Act and Model Rules, which has been published annually since 1977. The Model Act provides state boards of pharmacy with model language that may be used when developing state laws or board rules. The 2005 edition contained NABP's Model Rules for Pharmacy Interns, Institutional Pharmacy, Pharmaceutical Care, Nuclear/Radiologic Pharmacy, and Sterile Pharmaceuticals.

1974   The Department of Health, Education, and Welfare enacted a drug regimen review regulation for nursing homes in an attempt to improve the quality of drug prescribing in that health-care setting. Hammond et al. noted that a subsequent study indicated that "patients in the group managed by pharmacists had significantly fewer deaths, were discharged more often to lower levels of care, and were prescribed fewer drugs than the patients in the traditional care group."

1976   The Vitamins and Minerals Amendments (Proxmire Amendments) stopped the FDA from establishing standards limiting potency of vitamins and minerals in food supplements or regulating them as drugs based solely on potency.

1977   California Assembly Bill 717 authorized drug therapy management by specially trained pharmacists. Hammond et al. write, "The project was so successful in saving health-care dollars, that legislation was passed in 1981 allowing all pharmacists practicing in California-licensed acute and intermediate health care facilities to provide drug therapy management." In subsequent years, the law was expanded to include clinics and managed care organizations.

1979   The state of Washington was the first to authorize pharmacist participation in drug therapy management under protocol.

1982   Tamper-resistant packaging regulations were issued by the FDA to prevent poisonings such as deaths from cyanide placed in Tylenol capsules.

1983   The Orphan Drug Act passed, enabling the FDA to promote research and marketing of drugs needed for treating rare diseases.

Also in 1983, the Federal Anti-Tampering Act passed, making it a crime to tamper with packaged consumer products, including drugs.

1984 The Drug Price Competition and Patent Term Restoration Act (also known as the Hatch-Waxman Act) expedited the availability of less costly generic drugs by permitting the FDA to approve applications to market generic versions of brand-name drugs without repeating the research done to prove them safe and effective, essentially creating the generic drug industry. At the same time, the brand-name companies could apply for up to five years of additional patent protection for the new medicines they developed to make up for time lost while their products were going through the FDA's approval process.

1986 The Anti-Drug Abuse Act of 1986 banned all "designer drugs" and all possible variations of current and future controlled substances, creating a new class of substances: controlled substance analogues—substances that are not controlled substances but may be found in the illicit traffic. They are structurally or pharmacologically similar to Schedule I or II controlled substances and have no legitimate medical use. A substance that meets the definition of a controlled substance analogue and is intended for human consumption is treated under the Controlled Substances Act of 1970 (CSA) as if it were a controlled substance in Schedule I. Designer drugs are created by changing the molecular structure of an existing drug to create new drugs with similar pharmacological effects and began appearing as a way to circumvent the CSA.

Also in 1986, the Florida legislature authorized pharmacists to provide drug therapy to patients with acute illness, using drugs only from a specified formulary, which did not include narcotics or injectibles. This would be revised in 1997 to include all types of drugs.

1987 The FDA revised investigational drug regulations to expand access to experimental

drugs for patients with serious diseases with no alternative therapies.

1988 The Prescription Drug Marketing Act banned the diversion of prescription drugs from legitimate commercial channels. Congress found that the resale of such drugs leads to the distribution of mislabeled, adulterated, subpotent, and counterfeit drugs to the public. The new law required drug wholesalers to be licensed by the states; restricted reimportation from other countries; and banned sale, trade, or purchase of drug samples and traffic or counterfeiting of redeemable drug coupons.

1991 The FDA published regulations to accelerate reviews of drugs for life-threatening diseases. (See also Drug Discovery and Development, p. lii.)

1992 The Generic Drug Enforcement Act imposed debarment and other penalties for illegal acts involving abbreviated drug applications.

Also in 1992, the Prescription Drug User Fee Act (PDUFA) required drug and biologics manufacturers to pay fees for product applications and supplements and other services. The act also required the FDA to use these funds to hire more reviewers to assess applications. This legislation expedites the review of new drugs for the treatment of serious or life-threatening conditions, streamlines clinical research on drugs, establishes scientific advisory panels to provide scientific advice about clinical investigations, requires manufacturers to notify the FDA at least six months before a drug is discontinued, and creates expanded access to investigational therapies.

1993 The FDA established the MedWatch program to simplify the reporting of serious adverse events with any FDA-regulated medical product. The single form replaced a confusing system of five different forms for manufacturers and health professionals. By 1998, MedWatch online reporting was available at http://www.fda.gov/medwatch/—allowing health care professionals and consumers to report serious problems that they suspect are associated with the medical products they prescribe, dispense, or use. These reports, along with follow-up investigations, help to identify important safety concerns.

1994 The FDA announced it could consider regulating nicotine in cigarettes as a drug in response to a citizen's petition by the Coalition on Smoking OR Health.

Also in 1994, the Uruguay Round Agreements Act extended the patent terms of U.S. drugs from 17 to 20 years.

1995 The FDA declared cigarettes to be "drug delivery devices." Restrictions were proposed on marketing and sales to reduce smoking by young people.

Also in 1995, the Veterans Health Administration began allowing pharmacists with advanced training to participate in Collaborative Drug Therapy Management (CDTM), a collaborative practice agreement between one or more physicians and pharmacists wherein qualified pharmacists perform patient assessments, order drug therapy–related laboratory tests, and select, initiate, monitor, continue, and adjust drug regimens.

1997 The Food and Drug Administration Modernization Act reauthorized the Prescription Drug User Fee Act of 1992 and mandated the most wide-ranging reforms in agency practices since 1938. Provisions included measures to accelerate review of devices, to allow firms to disseminate peer-reviewed articles about unapproved uses of approved drugs and devices, expanded procedures under which the FDA could authorize health claims for foods in agreement with published data by a reputable public health source, and establish procedures for the development of good guidance practices for agency decision making.

1998 The United States Pharmacopeia (USP) began the Medmarx program—an Internet-accessible, anonymous medication error–reporting database specific to hospitals and health systems. It is available through an annual subscription service. The USP publishes annual summary information of the medication error records to contribute to health care's knowledge of the nature and incidence of medication errors, risk assessment, and prevention.

2001 The Best Pharmaceuticals for Children Act reauthorized the pediatric studies provision of the Food and Drug Administration Modernization and Accountability Act of 1997 to improve the safety and efficacy of pharmaceuticals for children. It encouraged pharmaceutical companies to conduct pediatric studies of on-patent drugs that are used in pediatric populations, but are not labeled for such use, by extending their market exclusivity for six months.

2002 The FDA suspended for two years a 1997 rule requiring pediatric studies of medicines for children, drawing criticism from a former FDA commissioner and the American Academy of Pediatrics, among others, who argued that voluntary testing would once again leave doctors guessing about which medications are safe to give children and that there would be no guarantee that tests for children would be carried out—or if they were, that any information would be included in the product's label. The FDA's decision reportedly stemmed from lawsuits challenging the FDA's authority to order pediatric drug trials if a manufacturer did not want to market its product specifically for children. Medical groups complained that the "Rule" added significant cost to the drugs and delayed new drugs from entering the marketplace. The FDA said safety concerns of drugs used for pediatrics were considered addressed by the incentive offered under Best Pharmaceuticals for Children Act. Industry people said their companies routinely did pediatric trials and that the incentive was sufficient.

The Public Health Security and Bioterrorism Preparedness and Response Act included the

Prescription Drug User Fee Amendments of 2002 (PDUFA III), reauthorizing user fees through fiscal year 2007.

2003 The Medicare Prescription Drug, Improvement, and Modernization Act, the largest overhaul to the Medicare Program since its inception, created a historic prescription drug benefit for Medicare beneficiaries, plus made significant payment changes to Medicare Part A and Part B and Medicaid. It established a new Medicare Advantage program to replace the current Medicare+Choice program. The prescription drug benefit, which began in 2006, is voluntary; beneficiaries pay a monthly premium after enrolling. Until that time, beneficiaries had access to a drug discount card to obtain discounts on their drug purchases under the Medicare-Endorsed Prescription Drug Discount Card & Transitional Assistance Program. A Centers for Medicare & Medicaid Services (CMS) Legislative Summary of the complete bill is posted at http://www.cms.hhs.gov/mmu/HR1/PL108–173summary.asp.

On March 28, the U.S. District Court for the District of Columbia ruled that for Michigan's preferred drug list (PDL), prior authorization and supplemental rebate policies were acceptable under federal law. The court decision rejected legal claims brought by manufacturers and permitted the Michigan program and similar laws in at least a dozen states to remain in place. In December, a Michigan state court also ruled in favor of the program. By the end of 2004, 37 state Medicaid programs had implemented, or had pending, PDL programs designed to better manage increasing prescription drug costs.

2004 Department of Health & Human Services (HHS) approved plans by five states (Michigan, Vermont, New Hampshire, Alaska, Nevada) to pool their collective purchasing power to gain deeper discounts on prescription medicines for their state Medicaid programs. It was the first time in the history of the Medicaid program that states have worked together in this manner. While states are not required to offer prescription drugs through Medicaid, all states do.

In March, the FDA issued a major report that identified both the problems and the potential solutions for bringing more breakthroughs in medical science to patients as quickly and efficiently as possible. The report, *Innovation or Stagnation? Challenge and Opportunity on the Critical Path to New Medical Products,* examined the crucial steps that determine whether and how quickly a discovery leads to a reliable treatment for patients. It looked at the development processes for drugs, biologics, and medical devices, calling for a joint effort of industry, academic researchers, product developers, patient groups, and the FDA to identify key problems and to develop solutions.

2005 Formation of the Drug Safety Board is announced, consisting of FDA staff and representatives from the National Institutes of Health and the Veterans Administration. The board advises the director, Center for Drug Evaluation and Research, FDA, on drug safety issues and works with the agency in communicating safety information to health professionals and patients.

Three final guidances were published to fulfill the FDA's commitment to the risk-management performance goals that were part of the 2002 reauthorization of PDUFA: premarketing risk assessment, development and use of risk minimization action plans, and good pharmacovigilance practices and pharmacoepidemiologic assessment.

2006 FDA approves final rule, Requirements on Content and Format of Labeling for Human Prescription Drug and Biological Products. New content and format requirements make it easier for health care professionals to access, read, and use information in FDA-approved labeling.

Hamilton, Donna. "A Brief History of the Center for Drug Evaluation and Research." FDA History Office, November 1997.

Hammond, Raymond W., et al. "Collaborative Drug Therapy Management by Pharmacists—2003." *Pharmacotherapy* 23, no. 9 (September 2003): 1,210–1,225.

Swann, John P. "History of the FDA." U.S. Food and Drug Administration. Available online. URL: http://www.fda.gov/oc/history/historyoffda/full-text.html. Downloaded on July 8, 2005.

Swann, John P. "The 1941 Sulfathiazole Disaster and the Birth of Good Manufacturing Practices." *PDA Journal of Pharmaceutical Science and Technology* 53, no. 3 (May–June 1999): 148–153.

Drug Discovery and Development

As they did in the very beginning of healing properties, plants continue to play a role in pharmaceutical drugs. In *Medicines by Design*, National Institute of Health experts explain their importance today: "Approximately 60 percent of the world's population still relies entirely on plants for medicines, and plants supply the active ingredients of most traditional medical products. Plants have also served as the starting point for countless drugs on the market today. Researchers generally agree that natural products from plants and other organisms have been the most consistently successful source for ideas for new drugs, since nature is a master chemist. Drug discovery scientists often refer to these ideas as 'leads,' and chemicals that have desirable properties in lab tests are called lead compounds."

Drug discovery is the term used to describe the research stage of coming up with a new drug, and *drug development* is the testing stage. Henderson and Cockburn wrote, "The goal of the research phase is to find a chemical compound that has a desirable effect in a 'screen' that mimics some aspect of a disease state in man, while the goal of the drug development process is to ensure that compounds identified through the research process are safe and effective in humans."

Every new medicine is the result of an intensive and focused research process. Thousands of ideas are tested, with only a tiny fraction surviving the rigorous testing necessary to become an approved drug. Drug discovery and development take time—and money. DiMasi et al. of the Tufts Center for the Study of Drug Development looked at the research and development costs of 68 randomly selected new drugs that were obtained from a survey of 10 pharmaceutical firms. Among their findings:

- total time was 15 years (on average) per new drug in the pharmaceutical industry
- the average out-of-pocket cost per new drug was $403 million (2000 dollars)

However, Angell cautioned that the "Tufts analysis was restricted to NMEs [new molecular entities; not new versions of drugs already on the market] developed entirely within drug companies. . . . But these constitute only a tiny percentage of all new drugs (and) cost companies more to develop than the others. It is cheaper to license a drug from someone else or make a new version of an old drug."

- Drug development firms have become better at weeding out failures early in the development process, with only 21.5 percent of drugs beginning Phase I clinical trials actually getting to market. Of 5,000 compounds evaluated, on average, five enter clinical trials, and of those one is approved by the Food and Drug Administration.
- During the 1990s, it took, on average, 90.3 months to go from the start of clinical testing to regulatory approval, a decline from the 98.9 months required in the 1980s.

Research procedures for new drugs

According to AstraZeneca, an international pharmaceutical company, drug development typically proceeds along the following time line. Although the general categories described here are fairly uniform across most large pharmaceutical companies, some companies may use different language to describe each step in the discovery process, and at a more detailed level, the actual processes and technologies may differ. Past the candidate drug stage, the clinical trial phases are all universal, as those procedures are required by regulatory bodies. Regulatory approval is needed by all companies in the countries where they hope to sell their final product.

FOUR TO FIVE YEARS—PRECLINICAL PHASES (TARGET IDENTIFICATION THROUGH CANDIDATE DRUG PRENOMINATION)

Preclinical studies take place before any testing in humans is done; their purpose is to find out if a drug, procedure, or treatment is likely to be useful and is reasonably safe for use in initial, small-scale clinical studies. Depending on whether the compound has been studied or marketed previously, the sponsor may have several options for fulfilling this requirement: (1) compiling existing nonclinical data from past laboratory or animal studies on the compound; (2) compiling data from previous clinical testing or marketing of the drug in the United States or another country whose population is relevant to the U.S. population; or (3) undertaking new preclinical studies designed to provide the evidence necessary to support the safety of administering the compound to humans.

During preclinical drug development, a sponsor evaluates the drug's toxic and pharmacologic effects through in vitro (taking place in a test tube, culture dish, or elsewhere outside a living organism) and in vivo (taking place in a living organism) laboratory animal testing. Genotoxicity screening (to test its potential to cause damage to a cell's DNA) is performed, as well as investigations on drug absorption, distribution, metabolism, elimination, and toxicity of the drug and its metabolites.

Target identification The "drug hunting" process begins by focusing on areas of unmet medical need and identifying biological targets that have the potential to be starting points for successful and commercially viable treatments. When the screening begins, there are, on average, 1 million substances to test.

Hit identification A selection is made from the possible targets to determine which to submit for High Throughput Screening (HTS). High Throughput Screening is an automated system for testing tens or even hundreds of thousands of compounds extremely rapidly and is highly effective for eliminating ineffective compounds and identifying potentially useful ones.

The result of this phase is the identification of "hits"—compounds that are active in primary and secondary screens that have an element of selectivity and have characteristics that make them suitable to be made into drugs. Those compounds, or hits, judged to be most interesting in this phase are now singled out for further examination. In the hit identification phase, the number of substances to be tested has decreased from 1 million to, on average, 1,000.

Lead identification In this phase, the hits, or positive results, acquired from High Throughput Screening are further analyzed to determine their potential as drugs. Typically, the number of hits entering this phase will be in the hundreds.

Through hit-to-lead chemistry, these hits are converted into a significantly lower number of lead compounds, which are chemicals that have proven to influence the target in a way that gives them the potential to become effective treatments. From 1,000 substances to be tested in the hit identification phase, the number has now decreased to, on average, 200.

Lead optimization Here, the lead compounds are further refined, and a smaller number of potential leads are identified. These optimized leads are tested for such attributes as absorption, duration of action, and delivery to the target. The results of these tests determine whether the leads have the potential for concept testing in humans and have the qualities to become fully fledged candidate drugs. The screening goes on, and the company is now down to testing, on average, 17 substances.

Candidate drug prenomination   To this point, the scientists have produced a large amount of data on a candidate drug. It is now time to take stock and make a critical decision. Does the compound meet the required quality threshold to be a successful drug?

Compounds that have been selected by the previous screening process are scrutinized with regard to safety (Will the drug harm man?), method of drug administration (How will the patient take the product?), bioavailability (How much of the drug will be active in the body?), and the potential needs for scale-up chemistry (Can the company make enough at an acceptable cost?).

Several different scientists are involved in a collaborative effort during this phase. An integrative bioscientist plans and designs animal studies, aiming to test if the substance is active and has the desired effect on relevant organs and the whole body. A pharmacokineticist looks at how quickly the drug is likely to be removed from the body, in what forms and via which routes, and once metabolites are identified, studies if they are biologically active. A pharmaceutical scientist advises colleagues on appropriate formulations (such as tablets, inhalers, or injectable solutions) for their work and starts to consider the lead compounds' phsical and chemical properties to ensure that the compounds can be developed into products. A clinical researcher does preliminary planning for clinical testing that may take place in the future.

The final result of this phase is the selection of a candidate drug that has thus far been shown to be safe in laboratory and animal testing and has the potential to be developed into a successful and commercially viable drug. Once a candidate drug has been chosen, then all the preclinical results are submitted to health authorities to apply for permission to conduct clinical studies in volunteers.

The screening goes on, and the number of substances to be tested is now reduced to, on average, 12 from the original 1,000,000 substances.

(See The Investigational New Drug Application under The FDA's Drug Approval Process, p. lvi.)

SIX YEARS—CLINICAL TRIAL PHASES (CONCEPT TESTING AND DEVELOPMENT FOR LAUNCH)

A clinical trial is a research study to answer specific questions about vaccines or new therapies or new ways of using known treatments. Clinical trials (also called medical research and research studies) are used to determine whether new drugs or treatments are both safe and effective. Carefully conducted clinical trials are the fastest and safest way to find treatments that work in people.

These clinical trials are in four phases (Phase IV continues beyond drug approval):

Concept testing   This is Phase I, where the decision is taken to test the candidate drugs in humans. Typically, no more than a few candidate drugs make it to this phase for any given disease.

A candidate drug is first tested in a small group of generally healthy volunteers who are very closely monitored. The purpose is to determine the metabolism and pharmacologic actions of drugs in humans, how well the drug is tolerated, and if it has the desired effect in humans and to learn about suitable dosage (the effects and side effects associated with increasing doses)—generally, to learn if the drug has characteristics that would allow it be made into a medicine. The total number of subjects included in Phase I studies is generally in the range of 20 to 80. There are now, on average, only nine substances left to test.

Development for launch   These controlled clinical studies (Phase II) are conducted to evaluate the effectiveness of the drug for a particular indication(s) in patients with the disease or condition under study and to determine the common short-term side effects. Phase II studies usually involve several hundred people.

At the end of Phase II, the company starts preparing a full business plan, which includes endorsement by their marketing companies, target product claims, financial assessment, commercial manufacturing strategy, trademark, publication of data, and detailed launch plans.

This is also the time when the company begins large-scale clinical Phase III trials, which expand the study to an even larger group of people. These are controlled and uncontrolled trials after preliminary evidence suggesting effectiveness of the drug has been obtained and are intended to gather additional information to evaluate the overall benefit-risk relationship of the drug, provide an adequate basis for extrapolating the results to the general population, and provide an adequate basis for physician labeling. Phase III studies usually include several hundred to several thousand people.

The results from these trials provide the basis for the final decision to continue or to abandon the project. Through continuous screening, the number has now been decreased to, on average, 2.2 substances to be tested.

1.5 years—launch phase
All the data from all the preclinical and clinical studies are collated and sent for review by regulatory agencies. After studying the existing competition, the marketing companies produce strategic plans for releasing the drug to the markets, including the details of product positioning and product support. There are now, on average, only 1.3 substances left to test.

Continuously ongoing—life cycle support
Life cycle management is more of a business concept, but is something all companies must do to varying degrees (especially Phase IV monitoring). If the drug is approved by regulatory agencies (e.g., FDA), it will be launched as rapidly as possible. In this phase, strategies and opportunities for the drug's life cycle are defined, assessed,

and funded as appropriate. Clinical Phase IV trials, which take place after the drug or treatment has been licensed and marketed, are intended to examine the long-term side effects and health economic aspects—to delineate additional information including the drug's risks, benefits, and optimal use.

New indications are closely examined, and studies are developed to examine possible new formulations of the substance. Drugs originally intended for treatment of one disease are sometimes found to have beneficial effects for others. Life cycle support focuses on finding ways to deliver the drug to treat more disease types. There is now only one substance left out of a million tested substances; this substance is the new medicine.

The FDA's drug approval process
The mission of the FDA's Center for Drug Evaluation and Research (CDER) is to assure that safe and effective drugs are available to the American people. While various industry estimates for drug discovery and development range from six years to 15 years, the FDA estimates that, on average, it takes 8.5 years to study and test a new drug before it can be approved for the general public. The FDA plays a key role at three main points in this process:

- determining whether the benefits of a new treatment outweigh the risks
- once clinical trials begin, deciding whether they should continue, based on reports of the treatment's side effects and effectiveness against disease
- when clinical trials are completed, deciding whether the treatment should be sold to the public and, if so, what claims the drug manufacturer can make and what the label should say about directions for use, side effects, and warnings

To make these decisions, the FDA must review studies submitted by the drug's sponsor (which is usually the company that makes the drug), evaluate any reports of side effects or complications (called adverse events) from preclinical studies and clinical trials, and review the adequacy of the chemistry and manufacturing.

Preclinical studies   At the preclinical stage, the FDA will generally ask, at a minimum, that sponsors: (1) develop a pharmacological profile of the drug, (2) determine the acute toxicity of the drug in at least two species of animals, and (3) conduct short-term toxicity studies in animals ranging from two weeks to three months, depending on the proposed duration of use of the substance in the proposed clinical studies.

By law, the FDA must review all test results for new treatments to ensure that products are safe and effective for specific uses. *Safe* does not mean that the treatment is free of possible adverse side effects; rather, it means that the potential benefits have been determined to outweigh any risks.

The Investigational New Drug application   If a treatment proves promising in the lab, the drug company or sponsor must apply for FDA approval to test it in clinical trials with people. The application is called an Investigational New Drug (IND) application. For drugs and recombinant proteins (made through genetic engineering, also called gene splicing [e.g., cytokines and monoclonal antibodies]), sponsors submit the IND to CDER. For other biologics, including gene therapies and vaccines, sponsors submit the IND to the Center for Biologics Evaluation and Research (CBER). Once the IND is approved by CDER or CBER, clinical trials can begin.

The main purpose of an IND application is to provide the data showing that it is reasonable to begin tests of a new drug on humans. Also, current federal law requires that a drug be the subject of an approved marketing application before it is transported or distributed across state lines. Because a sponsor will probably want to ship the investigational drug to clinical investigators

in many states, it must seek an exemption from that legal requirement. The IND is the means through which the sponsor technically obtains this exemption from the FDA.

The New Drug Application review process   If the treatment makes it through the clinical trials process—the studies show the treatment is safe and effective—the sponsor may submit to the FDA another application. For drugs, this is a New Drug Application (NDA); for biologics, it is a Biologics License Application (BLA). The application must include the following:

- the exact chemical makeup of the drug or biologic
- results of animal studies
- results of clinical trials
- how the drug or biologic is made, processed, and packaged
- quality control standards

Once the FDA receives the NDA, the formal New Drug Application review process begins—a process that has included every new drug in the United States since 1938. The NDA is the vehicle through which drug formally propose that the FDA approve a new pharmaceutical for sale and marketing in the United States. The data gathered during the animal studies and human clinical trials of an IND become part of the NDA. Today's NDAs require more than 4,000 patients for testing, compared with 1,300 typically needed during the mid-1980s, in an effort to discover more side effects. The goals of the NDA are to provide enough information to permit the FDA reviewers to reach the following key decisions:

- whether the drug is safe and effective in its proposed use(s), and whether the benefits of the drug outweigh the risks
- whether the drug's proposed labeling (package insert) is appropriate, and what it should contain

- whether the methods used in manufacturing the drug and the controls used to maintain the drug's quality are adequate to preserve the drug's identity, strength, quality, and purity

The documentation required in an NDA is supposed to tell the drug's whole story, including what happened during the clinical tests, what the ingredients of the drug are, the results of the animal studies, how the drug behaves in the body, and how it is manufactured, processed, and packaged. During the NDA review process, a physician, a statistician, and a pharmacologist, among others, generate lengthy review documents.

Fast Track, Priority Review, and Accelerated Approval *Fast Track* refers to a process for interacting with the FDA during drug development. *Priority Review* applies to the time frame the FDA targets for reviewing a completed application. *Accelerated Approval* (Subpart H) applies to the design and content of the studies used to support a marketing claim.

Fast Track is a formal mechanism to interact with the FDA using approaches that are available to all applicants for marketing claims. The Fast Track mechanism is described in the Food and Drug Administration Modernization Act of 1997 (FDAMA). The benefits of Fast Track include scheduled meetings to seek FDA input into development plans, the option of submitting a New Drug Application in sections rather than all components simultaneously, and the option of requesting evaluation of studies using surrogate endpoints (see Accelerated Approval below). The Fast Track designation is intended for the combination of a product and a claim that addresses an unmet medical need but is independent of Priority Review and Accelerated Approval. An applicant may use any or all of the components of Fast Track without the formal designation. Fast Track designation does not necessarily lead to a Priority Review or Accelerated Approval.

Priority Review is a designation for an application after it has been submitted to the FDA for review for approval of a marketing claim. Under FDAMA, reviews for New Drug Applications are designated as either Standard or Priority. A Standard designation sets the target date for completing all aspects of a review and the FDA's taking an action on the application (approve or not approve) at 10 months after the date it was filed. A Priority designation sets the target date for the FDA action at 6 months. A Priority designation is intended for those products that address unmet medical needs. Internal FDA procedures for the designation and responsibilities for a Priority Review are detailed in the Manual of Policies and Procedures.

Accelerated Approval, or Subpart H Approval, is a program described in the NDA regulations that is intended to make promising products for life-threatening diseases available on the market on the basis of preliminary evidence prior to formal demonstration of patient benefit. The studies are designed to measure, and the FDA evaluation is performed on the basis of, a surrogate marker (a measurement intended to substitute for the clinical measurement of interest, usually prolongation of survival) that is considered likely to predict patient benefit. The approval that is granted may be considered a provisional approval with a written commitment to complete clinical studies that formally demonstrate patient benefit. Without having a formal demonstration of patient benefit, a risk benefit assessment cannot be made. Accelerated Approval designation does not necessarily lead to a Priority Review.

The Abbreviated New Drug Application Rather than requiring a generic manufacturer to repeat the costly and time-consuming NDA process, the company requesting approval for a generic drug may file an Abbreviated New Drug Application (ANDA), which incorporates data that the "pioneer" manufacturer has already submitted to the FDA regarding the branded drug's safety and efficacy (its ability to produce the desired effect). The objective of the ANDA process is to demonstrate that the generic drug is "bioequivalent" to the relevant branded product. The ANDA must contain, among other things, a certification regarding each patent listed in *Approved Drug Products with Therapeutic Equivalence*, called the Orange Book. Known as a "Paragraph IV certification," the ANDA applicant certifies that the patents listed in the Orange Book either are no longer valid or will not be infringed by the manufacture, use, or sale of the drug products for which the ANDA is submitted.

A generic drug is the same as a brand-name drug in dosage, safety, effectiveness, strength, quality, the way it works, the way it is taken, and the way it should be used. However, U.S. trademark laws do not allow generic drugs to look exactly like the brand-name drug. Although the generic drug must have the same active ingredients, such things as color, flavor, shape, packaging, and, within certain limits, package labeling may be different. But these things do not affect the way the drug works and how the drug is scrutinized by the FDA.

Labeling of drugs   In addition to approving the safety of drugs, the FDA determines (from the information provided in the NDA) whether the drug's proposed labeling (package insert) is appropriate and what it should contain. The United States Pharmacopeia (USP) sets various standards for drug packaging, storage, expiration dating, labeling, and other drug standards that pharmacists, drug manufacturers, wholesalers, hospitals, and others must follow to ensure that medications patients receive provide the benefit they are intended to provide. The FDA regulates those standards.

The package insert, which is printed in plain black type on both sides of a folded sheet of white paper, provides extensive drug information for physicians and pharmacists. Newspaper and magazine articles and television newscasters will often refer to the package insert simply as the drug's "label." As explained by the Harvard Health Letter, "Package inserts follow a standard format, explaining the drug's chemical makeup, its mechanism of action, when (and when not)

to use it, whether it carries a risk of dependence or abuse, dosage information, and hazards and side effects." Two package insert headings receive especially close scrutiny:

- *black-box designation* A black-box warning is the most extreme warning placed in the labeling of a prescription medication and is mandated by the FDA. The black-box designation refers to a black outline surrounding a section of the label, reserved for only the most serious side effects. The warnings help health care professionals to prescribe a drug that may be associated with serious side effects in a way that maximizes its benefits and minimizes its risks.

- *beyond-use dating* The beyond-use date is the date that defines how long a prescription drug can be used after it has been dispensed by a pharmacist—often incorrectly referred to as an expiration date. The nature of drug dispensing within hospitals in particular has made unit-dose packaging useful and convenient; however, repackaging into unit-doses raises questions concerning their appropriate expiration dating by hospital or community pharmacies. In May 2005, the FDA issued a guidance document suggesting that the USP standards be followed. The USP directs dispensers of prescription drug products to place on the label of the prescription container a suitable beyond-use date to limit the patient's use of the product. The beyond-use date cannot be later than the expiration date on the manufacturer's container. The USP states:

For nonsterile solid and liquid dosage forms that are packaged in single-unit and unit-dose containers, the beyond-use date shall be one year from the date the drug is packaged into the single-unit or unit-dose container or the expiration date on the manufacturer's container, whichever is earlier, unless stability data or the manufacturer's labeling indicates otherwise.

After drug approval

As a drug is marketed and while Phase IV clinical trials continue, the manufacturer must inform the FDA of any unexpected side effects or toxicity that comes to its attention. If new evidence indicates that the drug may present an "imminent hazard," the FDA can withdraw approval for marketing or add new information to the drug's labeling—such as a black box.

A new drug is protected by a drug patent, which protects the company that made it first. Most drug patents are protected for 20 years. The patent does not allow anyone else to make and sell the drug during its protected period. When the patent expires, other drug companies can start selling the generic version of the drug. But, first, they must test the drug and the FDA must approve it (see The Abbreviated New Drug Application, p. lvii).

Angell, Marcia. *The Truth About the Drug Companies.* New York: Random House, 2004.

AztraZeneca International. "Seeking New Medicines." Available online. URL: http://www.astrazeneca.com/article/502178.aspx. Downloaded on July 18, 2005.

DiMasi, J. A., R. W. Hansen, and H. G. Grabowski. "The Price of Innovation: New Estimates of Drug Development Costs." *Journal of Health Economics* 22, no. 2 (March 2003): 151–185.

Harvard Health Letter. "Finding Out about the Side Effects of Your Prescription Drugs." Harvard Health Publications, April 2005. Available online. URL: http://www.health.harvard.edu/newsweek/Finding_out_about_the_side_effects_of_your_prescription_drugs.htm.

Henderson, Rebecca, and Iain Cockburn. "Scale, Scope, and Spillovers: The Determinants of Research Productivity in Drug Discovery." *Rand Journal of Economics* 27, no. 1 (Spring 1996): 32–59.

National Institute of General Medical Sciences. *Medicines by Design.* Bethesda, Md.: National Institutes of Health, revised October 2003.

Prescription Drug Types and Classification

The industry uses several terms to further delineate types of drugs.

Novel drugs are new classes of chemical compounds that require extensive testing before being approved as novel treatments in humans. Similarly, novel drug delivery systems take advantage of improved scientific understanding about how individuals' genetic makeups impact the effectiveness of the medications they are taking (pharmacogenomics).

Innovator drug (also brand-name drug) is a drug that receives a patent on its chemical formulation or manufacturing process, obtains approval from the Food and Drug Administration (FDA) after extensive testing, and is sold under a brand name.

Blockbuster drugs are meant for tens of millions of patients. Drugs reach blockbuster status when they achieve sales of $1 billion or more. Megablockbusters are drugs with sales of $1 billion plus in their first year.

Generic drug is a copy of an innovator drug, containing the same active ingredients, that the FDA judges to be comparable in terms of such factors as strength, quality, side effects, and therapeutic effectiveness. Generic drugs may be sold after the patent on a brand-name drug has expired, usually after 20 years. All drugs have generic names. When a pharmaceutical company first develops a new drug, it gives the drug a chemical (or generic) name, then gives the drug a brand name as part of its marketing plan. Generic drugs are generally sold under their chemical names, although sometimes manufacturers will market the generic form of a drug under a new trade name to help identify it in the marketplace.

Off-patent drugs are drugs whose patents have expired. Because drugs that are off-patent have low profit margins for their original manufacturers, there is little incentive for the original companies to pursue additional investigations on them, such as clinical testing in pediatric populations. In 2003 and 2004, the FDA created a list of 24 off-patent drugs needing pediatric clinical testing and issued nine written requests asking pharmaceutical companies if they would do the work. When companies decline, which is often the case, the National Institutes of Health's (NIH) National Institute of Child Health and Human Development steps in to fund the work.

Breakthrough drug is the first brand-name drug to use a particular therapeutic mechanism of action—that is, to use a particular method of treating a given disease. With a breakthrough drug, there are no comparable therapies, whereas a novel drug offers a substantial improvement over older therapies. According to Grau and Serbedzija, the classical ideal of drug development is to create a new chemical entity working through a brand new mechanism of action. "Obviously, this generates the highest level of novelty; however, it also has the highest level of associated risk." Although breakthrough drugs are riskier, they generally yield higher rewards because they have the potential to fundamentally change the way a disease is treated.

Me-too drugs are brand-name drugs that use the same therapeutic mechanism of action as a breakthrough drug and therefore compete with it directly. Grau and Serbedzija note, "Although this approach usually offers only an incremental benefit over already marketed therapies, it shields a company from the risks associated with developing a new target."

Redesigner drugs are drugs that have gone off patent and have been improved sufficiently to be newly patented. The redesigned drugs may have improved absorption and distribution and/or may have fewer side effects compared to the original drug. According to Dove, "The chief appeal of redesigning existing drugs is low risk. Rather than wondering whether the target is valid or whether the market will materialize, drug redesigners can follow a well-trodden path to profit, making this approach popular with investors and entrepreneurs alike. Since a reengineered compound is treated as a new chemical by regulatory agencies, most of these products enjoy the same brand-name exclusivity and profit potential as wholly new drugs. By eliminating harmful side effects, they may also save lives."

Repurposed drugs are existing or abandoned drugs for which companies have found new or expanded indications (uses). Grau and Serbedzija explain, "The repurposing approach uses new biological understanding to discover new mechanisms of action for existing compounds or new relevance for an existing target in a new disease area. The repurposing approach has the potential to identify new first-in-class mechanisms to treat disease, while at the same time, avoiding some of the challenges associated with the development of a new chemical entity."

Single-source drugs are drugs for which no generic or competitive brand is available; thus, they are available from only one manufacturer.

Multiple-source drug is a drug available in both brand-name and generic versions from a variety of manufacturers.

Niche drugs target small patient populations whose conditions are relatively uncommon, such as multiple sclerosis, rheumatoid arthritis, and hepatitis C. Many smaller companies in the pharmaceutical industry are referred to as niche companies because they specialize in developing pharmaceutical products for these smaller markets. Some niche drugs qualify as *orphan* drugs.

Orphan drugs are drugs that treat rare diseases and conditions that, in the United States, affect fewer than 200,000 people or, in the European Union, affect five or fewer per 10,000 people. Because sales of orphan drugs are likely to be small compared to their development costs, there is little financial incentive for the pharmaceutical industry to develop medications for these diseases or conditions. Orphan drug status, however, gives a manufacturer specific financial incentives to develop and provide such medications, including exclusive rights to market these medicines for a period of time. This exclusivity differs from a patent. A patent protects against competition from a drug with the same chemical structure. Market exclusivity as implemented by the Orphan Drug Act (1983) grants protection for seven years against competition from any drug with a similar effect. According to the FDA's Office of Orphan Products Development (OOPD), more than 200 drugs and biological products for rare diseases have been brought to market since 1983. In contrast, the decade prior to 1983 saw fewer than 10 such products come to market.

Over-the-counter (OTC) drugs are those drugs that are available to consumers without a prescription. According to the *Center for Drug Evaluation and Research (CDER) Handbook,* more than 100,000 OTC drug products are marketed, encompassing about 800 significant active ingredients and more than 80 therapeutic categories, ranging from acne drug products to weight control drug products. As with prescription drugs, CDER oversees OTC drugs to ensure that they are properly labeled and that their benefits outweigh their risks. OTC drugs generally have these characteristics:

- Their benefits outweigh their risks.
- The potential for misuse and abuse is low.
- The consumer can use them for self-diagnosed conditions.
- They can be adequately labeled.
- Health practitioners are not needed for the safe and effective use of the product.

Most OTC drug products have been marketed for many years prior to the laws that require proof of safety and effectiveness before marketing. For this reason, the FDA has been evaluating the ingredients and labeling of these products as part of "The OTC Drug Review Program." The goal of this program is to establish OTC drug monographs for each class of products. OTC drug monographs are a kind of "recipe book" covering acceptable ingredients, doses, formulations, and labeling. Products conforming to a monograph may be marketed without further FDA clearance, while those that do not must undergo separate review and approval through the New Drug Approval (NDA) system. The NDA system—and not the monograph system—is also used for new ingredients entering the OTC marketplace for the first time. For example, the newer OTC products (previously available only by prescription) are first approved through the NDA system, and their "switch" to OTC status is approved via the NDA system. The

FDA's review of OTC drugs is primarily handled by CDER's Division of Over-the-Counter Drug Products in the Office of Drug Evaluation IV.

Prescription drugs—classifications

Drugs may be classified in several ways, such as by chemical group (e.g., alkaloids or barbiturates); by the way they work in the body or their mechanism of action (pharmacologically); or according to their therapeutic uses (purpose). Pharmacological and therapeutic classifications sometimes have considerable overlap, because drugs that act upon the body in different ways may bring about the same desired therapeutic result. Also, classification by therapeutic usage is complicated by the fact that a given drug may be used to treat more than one disease or ailment; for example, many antidepressants are helpful in controlling anxiety as well as depression. Drugs judged to have abuse potential are classified according to schedules (I–V) of controlled substances by the Drug Enforcement Agency (DEA).

Within various classes of drugs, clinicians and pharmaceutical companies may further delineate drugs according to how they are used or their duration of use. For example:

Rescue drugs are short-acting or quick-relief medications that are intended to relieve an acute symptom. For example, albuterol and ipratropium can be used as rescue drugs for asthma sufferers, and corticosteroids can be used for the short-term treatment of inflammatory and allergic reactions.

Maintenance drugs, on the other hand, treat chronic conditions that are of longer duration, such as high blood pressure, diabetes, or epilepsy. Maintenance medicines must be taken on a regular, recurring basis.

Companion drugs are used in tandem with a standard drug treatment for certain diseases to enhance the main drug's effectiveness or to treat side effects of the standard drug, among other reasons. For example, the use of ethionamide alone in the treatment of tuberculosis results in rapid development of resistance. It is essential, therefore, to administer along with ethionamide a suitable companion drug or drugs to which the organism is known to be susceptible. Also, in the treatment of HIV, delavirdine is used as part of a three- or four-drug combination that includes nucleoside analogue drugs and/or protease inhibitors. These companion drugs are critically needed to enhance its antiviral activity and the duration of the treatment effect. Two or more drugs used in the treatment of HIV/AIDS is also called combination therapy. According to the American Foundation for AIDS Research (AmFAR™), "Typically, at least three drugs from two different classes are used. An example of combination therapy is two nucleoside analogs (such as 3TC and AZT) plus either a protease inhibitor or a non-nucleoside reverse transcriptase inhibitor." Treatment using only a single drug is called monotherapy.

Drug combinations that have independent modes of action are seen as a way of enhancing efficacy while ensuring mutual protection against resistance. Although evidence shows that combinations improve efficacy without increasing toxicity, the usual warnings, precautions, and dosage regimens for these companion drugs need to be observed. Researchers have noted that the absolute cure rates achieved by drug combinations vary widely and depend on the level of resistance of the standard drug.

Specialty pharmaceuticals represent a relatively new area of prescription medications, one with a small market in terms of patient populations. Primarily injectables, specialty pharmaceuticals are generally expensive and used to treat patients with chronic and progressively severe diseases, ranging from common illnesses that affect large patient populations serviced by multiple drugs, such as HIV/AIDS, multiple sclerosis, and cancer to "orphan" diseases serviced by a single therapy, such as growth hormones. The annual cost for specialty pharmaceuticals may range from $10,000 to as high as $250,000. Seventy-five percent of specialty drug spending is among the following five categories: oncology,

HIV/AIDS, renal disease, transplant (antirejection) medications, and hemophilia.

Pharmaceutical equivalent drugs contain the same active ingredient(s) in the same dosage form and route of administration and are identical in strength or concentration. Although they meet the same standards (i.e., strength, quality, purity, and identity), they may differ in characteristics such as shape, scoring configuration, release mechanisms, packaging, excipients (including colors, flavors, preservatives), expiration time, and, within certain limits, labeling.

Pharmaceutical alternative drugs contain the same therapeutic moiety (the part of a drug that makes the drug work the way it does) but are different salts, esters, or complexes of that moiety or are different dosage forms or strengths. Data are generally not available for the FDA to make the determination of tablet to capsule bioequivalence. Different dosage forms and strengths within a product line by a single manufacturer are thus pharmaceutical alternatives, as are extended-release products when compared with immediate- or standard-release formulations of the same active ingredient.

Therapeutic equivalent drugs are considered to be therapeutic equivalents only if they are pharmaceutical equivalents and if they can be expected to have the same clinical effect and safety profile when administered to patients under the conditions specified in the labeling. The FDA classifies as therapeutically equivalent those products that meet the following general criteria: (1) They are approved as safe and effective; (2) they are pharmaceutical equivalents in that they (a) contain identical amounts of the same active drug ingredient in the same dosage form and route of administration, and (b) meet compendial or other applicable standards of strength, quality, purity, and identity; (3) they are bioequivalent in that (a) they do not present a known or potential bioequivalence problem, and they meet an acceptable in vitro standard, or (b) if they do present such a known or potential problem, they are shown to meet an appropriate bioequivalence standard; (4) they are adequately labeled; and (5) they are manufactured in compliance with Current Good Manufacturing Practice regulations.

Many times, therapeutic alternatives are selected because they are equally as effective as the originally prescribed drug, but they cost less or are the preferred drug on the prescription benefits formulary. A formulary is a list of generic and brand-name prescription drugs that are covered by a health benefits plan. The study of the cost-benefit ratios of drugs with other therapies or with similar drugs, where costs include both financial and quality-of-life measures, is called pharmacoeconomics.

Bioequivalent drugs are pharmaceutical equivalent or alternative drugs that display comparable bioavailability when studied under similar experimental conditions. Bioavailability refers to the rate and extent to which the active ingredient or therapeutic ingredient is absorbed from a drug product and becomes available at the site of drug action. Under the Drug Price Competition and Patent Term Restoration Act of 1984, manufacturers seeking approval to market a generic drug product must submit data demonstrating that the drug product is bioequivalent to the pioneer (innovator) drug product.

Bioequivalence refers to equivalent release of the same drug substance from two or more drug products or formulations. This leads to an equivalent rate and extent of absorption from these formulations. Underlying the concept of bioequivalence is the thesis that if a drug product contains a drug substance that is chemically identical and is delivered to the site of action at the same rate and extent as another drug product, then it is therapeutically equivalent and, therefore, can be substituted for (or interchangeable with) that drug product.

Dove, Alan. "Redesigner Drugs." *Nature Biotechnology.* Available online. URL: http://www.nature.com/news/2004/040726/pf/nbt0804–953_pf.html. Published online July 27, 2004.

Grau, Daniel, and George Serbedzija. "Innovative Strategies for Drug Repurposing." *Drug Discovery & Development* 8, no. 8 (May 2005): 56–61.

Marketing of Drugs and Issues Raised

Critics of the industry say that pharmaceutical firms' revenues are often not fully reinvested in research and development (R&D) but are shifted to marketing current drugs. According to Families USA, a consumer advocacy group, eight of the nine largest firms spend twice as much on advertising as they do on R&D. However, a U.S. Government Accountability Office (GAO) report to Congress (2002) stated, "Pharmaceutical companies spend more on research and development initiatives than on all drug promotional activities. According to industry estimates, pharmaceutical companies spent $30.3 billion on research and development and $19.1 billion on all promotional activities in 2001." The GAO report did say that pharmaceutical companies have increased spending on direct-to-consumer advertising (or DTC ads, as they are referred to in the trade) more rapidly than they have increased spending on R&D. The Pharmaceutical Research and Manufacturers Association (PhRMA) statement on the issue is: "In 2003, PhRMA member companies alone spent much more on R&D—an estimated $33 billion—than the entire industry spent on all combined drug promotional activities, $25.3 billion. Of this amount, pharmaceutical companies distributed over $16 billion worth of free samples to office-based physicians." Pharmaceutical firms also argue that marketing increases sales and return on investments, which increases the opportunity for more R&D.

Other critics blame marketing expenditures for the rising costs of drugs, noting that as pharmaceutical marketing has escalated, so has the cost of drugs to consumers. According to a study by the GAO, drug prices rose 21.8 percent between 2000 and 2004, or three to four times the rate of inflation.

Historically, drug manufacturers concentrated their marketing efforts on reaching the people who made most medical decisions, such as which drugs to prescribe—the physicians. However, toward the end of the 20th century, consumers began taking a more active role in managing their own health—not only questioning medical decisions, but being proactive in discussing and even suggesting possible treatments with their doctors. Braman, a social science analyst in the FDA's Division of Drug Marketing, Advertising, and Communications (DDMAC), explains, "Pharmaceutical companies recognized this trend and started advertising directly to consumers (DTC) in magazines and newspapers in the 1980s."

Even with the surge in DTC advertising, the industry still invests more heavily in efforts to reach the prescribing physicians. Spending on DTC advertising surpassed $3.8 billion in 2004 (Nielsen Monitor-Plus), while drug companies spent more than $7 billion (not including drug samples) in 2003 on one-on-one marketing to doctors (Consumers Union).

Whether targeting the health care community or consumers, each form of drug marketing has its own issues.

Detailing

Detailers are pharmaceutical salespersons, once called detail men, although more than half now are women. Detailing refers to the function performed by the sales representative who is employed by a pharmaceutical manufacturer for the purpose of promotion of pharmaceutical drugs or related products, education about pharmaceutical drugs or related products, or to provide samples of pharmaceutical drugs, related products, or related materials. According to the Foundation for Taxpayer and Consumer Rights, "From 1996 to 2001, industry-wide spending on detailing rose from $4.9 billion to $9 billion. In a similar period, the number of sales representatives more than doubled, from about 42,000 to 90,000. Currently, there are between 80,000 and 100,000 detailers in the United States, and about 500,000 doctors. Doctors can get five or six visits per day from sales reps."

Among the issues raised by consumer and medical groups regarding this long-time drug marketing strategy: (1) Detailers push the latest and most expensive drugs even though these drugs may not be the best in their category according to the medical evidence; (2) companies often buy data about the prescribing patterns of individual physicians and then use detailers to shift those patterns; and (3) the more doctors rely on drug detailers for information about prescription medicines, the less likely they are to prescribe drugs in a manner consistent with patient needs, according to numerous medical studies.

E-detailing

Detailing is evolving into "e-detailing," the digital equivalent of a personal sales representative visit, using Internet-enabled technology in the sales detailing process to supplement and reinforce other offline marketing efforts. According to PharmWeb.com, the industry-sponsored portal for the pharmaceutical sector, "Solutions vary in interactivity from those that provide relatively static product information online to those that require doctors to go through interactive product materials online to those that involve the physician in a 'face-to-face' video detail via the computer." Among industry concerns with e-detailing is that doctors will miss the "personal touch" associated with the present system, the sense that they are dealing with someone they know and trust. E-detailing also requires the physician to take the initial step to obtain drug information, with both drug companies and consumers expressing concern that not all physicians will have the time or the inclination to do this sufficiently. So although e-detailing has made inroads into drug marketing, industry watchers do not expect it to replace traditional detailing for at least 10 to 15 years.

Publishing and advertising in medical journals

Publication of study results in peer review journals is important for the marketing of a new drug and for physicians to become aware of and familiar with it. (Peer review means that expert scientists have reviewed the manuscript for scientific merit and ethical considerations.) Marketing observers have noted that getting studies published occurs early in the drug development cycle in order to create a "buzz" about the drug in the medical community as well as to educate physicians on the drug's clinical merits. In many, if not most, cases, the published studies have been sponsored by the drug's manufacturer—a concern of many, including Richard Smith, a former editor of the *British Medical Journal*. Others question the journals' reliance on drug advertising. Smith elaborates on the two issues:

> The most conspicuous example of medical journals' dependence on the pharmaceutical industry is the substantial income from advertising, but this is, I suggest, the least corrupting form of dependence. The advertisements may often be misleading and the profits worth millions, but the advertisements are there for all to see and criticize. Doctors may not be as uninfluenced by the advertisements as they would like to believe, but in every sphere, the public is used to discounting the claims of advertisers.
>
> The much bigger problem lies with the original studies, particularly the clinical trials, published by journals. Far from discounting these, readers see randomized controlled trials as one of the highest forms of evidence. A large trial published in a major journal has the journal's stamp of approval (unlike the advertising), will be distributed around the world, and may well receive global media coverage, particularly if promoted simultaneously by press releases from both the journal and the expensive public-relations firm hired by the pharmaceutical company that sponsored the trial. For a drug company, a favorable trial is worth thousands of pages of advertising, which is why a company will sometimes spend upwards of a million dollars on reprints of the trial for worldwide distribution.

> The doctors receiving the reprints may not read them, but they will be impressed by the name of the journal from which they come. The quality of the journal will bless the quality of the drug.

While drug company sponsorship should always potentially be looked at as a limitation of the study, the reality is that most of the landmark clinical trials with drugs that improve survival today would have never been done without the support of the industry. And while the company-sponsored trials are not negated simply because of their support, we need to be critical as we read them to see if there is any potential for company influence.

Direct-to-consumer advertising

Direct-to-consumer advertising initially was concentrated in print media because of the FDA requirement that ads for prescription drugs extolling the product's benefits must also give information about the product's risks, especially side-effects. This is easy to do within the space allowed in print media, but difficult to do in a 30- to 60-second television commercial. However, in 1997, the FDA clarified the rules when they presented draft guidance describing how companies could satisfy this requirement for prescription drug ads on broadcast media. According to this guidance, drug companies can fulfill their obligations for informing consumers about prescription drugs by stating in the commercials themselves where listeners or viewers can obtain more risk information than what is contained in the radio or TV ad itself. For example, the commercials would say to visit a particular Web site, call a toll-free telephone number, or see a particular magazine ad that provides full risk information, or would encourage the viewer/listener to visit a doctor. Braman adds, "Despite the sometimes-common misconception that the FDA relaxed the rules, in fact the guidance was simply a clarification of how companies could fulfill the requirement of the existing laws."

The 2002 GAO report expressed concern that DTC advertising

> appears to increase prescription drug spending and utilization (the number of prescriptions dispensed). Drugs that are promoted directly to consumers often are among the best-selling drugs, and sales for DTC-advertised drugs have increased faster than sales for drugs that are not heavily advertised to consumers. Most of the spending increase for heavily advertised drugs is the result of increased utilization, not price increases. For example, between 1999 and 2000, the number of prescriptions dispensed for the most heavily advertised drugs rose 25 percent, but increased only 4 percent for drugs that were not heavily advertised. Over the same period, prices rose 6 percent for the most heavily advertised drugs and 9 percent for the others. The concentration of DTC spending on a small number of drugs for chronic diseases that are likely to have high sales anyway and the simultaneous promotion of these drugs to physicians may contribute to increased utilization and thereby increase sales of DTC-advertised drugs. In addition, consumer surveys have consistently found that about 5 percent of consumers (or, by our estimate, about 8.5 million consumers annually) have both requested and received from their physician a prescription for a particular drug in response to seeing a DTC advertisement.

While critics have charged that DTC leads to overprescribing, proponents have countered that it helps avert underuse of effective treatments, especially for conditions that are poorly recognized or stigmatized. Kravitz et al. concluded it probably does both. "Patients' requests have a profound effect on physician prescribing in major depression and adjustment disorders. Direct-to-consumer advertising may have competing effects on quality, potentially both averting underuse and promoting overuse."

Consumer and medical groups alike have complained about the content of some DTC ads, suggesting that rather than focusing on education and awareness, as the Federal Trade Commission (FTC) rules intended, their focus is too often on selling and "pushing pills." One

misconception by the public is that the FTC approves drug advertising. Rather, the FDA's Division of Drug Marketing, Advertising, and Communications (DDMAC) *oversees* marketing and advertising and can issue warnings only after the fact when claims of inappropriate wording are made. Braman explains, "Companies must submit their ads to DDMAC at the time they first show them on TV or print them in magazines or newspapers. In most instances, we have no authority to pre-approve ads before they go on the air. Companies have the option to submit proposed ads to us ahead of time. We are happy to provide comments before the ads are shown to the public." Rados explains, "It's the FDA's job to make sure that consumers are not misled or deceived by advertisements that violate the law."

According to Gallagher and Oransky, "In 2004, the FDA's division that monitors DTC ads sent 12 warning letters to companies whose ads they found misleading. That compares with an average of four or five letters in previous years, according to an FDA spokesperson, and is a sign of stepped-up enforcement."

Rados notes that "advertisements cannot be false or misleading and cannot omit material facts. FDA regulations also call for 'fair balance' in every product-claim ad. This means that the risks and benefits must be presented with comparable scope, depth, and detail, and that information relating to the product's effectiveness must be fairly balanced by risk information." In their review of prescription drug Web sites, applying the FDA's "fair-balance disclosure" provision, and specifically focusing on the quantity and quality of risk information, Huh and Cude determined that "even though most prescription drug Web sites provide both risk and benefit information, the two types of information are presented differently"—with more emphasis on the benefits and less on the risks.

Still others have voiced complaints concerning the number of DTC ads, especially on television. In their review, Brownfield et al. found that "Americans who watch average amounts of television may be exposed to more than 30 hours of direct-to-consumer drug advertisements each year, far surpassing their exposure to other forms of health communication."

In August 2005, the pharmaceutical industry announced new guidelines for consumer marketing of medicines, including pledges to educate doctors before beginning consumer advertising campaigns and to more clearly outline the risks involved in taking prescription drugs. Critics expressed doubt that the guidelines would have the necessary clout, since offenders would not be sanctioned by the industry and many of the new principles are already required by law.

Braman, Amie C. "Some Questions and Answers on Prescription Drug Advertising." *FDA Consumer* 38, no. 4 (July–August 2004): 40.

Brownfield, E. D., et al. "Direct-to-Consumer Drug Advertisements on Network Television: An Exploration of Quantity, Frequency, and Placement." *Journal of Health Communication* 9, no. 6 (November–December 2004): 491–497.

Gallagher, Richard, and Ivan Oransky. "How to Fix Drug Ads." *The Scientist* 19, no. 10 (May 23, 2005): 6.

Huh, J., and B. J. Cude. "Is the Information 'Fair and Balanced' in Direct-to-Consumer Prescription Drug Web Sites?" *Journal of Health Communication* 9, no. 6 (November–December 2004): 529–540.

Kravitz, R. L., et al. "Influence of Patients' Requests for Direct-to-Consumer Advertised Antidepressants: A Randomized Controlled Trial." *Journal of the American Medical Association* 293, no. 16 (April 27, 2005): 1,995–2,002.

Rados, Carol. "Truth in Advertising: Rx Drug Ads Come of Age." *FDA Consumer* 38, no. 4 (July–August 2004): 20–27.

Smith, Richard. "Medical Journals Are an Extension of the Marketing Arm of Pharmaceutical Companies." *PLoS Medicine* 2, no. 5 (May 2005): e138. Available online. URL: http://dx.doi.org/10.1371/journal.pmed.0020138.

U.S. General Accounting Office. *Prescription Drugs, FDA Oversight of Direct-to-Consumer Advertising Has Limitations,* GAO-03-177. Washington, D.C.: GAO, October 2002.

Other Drug Industry– and Prescription Drug–Related Issues

Discovery, manufacturing, and marketing may be the major links in the pharmaceutical drug chain, but a number of other issues are woven throughout that delivery chain, from preventing medication errors, to pricing of drugs, to patient privacy in today's electronic age.

Safety issues/medication errors

In 1992, the FDA began monitoring medication error reports it receives from the United States Pharmacopeia (USP), the Institute for Safe Medication Practices (ISMP), MedWatch, and manufacturers. A 1999 Institute of Medicine report disclosed that more than 7,000 deaths from medication errors occurred annually both in and out of hospitals—exceeding those from workplace injuries. This does not even include the cases of permanent disability, the unnecessary pain and suffering, the added costs, or the simple inconvenience caused by preventable medication errors. Medication errors can be traced to several causes.

Look-alike, sound-alike drugs According to the FDA, about 10 percent of all medication errors reported result from drug name confusion, which can occur between brand names, generic names, and brand-to-generic names such as Toradol and tramadol. One major medical center reported that as many as 20 percent of 32,000 prescription errors recorded over a 16-year period could be attributed to naming issues. Rados describes the problem further:

> Generic names are coined using an established stem, or group of letters, that represents a specific drug class. For example, the USAN (United States Adopted Names) stems include suffixes like -mab for monoclonal antibodies, such as infliximab, or prefixes like dopa- for dopamine receptor agonists. The arthritis medications celecoxib, valdecoxib, and rofecoxib are generic names containing the -coxib stem. Each belongs to a class of drugs known as the COX-2 inhibitors.

Names that include such stems, chemistry roots, or any other coded information are easier to remember, and give clues about what a drug is used for. These names, however, typically sound or look so much alike that they contribute to medication errors, especially if the products share common dosage forms and other similarities.

With more than 9,000 generic drug names and 33,000 trademarked brand names in use in the United States, similarities are bound to occur, even with FDA approval required for brand names. Rados explains,

To minimize confusion between drug names that look or sound alike, the FDA reviews about 400 brand names a year before they are marketed. About one-third are rejected. The last time the FDA changed a drug name after it was approved was in 2005, when the diabetes drug Amaryl was being confused with the Alzheimer's medication Reminyl, and one person died. Now the Alzheimer's medicine is called Razadyne.

Generic name confusion also has led to regulatory action, as well as to pharmacy practice recommendations. For example, the USP and the USAN changed the drug name "amrinone" to "inamrinone" after receiving reports of serious outcomes from medication errors involving the similarly named drug amiodarone. The generic drug industry also has responded to requests from the FDA to use a mixture of uppercase and lowercase letters to highlight differences in similar generic names, such as vinBLAStine and vinCRIStine. This step also encouraged manufacturers to supplement their new drug applications with revised labels and labeling that visually differentiated their generic names with the so-called "tall man" letters.

Decimal nomenclature and ambiguous abbreviations Abbreviations, acronyms, dose designations, and other symbols used in medication prescribing also have the potential for causing problems. "For example," Rados writes, "the abbreviation D/C means both 'discharge' and 'discontinue.' The National Coordinating Council for Medication Error Reporting and Prevention (NCCMERP) notes that patients' medications have been stopped prematurely when D/C—intended to mean discharge—was misinterpreted as discontinue because it was followed by a list of drugs." More than 60 abbreviations, symbols, and dose designations have been reported to the ISMP through the USP-ISMP Medication Errors Reporting Program as being frequently misinterpreted and involved in harmful medication errors. Among these:

1. The Latin abbreviations *Q.D.* (once daily), *Q.I.D.* (four times daily), and *Q.O.D.* (every other day) are sometimes mistaken for each other. The period after the *Q* can be mistaken for an *i* and the *O* can be mistaken for *I*. Instead, medical quality control guidelines now encourage writing out "daily," "four times daily," and "every other day."
2. *BT* (bedtime) is often mistaken as *BID* (twice daily).
3. *IU* (International Units) has been mistaken for *IV* (intravenous) or *10* (ten).
4. *HS* (half-strength) is sometime confused with *h.s.* (Latin abbreviation for bedtime).
5. *tiw* (used for 3 times a week) is easily confused with *t.i.d.* (Latin abbreviation for *ter in die*–"three times a day").
6. Abbreviations for morphine sulfate (MS and MSO4) and magnesium sulfate (MgSO4) can be confused for one another.
7. Trailing zeros and "naked" decimal points can lead to tenfold dosing errors. For example, *1.0* may be interpreted as *10* when the decimal point is not noticed (trailing zeros). Similarly, the number *.1* (naked decimal point) can and has been interpreted as a *1*.

(See also Appendix II—Common Medication Errors and Recommendations.)

Bad handwriting Prescribers' poor handwriting has long been a standing joke in our culture, but illegible handwriting on prescriptions can lead to serious medical errors, and it is a frequent problem. According to an ISMP *Medication Safety*

Alert, a 1979 study showed that it was difficult to interpret about half of all physicians' handwritten orders. For example, Rados writes, "Several errors have occurred involving mix-ups with the oral diabetes drug Avandia and the anticoagulant Coumadin. Although they don't look similar when typed or printed, the names have been confused with each other when poorly written in cursive. The first "A" in Avandia, if not fully formed, can look like a 'C,' and the final 'a' has appeared to be an 'n'."

A major initiative in recent years has been the transition from handwritten prescription orders to automated drug-ordering systems, sometimes via wireless handheld devices while the physician is meeting with the patient, with the order routed directly to the pharmacy. The technology is referred to as computerized physician order entry, or CPOE, or sometimes also known as provider order entry when nurses and other clinicians also enter orders. The Centers for Medicare and Medicaid Services (CMS) estimate that electronic prescriptions could eliminate up to 2 million medical errors a year. Many major hospitals have been using electronic medical records for a while, but individual doctors have been slow to adopt the new technology because of the cost. The Medicare Prescription Drug, Improvement and Modernization Act (MMA) of 2003 encourages the development of electronic prescribing systems by providing grants to help physicians invest in technology and by requiring the development and use of uniform standards for Medicare electronic prescribing. Electronic prescribing pilot projects were scheduled to begin January 1, 2006, with final standards due April 1, 2008, and implementation by April 1, 2009. The program is voluntary and includes safe harbors for group practices to make these technologies more widely available.

High-alert drugs Certain drugs have the greatest potential to cause serious harm when used incorrectly, such as insulin, opiates and narcotics, potassium chloride concentrate, and intravenous anticoagulants. Some high-alert medications also have a high volume of use, increasing the likelihood that a patient might suffer inadvertent harm. Though medication mishaps with these drugs are no more frequent than with other drugs, the consequences can be devastating. For this reason, safety groups such as the Veterans Health Administration's National Center for Patient Safety suggest several precautions medical centers can take, including:

- Reduce the number of concentrations and volumes.

- Remove high-alert drugs from critical areas.

- Have two individuals independently check the product to ensure it is correct, and communicate the results to each other. This is of particular importance when medications are received in bulk, and the packaging and labeling could misleadingly look similar to another drug.

Polypharmacy The term means "many drugs" and is used to refer to problems that can occur when a patient is taking many medications or more than are actually needed. The more drugs taken, the more likely adverse drug events may occur due to drug interactions. Because individuals react differently to drug combinations, the degree of side-effect impairment caused by polypharmacy may vary from patient to patient. With polypharmacy's strong but unpredictable potential to produce side effects, physicians who are aware of all the drugs a patient is taking can add new medications at the lowest dosage possible, counsel the patient to be alert to any impairing side effects, and adjust the dosages of individual medications as needed to achieve therapeutic effects with a minimum of impairment. Unfortunately, many medications prescribed by several different physicians and filled at different pharmacies may not be scrutinized adequately. Although the elderly are especially at risk for polypharmacy issues due to having multiple diseases and ailments, some clinicians blame direct-to-consumer advertising for a rise in "baby boomer" polypharmacy. (See also Adverse Drug Reactions/Events, p. lxxii.)

Polypharmacy also refers to the practice of intentionally prescribing two or more medications for the same disease. Pediatric polypharmacy for psychiatric symptoms in children is of particular concern to the American Academy of Child and Adolescent Psychiatry (AACAP), which issued a policy statement saying, "Anecdotally the prescribing of multiple psychotropic medications ('combined treatment'- 'polypharmacy') in the pediatric population seems on the increase. Little data exist to support advantageous efficacy for drug combinations, used primarily to treat co-morbid conditions."

See also Appendix II—Common Medication Errors and Recommendations for more extensive recommendations on medicine safety in various patient situations.

Potential solutions for helping minimize medication errors

Because of the number of documented medication errors from the various causes above, numerous steps have been taken by the medical community to encourage implementation of recommended safe practices to reduce the risk of as many errors as possible in the future.

National patient safety goals and drugs The Joint Commission on Accreditation of Healthcare Organizations (JCAHO), whose mission is to "continuously improve the safety and quality of care provided to the public through the provision of health care accreditation and related services that support performance improvement in health care organizations" has included several drug-related initiatives in its annual National Patient Safety Goals—which hospitals, nursing homes, and other health-care organizations must meet in order to retain accreditation. These goals have included the removal of specific high-alert medications from patient care units (2003); standardizing the abbreviations, acronyms, and symbols used throughout the organization, including a list of abbreviations, acronyms, and symbols not to use (2004); at a minimum, annually reviewing a list of look-alike

and sound-alike drugs used in their facility and taking action to prevent mix-ups (2005); and labeling all medications, medication containers (e.g., syringes, medicine cups, basins), or other solutions on and off the sterile field in perioperative and other procedural settings (2006).

NQF safe practices The National Quality Forum (NQF), a not-for-profit membership organization created in 1999 to develop and implement a national strategy for health-care quality measurement and reporting, approved 30 "safe practices" that should be universally used in health-care settings to reduce the risk of harm. Several are drug-related, including: "Pharmacists should actively participate in the medication-use process, including, at a minimum, being available for consultation with prescribers on medication ordering, interpretation and review of medication orders, preparation of medications, dispensing of medications, and administration and monitoring of medications."

Quality improvement organizations (QIOs) A national network of 53 organizations responsible for each U.S. state, territory, and the District of Columbia, supported by CMS. QIOs work closely with hospitals and others to improve care and review patient concerns in an attempt to make sure patients get the right care at the right time, particularly among underserved populations. CMS publicly discloses on their Web site how hospitals and other health-care providers across the country measure in meeting QIO goals, a number of which affect medication delivery and use. Hospitals, home health-care agencies, and nursing homes are not required to report their safety data, but their Medicare payments are reduced by 0.4 percent if they do not.

Automated dispensing Automated dispensing systems are drug storage devices or cabinets that electronically dispense medications in a controlled fashion and track medication use (e.g., Pyxis systems). Their principal advantage lies in permitting nurses to obtain medications for inpatients at the point of use. Most systems are linked to the pharmacy's computer order entry system, allowing review of orders by a pharmacist. Access to the medications requires user identifiers and passwords and is tracked by the device, providing a record of medications administered to the patient and usage data to the hospital's financial office for the patients' bills. Noting that "the invention and production of these devices brought hopes of reduced rates of medication errors," Murray wrote that early studies had not shown this to be the case:

> The evidence provided by the limited number of available, generally poor quality studies does not suggest that automated dispensing devices reduce medication errors. There is also no evidence to suggest that outcomes are improved with the use of these devices. Most of the published studies comparing automated devices with unit-dose dispensing systems report reductions in medication errors of omission and scheduling errors with the former. The studies suffer from multiple problems with confounding, as they often compare hospitals or nursing care units that may differ in important respects other than the medication distribution system.
>
> Human intervention may prevent these systems from functioning as designed. Pharmacists and nurses can override some of the patient safety features. When the turnaround time for order entry into the automated system is prolonged, nurses may override the system thereby defeating its purpose. Furthermore, the automated dispensing systems must be refilled intermittently to replenish exhausted supplies. Errors can occur during the course of refilling these units or medications may shift from one drawer or compartment to another causing medication mix-ups. Either of these situations can slip past the nurse at medication administration.

In their interviews with nurses, Stetina et al. found similar problems with reliance on automated medication dispensing machines (AMDMs): "Study participants described errors or potential errors caused by this reliance on assistive systems. In one instance, the section of the AMDM intended for ampicillin was filled with amoxicillin. The facility was unable to determine with complete certainty whether or not the incorrect medication had been administered. In another instance, an additional dose of an antibiotic was administered simply because an additional, erroneous scheduled time was present on the medication administration records (MAR). These examples of actual and potential errors demonstrate that over-reliance on any single system to prevent error may engender additional error potential."

Bar coding   The FDA rule on bar-code labeling means that as of April 26, 2006, most prescription drugs; biological products such as vaccines, blood and blood components; and over-the-counter (OTC) drugs that are commonly used in hospitals must carry a bar code similar to the bar codes on grocery store items. The bar-code rule is designed to reduce preventable medication errors in hospitals and encourage the facilities to adopt advanced technology systems, such as electronic medical records. The FDA requires that the bar code contain a product's National Drug Code, or NDC number, which represents the product's name, dosage form, and strength. With the new rule, any new drug products approved by the FDA must have a bar code on their packaging within 60 days of marketing approval. Products that were already on the market must be packaged with bar codes by April 2008.

Meadows explains how medicine bar coding works in hospitals that use a bedside point-of-care system that relies on bar-coded information: When patients enter a hospital, they receive bar-coded identification wristbands that can transmit information to the hospital's computer. Nurses have laptop computers and scanners on top of medication carts that they bring to patients' rooms. Nurses use the scanners to scan the patients' wristbands and the medications to be given. The bar codes provide unique, identifying information about drugs given at the patients' bedsides. Before giving medications, nurses use the scanner to pull up a patient's full name and social security number on the laptops, along with the medications. If there is not a match between the patient and the medication or some other problem, a warning box pops up on the screen.

The problem, according to Perry, "could be one or more of these common scenarios: wrong patient, wrong dose, wrong drug, wrong time to administer the drug, wrong route of administration, or the patient's chart has been updated and the prescribed medication has changed. Following this predicted chain of events, bar-coding could, for example, prevent a child from receiving an adult dose of a particular drug or prevent a patient from mistakenly receiving a duplicate dose of a drug received earlier."

Brown bag drug reviews   The term refers to pharmacies and medical clinics that have patients bring in all their medications, often during special community service events. These reviews have been successful not only in helping educate the patients on proper and safe medication use, but in discovering potential adverse drug reactions where patients have been prescribed medications by multiple physicians. Such reviews, which can also note OTC drugs being taken, can be more accurate than relying on a patient's medical record alone.

Pharmacy precautions   The FDA recommends also that pharmacists keep look-alike, sound-alike products separated from one another on pharmacy shelves, avoid stocking multiple product sizes together, and verify with the doctor any information that is not clear before filling a prescription. Also, medical safety experts suggest that doctors write both brand and generic names on prescriptions and also include the indication for the medication as part of the prescription order.

Adverse drug reactions/events   Although these terms are often used interchangeably, an adverse drug reaction (ADR) has been defined as a drug action that produces an undesirable effect, which may be expected or unexpected, on the body; and an adverse drug event (ADE) as any

undesirable symptom, occurrence, or reaction a trial subject experiences during the clinical trial; it may or may not be considered related to the study agent. Other terms used are adverse reaction, adverse experience (AE), and side effect.

The Institute of Medicine (IOM) defines an ADE as an injury resulting from a medical intervention related to a drug, which can be attributable to preventable and nonpreventable causes. Stucky adds, "Of these, adverse reactions to medications include those that are usually unpredictable, such as idiosyncratic or unexpected allergic responses, and those that are predictable, such as adverse effects or toxic reactions related to the inherent pharmacologic properties of the drug. In general, the number and severity of adverse medication reactions are directly related to the number of drugs administered to hospitalized patients. An allergic reaction to a medication can be an adverse reaction if there is no history of patient allergy, yet can be a medication error in that same case if the patient did have a documented history of allergies but that medical information was not available, not consulted, or overlooked." Although most serious adverse drug reactions are reported to be attributable to known side effects, incorrect dosage, and administration of drugs, they may also be related to multiple drugs, drug overuse or misuse, slowing of drug metabolism or elimination, or age-related chronic conditions or diseases, alcohol intake, and food-drug interactions.

Some studies and authors also include medication errors (see Safety Issues/Medication Errors, p. lxvii) as adverse drug reactions in their statistics. In that context, many serious adverse drug events occur because of unrecognized dosing errors; missed allergies, contraindicated drugs reaching patients, and drug interactions.

An FDA Center for Drug Evaluation and Research (CDER) learning module for physicians calls ADRs one of the leading causes of morbidity and mortality in health care:

The Institute of Medicine reported in January of 2000 that 44,000 to 98,000 deaths occur annually from medical errors. Of this total, an estimated 7,000 deaths occur due to ADRs. To put this in perspective, consider that 6,000 Americans die each year from workplace injuries.

However, other studies conducted on hospitalized patient populations have placed much higher estimates on the overall incidence of serious ADRs. These studies estimate that 6.7 percent of hospitalized patients have a serious ADR with a fatality rate of 0.32 percent. If these estimates are correct, then there are more than 2,216,000 serious ADRs in hospitalized patients, causing over 106,000 deaths annually. If true, then ADRs are the fourth leading cause of death—ahead of pulmonary disease, diabetes, AIDS, pneumonia, accidents, and automobile deaths.

These statistics do not include the number of ADRs that occur in ambulatory settings. Also, it is estimated that over 350,000 ADRs occur in U.S. nursing homes each year. The exact number of ADRs is not certain and is limited by methodological considerations. However, whatever the true number is, ADRs represent a significant public health problem that is, for the most part, preventable.

The report attributes the frequency of adverse drug reactions to several factors.

First, more drugs—and many more combinations of drugs—are being used to treat patients than ever before. To exemplify this point, 64 percent of all patient visits to physicians result in prescriptions.
Second, 2.8 billion prescriptions were filled in the year 2000. That is about 10 prescriptions for every person in the United States.
Finally, the rate of ADRs increases exponentially after a patient is on four or more medications.

Other authors and studies have suggested a wide range of ADR/ADE statistics, demographics, and causes, depending on each one's broadness of definition.

- According to WorstPills.org, the risk of an adverse drug reaction is about 33 percent

higher in people aged 50 to 59 than it is in people aged 40 to 49.

- In June 2004 congressional testimony, Janet Marchibroda, chief executive officer of eHealth Initiative, reported, "Adverse events occur in up to 3.7 percent of hospitalizations, with up to 13.6 percent of them leading to death. Studies show that adverse drug events occur in 5 to 18 percent of ambulatory patients."

- According to the American Heart Association, 1 billion prescriptions are taken incorrectly every year, resulting in 9 million adverse drug reactions a year.

- Jeff Donn, an Associated Press medical writer reported on April 17, 2005, "Hospital patients suffer seven hard-to-foresee adverse drug reactions and another three outright drug mistakes for every 100 admissions. That translates into 3.6 million drug misadventures a year."

- Doughton wrote, "Adverse drug reactions kill more than 100,000 Americans every year and cause serious side effects in 2.1 million others. A recent British study found that 10 percent of people hospitalized because of drug reactions were taking warfarin."

- Because seniors can take up to six to 10 medications at one time, they are especially at risk for potential adverse drug reactions. A 2004 *Washington Post* article said that according to the American Society of Consultant Pharmacists (ASCP), "Some 28 percent of hospitalizations among seniors are due to adverse drug reactions." The blame for this was attributed to "fragmentation of care. Frequently, doctors will put older adults on a new drug for a symptom—like impaired cognition, sleep patterns, balance or mobility—that is caused by other drugs."

- A hospice training module estimates that "5 to 15 percent of acute geriatric medical admissions are due to adverse drug events. Health care providers, patients, and caregivers can misinterpret these events because they appear to be disorders that are prevalent among older adults (e.g., falls, fatigue, cognitive impairment)."

- Fick et al. wrote, "Adverse drug events have been linked to preventable problems in elderly patients such as depression, constipation, falls, immobility, confusion, and hip fractures. A 1997 study of ADEs found that 35 percent of ambulatory older adults experienced an ADE and 29 percent required health care services (physician, emergency department, or hospitalization) for the ADE. Some two-thirds of nursing facility residents have ADEs over a four-year period. Of these ADEs, one in seven results in hospitalization."

The FDA/CDER learning module points out that many drug ADRs are not discernible until after they have been in the marketplace for some time:

> Most new drugs are approved with an average of 1,500 patient exposures and usually for only relatively short periods of time. However, some drugs cause serious ADRs at very low frequencies and would require many more exposures to detect the reaction. For example, bromfenac (Duract) was a non-steroidal anti-inflammatory agent (NSAID) that was removed from the market in 1998, less than one year after it was introduced. Bromfenac caused serious hepatotoxicity in only 1 in 20,000 patients taking the drug for longer than 10 days. To reliably detect the toxic effects of a drug with a 1 in 20,000 adverse drug reaction frequency, the new drug application database would have to include 100,000 patient exposures. A drug that is tested in a few thousand people may have an excellent safety profile in those few thousand patients. However, within a short time after entering the market, the drug may be administered to several million patients. That means that for drugs that cause rare toxicity, their toxicity can only be detected after, not before, marketing.
>
> If one case of hepatotoxicity is seen during pre-marketing testing, it can be difficult, if not impossible, to ascertain whether it was secondary to the drug or just the background rate of disease that is seen in the population.

> So, the safety profile for new drugs that come on the market is never totally defined because new drugs are studied only in relatively small and homogenous patient populations. The complete safety profile of a new drug will be defined only after it has been approved and is in use on the market. (*Note:* This is the purpose of Phase IV post-marketing studies.)

This point is reinforced by Bennett et al., who wrote, "Only half of newly discovered serious ADRs are detected and documented in the *Physicians' Desk Reference* within seven years of drug approval."

Complementary and alternative medicine (CAM) and drugs CAM is defined as a group of diverse medical and health care systems, practices, and products that are not presently considered to be part of conventional medicine. CAM includes herbal remedies, which when combined with certain prescription drugs can lead to adverse drug reactions or lessen the effect of the drugs. According to a National Institute of Health's National Center for Complementary and Alternative Medicine (NCCAM) survey released in May 2004, 36 percent of U.S. adults use some form of complementary and alternative medicine—with 19 percent using natural products (such as herbs, other botanicals, and enzymes)—yet only about 12 percent of adults seek care from a licensed CAM practitioner. Also, 55 percent of adults surveyed said they were most likely to use CAM because they believed that it would help them when combined with conventional medical treatments, with 26 percent using CAM because a conventional medical professional suggested they try it. Thirteen percent used CAM because they felt that conventional medicine was too expensive.

In June 2004, the World Health Organization (WHO) reported that adverse reactions and injuries from alternative treatments had more than doubled in three years. For example, Spencer reported, "Ginkgo biloba, an herb often taken to promote mental alertness, thins the blood." So a person already on warfarin, a prescription blood thinner, who also takes ginkgo biloba, would be at high risk for an ADR. Taking supplements that also affect clotting along with a blood thinner, such as warfarin, may lead to bleeding in the brain or gastrointestinal tract. "A major concern is the fact that consumers often fail to tell their doctors about the alternative treatments they are using, creating new health risks."

Autoimmune diseases experts have noted that the interaction vitamins or herbs can have with some pharmaceutical drugs is a particular concern for many chronic fatigue syndrome (CFS) and fibromyalgia (FM) patients, who are known to especially seek out a variety of means to manage their symptoms, from more traditional medications to natural supplements. For example, Addington writes, "Taking the herbs chaparral, comfrey, or coltsfoot with acetaminophen could result in a toxic liver condition. Various herbs including Saint-John's-wort, and dong quai, when paired up with NSAIDS, can cause increased sensitivity to the sun. Further, since NSAIDS alone can be tough on the stomach, caution should be used when combining with arginine, an amino acid that increases stomach acid."

Meadows emphasized the importance of patients keeping a list of all medications, including OTC drugs, dietary supplements, medicinal herbs, and other substances taken for health reasons, and reporting it to their health-care providers. "One National Institutes of Health study showed a significant drug interaction between the herbal product Saint-John's-wort and indinavir, a protease inhibitor used to treat HIV infection."

Off-label prescribing Many drugs that have gained FDA approval have uses other than those for which the drug was officially evaluated and approved. Once a drug has been approved for some particular use, it can be legally prescribed for any use because the FDA does not regulate the practice of medicine. As Ceccoli writes, "In the practice of medicine in the United States, physicians have the authority to prescribe medicines in any way they see fit." Approved uses are known as on-label uses (or used as described on the label and FDA-approved package inserts), whereas drugs prescribed for conditions other than those approved by the FDA are off-label uses. Manufacturers may disseminate information, either in literature to doctors or in advertisements to the public, about on-label uses, subject to restrictions. Many of the FDA's restrictions on dissemination of information related to off-label prescriptions were declared unconstitutional in 2000. But, Mehlman writes, "The agency's position does not specify the circumstances in which it will take action against a manufacturer for disseminating information about off-label uses, so the limits on off-label promotion remain unclear." Legal experts note that while off-label drug education is permitted, its promotion is not. Pelletier quotes Jane Chin, Ph.D., president of the Medical Science Liaison Institute, as cautioning, "The FDA doesn't regulate by job title. Sales reps need to know that medical science liaisons (MSLs) can only discuss off-label uses when a physician's request for the information is truly unsolicited."

Some drugs are used more frequently off-label than for their original, FDA-approved indications. An example is the use of tricyclic antidepressants to treat neuropathic pain. This old class of antidepressants is now rarely used for clinical depression due to side effects, but the tricyclics are often effective for treating neuropathic pain. In fact, off-label prescribing is most commonly done with older, generic medications that have found new uses but have not had the formal (and often costly) applications and studies required by the FDA to formally approve the drug for these new indications. However, there is usually extensive medical literature to support the off-label use. Mehlman adds, "Although there are no accurate data, estimates run as high as 60 percent of all drug prescriptions written in the United States in a given year, including a large proportion of chemotherapy and pediatric prescribing."

As prevalent as off-label prescribing is, it does raise issues. Ceccoli explains:

What makes off-label prescribing such a delicate issue is the potential connection between off-label prescribing and the occurrence of adverse drug reactions. On the one hand, such prescribing may offer the patient a clinical benefit that regulators may have been previously unaware of. For example, Lilly's leading-selling antidepressant drug, Prozac, was initially marketed as an appetite suppressant. Pfizer's anti-impotency drug, Viagra, was originally developed as a drug used in the treatment of hair loss. Additionally, the immunosuppressant drug, cyclosporine, which made the transplant of organs other than kidneys feasible in the early 1980s, was originally developed as a fungal antibiotic. In this sense, off-label prescribing has the potential to uncover all sorts of important (and unanticipated) therapeutic remedies.

On the other hand, off-label prescribing on the surface runs against all that goes into the approval of a medicine. In some cases, fairly safe drugs have been removed from the market because of adverse reactions that occurred, perhaps, as a result of the drug not being used in accordance with labeling instructions.

Noncompliance Medication compliance is the extent to which a patient takes his or her medications as prescribed by the health-care provider, including frequency, duration, proper dosage, and any food restrictions. Although the literature often uses *compliance*, Osterberg and Blaschke wrote, "The word 'adherence' is preferred by many health care providers, because 'compliance' suggests that the patient is passively following the doctor's orders and that the treatment plan is not based on a therapeutic alliance or contract established between the patient and the physician. Both terms are imperfect and uninformative descriptions of medication-taking behavior." Regardless of the term, drug companies and health-care providers struggle continuously to deal with patients' inability to follow medication directions. For example, the ongoing Minnesota Heart Survey finds that as many as half of patients prescribed a statin drug to lower their cholesterol stopped taking it after six months. According to reports, an estimated 125,000 lives could be saved annually with better compliance to heart disease medications alone. Compliance problems often are the result of confusion, misinterpretation, or unanswered questions about treatment information—but other factors also apply.

One in three adults who take prescription drugs on a regular basis have frequent problems complying with their treatment regimens, according to a *Wall Street Journal* Online/Harris Interactive health-care poll taken in March 2005 among a nationwide cross section of 2,507 adults. "The poll indicates that compliance problems are rampant in the United States for various reasons. When asked why they have failed in the last year to take their medicines as prescribed, two-thirds of those surveyed say they simply forgot. And nearly half say they have failed to do so because of concerns about the drugs themselves, including efficacy or potential side effects. Cost was also a factor in compliance, with 35 percent of those who take prescription drugs saying at least once or twice in the last year they have not taken a drug in order to save money, according to the survey."

A study carried out by the University of Michigan Health System and Cleveland Clinic and reported in the *Journal of General Internal Medicine* looked at 4,000 patients' compliance with their prescriptions for statins. The results showed the more patients had to pay out-of-pocket for their statins, the less likely they were to take the medications according to doctors' instructions. Yet the researchers found that only about 25 percent of doctors ever ask if the cost of medications is an issue.

In March 2004, the NQF established a national "safe medication use framework" aimed at increasing the effectiveness of prescription medication use by consumers, focusing especially on low-literacy and limited English–proficiency (LEP) populations. The project's goal is to make recommendations about the feasibility and appropriateness of establishing evidence-based safe medication use practices but not to endorse specific practices per se. "Poor adherence to prescription medication use recommendations is both common and costly. One study found a 76 percent discrepancy between what medicines patients were prescribed and what medicines (prescription and non-prescription) were actually taken. Noncompliance with recommended medication use has been found to be an underlying cause of up to 22 percent of hospitalizations. Not surprisingly, compliance in low-literacy and LEP populations is especially problematic because of the difficulty in understanding proper medication usage instructions."

Because they tend to be taking more medications, the elderly have also shown a high degree of noncompliance. Causes for noncompliance in the elderly include forgetfulness, misunderstanding of verbal directions, inability to purchase the medication, trouble with side effects, and difficulty in swallowing larger capsules and tablets.

Opiophobia   Opiophobia refers to a health-care provider's unfounded fear that patients will become physically dependent upon or addicted to opioids even when using them appropriately; it can lead to the underprescribing of opioids for pain management. Estimates are that more than 50 million Americans suffer from chronic pain. When treating pain, health-care providers have long wrestled with the dilemma of how to adequately relieve a patient's suffering while avoiding the potential for that patient to become addicted to pain medication.

Many health-care providers underprescribe opioid painkillers because they overestimate the potential for patients to become addicted to medications such as morphine and codeine. Although these drugs carry a heightened risk of addiction, research has shown that providers' concerns that patients will become addicted to pain medication are largely unfounded, according to the National Institute on Drug Abuse (NIDA).

Most patients who are prescribed opioids for pain, even those receiving long-term therapy, do not become addicted to the drugs. The few patients who do develop rapid and marked tolerance for and addiction to opioids usually have a history of psychological problems or prior substance abuse. Studies have shown that abuse potential of opioid medications is generally low in healthy, non-drug-abusing volunteers. A NIDA Research Report states, "One study found that only four out of about 12,000 patients who were given opioids for acute pain became addicted. In a study of 38 chronic pain patients, most of whom received opioids for four to seven years, only two patients became addicted, and both had a history of drug abuse."

The issues of underprescription of opioids and the suffering of millions of patients who do not receive adequate pain relief has led to the development of guidelines for pain treatment. These guidelines may help bring an end to underprescribing, but alternative forms of pain control are still needed. NIDA-funded scientists continue to search for new ways to control pain and to develop new pain medications that are effective but do not have the potential for addiction.

Drug shortages   Severe drug shortages are infrequent, but a minor supply problem creating a potential shortage usually arises about once or twice a month, according to the FDA, which oversees actual and potential problems through its Drug Shortage Program, a division of the CDER. The Drug Shortage Program was developed to respond to prescription, over-the-counter, and generic drug shortages that have significant impact on public health. Other products, such as vaccines, biologicals, veterinary drugs, devices, radiological products, and nutraceuticals, fall into the jurisdiction of other FDA centers.

Jensen et al. note that manufacturers often notify the Drug Shortage Program of potential or current shortages, although they are not legally required to do so. The program also learns of possible shortages from other FDA departments, health-care professionals, patients, and professional organizations. "Once we verify a shortage and are certain that it is not transient or self-limiting, the CDER review division that has the requisite scientific and medical expertise regarding the product is notified and consulted to determine whether the drug product is medically necessary. A medically necessary drug is defined as a product used to prevent or treat a serious or life-threatening disease or medical condition for which there is no other available source with sufficient supply of that product or alternative drug available."

CDER focuses on medically necessary drugs and other products because shortages of such items have the greatest potential to affect public health. "We do not usually investigate shortages that are expected to be temporary and self-limiting or those involving a specific strength or package size of a drug product because of finite resources and the transient nature of these shortages."

Once a drug shortage is identified, the FDA determines the cause of the shortage and takes steps to find alternative sources of the drug or control the distribution to make sure the most needy patients have access to it, working with the manufacturer(s) toward resolving the problem.

Some of the common causes of drug shortages include manufacturing problems, limited production capability, limited availability of the raw material from which the drug product is made, market concentration (such as company mergers, which may lead to fewer manufacturers producing the older products), increased clinical demand (such as may happen with natural disasters or influenza outbreaks), or company instability (when a product is manufactured by a few firms, one or more of which encounter difficulties). "The FDA has no authority over the business decisions made by drug manufacturers. Although the FDA does not have the authority to require a firm to produce a product, it can encourage a manufacturer to produce a drug in shortage by expediting the review of data supporting a new or generic drug."

Rarely, the FDA may allow temporary importation of a drug that is in acute short supply. In 2001, the FDA confirmed a nationwide shortage of naloxone hydrochloride injection (used to prevent or reverse the effects of opioids including respiratory depression, sedation, and hypotension), a shortage due to significant facility renovations and lack of inventory buildup. The shortage was expected to be a temporary situation lasting two to three months. Therefore, the FDA identified an alternate supplier in Canada, setting up the parameters for physicians and hospitals to obtain it from them.

The FDA maintains a Web page with tables showing Current Drug Shortages and Resolved Drug Shortages lists at http://www.fda.gov/cder/drug/shortages/default.htm.

Prescribing privileges   Also referred to as prescriptive privileges and prescriptive authority, the legal ability to prescribe medicines is not determined by the FDA but rather by individual state laws along with the various medical specialty and geographic medical boards. A physician may be licensed in the state but have his or her prescribing privileges revoked or suspended for any of various infractions. One exception to this is that in addition to being licensed by the state, in order to write prescriptions for any scheduled drugs (narcotics), one must also be licensed by the Drug Enforcement Administration, which has its own power to suspend or revoke certain prescribing privileges.

The "turf battle" over prescribing privileges has been ongoing in the United States for a number of years, with medical specialties other than physicians petitioning for and in some cases obtaining prescribing privileges with limitations. Gearon explains,

Pharmacists used to only make and hand out medications but today have authority to vaccinate patients in 37 states and can prescribe "morning after" emergency contraception in California, New Mexico, Alaska, and a handful of other places. Pharmacist prescribing generally is authorized under collaborative agreements with physicians but also allows pharmacists to monitor patients' ongoing conditions. In the late 1960s and 1970s, the prescription battle was waged between medical doctors (M.D.'s) and doctors of osteopathy (D.O.'s). Today, like M.D.'s, D.O.'s have unlimited, independent prescribing authority in every state. In the early 1980s, optometrists battled ophthalmologists for prescribing privileges. Now, optometrists can prescribe at least some eye-related medications in every state. Physician assistants (P.A.'s), a profession devised by physicians to work under their supervision, had a much easier time in the early 1990s obtaining the ability to write prescriptions under the auspices of M.D.'s. Nurse practitioners (N.P.'s) have gotten some level of prescribing privileges in most states.

In 2002, New Mexico became the first state to authorize licensed, doctoral-level psychologists who have completed a training and certification program the right to prescribe psychiatric medications. Prior to that, 12 states—Alaska, California, Connecticut, Florida, Georgia, Hawaii, Illinois, Louisiana, Missouri, Montana, Tennessee, and Texas—had rejected such legislation, some on multiple occasions. Then in 2004, Louisiana gave medical psychologists prescriptive authority only after obtaining the agreement of the primary or attending physician. Psychologists in other states continue to petition for prescribing privileges.

Importation/reimportation of drugs Although the terms are used interchangeably, *importation* precisely refers to patented drugs manufactured abroad and brought into the United States; *reimportation* refers to patented drugs manufactured in the United States and exported for sale abroad, then later returned to the United States for sale at a lower price, without the manufacturer's permission. Reimportation can be less costly to U.S. buyers because of price controls in other countries, which keep drug prices very low.

Federal law strictly regulates the importation and reimportation of pharmaceuticals into the United States to protect patient safety and, some argue, to protect drug companies' profits. Anderegg explains the issue: "Attempting to stretch health care dollars further, many U.S. consumers, and even some municipalities, are buying drugs (often via the Internet) from Canada at prices that can be 30 percent to 75 percent lower than in the United States. Manufacturers want this practice stopped, citing a decrease in revenues that results in smaller research budgets and a chilling effect on the development of innovative therapeutics."

The MMA of 2003 contained provisions that would permit the importation of prescription drugs into the United States if the secretary of the Department of Health and Human Services (HHS) certifies that drugs imported from Canada pose no additional risk to public health and safety and that such imports would provide significant cost savings to American consumers. The MMA also required the secretary to conduct a study on the importation of drugs. In December 2004, an HHS Task Force on Drug Importation released their report. Among their findings:

- Nearly 5 million shipments, comprising about 12 million prescription drug products with a value of approximately $700 million, entered the United States from Canada alone in 2003 via Internet sales and travel to Canada by American consumers. An equivalent amount of prescription drugs are currently coming in from the rest of the world, mostly through the mail and courier services.

- Some of the arriving products appear to have been made in the United States; however, many are not. The majority of these currently imported drugs are unapproved by the FDA and do not appear to conform in many aspects to the properly approved and manufactured products available in American pharmacies.

According to a Research and Markets report (May 2005), the volume of prescription drugs estimated to be imported into the United States on a daily basis is so great that neither the Customs and Border Protection (CBP) nor the FDA have mechanisms for keeping an accurate count. This was confirmed in the HHS Task Force report, which noted that of the 3,800 FDA employees assigned to field activities such as inspections, only 450 are involved in investigative import activities. "FDA managers have repeatedly noted that the large number of personal drug shipments coming into the international mail and courier facilities is overwhelming the available staff."

Although drugs entering the United States through the mail have historically come in via Canada, Ireland, or the United Kingdom, many pharmaceutical shipments are currently coming in from countries such as India, the Philippines, or Romania, which further exacerbates the safety debate. Related to the safety concerns is the issue that some drugs in other countries have different ingredients from drugs of the same name in the United States. Although Congress has twice approved importation so long as the FDA certifies that the foreign drugs are safe, U.S. health officials continue to warn that they cannot vouch for safety in a system they do not oversee.

Even if reimportation is approved, the HHS Task Force cautioned that drugs would need to be repackaged in order to meet FDA guidelines. "Repackaging may destroy the anti-counterfeiting measures used in the original packaging and labeling of the drug. It may also provide a point of entry for expired, adulterated, or counterfeit drugs into the distribution system because they may be repackaged in a way that makes them appear to be legitimate products. Finally, counterfeit and diverted product may be commingled with authentic product during the repackaging process, thereby finding its way to an end user."

The FDA maintains a Web page on drug importation at http://www.fda.gov/imported-drugs/ with links to regulatory actions and policy, government letters and testimony, and information of interest to consumers.

Counterfeit drugs   One concern about importing drugs from abroad is that it will lead to a rise in counterfeit drugs. In 2004, Hubbard reported, "Counterfeit drugs are still comparatively rare in the United States, but federal officials say the problem is growing. Throughout the 1990s,

the FDA pursued about five cases of counterfeit drugs every year. In each of the last several years, the number of cases has averaged about 20, but law-enforcement officials say that figure does not reflect the extent of the problem. Last year (2003), more than 200,000 bottles of counterfeit Lipitor (used to lower cholesterol) made their way onto the market. In 2001, a Sunnyvale, Calif., pharmacist discovered that bottles of Neupogen, an expensive stimulator of white blood cells prescribed for AIDS and cancer patients, were filled only with saltwater."

The following FDA table was included in "Combating Counterfeit Drugs: A Report of the Food and Drug Administration Annual Update," May 18, 2005.

Industry analysts have estimated that up to 10 percent of the U.S. drug supply is currently counterfeit, whereas in developing countries counterfeit drugs amount to as much as 50 percent of the supply. Although the true extent of the problem of counterfeit drugs is difficult to know or measure, the World Health Organization (WHO) has estimated that at least 8 to 10 percent of the world's total drug supply is counterfeit. Newspapers reported that an estimated 192,000 people died in China in 2001 because of counterfeit drugs.

It is not only the danger of unsafe ingredients in counterfeit drugs, but also their ineffectiveness that pose problems for consumers. For example, in February 2004, the FDA and Johnson and Johnson Co. of Raritan, New Jersey, warned the public about an overseas Internet site selling counterfeit contraceptive patches that contained no active ingredients. The counterfeit contraceptive patches were promoted as Ortho Evra transdermal patches, which are FDA approved and made by Johnson and Johnson's Ortho-McNeil Pharmaceutical, Inc. subsidiary. These counterfeit patches provided no protection against pregnancy.

The HHS Task Force reported that a number of anticounterfeiting technologies show potential for effectively assuring the authenticity of drugs and, thus, for combating the counterfeit-

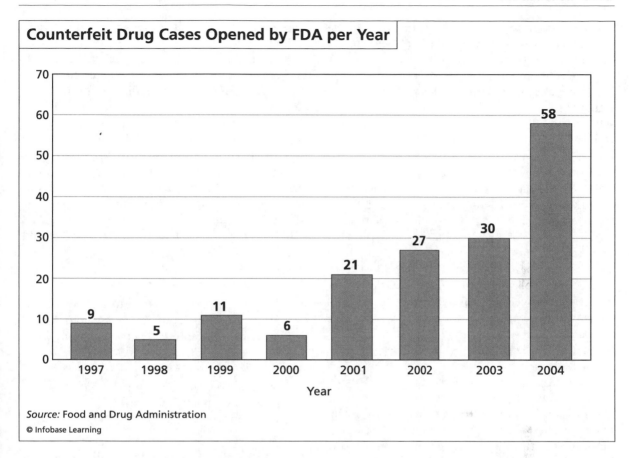

Counterfeit Drug Cases Opened by FDA per Year

Year

Source: Food and Drug Administration

© Infobase Learning

ing of drugs. Some examples include holograms, color shifting inks, and watermarks currently employed for U.S. currency. So-called track and trace technologies, such as radio-frequency identification (RFID) and sophisticated bar coding, can provide effective monitoring of a drug's movement from the point of manufacture and through the U.S. distribution chain. Others have cautioned that such safeguards can be easily duplicated and, therefore, must be changed on a periodic basis.

A 2004 FDA report, "Combating Counterfeit Drugs: A Report of the Food and Drug Administration," stated that adoption and widespread use of reliable track and trace technology is feasible by 2007. "This would help secure the integrity of the supply chain by providing an accurate drug 'pedigree,' a record documenting that the drug was manufactured and distributed under secure conditions. We particularly advocated for the implementation of electronic track and trace mechanisms and noted that RFID is the most promising technology to meet this need. RFID technology uses a tiny radio frequency chip containing essential data in the form of an electronic product code (EPC). Implementation of RFID will allow supply chain stakeholders to track the chain of custody (or pedigree) of every package of medication. By tying each discrete product unit to a unique electronic serial number, a product can be tracked electronically through every step of the supply chain."

The FDA maintains a Web page specifically for consumers with links to articles and information concerning counterfeit drugs at http://www.fda.gov/cder/consumerinfo/counterfeit_text.htm.

Internet and mail order sale of drugs   Purchasing medicines online has become convenient for consumers, but the FDA warns that it can be a hazardous proposition. Both consumers and legitimate pharmacies are now being threatened by fraudulent or disreputable Internet businesses that sell products illegally. While the FDA is working to combat these illegal sites, many are not based in the United States. Of particular concern are those Web sites selling medicine that are not U.S. state-licensed pharmacies or are not pharmacies at all, that give incorrect diagnoses and sell medicines not right for the patient or the condition, or that do not protect buyers' personal information. The FDA warns that some medicines sold online are counterfeit, are too strong or too weak, have dangerous ingredients, have expired (are out-of-date), are not FDA-approved or even guaranteed to be "FDA equivalent," are not made using safe standards, are not safe to use with other medicines or products being used by the patient, or are not labeled, stored, or shipped correctly.

According to Jupiter Research, a company that analyzes Internet sales, U.S. consumers ordered at least $1.4 billion worth of drugs over the Internet in 2004, which is double the amount spent in 2002. Spake noted that no one knows how many Internet sites sell prescription drugs. "One New York City investigative firm estimated that there are more than 1,400 Internet pharmacy sites. A consultant for Federal Express found 650,310 sites in a Web search where the FedEx brand was used on the same page as a list of the top 22 drug names. The Drug Enforcement Agency (DEA) says there are 537 sites selling controlled substances."

Some Internet drug sales are perfectly safe and legitimate. Among the precautions the FDA suggests consumers take is to make sure a Web site is a U.S. state-licensed pharmacy. Pharmacies and pharmacists in the United States are licensed by a state's board of pharmacy. Any state board of pharmacy can tell if a Web site is a state-licensed pharmacy and is in good standing. The National Association of Boards of Pharmacy (NABP) provides contact information for the various state boards of pharmacy at http://www.nabp.info.

The NABP also has a program to help consumers locate some of the legitimate pharmacies that are licensed to sell medicine online. Internet Web sites that display the Verified Internet Pharmacy Practice Sites™ Seal, (VIPPS® Seal) have been checked to make sure they meet state and federal rules. The main Web site for VIPPS is http://www.vipps.info, and a search page to locate verified Internet Web sites that sell drugs is at http://www.nabp.net/vipps/consumer/search.asp.

According to the FDA, a safe Web site should:

- be licensed by the state board of pharmacy where the Web site is operating

- have a licensed pharmacist to answer patient questions. NABP staff have verified that all Pharmacist-in-Charge licenses are in good standing for VIPPS-certified sites. This certification is reviewed annually.

- require a prescription from the patient's doctor or other health-care professional who is licensed in the United States to write prescriptions for medicine

- have a way for the patient to talk to a person if he or she has problems

- post privacy and security policies that are easy to find and easy to understand

- specifically state it will not sell your information unless you agree

Pharmaceutical arbitrage   Pharmaceutical arbitrage involves the buying of prescription drugs in one market, then selling in another market in order to profit from price differentials existing between those markets. Morais wrote, "No one really knows the size of this drug arbitrage business, since much of it takes place in the shadows. Where it is legal, few in the pharmaceutical industry—neither the arbitragers nor the manufacturers nor big wholesalers—want to talk about it on the record. But this much is clear: The business of arbitraging drugs is huge, fast-growing and constantly morphing around the globe according to local laws and customs. In Europe legal arbitrage of pharmaceuticals is already a $12 billion or so business." Called "parallel trade," it is "actively encouraged within the European Union (EU), but illegal for drugs coming from outside the EU."

Saul added, "The secondary pharmaceutical market includes purchases or resales outside the normal drug manufacturing channel. In some cases, wholesalers stock up on supplies of the drug, then hold them until manufacturers announce price increases, a form of arbitrage that financial analysts say has helped drive up pharmaceutical prices."

Costs of drugs According to a December 2004 U.S. government report, prescription drug costs are rising faster than any other area of medical care—15 percent higher in 2002 than the previous year. Among the various reasons given for the soaring costs are more expensive medicines today and increased numbers of Americans taking drugs—especially for psychiatric conditions, to lower their cholesterol, and to control asthma. While some place the blame for this increased use on direct-to-consumer advertising, others say it has much to do with the very method of testing drugs for FDA approval. Abboud explains:

> Clinical trials that companies do to get drugs approved aren't designed to provide the answers that doctors say they really need. For one, these trials don't compare one drug with another, because they are designed to show only whether a particular drug is effective against an illness. Thus, psychiatrists have little guidance on whether one drug works better than another or has fewer side effects than another.
>
> Also, at eight to 12 weeks long, drug-company trials are too short to reveal how patients fare or what side effects crop up long-term. And, in order to stay focused on a drug's efficacy on one illness, they exclude the sickest patients and people with co-existing diseases.
>
> In addition to comparing drugs, the trials are trying to fill another gap in the scientific litera-

ture: what to do with the many patients who don't get better on their first drug. Psychiatrists do a lot of switching patients from one antidepressant to another and tinkering with drug combinations. None of this is backed up with good evidence, and it can take months to find the right regimen. Practices and outcomes vary widely among doctors.

This point was also made during a May 2004 HHS Task Force hearing by Thomas Paul, chief pharmacy officer for Ovations, UnitedHealth Group's business that focuses on meeting the health-care needs of the over-50 population, who stated, "We think increased research on the comparative effectiveness of prescription drugs could have a much greater impact on reducing prescription drug costs, over the long run, than importation would have. More importantly, this type of research would allow us to address efficacy and quality first, not simply cost."

Continued escalation in the cost of providing prescription medicines has strained many state Medicaid budgets. Although states are not required to offer prescription drugs through Medicaid, all states do. In April 2004, HHS approved plans by five states—Michigan, Vermont, New Hampshire, Alaska, and Nevada—to pool their collective purchasing power to gain deeper discounts on prescription medicines for their state programs, the first time in the history of the Medicaid program that states had worked together in this manner.

Prescription drug abuse and misuse

Although many prescription drugs can be abused or misused, three classes of prescription drugs are most commonly abused: opioids—most often prescribed to treat pain; central nervous system depressants—used to treat anxiety and sleep disorders; and stimulants—prescribed to treat the sleep disorder narcolepsy, attention-deficit/hyperactivity disorder (ADHD), and obesity.

Several indicators suggest that prescription drug abuse is on the rise in the United States. According to the 2004 National Survey on Drug Use and Health, an estimated 2.8 million

Americans used prescription psychotherapeutics nonmedically for the first time in 2004. This represents a significant increase since the 1980s, when there were generally fewer than 500,000 first-time users per year. Use was defined as nonmedical if the drug was not prescribed for the respondent or if the respondent took the drug only for the experience or feeling it caused. Of those new users, 2.4 million used pain relievers, which included codeine, methadone, meperidine (Demerol), Percocet, hydrocodone (Vicodin), and oxycodone (Oxycontin). Also, 1.2 million used tranquilizers, 793,000 used stimulants, and 240,000 used sedatives. Some new users took more than one type of prescription drug nonmedically.

Although prescription drug abuse cuts across all parts of society without regard for race, religion, gender, age, or national origin, some trends of concern have been noted among older adults, adolescents, and women. In 2002, more than half (55 percent) of the new nonmedical pain-relief users were female. Also, lifetime non-medical use of sedatives increased significantly from 2002 to 2003 for males aged 12 to 17 (0.7 percent to 1.0 percent). Sedative choices listed in the survey were methaqualone, Nembutal, pentobarbital, Seconal®, secobarbital or butalbital, temazepam, Amytal, Butisol, chloral hydrate, Dalmane, Halcion, phenobarbital, Placidyl, and Tuinal.

Health-care professionals—including physicians, nurses, pharmacists, dentists, anesthesiologists, and veterinarians—may be at increased risk of prescription drug abuse because of ease of access as well as their ability to self-prescribe drugs. In spite of this increased risk, recent surveys and research in the early 1990s indicate that health-care providers probably suffer from substance abuse, including alcohol and drugs, at a rate similar to those in society as a whole, in the range of 8 to 12 percent.

In 2004, the Drug Abuse Warning Network (DAWN), a national surveillance system that collects data on drug abuse–related visits to emergency departments (EDs) and drug abuse–related deaths reviewed by medical examiners and coroners, reported several prescription drug statistics:

- In 2002, opioid pain relievers accounted for more than 119,000 ED mentions, or 10 percent of all the drug mentions in drug abuse–related ED visits. Oxycodone and hydrocodone were the most frequently named pain relievers, accounting for 40 percent (47,594 mentions) of the opioid pain relievers involved in these ED visits.

- In 1994, ED mentions of oxycodone numbered about 4,000 nationally. By 2002, ED mentions of oxycodone had increased to more than 22,000 mentions—an increase of 450 percent.

- In 1994, ED mentions of hydrocodone were more than twice as frequent as oxycodone, but that gap has narrowed. By 2002, ED mentions of hydrocodone had risen by 170 percent, from about 9,300 in 1994 to more than 25,000 in 2002.

- Approximately three-quarters of ED visits involving oxycodone and hydrocodone involved additional drugs (71 percent and 78 percent, respectively), while only 54 percent of all drug abuse–related visits involved multiple drugs.

Drug diversion

Along with this rise in prescription drug abuse and misuse has been an exponential rise in the diversion of legal prescription drugs for illicit purposes. In his September 2004 congressional testimony, Dr. Kenneth Varley, president/executive director of the Alabama Society of Interventional Pain Physicians, said, "The problem of prescription drug diversion has eclipsed illicit drug use as a public health and law enforcement challenge."

Through September 2003, the DEA had already registered 726 reported incidents of hospital/clinic drug loss amounting to 118,444 dosage units, with 466 different drug types diverted. Although hospital drug theft had long been viewed as an internal problem related to personal use, the escalating street value of prescription drugs has transformed it into more of a resale issue.

According to the National Drug Intelligence Center, pharmaceuticals usually are illegally obtained through theft, doctor shopping, prescription forgery, and improper prescribing practices by physicians. Pharmaceuticals are also stolen by pharmacy employees and others. Doctor shopping occurs when individuals, who may or may not have a legitimate ailment, visit numerous physicians to obtain drugs in excess of what should be legitimately prescribed. Prescription forgery occurs when dealers or abusers steal prescriptions from physicians or alter the writing on prescriptions that doctors have issued. Some unscrupulous physicians prescribe medications for individuals who do not have a legitimate need for the drug at the patient's request, sometimes for a fee. Legitimate prescription holders also divert portions of their prescriptions for abuse or financial gain.

In his congressional testimony, Varley said, "The DEA controls the manufacture and wholesale distribution of controlled pharmaceuticals through a nationwide database. The retail level, from the physician to the patient, however, is not constantly being monitored state by state and there is virtually no system in place to aid physicians in identifying unscrupulous patients trying to obtain medications under false pretenses. Some 15 to 21 states have some form of state prescription drug monitoring system. A monitoring system alone, however, will not give physicians the timely information needed to identify deceitful patients and stop diversion at its source."

Abboud, Leila. "The Next Phase in Psychiatry." *Wall Street Journal,* July 27, 2005, D1.

Addington, John. "Drug and Supplement Interactions: What CFS and Fibromyalgia Patients Need to Know." ImmuneSupport.com. Available online. URL: http://www.immunesupport.com/library/showarticle.cfm/ ID/3168/e/1/T/CFIDS_FM/. Posted on October 31, 2001.

Agnvall, Elizabeth. "The Druggist Is In; A New Type of Pharmacist Seeks to Help People Manage Complex Drug Regimens. The Catch: Someone Has to Pay." *Washington Post,* December 14, 2004, HE01.

Anderegg, Marcia A. "Drugs Spill Over Borders." *Mass High Tech,* August 1–7, 2005: 15, 21.

Ball, Judy, and Dana Lehder Roberts. "Oxycodone, Hydrocodone, and Polydrug Use, 2002." *The DAWN Report,* Office of Applied Studies, Substance Abuse and Mental Health Services Administration (SAMHSA), U.S. Department of Health & Human Services, July 2004.

Bates, D. W., et al. "The Costs of Adverse Drug Events in Hospitalized Patients. Adverse Drug Events Prevention Study Group." *Journal of the American Medical Association* 277, no. 4 (January 22–29, 1997): 307–311.

Bennett, Charles L., et al. "The Research on Adverse Drug Effects and Reports (RADAR) Project." *Journal of the American Medical Association* 293, no. 17 (May 4, 2005): 2,131–2,140.

Ceccoli, Stephen J. *Pill Politics: Drugs and the FDA.* Boulder, Colo.: Lynne Rienner Publishers, 2004.

Doughton, Sandi. "UW Researchers Identify Genetic Sensitivity to Drug." *Seattle Times,* June 2, 2005, B1.

Ellis, J. J., et al. "Suboptimal Statin Adherence and Discontinuation in Primary and Secondary Prevention Populations." *Journal of General Internal Medicine* 19, no. 6 (June 2004): 638–645.

Fick, Donna M., et al. "Updating the Beers Criteria for Potentially Inappropriate Medication Use in Older Adults." *Archives of Internal Medicine* 163, no. 22 (December 8, 2003): 2,716–2,724.

Gearon, Christopher J. "Medicine's Turf Wars." *U.S. News & World Report,* 31 January 2005: 57–64.

Hubbard, Gardiner. "Tiny Antennas to Keep Tabs on U.S. Drugs." *New York Times,* November 15, 2004, B3.

Jensen, Valerie, Lorene M. Kimzey, and Mark J. Goldberger. "FDA's Role in Responding to Drug Shortages." *American Journal of Health Systems Pharmacists* 59, no. 15 (August 2002): 1,423–1,425.

Meadows, Michelle. "Strategies to Reduce Medication Errors." *FDA Consumer* 37, no. 3 (May–June 2003): 21–27.

Mehlman, Maxwell J. "Bioethics: Off-Label Prescribing." Available online. URL: http://www.

thedoctorwillseeyounow.com/articles/bioethics/offlabel_11./ Posted May 2005.

Morais, Richard C. "Pssst . . . Wanna Buy Some Augmentin?" *Forbes,* 12 April 2004, 211.

Murray, Michael D. "Automated Medication Dispensing Devices." Chapter 11 in *Making Health Care Safer: A Critical Analysis of Patient Safety Practices.* Evidence Report/Technology Assessment: Number 43. AHRQ Publication No. 01-E058, July 2001. Agency for Healthcare Research and Quality, Rockville, Md. Available online. URL: http://www.ahrq.gov/clinic/ptsafety/.

Nordenberg, Tamar. "When a Drug Is in Short Supply." *FDA Consumer* 31, no. 6 (November–December 1997): 30–32.

Osterberg, Lars, and Terrence Blaschke. "Adherence to Medication." *New England Journal of Medicine* 353, no. 5 (August 4, 2005): 487–497.

Pelletier, Sue. "Off-Label, Off-Limits?" MeetingsNet. Available online. URL: http://mm.meetingsnet.com/ar/meetings_offlabel_offlimits/. Posted on March 1, 2005.

Perry, Leah E. "Bar Codes Expected to Be Adopted by Hospitals." *Drug Topics Health-System Edition,* 17 May 2004, HSE27.

Rados, Carol. "Drug Name Confusion: Preventing Medication Errors." *FDA Consumer* 39, no. 4 (July–August 2005): 35–37.

Saul, Stephanie. "Subpoenas Seek Data on Resales of Drugs." *New York Times,* April 9, 2005, C1.

Spake, Amanda. "Fake Drugs, Real Worries." *U.S. News & World Report,* 20 September 2004, 46, 48, 50.

Spenser, Jane. "Alternative-Medicine Usage Holds Risks, WHO Reports." *Wall Street Journal,* June 24, 2004, D5.

Stetina, P., M. Groves, and L. Pafford. "Managing Medication Errors—a Qualitative Study." *MEDSURG Nursing* 14, no. 3 (June 2005): 174–178.

Stucky, Erin R., et al. "Prevention of Medication Errors in the Pediatric Inpatient Setting." *Pediatrics* 112, no. 2 (August 2003): 431–436.

U.S. Food and Drug Administration, Center for Drug Evaluation and Research. "Preventable Adverse Drug Reactions: A Focus on Drug Interactions." Available online. URL: http://www.fda.gov/cder/drug/drugReactions/default.htm. Updated July 31, 2002.

WorstPills.org. "Adverse Drug Reactions." Available online. URL: http://www.worstpills.org/public/page.cfm?op_id=4&rint=1. Downloaded August 11, 2005.

Future of Prescription Drugs

Pharmacogenomics (the study of how a person's genome, or genetic inheritance, affects the body's response to drugs) is the word most often used by scientists and industry executives to project the future of drugs. Pharmacogenomics holds the promise that drugs might one day be tailor-made for individuals and adapted to each person's own genetic makeup. Although a number of factors (e.g., diet, age, health status, and other drugs being taken at the time) can influence how a person's body reacts to a particular drug, the person's genome is believed to be the real key to prescribing drugs most effectively. The FDA believes that the integration of pharmacogenomics into drug development will help identify sources of interindividual variability in drug response, which in turn will maximize effectiveness and minimize risk of drug treatment.

Several leaders from different areas of the drug industry offer specifically for this work their thoughts on the future of the drug industry.

Mario Ehlers, M.D., Ph.D., is chief medical officer for Pacific Biometrics, a Seattle, Washington, central lab that provides support for pharmaceutical and diagnostic product research. Dr. Ehlers has more than 11 years' experience in academic research and more than four years' biopharmaceutical industry experience in drug development, business development, and investor relations. Dr. Ehlers' comments:

The future of prescription drugs is the move towards targeted therapeutics. The era of the one-size-fits-all blockbuster is drawing to a close and will be replaced by drugs that are targeted at specific subpopulations of patients stratified on the basis of appropriate biomarkers that identify responders and non-responders. This trend will ultimately lead to true personalized medicine. These developments are being driven by advances in technology, heightened expectations by regulatory agencies, and consumer demand for safer and more effective medicines.

During the past decade, advances in molecular biology, structural biology, genomics, proteomics, and related gene-on-a-chip and protein-on-a-chip micro-array technologies have fueled a revolution in discovery of novel drug targets. Because of this, drug discovery is now accompanied by the co-development of related biomarkers that can serve as surrogate endpoints and eventual companion diagnostics during the clinical development of new drugs. These biomarkers—which can be genomic, proteomic, imaging, or conventional biochemical markers—are directly related to the targets modulated by drugs and can therefore preselect responders from non-responders, may be informative about which patients are at risk for adverse events, and can serve to monitor treatment efficacy. Use of such biomarkers will streamline clinical trials because investigational drugs will be tested only in likely responders. Post-approval, biomarkers will be used as companion diagnostics that target the drug to subpopulations that will respond, increasing the cost-effectiveness of the drug and reducing unnecessary exposure to potential adverse events. This approach—the combination of a therapeutic with a diagnostic, or using diagnostic testing to diagnose a disease, choosing the correct treatment regimen, and monitoring the patient's response to therapy—is called theranostics.

The FDA has issued several documents outlining its vision for the future of prescription drug development. In its *Critical Path Initiative*, the FDA highlighted the importance of new technologies, including biomarkers, that will streamline the drug development process. In addition, in a final guidance on pharmacogenomics, the FDA has suggested guidelines for the collection and submission of pharmacogenomic information during the drug approval process.

Consumer and patient advocacy groups are also driving this process as a result of high-profile drug failures and withdrawals, such as Vioxx, Tysabri, and Rezulin. Going forward, it will no longer be acceptable to develop drugs that are indiscriminately prescribed to all patients without attempting to preselect responders and non-responders and minimizing risks for adverse events by targeting drugs to appropriate patient subpopulations.

Targeted therapeutics and theranostics are exciting developments that will lead us one step closer to personalized medicine and will significantly improve the safety and efficacy of prescription drugs in the future.

John Rhodes is U.S. and global managing partner of Life Sciences for the Life Sciences & Health Care Practice of Deloitte & Touche USA. He has more than 20 years' experience working with pharmaceutical, biotech, medical products, and manufacturing industries, focusing on accounting and auditing, SEC reporting, business process and contracting issues, corporate compliance, strategic alliances, research and promotion collaborations, joint venture formations, and mergers and acquisitions. According to Mr. Rhodes, the following challenges face the pharmaceutical industry.

Pricing—The marketplace is driving more price constraints and public perception about the value of pharmaceuticals, and what should be paid is challenged by global conditions. Markets outside the United States have price controls, and importation issues are threatening the historic pricing model in the United States. This is also being challenged by the patent expiration pressures around certain blockbuster pharmaceutical products.

Manufacturing and Regulatory—With the increasing pressure from financial markets and stakeholders, pharmaceutical companies are looking at supply chain efficiencies and selective outsourcing of manufacturing operations. Supply chain refers to the entire process, from discovery to production to distributor to patient in the health care world, with the doctors playing an important role in prescribing.

Patent Uncertainty and Discovery—Discovery costs continue to grow, and companies are looking for ways to complete more effective and targeted researching-leveraging technology. Additionally, patent life is being challenged earlier in the life of a product by "within-patent" competition. Within-patent means that there is much more competition today while a prescription drug still has patent protection from other patented products that might treat the same condition. So patent exclusivity is great, but you could still have competition even before a generic launches later in the product life cycle.

Future alliances and technology convergence—Companies will continue to expand the number of alliances between pharmaceutical and biotech companies, and further relationships will develop among device, diagnostics and pharmaceutical companies as new medicines and treatments emerge.

William K. Sietsema, Ph.D., is vice president of clinical and regulatory strategic planning for Kendle International, a global contract research organization. He has been a scientist, drug developer, bone researcher, and director of clinical research for Kendle and Procter & Gamble. He is also adjunct professor of pharmaceutical sciences at the University of Cincinnati College of Pharmacy, where he teaches drug development principles to medical students, pharmacists, and industry representatives. Dr. Sietsema is author of *Strategic Clinical Development Planning: Designing Programs for Winning Products* (FDAnews, 2005), a guide for drug companies looking to streamline the trial process for faster FDA approvals and major cost savings. Dr. Sietsema's thoughts on the future of drugs with regard to pharmacogenomics:

As we learn more about how people's genetic makeup impacts the way in which drugs work, we find more and more examples of classes of drugs that work a little differently in some people than in others, which can be attributed to their genetic makeup. Speculation is that soon we'll have all of our DNA information on a credit-card size device that we give to the doctor, and he or she will then use that information to choose the best drugs to prescribe. I don't think this will be in place in the next five years, but it will be there eventually.

Personalized medicine is going to change the way we prescribe pills. Drug companies will shift from developing blockbusters to multibusters (a term the industry uses to differentiate the single drug blockbuster method of research from the search for smaller market, specialized drugs). For example, today we design one drug that is meant to fit all patients, such as COX-2 inhibitors. But before you give that drug to everyone, you really ought to understand the genomic differences associated with the use of that drug—and that might be differences in the way patients metabolize the drug, or it might be differences in the way patients eliminate the drug, or it might be differences in the way patients react to the drug. All those things are wrapped up into a genomic effect on how a patient responds to a drug. And the idea with multibusters is that instead of having one drug fits all, you understand what the differences are in how different patients respond to that drug, and if you have a group of patients with a receptor that's a little different than most other patients, then you might for those patients with that difference in the receptor, design a drug—adapted from that original drug—that's targeted especially to that altered receptor.

Right now drug companies spend a lot of time and effort making sure that a COX-2 inhibitor, for example, has a specific type of binding to the COX-2 receptor, but when they do that, they're using one COX-2 receptor isolated probably from one person. Whereas within the general population, there may be ten variations on the COX-2 receptor, with only slight differences from one person to the other. And one particular drug might bind better to one receptor type and another drug might bind better to another receptor type. So you could create a series of COX-2 inhibitors, each with very minor variations and structure, but which are designed to bind better to one receptor in particular. Then the challenge is that before a physician treats a patient, he or she finds out which variation of the COX-2 receptor the patient has, and prescribes the drug with the best binding affinity for that receptor.

This means that drug companies will need to combine the marketing of this series of products with a genomic diagnostic, if you will, that allows the physician to determine which of those receptors this patient has, or which variation of the receptor this patient has, and then to prescribe the COX-2 inhibitor that is the best match for that particular variant.

One of the future scenarios might be that a company develops six different variations all at the same time along with the diagnostic tool that helps the physician determine which COX-2 inhibitor would work best in a particular patient. One of the challenges in today's environment is that if six different companies produce those six different products, it becomes a little more difficult to coordinate the diagnostic versus what the physician actually prescribes, because each company, of course, wants their drug prescribed. Therefore, companies may actually try to block the preparation of a diagnostic because that could only detract from their sales.

When physicians are able to use genetic testing to perfectly pair patients with drugs, treatment will move away from today's trial and error prescribing, whereby the doctor tries one drug on a patient, and if it does not work, he or she will prescribe another drug to see if that one works, and then will eventually find one that does work. The general belief in the pharmaceutical industry is that good diagnostic and personalized medications will take trial and error out of the process. Each patient will leave the doctor's office with the right drug at the exact dosage he or she needs.

Jon Hess is a research and consulting project leader with Cutting Edge Information, a pharmaceutical consulting firm in Research Triangle Park, North Carolina. He has advised the industry's top firms on such areas as manufacturing, quality control, and recruitment and retention of study sites and patients for clinical trials. From this perspective, Mr. Hess offers his views on the future of the FDA drug approval process.

In light of the events involving Vioxx and concerns over the safety of a number of marketed drugs, I think we'll see the FDA shift to the conservative side a bit more, where they'll require more robust clinical trial data and more long-term studies to be done on the safety of a number of drugs. I also think the FDA's thinking and practices will rub off in Europe and in other major global markets, and we'll probably start seeing the same shift in philosophy there.

When it comes to conducting clinical trials, one of the greatest challenges the industry faces today is finding enough patients that meet their often stringent study protocol requirements to enroll in their studies. Some of our recent research has found that patient recruitment consumes the greatest portion of trial timelines—around 30 percent. Industry executives reported that patient recruitment also is the single most important area for the industry to focus on in terms of being able to shorten timelines and, therefore, bring products to market faster.

With the industry already facing this challenge, with competition—especially in the US—for patients already pretty fierce, and with the likelihood of the FDA requiring more/better clinical data, I think we'll see the patient recruitment struggle get worse before it gets better. I also think we'll see the clinical development side of the industry focusing more on ways to improve patient recruitment and to speed up trials.

One of the things that has helped alleviate this problem recently is that the industry has adopted the use of Web-based patient recruitment more over the past few years. Several specialized vendors have cropped up to meet this need, including Acurian and Veritas Medicine. Typically, recruiting patients via the Web is a cheaper, more predictable way to recruit patients (by comparison to traditional media, such as newspapers, TV and radio ads). Companies usually only rely on this avenue to get them 15–20 percent of the patients for a given trial, but oftentimes, they struggle to get that last chunk of patients, so this can be a big help.

Finally, I also think we'll see the FDA being more willing to use more data from trials conducted in Europe and other markets when evaluating the safety and efficacy of drugs in development. One trend that is continuing to build is that more companies are turning to eastern Europe, Asia, and South America to conduct clinical trials. Countries in these regions of the world offer relatively untapped patient populations, and the populations of many of these countries, such as India, are afflicted with many of the same diseases that are prevalent in the US.

Albert I. Wertheimer, Ph.D., M.B.A., PharmD., is director of the Center for Pharmaceutical Health Services Research at Temple University's School of Pharmacy. In addition to providing consulting services to institutions in the pharmaceutical industry, Dr. Wertheimer is the editor of the *Journal of Pharmaceutical Finance and Economic Policy*. He offers his thoughts on how pharmacoeconomics will influence prescription drugs in the coming years.

Pharmacoeconomics is going to have an enormous impact on drug development and drug use in the future all over the world.

In the realm of prescribing, in the United States, the tools used by managed care will be used by non-managed care organizations such as indemnity health insurers, the VA, Department of Defense facilities, and even state Medicaid programs. For example, there are about 18 beta blocker agents on the market. All lower blood pressure, but some do a better job with fewer (costly) side-effects, and the range of prices amongst them is wide. Pharmacoeconomic techniques will be used by nearly all purchasers of pharmaceuticals to determine the most "efficient" or cost-beneficial products, and it will be those products that will be seen on the formularies in the United States, and elsewhere as well.

In another example, there can be two antibiotic agents that have nearly identical prices, nearly identical effectiveness and other treatment characteristics, but one causes an 8 percent incidence of diarrhea while the other one is responsible for a 22 percent incidence. Those G.I. side effects often require physician visits, lab work and additional medications, making the drug responsible for the 22 percent rate of diarrhea undesirable for both its clinical profile as well as its pharmacoeconomic impact.

In Europe and in much of Asia, pharmacoeconomics are employed by pharmaceutical companies in presentations to the Ministries of Health or National Social Security Agencies who set drug prices for the country. A once-a-day dosage form that likely enhances compliance with the prescribed drug regimen can command a premium price over a tablet that must be taken three or four times a day. The companies present pharmacoeconomic data to bolster their price request. The national health insurance in those countries will only reimburse or pay for the drugs selected for the formulary, which are those that are the most efficient (have the best cost-benefit ratio).

This growth of the acceptance of pharmacoeconomic drug evaluation policies will have a halo effect on drug development subsequently. If a company knows that its product is no better or even inferior to existing products already on the market, it may choose to abandon the further development of the product. Today a product that offers no real advantage can be marketed and the strength of that firm's marketing muscle can create a success. In the future, the inferior product will probably be dropped. The equivalent product offering no clinical advantage may go forward and become successful by the strategy of a lower price than the existing products, thus introducing price competition, an always welcome event.

ENTRIES A TO Z

acid-suppressives　Medications that relieve acid indigestion (also called dyspepsia) and heartburn (also called pyrosis), which may lead to or be symptoms of gastric acid–related diseases. Acid indigestion involves an excess of hydrochloric acid (which helps break down food for digestion) in the stomach. Its symptoms can include discomfort or burning sensation in the upper portion of the stomach, nausea, abdominal bloating, or belching. Frequent occurrence of acid indigestion can lead to aggravation of the duodenum or to an aggravation of the lining of the stomach, both of which can play a role in the development of peptic ulcer disease, which can be life-threatening. Heartburn is a painful, burning sensation in the esophagus, just below the breastbone, caused by stomach (gastric) acid flowing back into the esophagus. The pain often rises in the chest and may radiate to the neck or throat. Heartburn may be a symptom of gastroesophageal reflux disease (GERD)—injury to the esophagus that develops from chronic exposure of the esophagus to acid coming up from the stomach.

The true incidence of GERD might be underestimated because of the relatively low proportion of individuals who seek medical attention for reflux symptoms. One report found that only 5 percent of patients with symptoms of heartburn and regurgitation had visited a physician because of this problem within the preceding year. Peptic ulcer disease is a sore or hole in the lining of the stomach or duodenum that is often caused by an infection with the bacterium *Helicobacter pylori*. Acid indigestion, gastric reflux, ulcers, and other digestive problems plague about a third of the U.S. population. In one study, approximately 3.6 million individuals, or 2 percent of U.S. adults, obtained medical care for dyspepsia during a single year. An estimated 100 million Americans experience heartburn every month; about 15 million battle it at least once a day.

Classes

Acid-suppressives are divided into three major drug classes according to their method of action.

- *Antacids* balance acids in the stomach. Available in over-the-counter (OTC) preparations, most antacids contain one or more of the following active ingredients: aluminum hydroxide, calcium carbonate, magnesium hydroxide, sodium bicarbonate. *Examples:* Di-Gel, Gaviscon, Maalox, Mylanta, Rolaids, and Tums.

- *H_2 receptor antagonists* (also called H_2RA, H_2-blockers, histamine H_2 antagonists, H_2-antagonists, histamine-2 blockers) reduce the amount of acid the stomach produces. Smaller doses of H_2-blockers are now available OTC; larger doses by prescription. *Examples:* cimetidine (Tagamet), famotidine (Pepcid), nizatidine (Axid), and ranitidine (Zantac).

- *Proton pump inhibitors* (PPIs) also stop the stomach from producing acid. All but one (Prilosec OTC) are available by prescription only. *Examples:* esomeprazole (Nexium), lansoprazole (Prevacid), omeprazole (Prilosec, Prilosec OTC), pantoprazole (Protonix), rabeprazole (Aciphex).

- Miscellaneous *stomach-lining protectors*. These do not suppress the formation of acid but do help to form a protective lining in the gut to protect it from the erosive effects of gastric acid. *Examples:* sucralfate (Carafate) and bismuth subsalicylate (Pepto-Bismol) (see ANTIDIARRHEALS).

How They Work

Antacids relieve indigestion and heartburn by neutralizing stomach acid. Calcium carbonate is the most effective at doing this, followed by sodium bicarbonate, magnesium hydroxide, and then aluminum hydroxide.

Histamine is a chemical produced naturally by the body that signals the stomach to make acid. H_2 receptor antagonists block the action of histamine on parietal cells in the stomach, decreasing acid production by these cells. They are used to treat conditions in which the stomach produces too much acid.

Compared to H_2 receptor antagonists, PPIs more completely inhibit acid secretion over a longer period of time by blocking the chemical "pump" needed for stomach cells to make acid. Because the proton pump is the final pathway for secretion of hydrochloric acid by the parietal cells in the stomach, its inhibition dramatically reduces acid secretion into the stomach and alters gastric pH. This provides excellent healing of inflammation of the esophagus, which is most often caused by GERD. PPIs reduce gastric acid secretion by up to 99 percent.

Bismuth subsalicylate coats the entire stomach lining, and sucralfate sticks to and covers gastric and duodenal ulcers.

Approved Uses

Antacids are used for temporary relief of acid indigestion, heartburn, and/or sour stomach. Antacids containing calcium carbonate are also used to treat calcium deficiency. Antacids containing aluminum hydroxide may also be used along with a low-phosphate diet to treat hyperphosphatemia (too much phosphate in the blood). Antacids containing magnesium hydroxide may be used to treat magnesium deficiencies.

H_2 receptor antagonists are used to treat gastric and duodenal ulcers (peptic ulcer disease) and GERD. OTC preparations are approved to treat only heartburn, sour stomach, and acid indigestion.

Proton pump inhibitors aid in the healing of gastric and duodenal ulcers and GERD and reduce the pain from indigestion and heartburn.

Sucralfate is approved for treating duodenal ulcers for up to eight weeks.

Off-Label Uses

Antacids with aluminum and magnesium can be effective at preventing stress ulcer bleeding. Antacids are also used to treat duodenal and gastric ulcers and may be used for initial treatment of GERD.

Cimetidine has been used to treat chronic viral warts in children.

Famotidine and ranitidine have been used to treat upper gastrointestinal (GI) bleeding and stress ulcers. They have also been found useful in preventing gastric acid from entering the lungs during surgery.

A three-part investigative series by Knight Ridder Newspapers in 2003 found that 21 percent of PPI prescriptions are for off-label uses such as difficulty swallowing, hernia, and pancreatitis.

Laryngitis caused by reflux can be treated with any of the PPIs.

Companion Drugs

H_2 receptor antagonists and PPIs may be combined with antibiotics to heal *Helicobacter pylori*–related peptic ulcers.

Administration

Antacids are available as effervescent tablets, chewables, or liquids. Generally, liquids work most quickly.

H_2 receptor antagonists are available by prescription as tablets, capsules, effervescent tablets, liquid, and injections. OTC formulations are available as tablets and chewables.

Proton pump inhibitors are available in delayed-release gelatin capsules containing enteric-coated granules (omeprazole, esomeprazole, and lansoprazole) or in delayed-release enteric-coated tablets (rabeprazole, pantoprazole, and Prilosec OTC). (An enteric coating prevents digestion of the medication until it reaches the small intestine.) Omeprazole is also available as a prescription in a powder for oral suspension. Prevacid is also available in orally disintegrating tablets and as granules for oral suspension. Omeprazole, lansoprazole, and esomeprazole should be taken 30 minutes to an hour before a meal. Pantoprazole and lansoprazole are also available as a powder for injection.

Cautions and Concerns

Aluminum hydroxide should be used with care in patients who have recently suffered massive upper gastrointestinal hemorrhage. Magnesium hydroxide should be used with caution in patients who have impaired kidney function.

H_2 receptor antagonists may mask the existence of a stomach malignancy. These drugs should be used with caution in patients with impaired kidney or liver function.

Ulcers treated with cimetidine may return when treatment is discontinued, with recurrence at a slightly higher rate than when healed with other forms of therapy.

Proton pump inhibitors should be used with caution in patients with severe liver disease.

In 2004, a Dutch study of more than 300,000 patients found that gastric acid suppression using H_2 receptor antagonists and PPIs is associated with an increased risk of community-acquired pneumonia. The highest risks occurred with PPIs. The acid in normal stomach fluids generally kills harmful bacteria. Suppressing the acid with drugs to treat heartburn and ulcers may make the body more hospitable to such germs, which may then infect the lungs and cause pneumonia, the researchers said. Although the apparent risk was small, it has been suggested that patients at higher risk of pneumonia, for example, the elderly, should be prescribed PPIs only at lower doses and only when necessary.

Also, people taking PPIs seem more prone to getting a potentially dangerous diarrhea caused by the bacterium *Clostridium difficile* (known as *C-diff* or *C-difficile*), according to research reported in December 2005. Dial et al. examined data on patients in the United Kingdom over a 10-year period. The incidence of *C-diff* increased from one per 100,000 in 1994 to 22 per 100,000 in 2004. Patients with prescriptions for PPIs were almost three times more likely to be diagnosed with *C-diff* than those not taking the drugs. The PPIs, which were widely used and heavily promoted during that period, reduce levels of gastric acid that can keep *C-diff* germs at bay. In a follow-up newspaper article, a U.S. Centers for Disease Control and Prevention researcher was quoted as saying PPIs had recently been implicated in a *C-diff* outbreak at a hospital and nursing homes in Maine.

Sucralfate releases small amounts of aluminum into the system, so caution is advised in patients with chronic kidney failure or who are receiving dialysis.

Warnings

Extended heavy use of calcium-containing antacids (20 grams or more daily for a prolonged period) may cause excess calcium in the blood, which can lead to kidney stones and reduced kidney function. People who already have impaired kidneys may develop milk-alkali syndrome (causing symptoms such as nausea, vomiting, mental confusion, and loss of appetite) with as little as 4 grams a day of these antacids.

Overuse of aluminum-containing antacids can weaken bones, especially in people with impaired kidney function, leading to conditions such as osteomalacia (softening of the bones, which causes symptoms such as tenderness, muscular weakness, and weight loss).

When Not Advised (Contraindications)

The Pediatric Gastroenterology, Nutrition and Hepatology Program at California Pacific Medical Center cautions against using antacids long term in young children. "Antacids are commonly used for short-term relief of intermittent gastroesophageal reflux symptoms in children and adolescents. Although there appears to be little risk to this approach, it has not been formally studied. In infants, treatment with aluminum-containing antacids significantly increases plasma aluminum levels. Because more convenient and safe alternatives are available, chronic antacid therapy is generally not recommended."

Because of their high sodium content, antacids containing sodium bicarbonate are not advised for people on a low-sodium diet or patients with congestive heart failure, kidney failure, edema, or cirrhosis. Antacids containing magnesium hydroxide are not recommended for patients with kidney failure.

H₂ receptor antagonists may not be appropriate for some people with liver, kidney, or immune system problems.

Proton pump inhibitors are not recommended for use in breastfeeding mothers.

Side Effects

The most common side effect of antacids is a chalky taste left in the mouth. Antacids containing magnesium may cause diarrhea. Those containing aluminum may cause constipation. Taking antacids containing both aluminum and magnesium (e.g., Mylanta or Maalox) may balance these effects. Prolonged use of antacids may result in nausea, headache, muscle weakness, or loss of appetite.

H₂ receptor antagonists cause relatively few side effects, which are usually reversible once the medication is stopped. Occasionally, they will cause headache, dizziness, diarrhea, constipation, drowsiness, or breast development in males. Breast development is most notable with cimetidine. Confusion and dizziness may occur in elderly people, especially those with liver or kidney problems. Less frequently, cimetidine used for longer than one month has led to agitation, anxiety, confusion, depression, disorientation, or hallucinations.

Proton pump inhibitors have few and infrequent side effects, though headache, nausea, diarrhea, abdominal pain, fatigue, and dizziness can occur. Less frequent side effects include rash, itching, flatulence, and constipation. The range and occurrence of side effects are similar for all of the PPIs, though they have been reported more frequently with omeprazole. This may be due to its longer availability on the market and greater clinical experience.

Sucralfate has been found to be generally well tolerated. Constipation is the most common side effect associated with the use of this drug. Bismuth subsalicylate can cause a black tongue.

Interactions

Antacids can affect the way a number of prescription medicines work or are used by the body. They may prevent or slow down some of the antibiotics from being absorbed by the stomach, thus decreasing their effects. Antacids can also interfere with the absorption of certain drugs for high blood pressure, kidney stones, tuberculosis, heart disease, and Parkinson's disease. With many medications, antacids need to be taken one to two hours before or after the other drug.

Cimetidine can affect the way the body breaks down a number of other medications, including warfarin, phenytoin, theophylline, ANTIARRHYTHMICS, ANTIDEPRESSANTS, and opioid ANALGESICS.

Proton pump inhibitors may increase blood levels of diazepam, warfarin, phenytoin, and digoxin and may interfere with the absorption of ketoconazole and itraconazole, thereby decreasing their effectiveness.

Aluminum accumulation and toxicity has occurred when sucralfate has been taken along with aluminum-containing antacids. Sucralfate may bind to and reduce the effectiveness of other drugs, including ANTICOAGULANTS, digoxin, quinidine, ketoconazole, fluoroquinolones, theophylline, and phenytoin. Therefore, to prevent this interaction, these medications should be taken at least two hours before the sucralfate.

Sales/Statistics

More than $10 billion is spent worldwide each year on acid-suppressives. *Chain Drug Review,* an industry trade magazine, reported in October

2005 that total sales for the year ending September 4, 2005, of OTC acid-suppressives in U.S. drug stores, supermarkets, and discount stores (excluding Wal-Mart stores) was $914.3 million (up 3.1 percent) and 141.7 million units (up 0.3 percent).

Kube wrote, "Zantac became the world's top selling medicine by 1986 but was later eclipsed by AstraZeneca's proton pump inhibitor (PPI) anti-ulcer drug Prilosec/Losec (omeprazole), the biggest selling PPI worldwide with peak annual global sales reaching $6 billion in 2001."

The Medco Health Solutions 2002 Drug Trend Report stated that spending on PPIs to treat heartburn and other GI disorders in children had increased by 660 percent over the prior five years.

Americans spent $13.5 billion on prescription PPIs in 2003, second only to cholesterol drugs. The RxList of Top 300 Prescriptions for 2004 showed 23,641,811 Nexium prescriptions, 23,628,587 Prevacid, 18,359,740 Protonix, 8,531,810 Aciphex, and 8,449,378 omeprazole (various brands).

According to a report from the IMS Institute for Healthcare Informatics (the public reporting arm of IMS, a pharmaceutical market intelligence firm), Nexium was the second-highest U.S. pharmaceutical product by spending in 2010, accounting for $6.3 billion. IMS also reported that generic omeprazole was the sixth most prescribed drug in the United States in 2010, with 53.4 million prescriptions dispensed. On their listings of top therapeutic classes, anti-ulcerants were ranked sixth in spending ($11.9 billion) and eighth in prescriptions dispensed (147.1 million).

Demographics and Cultural Groups

Asians have about 400 percent higher blood levels of omeprazole than Caucasians, and it is recommended to consider dosage adjustment in this particular population.

Using a national probability sample of the U.S. adult population, Rabeneck and Menke found that a predominance of women, individuals 65 years or older, and African Americans obtained care for dyspepsia.

Development History

Chalk (calcium carbonate) has been chewed for centuries to ease indigestion. The Sumerians have been credited with concocting the first antacids around 3500 B.C., experimenting with milk, peppermint leaves, and carbonates. Sodium bicarbonate (baking soda) was deemed to be the most effective. An understanding of the role of stomach acids by modern scientists prompted the development of antacids.

According to Goozner, the first industry scientist to conduct systematic studies on histamine blockers was the Glasgow pharmacologist James Black, whose team had developed the first beta-blocker, propranolol, for Great Britain's ICI Pharmaceuticals in 1962. Goozner writes,

> After moving on to Smith, Kline, and French, Black applied the same dual-receptor concept to the histamines that were unleashed by the presence of food and sent signals for the production of stomach acid. European academic researchers had shown that the first generation of antihistamines, while useful for allergic reactions, did not block the secretion of stomach acid. Positing there must be at least two receptors, Black began synthesizing analogues of a histamine blocker that might block only the histamine receptor that triggered action in the stomach. Eight years and seven hundred chemicals later, Black came up with his first drug for blocking the stomach histamine (H2) receptor. He spent several more years of fiddling before coming up with one that was useful as a drug. He called it cimetidine.

Cimetidine was introduced in 1977. Further work led to the development of other agents in that class with fewer side effects. Ranitidine was introduced in 1983 by Glaxo (now GlaxoSmithKline) in an effort to match the success of cimetidine by Smith, Kline and French (also now GlaxoSmithKline). In addition to fewer side effects, ranitidine was found to have longer-lasting action and 10 times the activity of cimetidine. Famotidine was developed by Merck & Co. and was first marketed in 1985. Famotidine proved to be 30 times more active than cimetidine. Nizatidine was developed by Eli Lilly and was first marketed in 1987. It is considered to be as potent as ranitidine. Nizatidine proved to be the last new H_2 receptor antagonist introduced prior to the advent of PPIs.

Goozner describes the discovery of PPIs:

> Academic scientists began looking for the engines in the stomach cells that actually produced the acid. In 1977, George Sachs, a Scottish physician who taught at the University of Alabama at Birmingham, attended a symposium in Sweden, where he presented his work on the ion-exchange mechanism in stomach cells that produced acid. He called it the proton pump. After his talk, a young scientist from Astra Pharmaceuticals approached the podium. "This Swedish person asked me a question that was intriguing," Sachs recalled. "He had found a compound that inhibited the gastric pump in rats. They sent me a couple of compounds. My lab discovered the acid pump was the target. We also discovered that the drugs were converted into active form by the acid. In 1978, we went there, told them the mechanism, and started a tight collaboration that resulted in the synthesis of omeprazole as a candidate drug."

Omeprazole was approved by the FDA in 1989, lansoprazole in 1995, rabeprazole in 1999, pantoprazole in 2000, and esomeprazole in 2001.

Dial, Sandra, J. A. Delaney, Alan N. Barkun, and Samy Suissa. "Use of Gastric Acid-Suppressive Agents and the Risk of Community-Acquired *Clostridium difficile*–Associated Disease." *Journal of the American Medical Association* 294, no. 23 (December 21, 2005): 2,989–2,995.

Goozner, Merrill. *The $800 Million Pill: The Truth behind the Cost of New Drugs.* Los Angeles: University of California Press, 2004.

Kube, D. M. "Profiles of Blockbuster Drugs and Effective Drug Targets." *Drug Discovery & Development* 6, no. 6 (March 2003): 73.

Pediatric Gastroenterology, Nutrition and Hepatology Program. "Pharmacotherapy for GERD (Gastroesophageal Reflux Disease)." California Pacific Medical Center. (February 2004) Available online. URL: http://www.cpmc.org/advanced/pediatrics/physicians/pedpage-204GI.html. Accessed February 2011.

Rabeneck, Linda, and Terri Menke. "Increased Numbers of Women, Older Individuals, and Blacks Receive Health Care for Dyspepsia in the United States." *Journal of Clinical Gastroenterology* 32, no. 4 (April 2001): 307–309.

alpha agonists/alpha blockers See ANTIHYPERTENSIVES.

amphetamines See CENTRAL NERVOUS SYSTEM (CNS) STIMULANTS.

analgesics Medications that relieve pain, usually temporarily, without causing the patient to lose consciousness; also referred to as painkillers and pain pills. More than 100 different analgesics are available in the United States.

Classes

Analgesics are divided into two main classes— narcotics (for severe pain) and non-narcotics (for mild pain)—with a few subclasses within these.

Narcotic analgesics, also known as opioids or opiates, are available only with a prescription and are controlled substances (see Governmental Oversight of Drugs, p. xliii). They relieve pain and cause drowsiness or sleep. Narcotics may include opium and the natural opium derivatives codeine and morphine, synthetic derivatives of morphine such as heroin, and synthetic drugs such as meperidine and propoxyphene hydrochloride. Codeine and hydrocodone can also be used to suppress cough. Some of these medications can be found in combination with non-narcotic drugs such as acetaminophen, aspirin, or cough syrups.

Examples of narcotics include codeine, codeine combined with acetaminophen (Tylenol #2, #3, and #4), hydrocodone with acetaminophen (Vicodin, Lorcet), fentanyl (Sublimaze, Actiq, Duragesic), hydromorphone (Dilaudid), levorphanol (Levo-Dromoran), meperidine (Demerol), methadone (Dolophine), morphine (Roxanol, MS Contin), oxycodone (Roxicodone), oxycodone combined with acetaminophen (Percocet, Roxicet, Tylox), oxycodone combined with aspirin (Percodan, OxyContin), oxycodone combined with ibuprofen (Combunox), and oxymorphone (Numorphan).

Non-narcotic analgesics range from simple analgesics such as acetaminophen, aspirin, and ibuprofen to prescription-only medications. Some of these drugs can also reduce fever and inflammation. Non-narcotic analgesics include:

- *Acetaminophen* (Tylenol), used in more than 100 products, is the most widely used pharmaceutical analgesic and antipyretic agent in the United States and in the world. Acetaminophen has been marketed in the United States as an over-the-counter (OTC) antipyretic/analgesic agent since 1960. It is widely available in a variety of strengths and formulations for children and adults as a single-ingredient product and can also be found in numerous combination OTC and prescription drug products. Because it has no anti-inflammatory properties, acetaminophen is not a member of the class of drugs known as nonsteroidal anti-inflammatory drugs (NSAIDs). Unlike opioid analgesics, acetaminophen does not cause euphoria or alter mood in any way. Acetaminophen relieves mild-to-moderate pain and reduces fever.
- *Nonsteroidal anti-inflammatory drugs* are widely used in both OTC and prescription medicines to control pain and reduce inflammation. Their use is widespread, with more than 70 million prescriptions being dispensed and billions of nonprescription pills being purchased annually in the United States. Because NSAIDs are not narcotics, their use does not result in drug tolerance or physical dependence. There are several classes of NSAIDs: salicylates, nonselective cyclooxygenase (COX) inhibitors,

selective COX-2 inhibitors, and preferential COX-2 NSAIDs.

- *Salicylates* are derivatives of salicylic acid, with the best known being acetylsalicylic acid, or aspirin (Bayer, Bufferin, Ecotrin). Originally derived from salicin, an active ingredient extracted from willow bark and used since antiquity to relieve pain, salicylates are now usually produced synthetically. Salicylates are less potent than the narcotics and are nonaddictive. They are often used to reduce pain resulting from inflammation.
- *Nonselective COX inhibitors,* or traditional NSAIDs, are effective in controlling pain and reducing the symptoms of inflammation, including pain, redness, warmth, and swelling, with the most widely used being ibuprofen (Advil, Motrin) and naproxen (Aleve, Anaprox, Naprelan, Naprosyn). Other nonselective NSAIDs include diclofenac (Catalfam, Voltaren), indomethacin (Indocin), ketoprofen, ketorolac (Toradol), oxaprozin (Daypro), piroxicam (Feldene), and sulindac (Clinoril).
- *Selective COX-2 inhibitors* (also known as coxibs) were introduced beginning in 1998, the first three being celecoxib (Celebrex), rofecoxib (Vioxx), and valdecoxib (Bextra). These COX-2 inhibitors are similar in efficacy to traditional NSAIDs but are believed to have a lower incidence of gastrointestinal (GI) side effects. Because of the lower incidence of GI side effects, COX-2 inhibitors were heralded as a welcome alternative to traditional NSAIDs. As the use of COX-2 inhibitors became widespread, however, a clearer profile of the potential side effects emerged, with Vioxx and Bextra being withdrawn from the market in 2004 and 2005, respectively.
- *Preferential COX-2 NSAIDs* are drugs that are less potent COX-2 inhibitors but still inhibit COX-2 more than COX-1. While some researchers refer to all NSAIDs that

inhibit COX-2 more than COX-1 as being COX-2 selective, others reserve the term COX-2 selective for NSAIDs that inhibit COX-2 more than COX-1 by a factor of 100 or more. *Examples:* etodolac (Lodine), meloxicam (Mobic), nabumetone (Relfen), and salsalate (Salflex, Amigesic).

- *Peptide channel blockers* are a synthetic version of sea snail venom first approved for use in the United States as a new class of drugs in December 2004. These drugs have their own unique mechanism of action: blocking N-type calcium channels. Candidates for these drugs are mostly people with diseases such as cancer or AIDS who have failed to get relief from other drugs, such as morphine. *Example:* ziconotide (Prialt) is the equivalent of the naturally occurring venom that tropical sea snails use to incapacitate prey; it is 1,000 times more potent than morphine and is not addictive.

In December 2004, the Food and Drug Administration (FDA) approved pregabalin (Lyrica) for the management of neuropathic pain associated with diabetic peripheral neuropathy and postherpetic neuralgia. Lyrica is the first FDA-approved treatment for both of these neuropathic pain states, which are distinctly different from arthritis or musculoskeletal pain. Lyrica is classified as a controlled substance in a category with lower potential for misuse or abuse relative to controlled substances in other categories.

How They Work

Narcotics provide relief for moderate-to-severe pain by acting on specific structures, called receptors, located on the nerve cells of the spinal cord or brain, altering the perception of pain. Narcotics depress neurotransmitter functioning, and those patients very sensitive to the effects of narcotics can become very drowsy. Tolerance to these drugs develops quickly, and first-time doses are much more likely to produce cognitive impairments than subsequent doses.

Acetaminophen's exact mechanism of action is not known. Its effectiveness as a fever reducer has been attributed to its effect on the hypothalamic heat center (the "thermostat" of the brain), while its pain-relieving effect is due to its ability to raise the pain threshold (by requiring a greater amount of pain to develop before it is felt by a person).

Salicylates work by decreasing the production of prostaglandins, which are hormonelike substances found in many tissues in the body. Prostaglandins produce a wide range of effects, including pain impulses and inflammation (redness, swelling) in damaged tissue. The overall process of decreasing prostaglandin formation decreases pain and inflammation. These agents also act on the brain's heat-regulating center to reduce fever.

In the course of the search for a specific inhibitor of the negative effects of prostaglandins but one that would not affect other actions of prostaglandins, such as clotting, it was discovered that prostaglandins could be separated into two general classes. These classes could loosely be regarded as "good prostaglandins" and "bad prostaglandins." Csuka explains, "The 'bad' prostaglandins are produced in response to injury, and act as mediators of inflammation and, hence, of pain. Inhibiting the production of these prostaglandins has demonstrated a reduction in inflammation and pain in both animal and human studies. The 'good' prostaglandins help to maintain the integrity of the lining of the stomach, promote clotting by platelets to prevent excessive bleeding and maintain kidney blood flow. Until recently, all NSAIDs were nonselective. In order to inhibit the 'bad' prostaglandins responsible for pain, one had to accept some inhibition of the 'good' prostaglandins."

More recent work has shown that there are at least two different types of COX: COX-1 and COX-2. Aspirin and the traditional NSAIDs inhibit both of them. Prostaglandins whose synthesis involves COX-1 are responsible for maintenance and protection of the gastrointestinal (GI) tract, while prostaglandins whose synthesis involves COX-2 are responsible for inflammation and pain.

Newer NSAID drugs called selective COX-2 inhibitors were then developed that inhibit only COX-2, with the hope that this would reduce the GI side effects. Older nonselective NSAIDs also block COX-1, which is why they can cause stomach problems. A search for selective COX-2 inhibitors resulted in promising candidates such as celecoxib, rofecoxib, and valdecoxib, marketed under the brand names Celebrex (1998), Vioxx (1999), and Bextra (2001), respectively. Celebrex is approximately 10 to 20 times more selective for COX-2 inhibition over COX-1. Bextra and Vioxx were about 300 times more potent at inhibiting COX-2 than COX-1, suggesting the possibility of relief from pain and inflammation without GI irritation. This promised to be a boon for those who had experienced such side effects previously or had comorbidities that could lead to such complications.

Although individual reactions to particular NSAIDs vary, in general the efficacy of selective COX-2 inhibitors has proved similar to that of other NSAIDs, as expected since both classes of drug inhibit the desired target, the action of COX-2 prostaglandins.

Researchers believe ziconotide works by blocking calcium channels on the nerves that transmit pain signals to the brain.

Pregabalin has a newly defined mechanism of action that is believed to work by calming hyperexcited neurons. It binds to the subunit of a voltage-gated calcium channel in the brain and spinal cord. This reduces flow of calcium into the axon during depolarization (firing) of the neuron, thereby reducing neurotransmitter release from that neuron.

Approved Uses

Narcotic analgesics generally are used to alleviate pain not relieved by the non-narcotic analgesics. They are used also as preoperative medication, for support of anesthesia, for relief of obstetrical pain, in patients undergoing major surgery, and for relief of anxiety in patients with dyspnea (shortness of breath) associated with acute left-ventricular failure and pulmonary edema.

Fentanyl skin patches are indicated for management of persistent, moderate-to-severe chronic pain that require continuous, around-the-clock opioid administration for an extended period of time, but which cannot be managed by other means such as nonsteroidal analgesics, opioid combination products, or immediate-release opioids.

Because oxymorphone hydrochloride causes little depression of the cough reflex, it is particularly useful in postoperative patients. Oxymorphone suppositories are used in older or debilitated patients unable to tolerate injectable analgesics but who need a potent, rapid-acting analgesic, such as for the control of cancer pain or following surgery.

Acetaminophen is used to treat mild-to-moderate pain due to headache, muscular aches, backache, toothache, minor arthritis pain, and menstrual cramps. It is the initial drug of choice for the treatment of pain associated with osteoarthritis (OA). The combination of acetaminophen, aspirin, and caffeine (Excedrin ES, Excedrin Migraine) is approved for acute treatment of migraines, including menstrually related migraines.

Salicylates, especially aspirin, are used to reduce fever and inflammation and to relieve headache, menstrual pain, and pain in muscles and joints. Because of the effects of salicylates on blood platelets and clotting, aspirin is often prescribed to prevent a first-time episode of stroke or heart attack in those who may be at risk for these events (primary prevention), as well as to prevent another episode of stroke or heart attack in those who have already experienced one of these conditions (secondary prevention).

Traditional NSAIDs treat lower back pain, minor injuries, and soft tissue rheumatism. Many prescription NSAIDs are approved for short-term use in the treatment of pain and primary dysmenorrhea (menstrual discomfort) and for longer-term use to treat the signs and symptoms of OA and rheumatoid arthritis (RA).

Celecoxib is used in the treatment of OA, RA, acute pain, ankylosing spondylitis, and primary dysmenorrhea and to reduce numbers of growths (polyps) in the colon and rectum in patients with familial adenomatous polyposis.

Meloxicam is popular in Europe for treatment of RA and was approved in the United States in 2004 for use in treating OA.

Ziconotide is approved for the management of severe chronic pain in patients for whom intrathecal (IT) therapy (spinal injection) is warranted and who are intolerant of or resistant to other treatment, such as systemic analgesics or IT morphine.

Pregabalin is approved for treatment of pain that occurs with both diabetic peripheral neuropathy and postherpetic neuralgia—two of the most common forms of nerve pain.

Off-Label Uses

Both narcotics and NSAIDs are frequently prescribed for children even when they have not been tested in nor approved for pediatric use. Acetaminophen is given to children for the treatment of fever or pain in general.

Several small studies have concluded that low-dose aspirin may reduce the risks of preeclampsia (previously called toxemia), a hypertensive disorder of pregnancy, and severe low birth weight, with no observed risk to the mother or baby. Although these studies have shown as much as 65 percent reduction in high blood pressure and 44 percent reduction in episodes of severe low birth weight infants, larger studies are needed.

Naproxen, ibuprofen, and indomethacin have been used to treat juvenile RA. Indomethacin has also been used clinically to delay premature labor by blocking the production of prostaglandins, which contribute to uterine contractions. However, prolonged use beyond 24 to 48 hours or during the last two months of pregnancy is not recommended because of possible effects on fetal heart development. Indomethacin can also be used to close a patent ductus arteriosus in newborns.

Administration

Narcotics may be taken by mouth, by injection into the muscle (intramuscularly), by injection through a vein (intravenously), or by rectal suppository. Methods of giving narcotics for more continuous pain relief also are available, such as fentanyl patches or intraspinal (e.g., implanted morphine pumps). Oral formulations can be given chronically for continuous pain relief as well. In the hospital setting, IV infusions can be given for continuous pain relief. Not all narcotics are available in each of these forms.

Extended- or controlled-release opioid tablets should never be crushed or chewed, as doing so may cause the patient to absorb a large dose rapidly, resulting in an overdose. Patient-controlled analgesic techniques can also be used, whereby patients have the option of injecting small quantities of narcotic type analgesics to control their own pain.

Acetaminophen is taken orally or via suppositories. The oral formulations are available in several strengths of tablets, caplets, gelcaps, and capsules as well as liquid and drops.

Aspirin is available in tablets, chewable tablets, gum tablets, and suppositories.

NSAIDs can be administered in any of several ways. Most widely used is the oral form of tablets or capsules. Pediatric versions are available as chewable tablets or as syrups or drops. These drugs should be taken with food or milk to minimize the GI distress. Some NSAIDs (e.g., ketorolac) are given as intramuscular or intravenous injections, particularly following surgical procedures. Indomethacin is available as suppositories, which are often used for pain following surgery and sometimes for chronic pain when the patient is unable to take medication by mouth. Celecoxib is available in capsules that are taken once or twice a day.

Ziconotide is released into the fluid surrounding the spinal cord by an internal or external pump. A major benefit is that it can be used long-term without the dose wearing off and without the dose having to be increased significantly. By contrast, narcotic analgesics, in addition to being addictive, make patients drowsy and lose their effect if administered long-term.

Pregabalin is available in capsules in a wide range of doses to allow physicians to choose the best dose for their patients. It can be taken with or without food.

Cautions and Concerns

Narcotic analgesics must be taken only as directed by a doctor or pharmacist because they may be habit-forming and can cause serious side effects when used improperly. Caution is required when motor skills are needed, including operating machinery and driving.

Normal doses of salicylates can cause GI disturbances in sensitive patients, and large doses can be toxic or fatal, especially to children.

Caution should be used when using blood thinners (e.g., warfarin) and aspirin together because this combination can increase bleeding.

A small but important proportion of patients with prolonged use of traditional NSAIDs may develop GI side effects, such as bleeding and ulcers, and perforation of the stomach or intestines, which can be fatal. These events can occur at any time during use and without warning symptoms. Ulcer complications from traditional NSAID use have been estimated to contribute to as many as 103,000 hospitalizations and 16,500 deaths each year. Elderly patients are at a greater risk for serious GI events.

In December 2004, the FDA issued an advisory following the decision by the National Institutes of Health to halt a five-year study, called the Alzheimer's Disease Anti-Inflammatory Prevention Trial. That study aimed to test both Aleve and Celebrex as preventatives for Alzheimer's disease. Preliminary information from the study showed naproxen elevated the risk of heart attack and stroke by 50 percent. The FDA advised patients taking OTC naproxen products to carefully follow the instructions on the label, avoid exceeding the recommended doses for naproxen (220 milligrams twice daily), and take naproxen for no longer than 10 days unless a physician directs otherwise. The public health advisory was an interim measure, pending further review by the FDA of data that continue to be collected.

Ziconotide can cause serious problems that patients should tell their doctors or health care professionals about immediately, such as severe psychiatric symptoms or neurological impairment, unconsciousness or reduced mental alertness, meningitis or other infections, or serious muscle damage.

In controlled studies, a higher proportion of patients treated with pregabalin reported blurred vision (6 percent) than did patients treated with placebo (2 percent), which resolved in a majority of cases with continued dosing. Although the clinical significance of the ophthalmologic findings is unknown, patients should notify their physicians if changes in vision occur. Also, when discontinuing pregabalin, the patient needs to taper off gradually over a minimum of one week. Abrupt or rapid discontinuation may result in insomnia, nausea, headache, or diarrhea.

Warnings

Propoxyphene carries an FDA-required black-box warning that in high doses, taken by itself or in combination with other drugs, it has been associated with drug-related deaths. Propoxyphene should not be taken in combination with other drugs that cause drowsiness: alcohol, tranquilizers, sleep aids, antidepressant drugs, or antihistamines. It also should not be taken in larger doses, more often, or for a longer period than prescribed by a physician.

Using damaged or cut fentanyl patches can lead to the rapid release of the contents of the patch and absorption of a potentially fatal dose of fentanyl. Because deaths and overdoses have occurred in patients using both the brand name product (Duragesic) and the generic fentanyl patches, the FDA issued a health advisory in July 2005 warning that directions for using the fentanyl skin patch must be followed exactly to prevent death or other serious side effects from overdose.

NSAIDs may cause an increased risk of serious cardiovascular thrombotic events, heart attack, and stroke, which can be fatal. This risk may increase with duration of use. Patients with cardiovascular disease or risk factors for cardiovascular disease may be at greater risk.

In September 2004, Merck & Co. voluntarily withdrew Vioxx (rofecoxib) from the market after a long-term study of the drug showed an increased risk of serious cardiovascular events, including heart attacks and strokes, among study patients taking Vioxx. This was followed in April 2005 by the FDA asking Pfizer, Inc. to withdraw Bextra (valdecoxcib) from the market because the overall risk versus benefit profile for the drug was unfavorable.

Also in September 2004, the FDA asked manufacturers of all marketed prescription NSAIDs, including celecoxib (Celebrex), the only selective COX-2 NSAID remaining on the U.S. market, to revise the labeling (package insert) for their products to include a boxed warning and a Medication Guide. The boxed warning is to highlight the potential for increased risk of cardiovascular events with these drugs and the well-described, serious, and potentially life-threatening GI bleeding associated with the use of traditional NSAIDs.

When Not Advised (Contraindications)

Because serious or life-threatening hypoventilation (abnormally slow and shallow breathing) could result, the fentanyl pain patch is contraindicated for use on an as-needed basis for the management of postoperative or acute pain or in patients who are not opioid-tolerant or who require opioid analgesia for only a short period of time.

Children and teenagers should not use salicylates when they have chickenpox. Because there appears to be a connection between aspirin and Reye's syndrome, aspirin and aspirin-containing drugs are no longer used to control flulike symptoms in children.

Celecoxib should not be given to patients who have experienced asthma or allergic-type reactions, such as hives, after taking aspirin or other NSAIDs. Celecoxib should also not be given to those with an allergy to sulfa drugs. Traditional NSAIDS should not be given to patients who have experienced asthma or allergic-type reactions, such as hives, after taking aspirin.

Ziconotide is contraindicated in patients with a preexisting history of psychosis or for those with infection or bleeding at the injection site.

Side Effects

Narcotics all have similar side effects, including drowsiness, constipation, nausea and vomiting, itching, and dry mouth. Constipation can usually be minimized by starting the patient with low doses. Some people also might experience dizziness, mental effects (nightmares, confusion, hallucinations), a moderate decrease in rate and depth of breathing, or difficulty in urinating.

Taking more than the maximum daily amount of acetaminophen may cause serious and possibly fatal liver problems.

Aspirin can cause upset stomach, and although coated tablets may be easier on the stomach, they can take longer to work.

NSAIDs can cause bleeding ulcers, high blood pressure, edema, and stomach irritation.

Celecoxib can cause serious problems such as bleeding ulcers, liver damage, sudden kidney failure or worsening of kidney problems, and fluid retention and swelling. Fluid retention can be a serious problem in patients with high blood pressure or heart failure. In addition to these serious side effects, some common but less serious side effects with celecoxib may include headache, indigestion, upper respiratory tract infection, diarrhea, sinus inflammation, stomach pain, or nausea.

The most common side effects of ziconotide are dizziness, nausea, confusion, headache, drowsiness, problems with vision, weakness, and difficulty walking.

The most common side effects of pregabalin are dizziness, drowsiness, dry mouth, edema, blurred vision, weight gain, and difficulty concentrating.

Interactions

Alcohol increases the sedative effects of narcotic analgesics and thus should not be taken while the narcotics are in one's system. Also, persons drinking three or more alcoholic beverages per day may be at increased risk of developing stomach ulcers when taking NSAIDs.

A study of 22,071 males taking aspirin to prevent a first heart attack found that those also taking other NSAIDs, such as ibuprofen, for more than 60 days a year more than doubled their risk of heart attack compared to those taking aspirin alone.

In addition, University of Utah College of Pharmacy researchers reported in November 2005 that patients who took OTC pain relievers such as ibuprofen or naproxen along with aspirin were at a two to three times higher risk of developing stomach ulcers, perforations, and bleeding compared to individuals who took the NSAIDs without aspirin.

Patients who are on anticancer drugs that may cause bleeding, such as cyclophosphamide or tamoxifen, should avoid NSAIDs.

Concomitant use of blood thinners (e.g., warfarin) and NSAIDs or aspirin can increase the risk of bleeding.

There may be an increased risk of bleeding when taking ginkgo biloba, ginger, or garlic with aspirin or blood thinners (e.g., warfarin).

Sales/Statistics

The use of all classes of NSAIDs has been increasing. Between 1995–96 and 2001–02, NSAID use associated with medical visits among adults increased from 20 to 27 visits per 100 population. Historically, women have higher NSAID use than men. In 2001–02, the rate of NSAID use was about 50 percent higher for women than men.

Although celecoxib was the 13th most frequently dispensed drug in the United States in 2003, with retail sales exceeding $2.2 billion, the business press reported in 2005 that demand for Celebrex dropped 44 percent after the warning of heart risks was added to the drug's label.

In the six months following the removal of Vioxx from the market, prescriptions for relatively expensive Mobic increased by 136 percent—the most of any alternative to Vioxx—while prescriptions for low-cost ibuprofen rose 28 percent, according to an analysis by *Consumer Reports Best Buy Drugs*.

When Tylenol reached its 50th anniversary on November 1, 2005, newspapers reported that the venerable pain reliever was in 70 percent of U.S. households and that sales had grown by "double digits" over the previous year. This growth spurt was attributed to concern over the risks of NSAIDs. According to Chicago research firm Information Resources Inc., Tylenol sales in 2004 totaled $786.5 million, but that did not include sales to hospitals, nursing homes, or Wal-Mart stores, which IRI does not track.

According to a report from the IMS Institute for Healthcare Informatics (the public reporting arm of IMS, a pharmaceutical market intelligence firm), narcotic analgesics were the third most prescribed therapeutic class in the United States in 2010, with 244.3 million prescriptions dispensed. Narcotic analgesics ranked number 11 in prescription spending ($8.4 billion). Generic hydrocodone with acetaminophen was the most prescribed drug in 2010 (131.2 million prescriptions). Oxycontin was the 15th highest U.S. pharmaceutical product by spending in 2010, accounting for $3.1 billion.

Demographics and Cultural Groups

Disparities in prescribing of pain medication among different cultural groups as well as between men and women have been reported for a long time. Green et al. reviewed 180 previously published studies and determined that blacks and Hispanics are less likely to be given pain medications than whites, even when they report higher levels of suffering. Among the examples documented in the study: Hispanics with broken arms or legs were twice as likely as whites to go without pain medication during emergency room visits, while black cancer patients in nursing homes were 64 percent more likely not to get pain medication than whites.

Other studies over the years have found similar cultural disparities:

- A study of 281 Hispanic and nonwhite outpatients with recurrent or metastatic cancer showed that 65 percent of the patients with pain did not receive analgesic medication as recommended by World Health Organization guidelines.
- White patients are significantly more likely than black patients to receive analgesics (74 percent versus 57 percent) despite similar records of pain complaints.
- Black and Hispanic patients with severe pain are less likely than white patients to be able to obtain commonly prescribed pain medicines, because pharmacies in nonwhite communities typically do not carry adequate stocks of opioids.
- Women are commonly given sedatives instead of painkillers because their pain is perceived as "all in her head."

Although research has suggested that some of the blame for these disparities can be placed on physicians' preconceived notions about specific groups of people, evidence also has shown that some undertreatment of pain can be traced to the distrust of minorities for the medical community. Because of this distrust, minorities oftentimes provide too little information to medical staff to allow adequate evaluation and treatment. Also, communication problems inhibit proper treatment when different languages and terminologies come into play.

Development History

Aspirin was the first discovered drug in the class of NSAIDs. Pincock explains succinctly the development of analgesics. Points taken from his article:

- In the 19th century, the European beaver *(Castor fiber)* was headed toward extinction, which could be, in part, attributed to the search for pain relief. Beavers were hunted for, among other things, castoreum—a smelly secretion known to have analgesic and anti-inflamma-

tory properties. Castoreum's benefits, subsequent analysis has shown, came from salicin, which was derived from the willow bark in the beaver's diet.

- If willow bark is the root of one branch of the pain-relief tree, the other is the poppy. *Papaver somniferum,* also called the opium poppy, was first classified by Linnaeus in 1753, although the drug first appeared in the Greek pharmacopoeia during the 5th century B.C. and in Chinese medical writings during the 8th century A.D. Opium—the dried juice of the opium seedpod—is a mix of sugars, proteins, ammonia, latex, gums, and alkaloids. In fact, it contains more than 50 alkaloids—the most important of which are morphine, noscapine, papaverine, codeine, and thebaine. In 1803, Friedrich Wilhelm Serturner, a German pharmacist, identified and isolated the main ingredient of opium, morphine. He called this alkaloid "morphia," after Morpheus, the Greek god of dreams. Codeine was first isolated from opium by Pierre-Jean Robiquet in 1832.
- John R. Vane revealed the mechanism of acetylsalicylic acid (aspirin) in 1971, showing that it suppresses prostaglandins and thromboxanes by inhibiting cyclooxygenase. That work garnered him a Nobel Prize and a knighthood, and it opened the door for the development of the whole class of NSAIDs, including, more recently, selective COX-2 inhibitors.

Future Drugs

Licofelone (ML3000), a dual COX/5-lipoxygenase (5-LOX) inhibitor and the first member of this new class of analgesic and anti-inflammatory drugs is being developed by the German pharmaceutical company Merckle GmbH and partners. It is currently under evaluation as a treatment for OA. Although phase III trials have been successfully completed in OA patients, no dates for regulatory submission have yet been given. Licofelone differs from both conventional NSAIDs and selective COX-2 inhibitors in that it inhibits not only COX-1 and COX-2, but also 5-LOX, an enzyme associated with the production of proinflammatory and gastrotoxic leukotrienes. According to Merckle, evidence suggests that NSAID-induced GI toxicity may involve shunting arachidonic acid metabolism to the 5-LOX pathway, thereby increasing the production of gastrotoxic leukotrienes. Inhibition of 5-LOX may therefore offer a new approach to reducing the GI toxicity associated with NSAID use while retaining the analgesic and anti-inflammatory properties of NSAIDs and selective COX-2 specific inhibitors. Clinical studies that have compared licofelone with conventional NSAIDs and selective COX-2 specific inhibitors suggest that it is at least as effective as these agents in providing symptomatic relief from OA but generally better tolerated.

Arnst suggests that "Prialt's approval may pave the way for other pain treatments derived from poisons. Wex Pharmaceuticals Inc., a Vancouver startup, is in clinical trials with a drug called tetrodotoxin (Tectin), derived from the deadly toxin of the puffer fish, whose flesh is a risky delicacy known as fugu in Japan. Delivered by injection, tetrodotoxin blocks sodium channels that play a role in transmitting many types of pain signals. Another startup, AlgoRx Pharmaceuticals Inc., is testing a drug based on capsaicin—not a poison, but the substance in chili peppers that burns the skin. Capsaicin inhibits C neurons, the nerve cells responsible for dull, throbbing, continuous pain (as opposed to sharp, acute, temporary pain).

"Nicotine, the poisonous chemical found in tobacco, has also been shown to soothe pain in animals, but it is far too addictive for use in humans. As an alternative, Abbott Laboratories has spent a decade looking for drugs that target subsets of the nicotinic receptors, the nerve-cell proteins that suck up nicotine. The hope is that by homing in on just those receptors involved in pain, a drug will quiet overexcited nerve endings without risk of addiction. After several attempts, Abbott has a nicotinic receptor pill, ABT-894, in early human trials. It will be a few

years, however, before 894—or any of the novel pain drugs in development—are ready for FDA review."

Arnst, Catherine. "No Pain, Some Gain." *BusinessWeek.* Available online. URL: http://www.businessweek.com/magazine/content/05_03/b3916089_mz018.htm. Posted on January 17, 2005.

Csuka, M. E. "Living With—and Without—Pain." *Quest* 8, no. 4 (August 2001). Available online. URL: http://www.mdausa.org/publications/Quest/q84pain2.cfm. Downloaded on November 5, 2005.

Green, Carmen, et al. "The Unequal Burden of Pain: Confronting Racial and Ethnic Disparities in Pain." *Pain Medicine* 4, no. 3 (September 2003): 277–294.

New York Times News Service. "Over-the-Counter Painkillers Raise Bleeding Risks." InteliHealth. Available online. URL: http://www.intelihealth.com/IH/ihtIH/WSIHW000/333/7228/441573.html. Posted on November 2, 2005.

Pincock, Stephen. "The Quest for Pain Relief." *The Scientist* 19, Suppl. 1 (March 28, 2005): s31. Available online. URL: http://f1000scientist.com/article/display/15372/. Accessed August 12, 2011.

antianginals Medications used in the treatment of angina pectoris, a symptom of heart disease, which is often referred to simply as angina. Angina pectoris is Latin for "choking of the chest" and may appear as sudden severe pain, tightness, or heaviness in the area behind the breastbone, although the pain may extend to the neck or jaw or down the inner sides of either arm. Angina is not a heart attack but makes it more likely that the patient will have a heart attack in the future. According to 2003 Centers for Disease Control and Prevention/National Center for Health statistics, 6,500,000 people in the United States suffer from angina. An estimated 400,000 new cases of stable angina occur each year according to the Framingham Heart Study, funded primarily by the National Heart, Lung, and Blood Institute (NHLBI). The three types of angina are stable, unstable, and variant (Prinzmetal's or vasospastic). The NHLBI describes them as follows:

- *Stable angina* is the most common type. It occurs during or just after situations in which the heart must work harder and needs increased oxygen, such as climbing stairs, exercising, or eating a heavy meal. There is a regular pattern to stable angina. After several episodes, the patient learns to recognize the pattern and can predict when it will occur. The pain usually goes away in a few minutes after the patient rests or takes antiangina medicine.

- *Unstable angina* is a very dangerous condition that requires emergency treatment. It is a sign that a heart attack could occur soon. Unlike stable angina, it does not follow a pattern. It can occur without physical exertion and is not relieved by rest or medicine.

- *Variant angina,* which is due to a spasm of the coronary artery, is rare and usually occurs at rest. The pain can be severe and usually occurs between midnight and early morning.

Angina occurs when the heart's demand for oxygen exceeds the amount of oxygen being supplied to the heart. Antianginals increase the flow of oxygen into the heart or reduce the heart's need for oxygen.

Classes

Three classes of pharmacological agents are used in the treatment of angina.

- *Nitrates* include nitroglycerin (Nitro-Dur, Nitrolingual, Nitrostat, NitroQuick, Transderm-Nitro, Nitro-Bid), isosorbide dinitrate (Dilatrate-SR, Isordil), isosorbide mononitrate (Imdur, Ismo, Monoket), and amyl nitrite (Amyl Nitrite Aspirols, Amyl Nitrite Vaporole).

- *Calcium channel blockers* used to treat angina include amlodipine (Norvasc), diltiazem (Cardizem, Tiazac, Cartia XT, Dilacor XR, Diltia XT, Taztia XT), felodipine (Plendil), nicardipine (Cardene), nifedipine (Adalat CC, Procardia XL, Nifediac CC, Afeditab CR, Nifedical XL), and verapamil (Calan, Isoptin SR, Covera-HS, Verelan). (See ANTIHYPERTENSIVES.)

- *Beta-adrenergic antagonists* (beta-blockers) used to treat angina include atenolol (Tenormin), metoprolol (Lopressor, Toprol XL), nadolol (Corgard), and propranolol (Inderal). (See ANTIHYPERTENSIVES.)

- Miscellaneous: Ranolazine (Ranexa), a new molecular entity approved in January 2006, was the first drug approved to treat chronic angina in more than 10 years and represents the first new class of antianginal therapy in the United States in more than 25 years.

How They Work

Nitrates dilate (widen) the blood vessels that supply blood (and oxygen) to the heart. They also reduce the heart's demand for oxygen by decreasing the amount of stress on the walls of the heart. Short-acting nitrates can relieve an episode of angina within one to three minutes and maintain their effectiveness for 30 minutes. Long-acting nitrates act too slowly to relieve pain during an acute angina attack but are used on a chronic basis to help prevent angina attacks.

Calcium channel blockers dilate the blood vessels that supply blood (and oxygen) to the heart. They also reduce the heart's demand for oxygen by lowering blood pressure. Certain calcium channel blockers (e.g., diltiazem and verapamil) further reduce the heart's demand for oxygen by slowing the heart rate and decreasing the force of contraction of the heart.

Beta-blockers reduce the heart's demand for oxygen by slowing the heart rate, lowering blood pressure, and decreasing the force of contraction of the heart. These drugs do not affect the supply of blood (and oxygen) to the heart.

Although several pharmacological activities of ranolazine have been described, the FDA noted that the precise way the drug works is not fully understood.

Approved Uses

Nitrates can be used for the treatment of stable, unstable, and variant (vasospastic) angina. Nitroglycerin can be used to relieve the pain of angina when it is taken at the beginning of an attack. It can also be used to prevent pain when taken just before pain or discomfort is expected to occur (five to 10 minutes before activity known to cause angina). Isosorbide dinitrate or mononitrate can be used on a long-term basis to reduce the number of episodes of angina. Intravenous nitroglycerin is used to acutely relieve the pain of angina or to control severe cases of high blood pressure in a hospital setting.

Calcium channel blockers can be used for the treatment of stable, unstable, and variant (vasospastic) angina. These drugs are used on a long-term basis to treat angina. They are also used as antihypertensives.

Unlike nitrates and calcium channel blockers, beta-blockers are used only for the treatment of stable or unstable angina. They are not effective against variant (vasospastic) angina. Beta-blockers are used on a long-term basis for the treatment of angina. They are also used as antihypertensives.

Because nitrates, calcium channel blockers, and beta-blockers are each useful in the treatment of angina and work to increase oxygen supply and/or oxygen consumption by different mechanisms, they are sometimes used in combination.

Because ranolazine affects electrical conduction in the heart (prolongs the QT interval, or the length of the heart's electrical cycle), it should be used only by patients who have not responded to other antianginals. In fact, it should be used in combination with amlodipine, beta blockers, and nitrates.

Off-Label Uses

Nitroglycerin ointment has been used at reduced (0.2 percent) concentration as an effective treatment for anal fissure. The ointment can relax the sphincter muscle, thus allowing the healing to proceed. Nitroglycerin ointment applied directly to the fingers has also been tried with some success to treat Raynaud's disease.

Nitroglycerin has also been used during childbirth. Carvalho wrote, "Nitroglycerin may be useful in a setting where advanced labor and parturient movement during uterine contractions makes the placement of an epidural difficult and potentially dangerous. A number of studies and case reports describe the use of nitroglycerin in achieving rapid uterine relaxation. Nitroglycerin has been used as a tocolytic to reduce uterine hyperactivity, assist reduction of an inverted uterus, facilitate intrapartum external cephalic version, and manage preterm labor contractions."

Nitrates have been used in combination with other drugs to treat chronic heart failure and acute myocardial infarction (heart attack). Isosorbide dinitrate is used to relieve pain and difficulty in swallowing associated with diffuse esophageal spasm when there is no gastroesophageal reflux.

For off-label uses of calcium channel blockers and beta-blockers, see ANTIHYPERTENSIVES.

Administration

Nitroglycerin can be administered via a number of routes—intravenous, lingual (sprayed onto the tongue), sublingual (tablets dissolved under the tongue), intrabuccal (extended-release tablets placed between the lip or cheek and gum), oral (capsules), transdermal (skin patches), or topical (ointment).

Isosorbide dinitrate can be administered sublingually or orally as tablets (immediate- and extended-release) and extended-release capsules.

Isosorbide mononitrate is administered orally as immediate- or extended-release tablets.

Amyl nitrate is administered by inhalation; it has a very rapid onset and works for three to five minutes.

Nitrates that dissolve under the tongue or between the cheek and gum or that are sprayed onto the tongue work quickly and are used to acutely relieve an angina episode. Nitrates in the form of tablets, extended-release capsules, or skin patches are used on a long-term basis to prevent attacks of angina.

For administration of calcium channel blockers and beta-blockers, see ANTIHYPERTENSIVES.

Ranolazine is available as extended-release tablets.

Cautions and Concerns

Continuous or frequent exposure to nitrates may lead to the development of tolerance or diminished response to the drug. Nitrate-free periods of at least eight hours (e.g., overnight) are suggested to reduce the development of tolerance. Because nitrates may cause dizziness, caution should be taken when driving a car or operating machinery. Nitrates may worsen angina in patients with hypertrophic cardiomyopathy and should be used with caution. After normal use, there is enough residual nitroglycerin in discarded patches that they are a potential hazard to children and pets. When patients stop taking nitrates suddenly, a severe anginal attack could occur.

For cautions and concerns of calcium channel blockers and beta-blockers, see ANTIHYPERTENSIVES.

Because ranolazine may cause dizziness and lightheadedness, patients should exercise caution when operating an automobile or machinery or engaging in activities requiring mental alertness or coordination. Ranolazine may also increase blood pressure in patients with severe kidney dysfunction.

Warnings

Ranolazine has been shown to prolong the QT interval in a dose-related manner. While the clinical significance of the QT prolongation in the case of ranolazine is unknown, other drugs with this potential have been associated with torsades de pointes–type arrhythmias and sudden death.

When Not Advised (Contraindications)

Nitrates are not advised for people with severe anemia because the vasodilation will further increase the heart rate and may increase the work of the heart. Because nitrates may increase fluid pressure inside the eye, these drugs should be avoided in patients with glaucoma. Nitrates are not advised for people with brain injury, head trauma, or cerebral hemorrhage, because they may further increase intracranial pressure. Nitrates should not be used in people who are also taking phosphodiesterase-5 inhibitors, such as sildenafil, tadalafil, or vardenafil, as they may be at risk for a severe reduction in blood pressure. Topical nitroglycerin patches are not advised for people who are allergic to adhesives.

For contraindications of calcium channel blockers and beta-blockers, see ANTIHYPERTENSIVES.

Ranolazine should not be used in patients with preexisting QT prolongation or liver impairment or in those who are taking QT-prolonging medications or CYP3A inhibitors, such as ketoconazole, diltiazem, verapamil, erythromycin, clarithromycin, HIV protease inhibitors, or grapefruit juice.

Side Effects

Headache is the most common side effect of nitrates. Headaches may diminish or disappear with continued use; if not, a lower dosage may control the headaches. Other side effects of nitrates include a sudden fall in blood pressure after quickly standing up, rapid heart rate, dizziness, flushing, or fainting.

For side effects of calcium channel blockers and beta-blockers, see ANTIHYPERTENSIVES.

In clinical studies, common side effects of ranolazine included dizziness, headache, constipation, and nausea.

Interactions

Nitrates in combination with sildenafil (Viagra), vardenafil (Levitra), or tadalafil (Cialis) can result in profound and life-threatening lowering of blood pressure. Because nitrates can lower blood pressure, other medications that also lower blood pressure taken along with nitrates may produce an unwanted additive effect. Examples of such medications are drugs used to treat high blood pressure, some ANTIDEPRESSANTS, some ANTIPSYCHOTICS, benzodiazepines, and opiates. Alcohol may also intensify the blood pressure–lowering effect of nitroglycerin.

Dihydroergotamine may oppose the vasodilatory actions of nitrates and may precipitate angina. A similar effect can occur with the decongestant pseudoephedrine (Sudafed).

For interactions with calcium channel blockers and beta-blockers, see ANTIHYPERTENSIVES.

Ranolazine should *not* be used with any drug that prolongs the QT interval. Plasma levels of ranolazine may be significantly increased when taken along with potent CYP3A inhibitors (i.e., ketoconazole, diltiazem, verapamil, erythromycin, clarithromycin, HIV protease inhibitors, and grapefruit juice). Ritonavir and cyclosporine may increase the effects of ranolazine; therefore, these drugs should be used with caution in patients receiving ranolazine. Ranolazine may increase the effects of simvastatin, digoxin, tricyclic antidepressants, and several antipsychotics; therefore, the dosages of these drugs may have to be reduced when starting ranolazine therapy.

Sales/Statistics

According to NDCHealth Information Services, the following nitrates were among the 300 most dispensed medications in 2004 through retail and mail-order pharmacy channels (excluding Wal-Mart):

- isosorbide mononitrate (generic)—9,621,678 prescriptions
- NitroQuick (whether patch or capsules or both not noted)—2,909,494 prescriptions
- nitroglycerin (generic)—2,782,410 prescriptions

For calcium channel blocker and beta-blocker sales and statistics, see ANTIHYPERTENSIVES.

Demographics and Cultural Groups

Of the 6.4 million Americans who have angina pectoris, 3.3 million are women and 3.1 million are men. Angina tends to develop in women at a later age than in men.

The rates of angina pectoris in women older than 20 years are 3.9 percent in white women, 6.2 percent in black women, and 5.5 percent in Hispanic American women. The rates of angina pectoris for men in the same ethnic groups are 2.6 percent, 3.1 percent, and 4.1 percent, respectively.

Unstable angina occurs more often in older adults. People with variant angina are often younger than those with other forms of angina.

Development History

Nitroglycerin was discovered by the Italian chemist Ascanio Sobrero in 1847, but it was much too volatile for him to deal with. In the 1860s, Alfred Nobel mixed nitroglycerin with silica to form dynamite. William Murrell of Westminster Hospital in London further refined amyl nitrate and nitroglycerin in 1879 for transient relief of angina.

According to the National Academy of Sciences (www.nasonline.org), "Although nineteenth-century scientists understood why nitroglycerin was a potent explosive, they had no idea what made it an effective treatment for angina. Somehow it relaxed the smooth muscles that surround blood vessels, allowing the vessels to dilate so that more blood could flow to the starved heart muscle. The secret of nitroglycerin emerged at last in the 1970s, when researchers realized that it works by reacting in the body to form a messenger molecule called nitric oxide, or NO."

Nitroglycerin's antianginal effect on smooth muscle led researchers at Hoechst to develop the antispasmodic fenipirane in 1942, a prototype for what came to be identified as calcium channel antagonists, such as verapamil (1962) and diltiazem (1971).

Beta-blockers were developed during the early 1960s.

Future Drugs

On January 31, 2005, Angiogenix announced results from the recently completed Phase IIb clinical trial for Acclaim, its product candidate for the prevention of nitrate tolerance in chronic stable angina patients. Results demonstrated that Acclaim, a fixed-dose combination of sustained-release isosorbide mononitrate plus sustained-release L-arginine, is safe and well tolerated. Acclaim, the first proprietary oral nitrate therapy in over a decade, did not meet its primary endpoint of increased treadmill walking time (TWT) with statistical significance. Analysis of the data did reveal positive, nonstatistically significant trends for patients treated with Acclaim with regard to time of onset of angina (during treadmill walking) and ST-segment depression.

According to the Pharmaceutical Research and Manufacturers of America (PhRMA), two other antianginals are in Phase II clinical trials—one to treat unstable angina and one to treat stable exertional angina.

Carvalho, Brendan. "Nitroglycerin to Facilitate Insertion of a Labor Epidural." *Anesthesiology* 102, no. 4 (April 2005): 872.

antianxiety agents   Drugs used to suppress anxiety as well as reduce tension and irritability without causing excessive sedation; also called anxiolytics, sedatives, depressants, downers, or minor tranquilizers. Some antianxiety agents are also used as sleeping aids. About 60 million Americans a year have insomnia often or for extended periods, according to the National Institute of Neurological Disorders and Stroke. Antianxiety drugs are not intended to be used for the anxiety or tension that accompanies typical stressors of everyday life, but rather to calm and relax people who experience excessive anxiety, nervousness, or tension or for short-term control of social phobias. Antianxiety agents are also used in the management of generalized anxiety disorder (GAD). The *Diagnostic and Statistical Manual of Mental Disorders,* Fourth Edition *(DSM-IV)* lists two criteria for GAD: excessive anxiety and worry (apprehensive expectation) occurring more days than not for a period of at least six months and difficulty in controlling the worry. In clinical settings, 50 to 60 percent of those presenting with GAD are female; in epidemiological studies, approximately two-thirds are women. In a community sample, the one-year prevalence rate for GAD was approximately 3 percent, and the lifetime prevalence rate was 5 percent. Generalized anxiety disorder is the most common anxiety disorder and is second only to depression (see ANTIDEPRESSANTS) as the most common disorder diagnosed in primary care. According to Allen, "An estimated 15 percent of Americans suffer from one or another of the anxiety disorders. These include generalized anxiety, specific phobias, obsessive-compulsive disorder and flat-out panic attacks. As a group, anxiety disorders constitute the most common disorder in the country." All antianxiety drugs in the United States are available only by prescription.

Classes

Antianxiety agents generally are separated into the following classes according to their chemical structure:

- *Barbiturates*   Because barbiturates act as central nervous system (CNS) depressants, they produce a wide spectrum of effects, from mild sedation to anesthesia, thus crossing several drug groups. Some are also used as ANTICONVULSANTS. Barbiturates are derivatives of barbituric acid. Though very popular in the first half of the 20th century, concern about their addiction potential and the ever-increasing number of fatalities associated with them led to the development of alternative medications. More than 2,500 barbiturates have been synthesized, and at the height of their popularity, about 50 were marketed for human use. Today, about a dozen are in medical use, with less than 10 percent of all depressant prescriptions in the United States being for barbiturates. *Examples:* mephobarbital (Mebaral), pentobarbital (Nembutal), phenobarbital (Luminal), secobarbital (Seconal).

- *Benzodiazepines*   The first true class of antianxiety drugs to receive FDA approval, benzodiazepines exhibit hypnotic, anxiolytic, anticonvulsant, amnesic, and muscle relaxant properties. Long-term use can be problematic due to the development of tolerance and dependency. Introduced in 1960 as a replacement for barbiturates, they became widely prescribed for stress-related ailments in the 1960s and 1970s. Touted as much safer depressants with far less addiction potential than barbiturates, today these drugs account for about one out of every five prescriptions for controlled substances. Benzodiazepines have been the mainstay of anxiolytic drug therapy for many years. Although they are generally safe and effective, concerns have been expressed regarding their potential for abuse and addiction, cognitive and functional impairment, withdrawal symptoms, and interaction with alcohol. Benzodiazepines are commonly divided into three groups according to how quickly they produce an effect and how long those effects last. Short-acting compounds act for less than six hours and have few residual effects if taken before bedtime; however, rebound insomnia may occur, and they might cause wake-time anxiety. Intermediate-acting compounds have an effect for six to 10 hours and may have mild residual effects; however, rebound insomnia is not common. Long-acting compounds have strong sedative effects that persist. A big downside of this group of drugs is prolonged sedation, which can contribute to falls, especially in the elderly. *Examples: Short-acting:* midazolam (Versed), triazolam (Halcion). *Intermediate-acting:* alprazolam (Xanax), clonazepam (Klonopin), estazolam (ProSom), lorazepam (Ativan), oxazepam (Serax), temazepam (Restoril). *Long-acting:* chlordiazepoxide (Librium), clorazepate (Tranxene), diazepam (Valium), flurazepam (Dalmane), quazepam (Doral).

- *Nonbenzodiazepine sedative hypnotics* These drugs cause sedation and muscle relaxation and have antianxiety properties; some resources group them separately from antianxiety agents, but the FDA groups them as antianxiety drugs. One subclass is imidazopyridines, of which zolpidem (Ambien) has been approved (1999). Zolpidem is said to have

selectivity because it has little of the muscle-relaxant effect and more of the sedative effect; thus, it is used for the short-term treatment of insomnia (as a sleeping pill). It works quickly (usually within 15 minutes) and has a short half-life (two to three hours) but will last longer in patients with liver dysfunction. Another subclass is pyrazolopyrimidines, of which zaleplon (Sonata) has been approved (1999) for short-term treatment of insomnia. Eszopiclone (Lunesta), approved by the FDA in December 2004, is used in treatment of insomnia. Unlike zolpidem and zaleplon, which are recommended for only one week to 10 days, eszopiclone is approved for use up to six months. Trials suggest that patients do not get addicted to Lunesta. Ramelteon (Rozerem), approved by the FDA in July 2005, was the first prescription sleeping aid not to be classified as a controlled substance.

- *Azapirones* A unique class of psychotropic drugs, azapirones were the first effective alternative to benzodiazepines for the treatment of anxiety to have been introduced in nearly three decades. Buspirone (BuSpar), the first azapirone introduced into clinical practice, was approved in the United States in 1986. Other azapirones are still in clinical trials. While benzodiazepines are more suitable for intermittent or short-term use, buspirone is more useful long-term. Azapirones' effectiveness at relieving anxiety is similar to that of the benzodiazepines, with a better safety profile. Unlike the benzodiazepines, azapirones have no muscle-relaxant or anticonvulsant properties; no significant abuse potential or withdrawal effects; no cognitive, memory, or psychomotor impairment properties; no significant withdrawal symptoms; negligible overdose toxicity; and no respiratory depressant properties. Azapirones have the additional benefit of being well tolerated by elderly patients.

- *Miscellaneous antianxiety agents* The following are not benzodiazepines but have similar effects:

- Hydroxyzine (Vistaril) is an ANTIHISTAMINE approved by the FDA in 1957 that has sedative properties as one of its side effects, so is also used as an antianxiety drug.

- Meprobamate is a tranquilizing drug that acts as a depressant of the CNS that can be used in the treatment of anxiety. Although meprobamate is chemically unlike barbiturates and has lower toxicity, it has similar pharmacological effects, especially the ability to induce sleep and alleviate anxiety. Originally introduced in 1954, it is marketed under the trade name Miltown.

How They Work

The precise action of antianxiety agents is not fully understood, but it is believed that most antianxiety medications appear to affect the action of neurotransmitters (chemicals) in the brain. They may work by affecting the part of the brain associated with emotion.

Barbiturates work by depressing (slowing down) the central nervous system (the brain and spinal cord). They affect a neurotransmitter that normally acts as a brake on the electrical activity of the brain. Barbiturates increase the braking effects of this chemical, causing sedation.

Benzodiazepines are believed to act on the specialized receptors in the brain that are adjacent to receptors for a neurotransmitter called gamma-aminobutyric acid (GABA), which inhibits anxiety. It is possible that the interaction of benzodiazepines with these receptors expedites the anxiety-suppressing action of GABA within the brain.

Sedative-hypnotic drugs act by reducing brain-cell activity. They activate the same neuronal receptors as the benzodiazepines but have a different chemical structure than these drugs. Zaleplon interacts with the GABA receptor complex and shares some of the pharmacological properties of the benzodiazepines. Zolpidem works by enhancing the effect of GABA. It is not known exactly how eszopiclone works, but it is thought to have an effect on the GABA receptors

somewhere near the site where benzodiazepines produce their effect.

Ramelteon offers a completely new mechanism of action, specifically targeting two melatonin receptors in the brain, MT_1 and MT_2. The MT_1 and MT_2 receptors are located in the brain's suprachiasmic nuclei (SCN). The SCN is known as the body's "master clock" because it regulates the 24-hour sleep-wake cycle. Ramelteon mimics the action of melatonin, a naturally occurring hormone that regulates the sleep cycle and hastens onset of sleep.

Buspirone is thought to act by interfering with the function of the neurotransmitter serotonin in the brain, particularly by serving as a 5-HT_{1A} receptor partial agonist. Buspirone has moderate affinity for brain D_2-dopamine receptors. Some studies suggest that buspirone may have indirect effects on other neurotransmitter systems. It has no effect on GABA receptors.

Hydroxyzine's calming effects may be due to suppression of certain regions of the brain or by affecting other natural substances, such as acetylcholine or serotonin.

The exact mechanism by which meprobamate works is unknown, but it is believed to act in the brain to cause sedation, reduce anxiety, and relax the muscles.

Approved Uses

Barbiturates may be used to treat short-term insomnia, as they generally lose their effectiveness after two weeks. However, benzodiazepines have largely replaced barbiturates for treating anxiety or sleeplessness, with barbiturates now used mostly in the emergency treatment of convulsions.

Benzodiazepines are used in many situations, depending on their pharmacokinetics (how they are absorbed, distributed, metabolized, and excreted). The main use of the short-acting benzodiazepines is in insomnia, while anxiety responds better to medium- to long-acting substances that will produce their effects throughout the day. Certain benzodiazepines are also used as anticonvulsants (e.g., clorazepate, clonazepam, diazepam) and MUSCLE RELAXANTS (e.g., diazepam). Midazolam, which is available only as an injectable, is used for sedation in the hospital setting.

Nonbenzodiazepine sedative-hypnotic drugs are used both as sedatives to reduce anxiety and as hypnotics to induce sleep, although not all are approved for both. For example, zaleplon, zolpidem, eszoplicone, and ramelteon are approved only for the treatment of insomnia. They are not approved as antianxiety medications.

Buspirone is used to treat persons with generalized anxiety of a limited or moderate degree.

Hydroxyzine is used as a sleep aid; to induce sedation prior to medical procedures that lead to anxiety, such as dental work; and following general anesthesia.

Meprobamate is used to treat anxiety.

Off-Label Uses

Benzodiazepines have been used to relieve the symptoms of irritable bowel syndrome (IBS) and premenstrual syndrome (PMS).

Benzodiazepine drugs have also been reported to be effective in minimizing sleep disorders in fibromyalgia patients, in particular, clonazepam for reducing restless leg syndrome, a common symptom of fibromyalgia. However, when taken for longer than two weeks, benzodiazepines can worsen sleep patterns by shortening the length of restorative deep sleep and increasing the number of wake-up times each night. Lorazepam and alprazolam can also be used to treat muscle spasms that often go along with severe pain.

Companion Drugs

Buspirone is also useful as an augmenting agent for the treatment of depression when added to selective serotonin reuptake inhibitor (SSRI) ANTIDEPRESSANTS.

Administration

Benzodiazepines are available in several dosage forms: oral (taken by mouth—extended-release tablets, immediate release tablets, capsules, liquid concentrate), intramuscular injection (chlordiazepoxide, diazepam, lorazepam), and intravenous injection (diazepam, chlordiazepoxide, and lorazepam).

Non-benzodiazepine sedative hypnotics are available as tablets (eszopliclone, ramelteon, zolpidem) and capsules (zaleplon) to be taken by mouth. Zaleplon should be taken immediately before bedtime or after the patient has gone to bed and has experienced difficulty falling asleep.

Buspirone and meprobamate are available in tablet form.

Hydroxyzine can be administered orally or as an intramuscular injection.

Cautions and Concerns

Benzodiazepines induce physical dependence and are potentially addictive. An abrupt discontinuation of benzodiazepines may result in convulsions, confusion, psychosis, or effects similar to delirium tremens (colloquially, DTs, a condition associated with complete alcohol withdrawal in an individual with a reported history of long-term alcohol consumption). In addition, benzodiazepine withdrawal syndrome can be characterized by insomnia, anxiety, tremor, perspiration, loss of appetite, and delusions. Some of the withdrawal symptoms are identical to the symptoms for which the medication was originally prescribed. Because of this potential withdrawal syndrome, persons on long-term (four to six weeks or longer) or high dosage of any benzodiazepine should be carefully weaned off the drug. Onset of the withdrawal syndrome might be delayed as long as 10 days. Even withdrawal from short-acting benzodiazepines such as alprazolam taken less than three months may present withdrawal symptoms.

Older people demonstrate an increased response to benzodiazepines and sedative hypnotics.

Because meprobamate is highly addictive, those who have been using it for prolonged periods may be addicted and may need to be withdrawn slowly.

Hepatic (liver) dysfunction can affect the elimination of a number of benzodiazepines as well as the nonbenzodiazepine sedative hypnotics and barbiturates. Therefore, smaller dosages are recommended for patients with this condition.

Because eszopiclone's sedation effects may occur as soon as 10 minutes and may last up to six hours, it should be taken immediately before going to bed and only when the patient plans to sleep for at least eight hours.

Sleep disorder experts caution that sleep medications do not cure the causes of insomnia and do not make insomnia patients normal sleepers; when the patient stops taking the sleep aid, his or her insomnia will return. Reinberg quoted Gregg D. Jacobs, director of the Sleep Disorders Center at Boston's Beth Israel Deaconess Medical Center, as being worried about the long-term effects of taking sleeping pills: "We have no idea what the long-term effects are of taking a sleeping pill every night for six months or one year; we don't know what that does to brain functioning." Jacobs recommends cognitive behavior therapy to get to the root causes of insomnia, with sleeping pills used only for short-term insomnia.

Dr. Jerry Avorn of Harvard Medical School and Brigham and Women's Hospital in Boston was critical of the FDA approval of ramelteon (Rozerem), cautioning that it was approved on the basis of trials that found improvements over one or two nights only. Another study did not demonstrate a benefit in patients under the age of 65, he has stated.

Warnings

Depending on the dose, frequency, and duration of use, one can rapidly develop tolerance, physical dependence, and psychological dependence to barbiturates. With the development of tolerance, the margin of safety between the effective dose and the lethal dose becomes very narrow.

When Not Advised (Contraindications)

Alcohol should be avoided with all antianxiety drugs because of the additive sedative effects, which may result in depressed heart and breathing functions.

Because meprobamate is highly sedative, it is not advised for use in the elderly; in cases when it is prescribed, only the lowest possible dose should be used. In fact, most antianxiety agents should be used cautiously (and at the lowest possible dose) in the elderly due to the risk of falls.

Antianxiety agents should not be used by patients with preexisting depression because they can worsen the depression.

An increased risk of congenital malformations, specifically cleft lip or palate, associated with the use of minor tranquilizers such as chlordiazepoxide, diazepam and meprobamate during the first trimester of pregnancy has been suggested in several studies. Because use of these drugs is rarely a matter of urgency, their use during this period should almost always be avoided. The possibility that a woman of childbearing potential may be pregnant at the time of institution of therapy should be considered. Patients should be advised that if they become pregnant during therapy or intend to become pregnant they should communicate with their physicians about the desirability of discontinuing the drug.

Because ramelteon has not been studied in children, it is not known if it is safe and effective for children. Similarly, the safety and effectiveness of buspirone has not been established in patients ages six to 17 at doses recommended for use in adults.

Side Effects

All antianxiety and sedative/hypnotic drugs can impair the ability to drive vehicles and to operate machinery. The impairment is worsened by consumption of alcohol, because both act as depressants on the CNS.

More common side effects from barbiturates include clumsiness or unsteadiness, dizziness or lightheadedness, drowsiness, or feeling as if one has a hangover. Less common side effects include anxiety or nervousness, irritability, excitability, agitation, confusion, hallucinations, mental depression, liver damage, constipation, skin rashes, feeling faint, headache, fever, nausea or vomiting, insomnia, or nightmares. Children can experience irritability and hyperactivity.

Benzodiazepines have largely replaced barbiturates because they have a lower abuse potential and relatively lower incidence of adverse reactions and drug interactions. Still, drowsiness, ataxia (involuntary muscle movement), confusion, vertigo, impaired judgment, and memory impairment are common. Other side effects include depression, crying, lethargy, apathy, fatigue, amnesia, headache, slurred speech, irritability, inability to concentrate, skin rash, constipation, diarrhea, change in appetite, vomiting, difficulty in swallowing, incontinence, libido changes, menstrual irregularities, visual disturbances, behavior problems, depressed hearing, hiccoughs, or fever. The effects of long-acting benzodiazepines can linger over to the following day.

When taken for fewer than 10 days as recommended and at the dosages recommended, zolpidem has shown side effects of drowsiness, dizziness, and diarrhea. However, with higher than recommended doses or when taken over a longer period of time, other side effects have been reported. These include hallucinations, delusions, poor motor coordination, increased appetite, increased sex drive, poor judgment, and, following use, inability to remember events that took place while under the influence of the drug. Zolpidem can become psychologically addictive if taken for extended periods of time due to dependence on its ability to put one to sleep or to the unique sense of euphoria it can produce. Under the influence of the drug, it is common to take more zolpidem than is necessary; thus, prescriptions in small quantities are advised as well as advising users to restrict their own access to remaining pills.

The more common side effects for zaleplon are headache, muscle weakness, dizziness, lightheadedness, nausea, abdominal pain, or daytime drowsiness. Less frequently, zaleplon may cause hallucinations, abnormal behavior, or severe confusion. Because some of the more serious side effects appear to be dose-related, the lowest possible effective dose is recommended. Although zaleplon may cause amnesia, memory problems can usually be avoided if the patient can get more than four hours of sleep after taking it.

The most common side effects of eszopiclone are headache, dizziness, drowsiness when awake, loss of coordination, and unpleasant taste. In a controlled study, adults taking larger doses of ezopiclone reported a greater incidence of viral infection, dry mouth, dizziness, hallucinations, infection, rash, and unpleasant taste.

The most common side effects reported for ramelteon have been daytime drowsiness, fatigue, and dizziness; also reported have been headache, tiredness, nausea, worsening insomnia, and colds. The drug also has the potential to exacerbate symptoms of depression.

The most commonly noted side effects associated with buspirone are dizziness, nausea, headache, nervousness, lightheadedness, excitement, headache, fatigue, and insomnia.

The side effects of hydroxyzine are usually mild and include dry mouth and in rare cases muscle tremor and convulsions.

Side effects from meprobamate are not common, but they can occur. Those reported include drowsiness, upset stomach, vomiting, diarrhea, headache, difficulty coordinating movements, excitement, and muscle weakness.

Interactions

Consuming alcohol along with antianxiety agents can lead to various problems ranging from sleepiness to coma. Doses of benzodiazepines that are excessively sedating may cause severe drowsiness in the presence of alcohol, increasing the risk of household and automotive accidents. Since alcoholics often suffer from anxiety and insomnia and since many of them take morning drinks, this interaction may be dangerous. Acute or chronic alcohol consumption enhances the sedative effect of barbiturates at their site of action in the brain, sometimes leading to coma or fatal respiratory depression.

Taking zaleplon along with or immediately following a high-fat/heavy meal slows its absorption and may also slow its onset of action.

Buspirone used along with monoamine oxidase (MAO) inhibitors, which are used in psychotic disorders, may cause increased blood pressure. The combination of buspirone and a selective serotonin reuptake inhibitor (e.g., fluoxetine, sertraline) can increase the risk of developing serotonin syndrome. When taken while grapefruit juice is in the system, the effects of buspirone could increase as much as 400 percent.

Sales/Statistics

According to the Substance Abuse and Mental Health Services Administration (SAMHSA), antianxiety agents have exceeded other classes in sales and usage since the 1980s. Prescriptions for the popular anxiolytic benzodiazepines have more recently shifted from diazepam to shorter-acting compounds, particularly alprazolam and lorazepam. Additional changes include replacing the earlier long-acting hypnotic benzodiazepine flurazepam with the shorter-acting triazolam and temazepam. Overall, sales of benzodiazepine anxiolytics have decreased in more recent years. However, use of benzodiazepines as sleep-inducing hypnotics has increased or remained stable.

Also, SAMHSA stated that an estimated 95 percent of benzodiazepine prescriptions for older adults in this country are ordered for anxiety and insomnia, with 5 percent used as adjuncts for general anesthesia, as muscle relaxants, or as anticonvulsants.

The U.S. market for FDA-approved sleep medications was reported to be approximately $2.1 billion between November 2003 and October 2004, representing a 20 percent increase over the same period the previous year. Ambien accounted for 70 percent of those sales. *The Wall Street Journal* reported Lunesta to be off to one of the fastest sales starts on record, with 42,508 prescriptions sold during its first seven days of availability.

According to a report from the IMS Institute for Healthcare Informatics (the public reporting arm of IMS, a pharmaceutical market intelligence firm), tranquilizers were the 11th most prescribed therapeutic class in the United States in 2010, with 108.6 million prescriptions dispensed; hypnotics and sedatives were 20th, with 66 million prescriptions. IMS listed generic alprazolam as the 11th most prescribed drug in the United States, with 46.3 million prescriptions dispensed in 2010. Zolpidem ranked 15th, with 38 million prescriptions.

Demographics and Cultural Groups

In a survey by the Agency for Healthcare Research and Quality (AHRQ), hospitalized men with an accompanying but unrelated (to their primary disease or disorder) report of anxiety were more likely than women to be prescribed an antianxiety agent at discharge (48.4 percent vs. 5.9 percent). However, the opposite was observed among outpatients, among whom 56.8 percent of women with anxiety were prescribed antianxiety agents compared with 30.9 percent of men, suggesting that antianxiety agents are used for different purposes among inpatients and outpatients—to calm agitated men in the hospital and to reduce anxiety among women in the community.

A Duke University Center for the Study of Aging examined the usage of antianxiety medications over a 10-year period among racial groups in an aging population and found that whites were more likely to be taking these medications than African Americans. "Sedatives, hypnotics and antianxiety agents were used frequently by this cohort and, despite efforts to decrease the use of these medications in older adults, the use of antianxiety medications declined only slightly during our 10-year follow-up period. While benzodiazepines accounted for the majority of these medications prescribed, whites were two to three times more likely than African Americans to be taking non-benzodiazepines as well as benzodiazepines across all 10 study years. In controlled analyses, use of sedatives, hypnotics and antianxiety medications was associated with white race, female gender, depression, a higher number of visits to health care professionals, some impairment in physical functioning, and perceived health as fair or poor."

Development History

Historically, people of almost every culture have used chemical agents to induce sleep, relieve stress, and allay anxiety. While alcohol is one of the oldest and most universal agents used for these purposes, hundreds of substances have been developed that produce CNS depression.

Barbituric acid was discovered by the Belgian researcher Adolf von Baeyer on December 4, 1863, the day of St. Barbara; thus, he reportedly chose the name *barbituric* as a combination of St. Barbara and *urea*. Von Baeyer combined urea and malonic acid in a condensation reaction. Malonic acid has since been replaced by diethyl malonate. In 1903, barbitone, the first medicinal barbiturate, was synthesized from barbituric acid by the German scientists Emil Hermann Fischer and Joseph von Mering and marketed under the trade name Veronal. In 1912, phenobarbital was introduced under the trade name Luminal as a sedative hypnotic.

During the 1950s and 1960s, reports increased about side effects and dependence related to barbiturates, resulting in pentobarbital, secobarbital, amobarbital, butabarbital, phenobarbital, and barbital being classified as controlled drugs with the passage of the Comprehensive Drug Abuse Prevention and Control Act of 1970.

The first benzodiazepine, chlordiazepoxide (Librium) was discovered serendipitously in 1954 by the Austrian scientist Dr. Leo Sternbach working for the pharmaceutical company Hoffmann-La Roche. Initially, he discontinued his work on the compound Ro-5–0690, but he "rediscovered" it in 1957 when an assistant was cleaning up the laboratory. Although initially discouraged by his employer, Sternbach conducted further research that revealed Ro-5–0690 was a very effective tranquilizer.

Future Drugs

One area drug researchers are working on is helping people sleep throughout the night without next-day impairment. According to Neurocrine Biolsciences, the elderly population, which represents about 35 to 40 percent of prescriptions for sedative hypnotics, would especially benefit from a novel therapeutic with an improved safety profile, rapid onset, and decrease in memory impairment. Neurocrine has submitted a New Drug Application (NDA) to the FDA for indiplon, which is expected to help people fall asleep and then maintain sleep throughout the night.

Allen, Colin. "When Worry Takes Control." *Psychology Today* 36, no. 3 (June 10, 2003)

Blazer, Dan G., et al. "Sedative, Hypnotic, and Antianxiety Medication Use in an Aging Cohort over Ten Years: A Racial Comparison." *Journal of the American Geriatrics Society* 48, no. 9 (September 2000): 1,073–1,079.

National Women's Health Information Center. "FDA Taken to Task, Again." Available online. URL: http://www.4woman.gov/news/english/527841.htm. Posted on September 7, 2005.

Reinberg, Steven. "New Sleeping Pill Promises Long-Term Results." *HealthDay Reporter.* Available online. URL: http://www.healthfinder.gov/news/newsstory.asp?docID=525280. Posted on April 27, 2005.

antiarrhythmics Medications used to treat abnormal heart rhythms, called arrhythmias, resulting from a disturbance in the heart's electrical system. Common symptoms of arrhythmias include heart palpitations, irregular heartbeats, fast heartbeats, dizziness, fainting, chest pain, and shortness of breath. Abnormal heart rhythms may be too slow (bradycardia) or too fast (tachycardia) or may beat in a chaotic or irregular pattern (extra beats or fibrillation). Irregular heartbeats may be present from birth or may develop if part of the heart muscle tissue (myocardium) is irritated or damaged, leading to a disruption or "short circuit" in the heart's electrical system. Some arrhythmias are relatively harmless; others can be life-threatening, leading to cardiac arrest. The most serious arrhythmias contribute to nearly 500,000 deaths in the United States each year according to the American Heart Association, with annual deaths attributable to the condition rising steadily. HeartCenterOnline adds that of these, "one type of arrhythmia, ventricular fibrillation, causes most of the 340,000 sudden cardiac deaths (from cardiac arrest) that occur each year." Wattigney et al. found that the death rate (per 100,000 U.S. population) associated with atrial fibrillation among adults 45 years or older increased from 27.6 in 1980 to 69.8 in 1998.

Classes

Antiarrhythmics are available only by prescription and are typically grouped into classes according to their primary mechanism of action (the way they control a person's heart rhythm). However, many antiarrhythmic agents have multiple mechanisms of action and therefore cross classes.

- Class I antiarrhythmic medicines are sodium channel blockers. Class I is divided into three separate subclasses (IA, IB, and IC) according to their different effects on sodium channels. *Examples:* IA—disopyramide (Norpace), procainamide (Procanbid, Pronestyl), and quinidine (Quinaglute, Quinidex); IB—lidocaine (LidoPen, Xylocaine) and mexiletine (Mexitil); IC—flecainide (Tambocor), propafenone (Rythmol), and moricizine (Ethmozine).

- Class II antiarrhythmic medicines are beta-blockers. *Examples:* atenolol (Tenormin), metoprolol (Lopressor, Toprol), propranolol (Inderal). (See also ANTIHYPERTENSIVES.)

- Class III antiarrhythmic medicines are potassium channel blockers. *Examples:* amiodarone (Cordarone, Pacerone), dofetilide (Tikosyn), dronedarone (Multaq), ibutilide (Corvert), sotalol (Betapace).

- Class IV antiarrhythmic medicines are calcium channel blockers. *Examples:* diltiazem (Cardizem) and verapamil (Calan, Isoptin). (See also ANTIHYPERTENSIVES.)

- Miscellaneous antiarrhythmic medications work by other mechanisms. *Examples:* digoxin (Lanoxin) and adenosine (Adenocard).

How They Work

Antiarrhythmics can correct an irregular heartbeat by restoring normal rhythm. Also, by slowing down a heart that is beating too fast, antiarrhythmics enable the heart to work more efficiently. The pace at which the heart beats is controlled by electrical impulses (or signals) that begin in the sinoatrial (SA) node of the heart, which is located in the upper right chamber (atrium). This signal is generated by the flow of electrolytes through passageways in the heart called ion channels. Ions, or electrolytes, include sodium, potassium, magnesium, and calcium. The electrical signal spreads across the two upper chambers of the heart (atria), then to the atrioventricular (AV) node. The AV node connects to specialized fibers in the lower chambers (ventricles) of the heart that conduct the electrical impulses into the ventricles and cause them to contract. Arrhythmias develop when this control mechanism is disrupted. Antiarrhythmics work in a variety of ways to slow the electrical impulses in the heart so that the heart can resume a regular rhythm.

By blocking sodium channels in heart cells, Class I antiarrhythmics slow the conduction of electrical impulses from cell to cell in the heart. Class IA antiarrhythmics have a moderate effect on sodium channels and usually prolong the duration of repolarization—the time it takes to "recharge" the heart after every beat. Some of these drugs, such as quinidine, also reduce the force of heart muscle contractions. Class IB antiarrhythmics are the least effective at blocking sodium channels. They work by slowing nerve impulses in the heart. Usually, they shorten the duration of repolarization. Class IC antiarrhythmics are strong sodium channel blockers. They also slow nerve impulses in the heart but have little to no effect on repolarization.

Class II antiarrhythmics work by slowing conduction of electrical impulses through the SA and

AV nodes. They work primarily by interfering with hormonal influences (such as adrenaline [epinephrine]) on the heart's cells. By doing this, they also reduce blood pressure and heart rate.

By blocking the heart's potassium channels, class III antiarrhythmics primarily lengthen the duration of repolarization.

Class IV antiarrhythmics work like class II drugs but act by blocking the calcium channels in the heart.

Digoxin and adenosine slow conduction of electrical impulses through the AV node.

Because each kind of antiarrhythmic medicine works in a slightly different way, no single drug cures all arrhythmias in all patients. It may take trying a few different antiarrhythmics before finding which works best for a patient. Some patients may need extra monitoring or testing, either with a Holter monitor or electrophysiology studies (EPS) to help clarify what type of antiarrhythmic is best.

Approved Uses

Antiarrhythmic drugs are used to achieve any of four therapeutic goals, according to Lipicky: "(1) Prevent the first occurrence of an arrhythmia, supraventricular or ventricular; (2) convert the arrhythmia to normal sinus, supraventricular or ventricular; (3) allow a supraventricular arrhythmia to persist, but simply control ventricular rate; and (4) given normal sinus at the moment, lengthen the time to arrhythmia recurrence, supraventricular or ventricular."

All class I antiarrhythmics can be used to treat ventricular arrhythmias—abnormal heart rhythms that originate in the lower chambers (ventricles) of the heart. They include ventricular premature beats, ventricular tachycardia, and ventricular fibrillation. Class IA and class IC antiarrhythmics can also be used to treat atrial fibrillation or atrial flutter. Class IB antiarrhythmics are used only for the treatment of ventricular arrhythmias.

Class II antiarrhythmics are used to treat ventricular arrhythmias, including premature ventricular beats and ventricular tachycardia.

They are also used to slow the ventricular rate in patients with atrial fibrillation or atrial flutter and to treat paroxysmal supraventricular tachycardia.

Amiodarone (intravenous and oral) is approved only for the treatment of ventricular arrhythmias. Sotalol is approved for the treatment of ventricular arrhythmias as well as atrial fibrillation and atrial flutter. Ibutilide is approved only for the acute termination of atrial fibrillation or atrial flutter of recent onset. Dofetilide is approved only for the maintenance of sinus rhythm in individuals with atrial fibrillation or atrial flutter who have been converted to sinus rhythm and for the chemical cardioversion of atrial fibrillation or atrial flutter to sinus rhythm.

Dronedarone was approved for the prevention and treatment of atrial fibrillation and is intended for people who have had atrial fibrillation or atrial flutter in the last six months but who may currently have a regular heart rhythm or will have medical treatment to return to a regular rhythm.

Class IV antiarrhythmics are used to slow the ventricular rate in patients who have atrial fibrillation or atrial flutter and to treat paroxysmal supraventricular tachycardia.

Digoxin is used to decrease the ventricular rate in patients who have atrial fibrillation or atrial flutter and to treat paroxysmal supraventricular tachycardia. Adenosine is used to end episodes of paroxysmal supraventricular tachycardia.

In individuals suspected of suffering from a supraventricular tachycardia (SVT), adenosine is used to help identify the rhythm. Certain SVTs can be successfully terminated with adenosine. This includes any reentrant arrhythmias that require the AV node for the reentry, such as, AV reentrant tachycardia (AVRT) or AV nodal reentrant tachycardia (AVNRT). In addition, atrial tachycardia can sometimes be terminated with adenosine.

Off-Label Uses

Intravenous procainamide has been used effectively to treat arrhythmias associated with malignant hyperthermia, a life-threatening condition resulting from a genetic sensitivity of skeletal muscles to volatile anesthetics and depolarizing neuromuscular blocking drugs that occurs during or after anesthesia.

Mexiletine has been used with mixed results in the management of painful diabetic neuropathy.

Amiodarone has been used effectively to restore sinus rhythm in patients with atrial fibrillation or atrial flutter. Other unlabeled uses include atrial flutter, multifocal atrial tachycardia, paroxysmal atrial fibrillation, and paroxysmal supraventricular tachycardia. A three-part investigative series by Knight Ridder Newspapers in 2003 found that doctors wrote nearly 2.3 million off-label amiodarone prescriptions in the previous year—which was 82 percent of all the prescriptions for the drug.

Administration

Antiarrhythmics are available as capsules, tablets, and injections. Only procainamide, lidocaine, ibutilide, and amiodarone are available in an intravenous formulation.

Mexiletine, amiodarone, and dronedarone should be taken with food to minimize gastrointestinal side effects.

Cautions and Concerns

Antiarrhythmic drugs may cause new arrhythmias or more frequent occurrence of preexisting arrhythmias—referred to as proarrhythmia. A patient's serum potassium and magnesium levels should be normal before starting any antiarrhythmic agent to minimize this risk of proarrhythmia.

Warnings

Because of its potent anticholinergic effects, disopyramide should be used with extreme caution in patients with urinary retention, prostate problems, or glaucoma. It should also be used with caution in patients with impaired kidney or liver function.

Blood disorders (agranulocytosis, bone marrow depression, neutropenia, hypoplastic anemia, and thrombocytopenia) have been reported in patients receiving procainamide at a rate of approximately 0.5 percent. These disorders have been shown to occur in patients who have been receiving procainamide within the recommended dosage range. Fatalities have occurred (with approximately 20 to 25 percent mortality in reported cases of agranulocytosis). Because most of these events have been noted during the first 12 weeks of therapy, complete blood counts are recommended at weekly intervals for the first three months of therapy and periodically thereafter. Complete blood counts also are recommended if the patient develops any signs of infection (such as fever, chills, sore throat, or stomatitis), bruising, or bleeding. If any of these blood disorders occur, procainamide should be discontinued. Blood counts usually return to normal within one month of discontinuation. Caution is also recommended for patients with preexisting bone marrow failure, cytopenia of any type, or impaired kidney function.

Quinidine should be used with caution in patients with impaired liver function.

Lidocaine should be used with caution in patients with impaired liver function or heart failure.

Propafenone, flecainide, and moricizine should be used with caution in patients with impaired liver function.

Class II antiarrhythmics, propafenone, sotalol, and amiodarone should be used with caution in patients with asthma.

In June 2005, the Federal Drug Administration (FDA) began notifying physicians and pharmacists that a Medication Guide for patients must be distributed with each prescription for amiodarone. The FDA requires these guides for drugs that pose a serious public health concern. The guide explains to patients that amiodarone can cause lung damage and liver damage. Pulmonary (lung) toxicity and fibrosis has occurred at rates as high as 10 to 17 percent in studies and has been fatal in about 10 percent of those affected. Amiodarone should be used with caution in patients with preexisting pulmonary, liver, or thyroid dysfunction.

Dronedarone also has a required Medication Guide. Dronedarone may increase the risk of death in people who have severe heart failure. It also may cause liver problems, including life-threatening liver failure.

Due to the proarrhythmic potential of dofetilide, all patients being initiated on this antiarrhythmic must be hospitalized for at least three days. Dofetilide is available only to hospitals and prescribers who have undergone specific training in the risks of treatment with this drug. In addition, prescriptions for dofetilide can be filled only at pharmacies that are enrolled in a program through the manufacturer.

Sotalol and dofetilide should be used with caution in patients with impaired kidney function.

When Not Advised (Contraindications)

All of the antiarrhythmics, except for amiodarone and dofetilide, have negative inotropic effects (i.e., decrease the pumping action of the heart). Disopyramide has the most potent negative inotropic effects. Therefore, all antiarrhythmics, except for amiodarone and dofetilide, should be avoided in patients with heart failure.

Because long-term use of procainamide has been reported to result in a lupuslike syndrome (arthralgia, arthritis, pleuritis, pericarditis, fever, chills, myalgia, rash) in up to 30 percent of patients, it is not advised for use in patients diagnosed with systemic lupus erythematosus (SLE). Procainamide also may be contraindicated for patients with myasthenia gravis because of reports that it increases muscle weakness in these patients.

Extreme caution is advised with flecainide, propafenone, and moricizine in patients with an acute myocardial infarction (heart attack) because of the increased risk of death in this group.

Dronedarone should not be taken by patients with severe heart failure, who have been hospitalized recently for heart failure, who have second- or third-degree atrioventricular block or sick sinus syndrome (unless its use is in combination with a functioning pacemaker), who have bradycardia less than 50 beats per minute, who have severe liver problems, or who are pregnant or breast-feeding.

Dofetilide should be avoided in patients taking any of the following medications: verapamil, cimetidine, hydrochlorothiazide, trimethoprim, itraconazole, ketoconazole, prochlorperazine, or megestrol.

Adenosine should be avoided in people who have asthma.

Class IV antiarrhythmics should not be used in people with heart failure.

Side Effects

The most common side effects of disopyramide are dose-dependent and include urinary retention, dry mouth, and constipation. This drug can also cause or worsen heart failure. Disopyramide can also cause QT interval (length of the heart's electrical cycle) prolongation on the electrocardiogram.

Procainamide's more common side effects include diarrhea, nausea, rash, myalgia, and fever. Long-term use of procainamide has also been associated with the development of a lupuslike syndrome, which may be reversible once the drug is discontinued. Procainamide can also cause QT interval prolongation on the electrocardiogram.

Chronic use of quinidine, which is chemically similar to quinine (originally derived from the bark of the cinchona tree), can lead to cinchonism, a syndrome usually comprised of tinnitus, hearing loss, vertigo, blurred or double vision, diplopia, and headache. Outside of this syndrome (which is not all that common), quinidine is most commonly associated with diarrhea, nausea, vomiting, abdominal cramping, and lightheadedness. Quinidine can also cause QT interval prolongation on the electrocardiogram.

Lidocaine may cause dizziness, lightheadedness, insomnia, drowsiness, slurred speech, confusion, agitation, hallucinations, and blurred or double vision. In more severe cases, seizures or coma may occur.

The most frequently reported side effects of mexiletine are gastrointestinal-related, particularly nausea, vomiting, or heartburn. Other common side effects include tremor, dizziness, blurred vision, headache, coordination difficulties, nervousness, insomnia, and numbness.

The most frequently reported side effect of flecainide is dizziness, including lightheadedness, fainting, vertigo, and unsteadiness. Other common side effects include difficulty breathing, headache, nausea, fatigue, palpitation, chest pain, tremor, and abdominal pain.

Propafenone side effects most frequently reported are dizziness, nausea, vomiting, unusual taste, constipation, fatigue, difficulty breathing, angina, chest pain, palpitations, headache, and blurred vision.

Although side effects with moricizine are not common, the most frequently reported are dizziness, nausea, headache, fatigue, palpitations, and difficulty breathing.

Class II antiarrhythmics can cause spasm of the airways, impaired circulation, possible masking of low blood sugar levels, insomnia, shortness of breath, depression, Raynaud's syndrome, hallucinations, sexual dysfunction, and fatigue.

Amiodarone is associated with numerous side effects, as it affects nearly all the body's organs. Side effects occur in more than 75 percent of patients receiving amiodarone and are more likely to develop the longer patients receive this drug. Amiodarone can cause pulmonary fibrosis (scarring in the lungs), which is potentially life-threatening if the drug is not discontinued. It may also cause a blue-gray color to appear on the patient's skin, especially in areas exposed to the sun. Amiodarone can also cause sensitivity to sunlight, making patients sunburn more easily—even through a window or cotton clothing. Due to the iodine content of amiodarone, abnormalities in thyroid function are common. Amiodarone may also cause liver function abnormalities. Other common side effects include visual disturbances, abnormal taste and smell, malaise and fatigue, sleep disturbances, prickling or tingling sensation on the skin, lack of coordination, nausea, vomiting, constipation, and loss of appetite.

The most frequently reported side effects for dofetilide are headache, chest pain, and dizziness. Other side effects include respiratory tract infection, shortness of breath, nausea, flu syndrome, insomnia, accidental injury, back pain, diarrhea, rash, and abdominal pain. Dofetilide can also cause QT interval prolongation on the electrocardiogram.

The most common side effects of dronedarone are diarrhea, nausea, abdominal pain, vomiting, heartburn, weakness, rash, itching, and skin redness.

Common side effects of ibutilide include ventricular arrhythmias, palpitations, and headache. Ibutilide can also cause QT interval prolongation on the electrocardiogram.

The most common side effects of sotalol include a slow heart rate, chest pain, palpitations, fatigue, dizziness, lightheadedness, weakness, confusion, headache, nausea, vomiting, diarrhea, and shortness of breath. Sotalol can also cause QT interval prolongation on the electrocardiogram.

Class IV antiarrhythmics can cause diarrhea, flushing, dizziness, headache, low blood pressure, and swollen feet. Verapamil can also cause constipation.

High blood levels of digoxin can be associated with visual disturbances (blurred or green-yellow vision), weight loss, nausea, vomiting, and development of arrhythmias.

Adenosine can cause spasm of the airways, facial flushing, sweating, lightheadedness, or nausea.

Interactions

Drugs that prolong the QT interval should be avoided in patients receiving class IA or class III antiarrhythmics because of the potential for causing torsade de pointes, a lethal ventricular arrhythmia.

Ketoconazole, itraconazole, erythromycin, and verapamil may increase disopyramide and quinidine levels, while phenobarbital, rifampin, and phenytoin may decrease levels of these antiarrhythmics.

Cimetidine, fluoxetine, paroxetine, and ritonavir may increase procainamide levels.

Quinidine may increase levels of beta-blockers, paroxetine, risperidone, ritonavir, venlafaxine, warfarin, and amitriptyline.

Carbamazepine, phenobarbital, and rifampin may decrease levels of mexiletine. Mexiletine may increase levels of theophylline.

Milk may inhibit absorption of flecainide in infants. Cimetidine increases flecainide levels by 30 percent. Flecainide, paroxetine, and ritonavir may increase levels of flecainide and propafenone. Propafenone may increase digoxin levels.

Amiodarone may intensify the effects of ANTICOAGULANTS, such as warfarin, and cause bleeding problems unless a reduction in the anticoagulant dose is taken. Amiodarone increases the blood concentrations of digoxin, quinidine, cyclosporine, simvastatin, lovastatin, procainamide, flecainide, theophylline, and other drugs.

According to Drugs.com, a total of 440 drugs are known to interact with dronedarone; therefore, it is important that patients apprise doctors, nurses, and pharmacists about all the prescription and over-the-counter medications and herbal products they are taking. For example, ketoconazole, itraconazole, erythromycin, ritonavir, rifabutin, Saint-John's-wort, carbamazepine, phenytoin, and nefazodone can affect the removal of dronedarone from the body, which may affect dronedarone's effectiveness. Also, dronedarone can slow down the removal of other drugs from the body, such as atorvastatin, lovastatin, simvastatin, warfarin, tacrolimus, sirolimus, digoxin, and dabigatran. Grapefruit and grapefruit juice increase the amount of dronedarone the body absorbs, which may lead to side effects. Thus, any type of grapefruit, including supplements with grapefruit extract, must be avoided.

Sotalol, propafenone, and beta-blockers may affect how the body reacts to insulin or oral diabetes medicines.

The pharmacological effects of adenosine are blunted in patients who are taking methylxanthines (e.g., caffeine and theophylline).

Adenosine's effects may be increased in patients who are taking disopyramide.

Sales/Statistics

Al-Khatib et al. reported that the number of prescriptions for Class III antiarrhythmics more than doubled between 1995 and 2000 due primarily to an increase in the number of prescriptions for amiodarone.

According to a news release distributed by the pharmaceutical company AstraZeneca in October 2000, "The antiarrhythmic market has an estimated annual potential of $2.9 billion. Current sales of antiarrhythmics total $1.0 billion, of which $0.5 billion are attributable to ventricular antiarrhythmics and $0.5 billion to atrial antiarrhythmics."

The RxList of Top 300 Prescriptions for 2004 (retail and mail order, excluding Wal-Mart) included several antiarrhythmics: Lanoxin, 5,264,880; digoxin (various brands), 4,217,773; and amiodarone HCL (various brands), 2,657,941. A number of beta-blockers and calcium channel blockers used to treat arrhythmias were also on the list, but because they are used for a variety of indications in addition to arrhythmias, all of their prescriptions would not have been for the treatment of arrhythmias. These included atenolol (various brands), Toprol XL, metoprolol tartrate (various brands), verapamil HCl (various brands), diltiazem HCl (various brands), and Inderal LA.

See ANTIHYPERTENSIVES for additional sales and statistical information on beta-blockers and calcium channel blockers.

Demographics and Cultural Groups

Scientists supported by the National Heart, Lung, and Blood Institute have identified a gene variant that is associated with arrhythmia in African Americans. Mark Keating, M.D., of Children's Hospital, Harvard Medical School, and colleagues reported in the August 23, 2002 issue of *Science* that a variant of the cardiac sodium channel gene SCN5A produces a small increase in the risk of arrhythmia. When the variant is combined with other factors such as certain medications, low blood potassium (hypokalemia), or structural heart disease, the risk of life-threatening arrhythmias is increased, according to the researchers. Keating and study coauthors concluded that the gene variant, when combined with other risk factors, may one day be a useful marker for the prediction of arrhythmia. At present, there is no test generally available to identify this gene variant, which is present in an estimated 4.6 million African Americans.

Development History

Although several of the drugs used to treat cardiac arrhythmias have been used for many years (e.g., quinidine since the early 1900s), many of the drugs approved for this use have only been available for 25 years or so.

Lidocaine has been used as a local anesthetic since its approval by the FDA in 1948, but it was not until 1962 that the drug was first used to treat ventricular tachycardia or ventricular fibrillation.

Amiodarone was initially developed in 1961 in Belgium as a treatment for angina. Widely used throughout Europe as an antianginal, it was soon found to suppress arrhythmias. Fiji-born Dr. Bramah Singh, who was working on a Ph.D. degree at Oxford in the late 1960s, determined that amiodarone and sotalol belonged to a new class of antiarrhythmic agents. This new class would become the Class III antiarrhythmics, which would prolong repolarization of the cardiac action potential. Based on this, the Argentinian physician Dr. Mauricio Rosenbaum began using amiodarone to treat his patients who suffered from supraventricular and ventricular arrhythmias, with impressive results. Based on papers written by Dr. Rosenbaum, physicians in the United States began prescribing amiodarone to their patients with potentially life-threatening arrhythmias in the late 1970s. By that time, amiodarone was commonly prescribed throughout Europe for the treatment of arrhythmias. Because amiodarone was not approved by the FDA for use in the United States at the time,

physicians obtained the drug from pharmaceutical companies in Canada and Europe. According to *FDA Consumer,* more than 600 U.S. cardiologists treated some 20,000 patients with amiodarone before its approval.

The FDA was reluctant to officially approve the use of amiodarone because initial reports had shown increased incidence of serious pulmonary side effects. In the mid-1980s, the European pharmaceutical companies began putting pressure on the FDA to approve amiodarone by threatening to cut their supply to the American physicians. In December 1985, amiodarone was approved by the FDA for the treatment of ventricular arrhythmias. Oral amiodarone did not undergo traditional phase I–III FDA-approved clinical trials but instead received approval based on its widespread clinical use. This makes amiodarone one of the few drugs approved by the FDA without rigorous randomized clinical trials.

Approval dates for several other antiarrhythmics: procainamide, 1950; disopyramide, 1977; bretylium, 1978; flecainide, 1985; mexiletine, 1985; propafenone, 1989; adenosine, 1989; moricizine, 1990; sotalol, 1992; ibutilide, 1995; dofetilide, 1999; dronedarone, 2009.

Future Drugs

In December 2005, the Pharmaceutical Research and Manufacturers of America (PhRMA) reported that 13 medicines for arrhythmias were in development.

Efforts to develop new antiarrhythmic drugs have focused on Class III medications because they are less likely to adversely affect the heart's pumping ability, and they act on tissues in both the upper and lower chambers of the heart.

Al-Khatib, S. M., et al. "Outpatient Prescribing of Antiarrhythmic Drugs from 1995 to 2000." *American Journal of Cardiology* 91, no. 1 (January 1, 2003): 91–94.

Lipicky, Raymond John. "Antiarrhythmics: Indications, Claims, and Trial Design." In *Cardiovascular Drug Development: Protocol Design and Methodology,* edited by Jeffrey S. Borer and John C. Somberg, 137–140. New York: Marcel Dekker, 1999.

Wattigney, W. A., G. A. Mensah, and J. B. Croft. "Increased Atrial Fibrillation Mortality: United States, 1980–1998." *American Journal of Epidemiology* 155, no. 9 (May 1, 2002): 819–826.

antibacterials Among the most frequently prescribed medications in modern medicine, antibacterials are used to treat infections caused by bacteria, including strep throat, tuberculosis, urinary tract infections, skin infections, and pneumonia. Oftentimes, the term *antibiotic* is used in place of *antibacterial*; however, *antibiotic* may also encompass drugs that act on other organisms such as fungi (see ANTIFUNGALS), parasites, or viruses (see ANTIVIRALS). Overall, drugs used to treat infections generally may be referred to as anti-infectives or antimicrobials. Derived from the ancient Greek for *against life*, antibiotics are substances produced by or derived from one organism (such as a fungus or bacterium) that can in turn destroy or limit the growth of another microorganism, although today, some antibiotics are synthetics. After their development in the 1940s, antibacterials transformed medical care and dramatically reduced illness and death from infectious diseases. Today, more than 150 different antibacterials are available to doctors to cure infections ranging from minor discomforts to life-threatening infections. Before antibacterials, a simple scratch carried the risk of infection and death.

Classes

Antibacterials can be classified in several ways: by chemical structure, by mechanism of action (how they selectively attack bacterial cells), by the organisms against which they are effective, and by the type of infection for which they are used. Antibacterials are also classified as narrow-spectrum drugs when they are effective against a few types of bacteria and as broad-spectrum drugs when they are effective against a wider range of bacteria.

Typically, antibacterial drugs are grouped into families, with each family comprising many members. Among the most commonly used:

- *aminoglycosides* Broad-spectrum antibacterials. Those derived from species of *Streptomyces* have the suffix *-mycin*, and those derived from species of *Micromonospora* have the suffix *-micin*. *Examples:* amikacin (Amikin), gentamicin (Garamycin), kanamycin (Kantrex), neomycin (Neo-Fradin), paromomycin (Humatin), streptomycin, and tobramycin (Tobrex).

- *carbapenems* Broad-spectrum antibacterials. Also known as thienamycins, carbapenems are naturally produced by bacteria only in very small amounts, and while most antibacterials are made by fermentation, cfonamide-sarbapenems must be produced commercially through synthesis, which greatly increases their cost. *Examples:* ertapenem (Invanz), imipenem-cilastatin (Primaxin), and meropenem (Merrem).

- *cephalosporins* Broad-spectrum antibacterials similar to penicillins in structure but that generally can treat a broader range of infections. Cephalosporins are grouped into "generations" by their antimicrobial properties. The first cephalosporins were designated first generation, while the next, more extended spectrum cephalosporins were classified as second generation cephalosporins. Currently, four generations of cephalosporins are recognized. Each newer generation of cephalosporins has significantly broader range against gram-negative organisms (such as *Escherichia coli* and *Salmonella*) than the preceding generation. Conversely, the older generations of cephalosporins have greater gram-positive (staphylococcus and streptococcus) coverage than the newer generations. The newer cephalosporins have much longer half-lives resulting in a decrease of dosing frequency. Cephalosporins are the most frequently prescribed class of antibacterials. *Examples:* First generation: cefadroxil (Duricef), cefazolin (Ancef), cephalexin (Keflex), and cephradine (Velosef). Second generation: cefaclor (Ceclor), cefotetan (Cefotan), cefoxitin (Mefoxin), cefprozil

(Cefzil), cefuroxime (Ceftin, Zinacef), and loracarbef (Lorabid). Third generation: cefdinir (Omnicef), cefixime (Suprax), cefoperazone (Cefobid), cefotaxime (Claforan), cefpodoxime (Vantin), ceftazidime (Fortaz, Tazicef), ceftibuten (Cedax), ceftizoxime (Cefizox), and ceftriaxone (Rocephin). Fourth generation: cefepime (Maxipime).

- *cyclic lipopeptides* Broad-spectrum antibacterials; a new class of antibiotic isolated from *Streptomyces* soil bacteria. *Example:* daptomycin (Cubicin).

- *fluoroquinolones* Broad-spectrum antibacterials used to treat bacterial infections in many parts of the body. A newer class of antibacterials, they are generally well tolerated. Fluoroquinolones are synthetic agents, not derived from bacteria. *Examples:* ciprofloxacin (Cipro, Proquin XR), gatifloxacin (Tequin), gemifloxacin (Factive), levofloxacin (Levaquin), lomefloxacin (Maxaquin), moxifloxacin (Avelox), norfloxacin (Noroxin), and ofloxacin (Floxin).

- *glycylcyclines* Broad-spectrum antibacterials; a comparatively new class derived from the older tetracyclines and specifically designed to overcome two common mechanisms of tetracycline resistance. *Example:* tigecycline (Tygacil).

- *ketolides* Narrow-spectrum semisynthetic antibacterials structurally related to the macrolides, but with a broader spectrum. *Example:* telithromycin (Ketek).

- *lincosamides* Narrow-spectrum antibacterials derived from cultures of the bacterium *Streptomyces lincolnensis. Examples:* clindamycin (Cleocin) and lincomycin (Lincocin).

- *macrolides* Narrow-spectrum antibacterials produced naturally by *Streptomyces,* a type of aerobic bacteria, meaning they can grow and live in the presence of oxygen. *Examples:* azithromycin (Zithromax), clarithromycin (Biaxin), and erythromycin (E-Base, E-Mycin).

- *monobactams* Broad-spectrum synthetic antibacterials originally isolated from *Chro-*

mobacterium violaceum. Example: Aztreonam (Azactam).

- *nitrofurans* Broad-spectrum synthetic antibacterials. *Example:* nitrofurantoin (Furadantin, Macrobid, Macrodantin).

- *oxazolidinones* Narrow-spectrum antibacterials used against gram-positive pathogens. *Example:* linezolid (Zyvox).

- *penicillins* Narrow- to broad-spectrum antibacterials obtained from *penicillium* molds (those commonly found on bread or fruits) or produced synthetically; used in the treatment of various infections and diseases. Synthetic penicillins have a broader spectrum of activity than natural penicillins. *Examples:* amoxicillin (Amoxil), ampicillin (Principen), carbenicillin (Geocillin), dicloxacillin, nafcillin, oxacillin, penicillin G (Pfizerpen), penicillin V potassium (Veetids), piperacillin, and ticarcillin (Ticar). There are also several combination pencillins, which further expand the drug's spectrum of action. *Examples:* amoxicillin and clavulanate acid (Augmentin), ampicillin and sulbactam (Unasyn), piperacillin and tazobactam (Zosyn), and ticarcillin and clavulanate (Timentin).

- *polypeptides* Narrow-spectrum antibacterials that are generally too toxic to be used in the body, but are not toxic if used on the surface of the skin (topically). *Examples:* bacitracin and polymyxin B.

- *rifamycins* Broad-spectrum antibacterials originally isolated from a strain of the soil microorganism *Streptomyces mediterranei;* they may be synthesized synthetically. *Examples:* rifabutin (Mycobutin), rifampin (Rifadin), and rifapentine (Priftin).

- *streptogramins* Narrow-spectrum antibacterials produced semisynthetically by various *Streptomyces* species. *Example:* quinupristin/dalfopristin (Synercid), a combination of streptogramins A and B, is the only antibacterial in this class.

- *sulfonamides* Broad-spectrum synthetic antibacterials derived from sulfonic acid; also called sulfa drugs. *Examples:* sulfacetamide, sulfadiazine, sulfamethoxazole/trimethoprim (Bactrim), and sulfisoxazole (Gantrisin).

- *tetracyclines* Broad-spectrum antibacterials that led to the development of many chemically altered antibacterials, proving to be one of the most important discoveries made in the field of antibacterials. *Examples:* demeclocycline (Declomycin), doxycycline (Doryx, Vibramycin), minocycline (Minocin, Dynacin), oxytetracycline (Terramycin), and tetracycline (Achromycin, Sumycin).

- *miscellaneous* Individual drugs are available that are useful for treating specific infections. *Examples:* chloramphenicol (Chloromycetin), metronidazole (Flagyl), and vancomycin (Vancocin, Vancoled).

How They Work

There are a variety of methods by which antibacterials can destroy bacteria. Some impede the processes by which bacteria get energy, others interfere with bacteria genetics (DNA production), others disturb the structure of the bacterial cell wall, and still others interfere with the production of essential proteins. Some antibacterials actually kill the bacteria and are known as bactericidal. Others merely prevent the bacteria from multiplying until the patient's immune system can overcome them and are known as bacteriostatic. High concentrations of most bacteriostatic agents may also be bactericidal.

Aminoglycosides are bactericidal; they inhibit protein synthesis by binding to the 30S and 50S subunits of bacterial ribosome. The ribosome, a small, ball-like particle in the cell's cytoplasm, serves as a platform on which the cell's proteins are made. As protein synthesis is inhibited, cell death follows.

Carbapenems are bactericidal; they inhibit bacterial cell wall synthesis.

Cephalosporins are bactericidal; they inhibit bacterial cell wall synthesis.

Cyclic lipopeptides are bactericidal; they interfere with protein, DNA, and RNA synthesis.

Fluoroquinolones are bactericidal; they interfere with bacteria's ability to reproduce.

Glycylcyclines are bacteriostatic; their mechanism of action is similar to tetracycline antibacterials. Both classes bind to the 30S ribosomal subunit of the bacterial ribosome and prevent protein synthesis; however, the glycylcyclines appear to bind more effectively than the tetracyclines.

Ketolides are bacteriostatic; they prevent bacteria from growing by binding to the 50S subunit of the bacterial ribosome and subsequently blocking protein synthesis.

Lincosamides are bacteriostatic; they inhibit protein synthesis by binding to the 50S subunit of the bacterial ribosome.

Macrolides are bacteriostatic; they inhibit protein synthesis by binding to the 50S subunit of the bacterial ribosome.

Monobactams are bactericidal; they inhibit bacterial cell wall synthesis.

Nitrofurans may be bacteriostatic or bactericidal. Nitrofurantoin is bacteriostatic at low concentrations and bactericidal in higher concentrations; it works by inhibiting the protein and cell wall synthesis in bacteria.

Linezolid has exhibited both bactericidal and bacteriostatic activity; it inhibits protein synthesis by a mechanism that is different from that of all other antibacterial agents. It binds to bacterial 23S ribosomal RNA of the 50S subunit.

Penicillins are bactericidal; they inhibit bacterial cell wall synthesis.

Polypeptides are bactericidal. Bacitracin works by inhibiting bacterial cell wall synthesis, while polymyxin B works by damaging the cytoplasmic membrane of bacteria.

Rifamycins are bactericidal; they work by inhibiting bacterial RNA synthesis. Researchers had believed that rifamycins all killed bacteria in the same way, but in 2005, Artsimovitch et al. reported their discovery that these drugs remove a key component of the bacteria they attack and that different rifamycins bring about this same result in slightly different ways. The researchers noted that their findings help explain why bacteria that are resistant to one kind of rifamycin antibacterial might still be sensitive to another and may help to narrow down the search for new synthetic derivatives to conquer resistance altogether.

Streptogramins are bacteriostatic on their own and bactericidal when used in combination. Dalfopristin inhibits the early phase of protein synthesis in the bacterial ribosome, and quinupristin inhibits the late phase of protein synthesis. The combination of the two components acts synergistically and is more effective than each component alone.

Sulfonamides are bacteriostatic; they work by inhibiting the synthesis of folic acid, which interferes with bacterial growth.

Tetracyclines are bacteriostatic; they work by binding to the 30S subunit of the bacterial ribosome to prevent protein synthesis.

Chloramphenicol is bacteriostatic; it inhibits protein synthesis by binding to the 50S subunit of the bacterial ribosome.

Metronidazole is bactericidal; it works by interfering with bacterial DNA synthesis.

Vancomycin is bactericidal; it works by inhibiting bacterial cell wall synthesis.

The effectiveness of individual antibacterials varies with the location of the infection, the ability of the antibacterial to reach the site of infection, and the ability of the bacteria to resist or inactivate the antibacterial agent.

Approved Uses

Antibacterials are very powerful medications and should be used only when prescribed by a doctor to treat bacterial infections, such as pneumonia, meningitis (inflammation of the membranes [meninges] covering the brain and the spinal cord), urinary tract infections (UTI), otitis media (inflammation of the middle ear), cellulitis (inflammation of the connective tissue underlying the skin), Lyme disease, and tuberculosis.

Aminoglycosides are used to treat life-threatening infections caused by aerobic, gram-negative bacteria—especially bone infections, skin and soft tissue infections, UTIs, respiratory tract infections, meningitis, septicemia (blood poisoning), intra-abdominal infections, endocarditis (an inflammation of the inner layer of the heart), eye infections, and otitis externa (also called swimmer's ear). Kanamycin and streptomycin are also effective against mycobacteria, the bacteria responsible for tuberculosis. Topical gentamicin is used to treat skin infections such as impetigo as well as infected abscesses and cysts and infected contact dermatitis (including poison ivy). Inhaled tobramycin is used in the management of cystic fibrosis patients who have *Pseudomonas aeruginosa* in their lungs.

Carbapenems are used to treat infections that are resistant to traditional antibacterials. They are useful for respiratory tract infections, intra-abdominal infections, septicemia, endocarditis, meningitis, skin and skin structure infections, bone and joint infections, gynecological infections, and UTIs.

All cephalosporins can be used to treat most common UTIs and upper respiratory tract infections such as pharyngitis (throat inflammation) and tonsillitis. First-generation cephalosporins are also used to treat otitis media, bone infections, and skin and soft tissue infections. Cefazolin is also used preoperatively to prevent infections following surgery. Second-generation cephalosporins are also used to treat lower respiratory tract infections such as pneumonia and bronchitis, otitis media, skin and skin structure infections, intra-abdominal infections, gynecological infections, septicemia, bone and joint infections, gonorrhea, and Lyme disease. Third-generation cephalosporins are also used to treat a broad number of bacterial infections, including lower respiratory tract infections, gonorrhea, skin and skin structure infections, sinusitis, septicemia, intra-abdominal infections, meningitis, gynecological infections, and bone and joint infections. Ceftriaxone and cefotaxime are also used preoperatively to prevent infections following surgery. The fourth-generation cephalosporin, cefepime, is also used to treat skin and skin structure infections, pneumonia, febrile neutropenia, and intra-abdominal infections.

Daptomycin, the first cyclic lipopeptide, is used to treat skin and skin structure infections caused by gram-positive bacteria such as methicillin-resistant *Staphylococcus aureus* (MRSA) and *Enterococcus faecalis* (only those strains sensitive to vancomycin).

Fluoroquinolones treat pneumonia and other respiratory illnesses, such as acute bronchitis, as well as UTIs in people over the age of 18. They also are used to treat bone and joint infections, as well as infections in the gastrointestinal tract. Specifically, ciprofloxacin is used in lower respiratory tract infections, bone and joint infections, sinusitis, UTIs, prostatitis, gonorrhea, skin and skin structure infections, typhoid fever, septicemia, Legionnaires disease, febrile neutropenia, intra-abdominal infections, infectious diarrhea, and to prevent the development of progression of anthrax in people following inhalational exposure to anthrax. Ophthalmic ciprofloxacin can be used to treat corneal ulcers and conjunctivitis. Gatifloxacin is used in lower respiratory tract infections, sinusitis, skin and skin structure infections, UTIs, and gonorrhea. Ophthalmic gatifloxacin can be used to treat conjunctivitis. Gemifloxacin is used to treat lower respiratory tract infections. Levofloxacin is used in lower respiratory tract infections, sinusitis, prostatitis, skin and skin structure infections, UTIs, and to prevent the development of inhalational anthrax following exposure. Ophthalmic levofloxacin can be used to treat corneal ulcers and conjunctivitis. Lomefloxacin is used in bronchitis, UTIs, and prior to urologic surgeries to prevent infections. Moxifloxacin is used in lower respiratory tract infections, sinusitis, skin and skin structure infections, and intra-abdominal infections. Ophthalmic moxifloxacin can be used to treat conjunctivitis. Norfloxacin is used in UTIs, gonorrhea, and prostatitis. Ofloxacin is used in lower respiratory tract infections, sexually transmitted diseases (STDs), UTIs, skin and skin structure infections, gynecologic infections, and prostatitis. Ophthalmic ofloxacin can be used to treat corneal ulcers and conjunctivitis. Otic ofloxacin can be used to treat otitis externa and otitis media.

Tigecycline, the first glycylcycline available for clinical use, is effective in treating intra-abdominal and skin and skin structure infections. It can also fight the hard-to-treat bacterium called MRSA. Once spread mostly in hospitals, MRSA now is increasingly spread in the community as well, such as between athletes.

Telithromycin, the first ketolide, is used to treat lower respiratory tract infections and sinusitis.

Lincosamides are used to treat serious infections in patients who are allergic to penicillin or when penicillin is inappropriate. Clindamycin is preferred because it is better absorbed and more potent than lincomycin. Clindamycin is used to treat infections caused by anaerobic bacteria or gram-positive cocci (streptococci, staphylococci). It can be used to treat respiratory tract infections, skin and soft tissue infections, serious bone and joint infections, septicemia, gynecologic infections, and intra-abdominal infections. Topical clindamycin can be used to treat severe acne.

Macrolides are used to treat upper and lower respiratory tract infections, sinusitis, otitis media, gastrointestinal tract infections, and skin and skin structure infections. The macrolides are often used to treat infections in patients who are allergic to penicillin. Erythromycin is also used to treat pertussis (whooping cough), diphtheria, and Legionnaire's disease. Ophthalmic erythromycin can be used to treat corneal ulcers and conjunctivitis. Topical erythromycin is used to treat acne. Both erythromycin and azithromycin can be used to treat STDs and gynecologic infections. Clarithromycin and azithromycin can be used to treat and prevent Mycobacterium avium complex (MAC) disease in patients with advanced human immunodeficiency virus (HIV) infection. Clarithromycin can also be used to treat duodenal ulcer disease associated with *Helicobacter pylori (H. pylori)* infection (in combination with other antibiotics and/or antiulcer drugs).

Aztreonam, the sole monobactam, is used to treat UTIs, lower respiratory tract infections, septicemia, skin and skin structure infections, intra-abdominal infections, and gynecologic infections. It is often used in patients who have an allergy to penicillins.

Nitrofurantoin, the only nitrofuran available in the United States, is used to treat UTIs.

Linezolid, the first commercially available oxazolidinone, is usually reserved for the treatment of serious bacterial infections when older antibiotics have failed due to antibiotic resistance. It is used to treat pneumonia and skin and skin structure infections, including diabetic foot infections caused by gram-positive bacteria. It can be used to treat infections caused by MRSA or those caused by vancomycin-resistant *Enterococcus faecium* (commonly called VREF).

Penicillins are used to treat syphilis, meningitis, endocarditis, upper and lower respiratory tract infections, otitis media, sinusitis, septicemia, skin and soft tissue infections, bone and joint infections, and UTIs as well as to prevent rheumatic fever. Amoxicillin is also used to treat duodenal ulcer disease associated with *Helicobacter pylori (H. pylori)* infection (in combination with other antibiotics and/or antiulcer drugs).

Polypeptides are primarily used topically for the treatment of or prevention of skin infections in minor cuts and abrasions as well as for eye infections.

Rifamycins are particularly effective against mycobacteria. Both rifampin and rifapentine are used in combination with other drugs to treat tuberculosis. Rifampin can also be used to prevent meningitis in people who have been exposed to a *Neisseria meningitidis* infection. Rifabutin is used to treat and prevent MAC disease in patients with advanced HIV infection.

The streptogramin, quinupristin/dalfopristin, is used to treat serious or life-threatening infections associated with VREF bacteremia. It is also approved to treat skin and skin structure infections caused by gram-positive organisms (not including MRSA).

Sulfamethoxazole/trimethoprim is used to treat UTIs, otitis media, bronchitis, and traveler's diarrhea, as well as to treat and prevent *Pneumocystis jiroveci* pneumonia (PCP). Sulfadiazine is used to treat UTIs, malaria, and toxoplasmosis. Sulfisoxazole is used to treat UTIs and otitis media. Sulfacetamide can be used ophthalmically to treat corneal ulcers and conjunctivitis and topically to treat various bacterial skin infections, including acne.

Tetracyclines may be used in the treatment of upper and lower respiratory tract infections, sinusitis, UTIs, STDs, gynecologic infections, Rocky Mountain spotted fever, typhus fever, and eye infections. Tetracycline, doxycycline, and minocycline are used as adjunctive therapy to treat severe acne. Tetracycline is also used to treat duodenal ulcer disease associated with *H. pylori* infection (in combination with other antibiotics and antiulcer drugs). Doxycycline is used to reduce the incidence or progression of disease following exposure to anthrax. Minocycline can also be used to prevent meningitis in people who have been exposed to a *Neisseria meningitidis* infection. Tetracyclines are often prescribed for people who are allergic to penicillin.

Chloramphenicol is effective against a wide variety of microorganisms, but due to serious side effects (see *Warnings*), it is usually reserved for the treatment of serious and life-threatening infections such as typhoid fever, meningitis, and Rocky Mountain spotted fever.

Systemic metronidazole is used to treat the following infections that are caused by anaerobic bacteria or protozoa: intra-abdominal infections, skin and skin structure infections, pseudomembranous colitis (often associated with the use of antibiotics), gynecologic infections, STDs, bone and joint infections, lower respiratory tract infections, septicemia, meningitis, brain abscesses, and endocarditis. Systemic metronidazole is also used to treat duodenal ulcer disease associated with *H. pylori* infection (in combination with other antibiotics and antiulcer drugs). Topical metronidazole is used to treat rosacea, and the vaginal gel is used to treat bacterial vaginosis.

Vancomycin is used to treat serious or severe infections caused by gram-positive bacteria. It is often used after treatment with other antibacterials have failed or in patients who are allergic to penicillins and cephalosporins. These infections may include endocarditis, meningitis, bone infections, respiratory tract infections, septicemia, and skin and skin structure infections. Oral vancomycin therapy is used only in the treatment of pseudomembranous colitis; oral use is not effective against other types of infection.

Off-Label Uses

Amikacin may be used as part of a multidrug regimen for MAC. Gentamicin is used as an alternative treatment for pelvic inflammatory disease.

Imipenem-cilastatin and meropenem are used alone or with other antibacterials to treat presumed bacterial infections in patients with febrile neutropenia.

Among the cephalosporins, ceftriaxone has been shown to be effective in treating arthritis and carditis (inflammation of the muscle tissue of the heart) associated with Lyme disease in patients with penicillin resistance.

The cyclic lipopeptide, daptomycin, may be used to treat infective endocarditis caused by MRSA or vancomycin-resistant enterococci.

Fluoroquinolones are used to treat pediatric patients with febrile neutropenia. Ciprofloxacin has been used to treat acute pulmonary exacerbations in children with cystic fibrosis. Ciprofloxacin and norfloxacin have been used to treat gastroenteritis in children. Levofloxacin, gatifloxacin, and moxifloxacin can be used as alternative agents for the treatment of tuberculosis. Although the ophthalmologic formulations of both moxifloxacin and gatifloxacin are approved only for treatment of conjunctivitis, off-label use for other eye infections such as microbial keratitis and protective treatment for eye surgery has been reported.

Systemic clindamycin is an alternative treatment for anthrax, toxoplasmosis, pharyngitis, and tonsillitis plus is used prior to surgery to prevent infections. Topical clindamycin is used off-label to treat infected eczema and rosacea.

The macrolides have a number of off-label uses. Among them: Azithromycin or clarithromycin can be used to not only prevent infective endocarditis in at-risk patients undergoing dental or surgical procedures who are allergic to penicillin but also to treat early Lyme disease and pertussis. Erythromycin can also be used to treat early Lyme disease as well as gastroparesis (paralysis of stomach muscles, which results in delayed emptying of food from stomach to small intestine).

The polypeptide bacitracin has been used successfully in treating antibiotic-associated colitis.

Among the rifamycins, rifampin is used alone for prophylaxis of *Haemophilus influenzae* type B infection and in combination with other antibacterials to treat a number of infections, such as bone and joint infections and meningitis.

Tetracycline is used off-label in the treatment for early Lyme disease, malaria, and ocular rosacea. Doxycycline is used in the treatment of malaria, ocular rosacea, traveler's diarrhea, and early Lyme disease. Doxycycline is also used as a malaria preventive for travelers. Minocycline is used in the treatment of rheumatoid arthritis.

Chloramphenicol is used as an alternative treatment of anthrax, plague, and bat-bite fever.

Systemic metronidazole is used along with ciprofloxacin to treat Crohn's disease. Topical metronidazole has been used to treat bed sores and perioral dermatitis (a condition related to acne, consisting of red superficial pustules around the mouth).

Administration

Some antibacterials are available in pill form, and some as ointments or eye drops, but more serious infections may be treated with intravenous antibacterials.

Aminoglycosides are generally administered via intravenous or intramuscular injection. Oral aminoglycosides are poorly absorbed and therefore are used primarily for suppression of gastrointestinal flora either for patients prior to bowel surgery (e.g., neomycin) or patients with hepatic encephalopathy, a complication of cirrhosis of the liver (e.g., neomycin, paromomycin). Some aminoglycosides may be given by irrigation (applying a solution to the mucous membrane or washing out a body cavity) or by inhalation into the lungs using a nebulizer (also called an atomizer). Gentamicin is available as an ointment and cream for use on skin infections as well as an ophthalmic ointment and solution for eye infections.

Carbapenems are administered via intravenous or intramuscular injection.

Cephalosporins are administered orally (capsules, tablets, chewable tablets, extended-release tablets, suspension) or via intravenous or intramuscular injection (cefazolin, cefotetan, cefoxitin, cefuroxime [also available orally], cefoperazone, cefotaxime, ceftazidime, ceftizoxime, ceftriaxone, cefepime). Cefaclor extended-release tablets should be taken with food to increase absorption of the medicine (other formulations can be taken without regard to meals). Cefpodoxime tablets should also be taken with food to increase absorption of the medicine (oral suspension can be taken without regard to meals). Cefuroxime oral suspension should also be taken with food (tablets can be taken without regard to meals). Ceftibuten oral suspension should be taken on an empty stomach, at least two hours before or one hour after a meal (capsules can be taken without regard to meals). Loracarbef should also be taken on an empty stomach, either one hour before or at least two hours after a meal.

The cyclic lipopeptide, daptomycin, is administered by intravenous injection.

Fluoroquinolones are administered orally (tablets, extended-release tablets, suspension, solution) or via intravenous injection (ciprofloxacin, gatifloxacin, levofloxacin, moxifloxacin). Ciprofloxacin, gatifloxacin, levofloxacin, moxifloxacin, and ofloxacin are also available as an ophthalmic solution or ointment (ciprofloxacin) for eye infections. Ofloxacin is also available as an otic solution for ear infections. Levofloxacin oral solution should be taken on an empty stomach, either one hour before or two hours after a meal (tablets can be taken without regard to meals). Lomefloxacin and norfloxacin should

also be taken on an empty stomach, either one hour before or at least two hours after a meal.

Tigecycline, currently the only glycylcycline available, is used intravenously.

Telithromycin, currently the only ketolide available, is available as tablets.

The lincosamides, clindamycin and lincomycin, can both be administered via intramuscular or intravenous injection. Clindamycin is also administered orally (capsules, solution) and topically (available as a foam, gel, lotion, solution, swabs, and vaginal cream or suppositories).

The macrolides are available orally (tablets, extended-release tablets, suspension, extended-release suspension) or intravenously (azithromycin, erythromycin). Azithromycin extended-release suspension should be taken on an empty stomach, at least one hour before or two hours after a meal (tablets and immediate-release suspension can be taken without regard to meals). Clarithromycin extended-release tablets should be taken with food to increase absorption of the medicine (immediate-release tablets and suspension can be taken without regard to meals). Erythromycin is also available as a gel, ointment, and solution for skin infections as well as an ophthalmic ointment for eye infections.

The monobactam, aztreonam, is given by intravenous or intramuscular injection.

The nitrofuran, nitrofurantoin, is administered orally as a suspension or capsules. It should be taken with food to increase absorption of the medicine.

The oxazolidinone, linezolid, is administered orally (tablets, suspension) or via intravenous injection.

Penicillins are given by intravenous or intramuscular injection (ampicillin, nafcillin, oxacillin, penicillin G, piperacillin, ticarcillin, ampicillin/sulbactam, piperacillin/tazobactam, ticarcillin/clavulanate) and orally via tablets, capsules, chewable tablets, extended-release tablets, solution, or suspension. Ampicillin, dicloxacillin, and penicillin VK should be taken on an empty stomach, either one hour before or at least two hours after a meal. Amoxicillin/clavulanate extended-release tablets should be taken with food to increase absorption of the medicine (other formulations can be taken without regard to meals).

Among the polypeptides, systemic bacitracin is administered by intramuscular injection and systemic polymyxin by intravenous or intramuscular injection, although intramuscular is not used routinely because of severe pain at injection sites, especially in infants and children. Polypeptides are also available as an ophthalmic ointment or solution for eye infections. Topical bacitracin used to prevent infection in minor wounds is available over-the-counter (OTC) as an ointment or powder.

The rifamycins may be administered orally in tablets or capsules or by intravenous injection. Rifampin should be taken on an empty stomach, either one hour before or two hours after a meal, and with a full glass of water.

The streptogramin quinupristin/dalfopristin is administered by intravenous injection.

Sulfonamides are administered orally (tablets, suspension) or via intravenous injection (sulfamethoxazole/trimethoprim). Sulfacetamide is also available as a cream, foam, gel, or lotion for skin infections and as an ointment and solution for eye infections.

Tetracyclines are administered orally via capsules, delayed-release capsules, tablets, delayed-release tablets, suspension, and syrup and via intramuscular or intravenous injection. Demeclocycline and tetracycline should be taken on an empty stomach, either one hour before or two hours after a meal.

Chloramphenicol is intended for intravenous injection only.

Systemic metronidazole is administered orally (tablets, extended-release tablets, capsules) and intravenously. Extended-release tablets should be taken on an empty stomach, either at least one hour before or two hours after a meal. Topical metronidazole is available as a lotion, cream, gel, and vaginal gel.

Vancomycin is given intravenously for systemic therapy since it does not cross through the intestinal lining when given orally. It may be given orally as capsules to treat colitis, or, alternatively, an oral solution can be prepared using the IV product.

It is very important that patients taking antibacterials complete the full course even if symptoms improve; otherwise, the antibacterials are not given enough time to work on the infection completely, which can cause a relapse. Also, the bacteria can become so resistant that the antibacterials no longer work for that patient the next time.

Double doses should not be taken to make up for missed ones. Rather, the missed dose should be taken at once, unless it is time for the next dose; then the next dose should be taken and the earlier missed dose simply skipped.

Antibacterials should not be shared with anyone, and any leftover antibacterials should be discarded—not saved for later use.

Cautions and Concerns

A major concern with the use of antibacterials is antibiotic resistance, also known as antimicrobial resistance, which occurs when bacteria change in a way that reduces or eliminates the effectiveness of antibacterials. Every time a person takes antibacterials, sensitive bacteria are killed, but resistant germs may be left to survive, grow, and multiply. Resistant bacteria do not respond to the antibacterials and continue to cause more harm, such as a longer illness, more doctor visits, and a need for more expensive and more toxic antibacterials.

The cycle is repeated each time a patient takes an antibacterial unnecessarily or improperly, increasing his or her chances of developing drug-resistant bacteria. Antibiotic resistance can cause significant danger and suffering for people who have common infections that once were easily treatable with antibacterials. Some resistant bacteria may even cause death.

Antibiotic resistance is not a new phenomenon. Within four years of the first widespread use of penicillin, microbes began appearing that could resist this antibacterial. However, experts warn that antibiotic resistance is now one of the world's most pressing public health problems.

According to the Centers for Disease Control (CDC), half of the 100 million antibacterial prescriptions a year written by office-based physicians in the United States are unnecessary because they are prescribed for the common cold and other viral infections, which antibacterials are not active against. Unnecessary use of antibacterials in hospitals is also reportedly common. This overprescribing may contribute to the development of drug-resistant bacteria.

Regarding the use of antibacterials while breast-feeding, Bar-Oz et al. write, "The use of most antibiotics is considered compatible with breast feeding. Penicillins, aminopenicillins, clavulanic acid, cephalosporins, macrolides and metronidazole at dosages at the low end of the recommended dosage range are considered appropriate for use for lactating women."

Because of their potential for damage to the ears and kidneys, intravenous aminoglycosides are administered in doses based on body weight. Blood levels of the drug and serum creatinine need to be monitored during the course of treatment to avoid potentially toxic levels and potential harm to the kidneys. Benzyl alcohol is contained in some aminoglycosides as a preservative, which has been associated with a fatal "gasping syndrome" in premature infants. Some of the drugs in this class also contain sulfites that may cause life-threatening allergic-type reactions in susceptible persons.

Organ system functions, including kidney and liver, need to be monitored for any toxicities during prolonged treatment with carbapenems. Dosage adjustments may be necessary for patients with impaired kidney function.

Diabetic patients should be aware that cephalosporins may cause false test results with some urine sugar tests. Dosage adjustments may be necessary for elderly patients with impaired kidney function. The names of many cephalosporins are quite similar and easily confused.

Patients receiving the cyclic lipopeptide, daptomycin, need to be monitored for the development of muscle pain or weakness. Unexplained muscle pain, tenderness, weakness, numbness or tingling may be early signs of muscle or nerve problems. Serum creatinine phosphokinase (CPK) levels should be monitored weekly in patients receiving daptomycin, as these levels could be elevated. Symptoms of muscle pain or weakness usually resolve within three days, and CPK levels usually return to normal within seven to 10 following discontinuation of therapy. In clinical trials of daptomycin, adverse events were more common in elderly patients compared with those younger than 65.

Fluoroquinolones may exacerbate the signs of myasthenia gravis and lead to life-threatening weakness of the respiratory muscles. Blood glucose disturbances (both hypoglycemia and hyperglycemia) have been reported in diabetic patients taking fluoroquinolones. Close blood glucose monitoring should be performed in these patients. Dosage adjustments may be necessary for patients with impaired kidney function. Fluoroquinolones may cause photosensitivity reactions; susceptible individuals should wear protective clothing and use sunscreens when exposed to ultraviolet light or sunlight.

The safety and effectiveness of glycylcyclines in patients below age 18 have not been established. Tigecycline should be used with caution in patients with impaired liver function.

Telithromycin may cause visual disturbances, including blurred vision, double vision, or trouble focusing. Although most such instances are mild to moderate, patients exhibiting such symptoms should avoid driving, operating machines, or engaging in other potentially dangerous activity. The safety and effectiveness of this drug in patients below age 18 and in breast-feeding women have not been established. Telithromycin should be used with caution in patients with impaired liver function. Dosage adjustments may be necessary for patients with impaired kidney function. Telithromycin may exacerbate the signs of myasthenia gravis and lead to life-threatening weakness of the respiratory muscles.

During prolonged therapy with lincosamides, liver/kidney function tests and blood counts should be monitored. Lincosamides should be used cautiously in patients with gastrointestinal (GI) disease, particularly colitis. Some lincosamide products contain benzyl alcohol, which has been associated with fatal "gasping syndrome" in premature infants. Clindamycin topical solution, suspension, and lotion have an alcohol base that will burn and irritate the eye. The vaginal cream may also cause burning or irritation in the eyes. Patients receiving intravaginal clindamycin should not engage in vaginal intercourse and should not use douches or tampons at any time during therapy. Condoms or vaginal contraceptive diaphragms are weakened by ingredients in vaginal cream and suppositories and may not be effective as contraceptives and/or microbial barriers if used within 72 hours following intravaginal clindamycin.

Because azithromycin is principally eliminated via the liver, caution should be exercised in patients with impaired liver function. Local intravenous site reactions (pain and inflammation) have been reported with the intravenous administration of azithromycin.

Liver-function tests should be periodically monitored during treatment with monobactams. Dosage adjustments may be necessary for patients with impaired kidney function.

Lactic acidosis, characterized by repeated episodes of nausea and vomiting, has been reported in patients taking the oxazolidinone, linezolid. Peripheral and optic neuropathy, even loss of vision, have also been reported in patients treated with linezolid, but in most cases, treatment was for longer than the maximum recommended 28 days.

As many of the penicillins are eliminated by the kidneys, dosage adjustments may be necessary for many of these drugs in patients with impaired kidney function.

Systemic bacitracin has caused rash and anaphylactic reactions ranging from generalized itching, swelling of the face, sweating, and tightness of the chest to hypotension, unconsciousness, and cardiac arrest. If signs of sensitivity occur, the use of bacitracin should be discontinued.

The rifamycins can cause certain bodily fluids, such as urine, semen, sweat, sputum, and tears, to be become orange-red in color. This may permanently stain soft contact lenses. It also may be excreted in breast milk. Therefore breast-feeding should be avoided. These drugs should be used with caution in patients with impaired liver function.

Episodes of severe joint or muscular pain have been reported in patients treated with the streptogramin quinupristin/dalfopristin. Reducing dose frequency has resulted in improvement for some patients. Quinupristin/dalfopristin should be used with caution in patients with impaired liver or kidney function.

Sulfonamides may cause photosensitivity reactions (exaggerated sunburn reaction); susceptible individuals should wear protective clothing and use sunscreens when exposed to ultraviolet light or sunlight. These drugs should be used with caution in patients with impaired liver or kidney function. Patients with diabetes may have an increased risk of developing low blood sugar when receiving a sulfonamide antibacterial. These drugs should also be used with caution in patients with possible folate deficiency (e.g., malnourished, chronic alcoholics, elderly), as they may cause a worsening of this condition. Injectable sulfamethoxazole/trimethoprim contains benzyl alcohol, which has been associated with fatal "gasping syndrome" in premature infants.

Tetracyclines become dangerous past their expiration dates. While most prescription drugs lose potency after their expiration dates, tetracyclines are known to become toxic over time; expired tetracyclines can cause serious damage to the kidneys. Because lightheadedness, dizziness, or vertigo may occur with tetracyclines, patients taking them should observe caution while driving or performing other tasks requiring alertness. Tetracyclines may cause photosensitivity reactions; susceptible individuals should wear protective clothing and use sunscreens when exposed to ultraviolet light or sunlight. Some tetracycline products contain sulfites that may cause allergic reactions in certain susceptible people.

Chloramphenicol should not be used longer than necessary to produce a cure. Blood studies should be evaluated approximately every two days during therapy, as chloramphenicol has been associated with bone marrow suppression with long-term use. Chloramphenicol should be used with caution in patients with impaired liver or kidney function.

Metronidazole should be used with caution in patients with impaired liver function. For such patients, doses below those usually recommended should be administered cautiously. Metronidazole vaginal gel contains ingredients that may cause burning and irritation of the eye.

Since vancomycin is eliminated by the kidneys, dosage adjustments may be necessary in patients with impaired kidney function.

Antibacterial topical products are for external use only; eye contact should be avoided.

Warnings

In rare cases, antibacterials can cause a severe diarrhea known as pseudomembranous colitis. Patients with this disorder have severe watery diarrhea (not simply loose stools). When this occurs, patients need to notify their doctors and not attempt to treat themselves with antidiarrheal medications or wait for it to go away.

Aminoglycosides have the potential for a toxic effect on the ear, especially on its nerve supply, as well as on the kidneys. Auditory changes are irreversible. Damage to the kidneys may also be irreversible. Safety for treatment periods longer than 14 days has not been established.

Serious and occasionally fatal hypersensitivity (anaphylactic) reactions have been reported in patients receiving antibiotics, particularly beta-lactam therapy (carbapenems, cephalosporins, monobactams, penicillins). There is also a risk of cross-sensitivity to these beta-lactam drugs.

The carbapenems should be used with caution in patients with a history of seizures because of their potential for causing seizures in these patients. Seizures from these drugs have occurred most commonly in patients with central nervous system (CNS) disorders.

Several cephalosporins have been associated with seizures. This is more likely to occur in patients with renal impairment when the dosing regimen was not appropriately adjusted. Cefoperazone, cefotetan, and cefoxitin may be associated with a fall in prothrombin activity and problems in poor blood clotting. Those at risk include patients with kidney or liver impairment, cancer, or poor nutritional state as well as patients receiving a protracted course of antimicrobial therapy and patients previously stabilized on anticoagulant therapy. Prothrombin time should be monitored in patients at risk, with vitamin K given as needed. Some cephalosporins may cause kidney toxicity.

Since late 2004, fluoroquinolones have been required by the FDA to carry the following risk warnings or precautions: irreversible peripheral neuropathy (nerve damage), tendinitis including spontaneous tendon rupture both during and after therapy, seizures, pseudomembranous colitis, and ventricular arrhythmias, including torsades de pointes. To minimize the risk of seizures, fluoroquinolones should be used with caution in patients with a history of seizures or other factors that may predispose them to seizure development (drug interactions, impaired kidney function). In February 2006, the FDA announced labeling changes for gatifloxacin to strengthen the previous warning of risks of low blood sugar and high blood sugar (see *Contraindications*).

Telithromycin may cause increased liver enzymes and hepatitis, with or without jaundice. These changes usually reverse when therapy is discontinued. In January 2006, FDA MedWatch issued a statement noting that three patients had experienced serious liver toxicity following administration of telithromycin. One of the patients died from liver failure, and another required a liver transplant. The statement read, "The FDA is continuing to evaluate the issue of liver problems in association with use of telithromycin in order to determine if labeling changes or other actions are warranted." Telithromycin has also been associated with prolongation of the QTc interval, which may predispose patients to the development of torsades de pointes. (The QT interval is the time between the start of the Q wave and the end of the T wave in the cardiac electrical cycle. The QTc is the QT interval corrected for heart rate.)

Lincosamides can cause severe and possibly fatal colitis, characterized by severe persistent diarrhea, severe abdominal cramps, and possibly by the passage of blood and mucous. These symptoms can begin up to several weeks following cessation of therapy.

Azithromycin has rarely been associated with allergic reactions, including swelling, anaphylaxis, and severe skin reactions. Although rare, fatalities have been reported. Despite initially successful treatment of the allergic symptoms, once treatment was discontinued, the allergic symptoms returned soon thereafter in some patients without further azithromycin exposure. These patients required prolonged treatment. If pregnancy occurs while taking clarithromycin, the patient should be apprised of potential hazard to the fetus. Macrolides (especially clarithromycin and erythromycin) have been associated with prolongation of the QTc interval, which may predispose patients to the development of torsades de pointes.

Rare cases of toxic epidermal necrolysis (a life-threatening skin condition) have been reported in association with the monobactam, aztreonam, in patients undergoing bone marrow transplant with multiple risk factors including sepsis, radiation therapy, and other concomitantly administered drugs associated with toxic epidermal necrolysis.

Nitrofurantoin has caused acute and more rarely chronic pulmonary reactions manifested by sudden and severe shortness of breath, chills, chest pain, fever, and cough. If a pulmonary reaction is suspected, nitrofurantoin should be discontinued immediately.

Myelosuppression, a reduction in the ability of the bone marrow to produce blood cells, has been reported in patients receiving the oxazolidinone, linezolid. Complete blood counts should be monitored weekly in patients who receive linezolid, particularly when treatment lasts longer than two weeks.

Cystic fibrosis patients have a higher incidence of side effects when treated with piperacillin.

In December 2004, the FDA announced important labeling changes regarding Bicillin CR (penicillin G benzathine and penicillin G procaine injectable suspension) and Bicillin LA (penicillin G benzathine injectable suspension), which included a new boxed warning against intravenous use plus a precautionary note for Bicillin CR explaining it is not for treatment of syphilis. Intravenous administration of Bicillin CR or Bicillin LA has been associated with serious adverse effects in postmarketing reports, including cardiorespiratory arrest and death. The CDC's 2002 Sexually Transmitted Diseases Treatment Guidelines recommend penicillin G benzathine for the treatment of syphilis infection, consistent with the labeled indications for Bicillin LA. However, the manufacturer, King Pharmaceutical, Inc., became aware of postmarketing reports from multiple STD clinics in the United States where Bicillin CR had been inappropriately used to treat patients infected with syphilis.

Intramuscular administration of polypeptides may cause kidney failure and should be used only when constant supervision of the patient is possible. Kidney function should be carefully monitored prior to and daily during intramuscular therapy. The recommended daily dose should not be exceeded and fluid intake and urinary output maintained at proper levels to avoid kidney toxicity. If toxicity occurs, the drug should be discontinued.

Rifamycins have been shown to produce liver damage, and fatalities associated with jaundice have occurred in patients with liver disease who were taking these drugs. Thus, patients with impaired liver function should be given rifamycins only in cases of necessity and then with caution and under strict medical supervision. In these patients, careful monitoring of liver function is necessary.

In rare cases, patients have experienced severe and life-threatening reactions to sulfonamides, including sudden, severe liver damage, serious blood dyscrasias (aplastic anemia, agranulocytosis), Stevens-Johnson syndrome (a severe inflammatory eruption of the skin and mucous membranes), and toxic epidermal necrolysis (a syndrome with red, blistering, peeling skin). Complete blood counts need to be monitored frequently, especially during prolonged administration.

Tetracyclines should be used with caution in those with liver impairment and may worsen renal failure (except doxycycline). Tetracyclines should be used with caution in patients with history of allergy, asthma, or hay fever, as they are more likely to experience sensitivity reactions. The use of tetracyclines during tooth development (from the last half of pregnancy through eight years of age) may cause permanent discoloration of teeth.

Serious and fatal blood dyscrasias (aplastic anemia, hypoplastic anemia, thrombocytopenia, and granulocytopenia) are known to occur after the administration of chloramphenicol. In addition, there have been reports of aplastic anemia attributed to chloramphenicol that later terminated in leukemia. Damage to the bone marrow may occur. Toxic reactions, including fatalities, have occurred in premature infants and newborns, most often when therapy was begun within the first 48 hours of life. The symptoms associated with these reactions have been referred to as the "gray syndrome."

Seizures and peripheral neuropathy (characterized mainly by numbness or pins-and-needles feeling of an extremity) have been reported in patients treated with metronidazole. If abnormal neurologic signs appear, metronidazole should be discontinued immediately. Metronidazole should be administered with caution to patients with central nervous system diseases. Also, metronidazole has shown evidence of carcinogenic activity with long-term use in a number of animal studies, but the risk to humans is unknown.

Rapid administration of vancomycin may be associated with abnormally low blood pressure, including shock and, rarely, cardiac arrest. Ototoxicity (damage to the ear) has occurred in patients receiving vancomycin, but mostly in those receiving excessive doses or who have an underlying hearing loss.

When Not Advised (Contraindications)

Colds, flu, and sore throats (except for those resulting from strep throat) are usually caused by viruses and should not be treated with antibacterials.

Broad-spectrum antibiotics should be prescribed with caution in individuals with a history of gastrointestinal disease, particularly colitis.

Antibacterials are not generally advised for women who are breast-feeding due to risk of alteration to the infant's intestinal flora and risk of masking infection in the infant.

With the exception of streptomycin for tuberculosis, aminoglycosides are generally not advised for long-term therapy because of potential for ear and kidney toxicity with extended use.

Because lidocaine HCl is used to dilute imipenem-cilastatin and ertapenem intramuscular administration, this use is contraindicated in patients with a known hypersensitivity to local anesthetics of the amide type. Carbapenems should not be used in patients with a history of immediate-type hypersensitivity (anaphylactic) reactions to penicillins or cephalosporins.

Some cephalosporins contain benzyl alcohol, which has been associated with neurological and other complications, even fatalities, in newborn infants; thus, benzyl alcohol–containing cephalosporins should not be used in newborns. Cephalosporins should not be used in patients with a history of immediate-type hypersensitivity reactions to penicillins or carbapenems.

Because fluoroquinolones may affect bone growth, they are not recommended in children or pregnant women, except for ciprofloxacin, which is indicated in children. Even ciprofloxacin should not be considered the drug of choice in children (except for anthrax). This applies more for systemic administration than for topical (ophthalmic, otic). Gatifloxacin is not recommended for use in diabetic patients because of the significant risk of hyperglycemia or hypoglycemia (see *Warnings*).

The glycylcycline tigecycline may cause fetal harm when administered to a pregnant woman. Also, its use during tooth development (last half of pregnancy, infancy, and childhood to the age of eight years) may cause permanent discoloration of the teeth (yellow-gray-brown).

The ketolide telithromycin is not recommended for use in patients with myasthenia gravis, as it may make the symptoms worse and potentially lead to life-threatening respiratory failure. Telithromycin is also not recommended in patients who may be at increased risk for developing ventricular arrhythmias, especially torsades de pointes. These patients include those with a prolonged QTc interval at baseline, abnormally slow heart rate, low blood levels of potassium or magnesium, or those receiving class Ia or III antiarrhythmic drugs. Pregnancy and breast-feeding is a caution with this drug; also, kidney disease is a caution.

Clindamycin should not be used by patients with a history of regional enteritis, ulcerative colitis, or antibiotic-associated colitis.

Clarithromycin should not be used in pregnant women except in clinical circumstances when no alternative therapy is appropriate.

Nitrofurantoin should not be used in persons with poor kidney function. Although its use has proved to be reasonably safe during pregnancy, nitrofurantoin should not be used near term or during labor or delivery, as it interferes with the immature enzyme systems in the red blood cells of newborns, damaging the cells and causing anemia. Because of this, nitrofurantoin should also not be used in infants less than one month of age.

Penicillins should not be used in any patient with a history of hypersensitivity reaction to any penicillin, cephalosporin, or carbapenem.

Sulfonamides are not recommended for individuals with hypersensitivity to chemically related drugs, such as thiazide and loop diuretics (except ethacrynic acid), carbonic anhydrase inhibitors, or sunscreens with PABA. Sulfonamides are also not recommended in patients with megaloblastic anemia due to folate deficiency. Because of the risk of kernicterus (form of brain damage caused by excessive bilirubin levels in the blood), sulfonamides are also not recommended in women who are pregnant (at term) or breast-feeding or in children less than two months of age.

Tetracyclines are not recommended for children under the age of nine or for pregnant women because of the potential for permanent tooth discoloration.

Chloramphenicol must not be used to treat trivial infections nor for prevention of infections.

Metronidazole should not be used in pregnant women with trichomoniasis during the first trimester and should be used in the second and third trimesters only after alternative treatment has inadequately controlled symptoms.

Side Effects

Side effects from antibacterials range from slight headache to a major allergic reaction. One of the more common side effects is diarrhea, which results from the antibacterial destroying the beneficial intestinal flora, the "good" bacteria necessary for digestion and protection against infection inside the human digestive system. Other side effects can include lightheadedness, headaches, cramps, vomiting, and stomach discomfort. It is important for patients to let their physicians know if any of these side effects persist or become serious.

Allergies may develop with the use of antibacterials. Such allergic reactions may range from rashes, hives, and itching to swelling of a person's throat, difficulty breathing, and potential death. The allergy usually does not occur until the patient's second exposure to a drug.

Side effects for aminoglycosides include kidney damage, hearing loss, headache, dizziness, clumsiness, unsteadiness, increased thirst, loss of appetite, numbness, difficulty breathing, and muscle twitching or paralysis. Streptomycin can also cause tingling or burning of the mouth or face. In addition, streptomycin injections are painful, and abscesses may form at injection sites.

The more common side effects for carbapenems include nausea, vomiting, diarrhea, constipation, bloated abdomen, phlebitis, low blood pressure, headache, fever, and rash.

Cephalosporins may cause allergic reactions such as rash, itching, or fever. More common side effects for cephalosporins include mild diarrhea, mild stomach cramps, nausea, chest pain, chills, cough, fever, painful or difficult urination, vaginal itching or discharge, shortness of breath, sore throat, swollen glands, unusual bleeding or bruising (more common for cefoperazone, cefotetan, and cefoxitin), headache, unusual tiredness or weakness, and sores, ulcers, or white spots on lips or in mouth.

The more common side effects with the cyclic lipopeptide, daptomycin, include constipation, nausea, diarrhea, injection site reactions, and headache.

The more common side effects for fluoroquinolones include nervousness, headache, dizziness, lightheadedness, drowsiness, insomnia, nausea, vomiting, rash, abdominal pain or cramping, and diarrhea. Fluoroquinolones may also make the skin extra sensitive to sunlight (see *Cautions and Concerns*).

The most common side effects of tigecycline are nausea, diarrhea, and vomiting. Nausea and vomiting are mild or moderate and usually occur during the first two days of therapy. Other side effects include pain at the injection site, swelling, and irritation. Tigecycline is similar to tetracyclines and therefore may have similar side effects such as increased sensitivity to sunlight.

Telithromycin's more common side effects include diarrhea, headache, nausea, vomiting, dizziness, visual disturbances, headache, and elevated liver function tests.

The most common side effects of lincosamides are gastrointestinal (diarrhea, nausea, vomiting, abdominal pain). Less common are skin rashes, vertigo, and pain following injection.

The most common side effects of the macrolides include abdominal pain, nausea, vomiting, diarrhea, rash, and jaundice. Gastrointestinal symptoms may be minimized by taking these drugs with food. Erythromycin may cause headache or dizziness. When given by injection, erythromycin may cause severe phlebitis (inflammation of the veins). Clarithromycin can also cause taste disturbances.

Common side effects of the monobactam aztreonam include diarrhea, nausea, vomiting, and rash. Less common are hypotension, flushing, confusion, headache, vertigo, and amnesia. Local reactions, such as phlebitis following intravenous administration and discomfort/swelling at the injection site following intramuscular administration, have also occurred.

The most common side effects with nitrofurantoin are gastrointestinal, including nausea and vomiting, loss of appetite, diarrhea, and abdominal pain—which can usually be avoided by taking the drug with food. Nitrofurantoin may also cause headache, dizziness, or drowsiness.

The most common side effects for the oxazolidinone linezolid include rash, diarrhea, nausea, vomiting, constipation, headache, insomnia, dizziness, and fever.

Common side effects for the penicillins include diarrhea, abdominal cramps, nausea, skin rash, and hives. Pain and inflammation at the injection site are also common.

Common side effects for polypeptides include facial flushing, dizziness, skin rashes, nausea, and vomiting.

The most common side effects of rifamycins are gastrointestinal disturbances (heartburn, nausea, vomiting, cramps, diarrhea), fever, headache, dizziness, fatigue, reddish-orange discoloration of bodily fluids (urine, semen, sweat, sputum, and tears), skin rashes, flushing, and sore tongue or mouth.

The more common side effects of the streptogramin quinupristin/dalfopristin include pain, burning, or inflammation at the infusion site, joint or muscle aches, nausea, diarrhea, vomiting, rash or itching, and headache.

The most common side effects of sulfonamides are diarrhea, nausea, vomiting, skin rashes, dizziness, headache, loss of appetite, and tiredness. These effects usually occur during the first few days as the body adjusts to the drug. Sulfonamides may also make the skin extra sensitive to sunlight (see *Cautions and Concerns*).

Tooth discoloration can occur with the use of tetracyclines (see *Warnings*). Tetracylines may also make the skin extra sensitive to sunlight (see *Cautions and Concerns*). Other common side effects of tetracyclines include upset stomach with nausea or vomiting and diarrhea.

Chloramphenicol side effects include nausea, vomiting, diarrhea, headache, and mild depression. (See also *Warnings*.)

Common side effects associated with metronidazole include headache, dizziness, nausea, metallic taste, dark urine, diarrhea, and abdominal pain. Topical metronidazole can cause local redness, dryness, and/or skin irritation plus eye watering if applied near the eyes.

Vancomycin may cause itching, wheezing, fever, nausea, or chills. A reaction called "red man syndrome" may also occur if the vancomycin is infused too quickly, when patients can develop flushing and a rash. This reaction is reversible if the rate of infusion is slowed down.

Interactions

Use of all antibacterials may temporarily reduce the effectiveness of birth control pills; alternative birth control methods should be used while taking these drugs.

The aminoglycosides can interact with a variety of other drugs causing increased toxicity and/or decreased effectiveness. Aminoglycosides may increase the effects of neuromuscular-blocking agents. Penicillins, cephalosporins, amphotericin B, and loop diuretics may exacerbate the potential for kidney toxicity associated with aminoglycosides.

The carbapenems should not be administered concurrently with probenecid, a drug used primarily in the treatment of gout. Imipenem-cilastatin should not be administered along with the antiviral ganciclovir, as generalized seizures have occurred with this combination.

Patients receiving cefoperazone or cefotetan should not drink alcoholic beverages or take other alcohol-containing preparations during treatment and for several days after stopping treatment. Alcohol in combination with these drugs may cause stomach cramps, nausea, vomiting, headache, fainting, fast or irregular heartbeat, difficult breathing, sweating, or redness of the face or skin. H_2 antagonists, iron supplements, and antacids may decrease the absorption of cefdinir and cefpodoxime. When antacids must be taken during treatment with these drugs, the cephalosporin should be taken two hours before or after the antacid. Probenecid may increase the effects of cephalosporins. Some cephalosporins may increase the effects of warfarin (see *Warnings*) and place the patient at an increased risk of bleeding.

Anticoagulant activity in patients receiving daptomycin and warfarin should be monitored for the first several days after initiating therapy with daptomycin. HMG-CoA reductase inhibitors may cause myopathy when taken along with daptomycin; therefore, temporarily discontinuing use of these drugs during daptomycin therapy should be considered.

Because fluoroquinolones interact with a large number of other medicines, patients taking them should provide their doctors with a list of all other medications they take on a regular basis, including OTC drugs and herbal preparations. The concomitant use of calcium, iron, zinc, sucralfate, didanosine (used to treat HIV infection), or antacids containing magnesium or aluminum may decrease the absorption of fluoroquinolones (administration should be separated by approximately two hours). Ciprofloxacin can increase levels of theophylline. Gatifloxacin taken along with glucose-altering medications can result in serious low blood sugar or high blood sugar. Fluoroquinolones may also increase the effects of antiarrhythmic agents, caffeine, and warfarin. Cimetidine may increase the effects of fluoroquinolones.

Tigecycline may decrease the elimination of warfarin, thereby increasing warfarin levels in blood.

The use of telithromycin with pimozide is not recommended because of the increased risk of ventricular arrhythmias, such as torsades de pointes. Telithromycin may increase the action and toxicity of atorvastatin, lovastatin, and simvastatin; thus the use of these statins should be suspended during telithromycin therapy. Telithromycin can increase the effects of alprazolam, midazolam, triazolam, carbamazepine, cyclosporine, sirolimus, tacrolimus, and metoprolol. The risk for torsades de pointes may be increased if telithromycin is administered with other drugs that prolong the QTc interval (class Ia and III antiarrhythmics, fluoroquinolones, antipsychotics). Telithromycin may increase digoxin concentrations as well as the effects of warfarin. The action of telithromycin may be increased by concurrent use of fluconazole, itraconazole, ketoconazole, calcium channel blockers, and human immunodeficiency virus (HIV) protease inhibitors. The action of telithromycin may be reduced by concurrent use of carbamazepine, phenobarbital, phenytoin, Saint-John's-wort, and rifampin.

Because the lincosamides have neuromuscular blocking properties, they should be used with caution in patients receiving neuromuscular-blocking agents.

Concurrent use of macrolides and warfarin in clinical practice has been associated with increased anticoagulant effects. Macrolides have elevated digoxin levels. Taking erythromycin and clarithromycin along with atorvastatin, simvastatin, or lovastatin can cause muscle damage. Concurrent use of clarithromycin with pimozide or ergot derivatives is not recommended because of the increased risk for toxicity. The risk for torsades de pointes may be increased if erythromycin or clarithromycin is administered with other drugs that prolong the QTc interval (class Ia and III antiarrhythmics, fluoroquinolones, antipsychotics). Other drugs that can interact with macrolides include fluconazole, itraconazole, ketoconazole, carbamazepine, calcium channel blockers, H_2 antagonists, phenytoin, rifampin, phenobarbital, benzodiazepines, cyclosporine, tacrolimus, sirolimus, sildenafil (and other similar drugs), HIV protease inhibitors, and theophylline.

Antacids may decrease the absorption of the nitrofuran, nitrofurantoin. Probenecid may increase the effects of nitrofurantoin.

The oxazolidinone linezolid is a weak monoamine oxidase inhibitor (MAOI) and cannot be taken along with foods or beverages with high tyramine content. Foods containing considerable amounts of tyramine include fish, chocolate, alcoholic beverages, and fermented foods such as cheese, soy products, sauerkraut, and processed meat. Linezolid also has the potential for interaction with adrenergic agents (e.g., dopamine and epinephrine) and serotonergic agents (e.g., fluoxetine, paroxetine, and sertraline).

Concurrent administration of bacteriostatic antibacterials (e.g., erythromycin, tetracycline) may diminish the bactericidal effects of penicillins by slowing the rate of bacterial growth. While most of the penicillins can increase the bleeding risks of warfarin, dicloxacillin and nafcillin have been associated with warfarin resistance.

Polypeptides used along with aminoglycosides may increase the risk of respiratory paralysis and kidney dysfunction.

Rifamycins accelerate the metabolism of anticonvulsants, antiarrhythmics, antifungals, beta-blockers, calcium channel blockers, chloramphenicol, clarithromycin, corticosteroids, cyclosporine, digoxin, hormonal contraceptives, dapsone, diazepam, doxycycline, fluoroquinolones, haloperidol, oral hypoglycemic agents (e.g., sulfonylureas), levothyroxine, narcotic analgesics, phenobarbital, progestins, quinine, tacrolimus, theophylline, tricyclic antidepressants, warfarin, and zidovudine. Dosages of these drugs may need to be increased when taken along with rifamycins.

Selected drugs that are predicted to have plasma concentrations increased by the streptogramin, quinupristin/dalfopristin, include (but are not limited to) anti-HIV drugs (delavirdine, nevirapine, indinavir, ritonavir), antineoplastic agents (vinblastine, docetaxel, paclitaxel), benzodiazepines (midazolam, diazepam), calcium channel blockers, HMG-CoA reductase inhibitors (lovastatin, simvastatin, atorvastatin), immunosuppressive agents (cyclosporine, tacrolimus), steroids (methylprednisolone), carbamazepine, quinidine, lidocaine, and disopyramide.

Among the drugs that may interact with sulfonamides are angiotensin-converting enzyme inhibitors, angiotensin II receptor antagonists, cyclosporine, carbamazepine, phenytoin, phenobarbital, glimepiride, glipizide, glyburide, pioglitazone, rosiglitazone, warfarin, fluoxetine, sertraline, amantadine, methotrexate, and potassium-sparing diuretics.

Antacids, iron, calcium supplements, and milk reduce the absorption of tetracyclines. Tetracyclines may increase the effects of benzodiazepines, calcium channel blockers, tacrolimus, HMG-CoA reductase inhibitors (lovastatin, simvastatin, atorvastatin), and warfarin. Phenobarbital, phenytoin, carbamazepine, and rifampin may decrease the effects of tetracyclines.

Phenobarbital and rifampin may decrease the effects of chloramphenicol. Chloramphenicol may increase the effects of warfarin and phenytoin.

Metronidazole may cause nausea, vomiting, headache, and possibly convulsions when taken in combination with heavy alcohol consumption. Alcohol should be avoided by patients during systemic metronidazole therapy and for three days after completion of treatment. Metronidazole has been reported to enhance the effects of warfarin and lithium. Phenobarbital and phenytoin may decrease the effects of metronidazole. However, cimetidine may increase the effects of metronidazole.

Administration of vancomycin along with anesthetic agents has been associated with reddening of the skin and histaminelike flushing in children.

Sales/Statistics

According to RiboNovix, Inc., a pharmaceutical firm founded in 2003 to discover and develop new antibiotic drugs that are refractory to antibiotic resistance, antibiotics are the second largest pharmaceutical market, with annual worldwide sales of about $25 billion, including $8 billion in the United States. RiboNovix reported that five antibacterials had revenues of more than $1 billion in 2001, and 15 have sales of more than $250 million annually. Those five antibacterials are Cipro, $2.2 billion; Augmentin, $2 billion; Zithromax, $1.5 billion; Rocephin, $1.3 billion; and Biaxin/clarithromycin, $1.2 billion. However, mortality from infectious disease in the United States increased 58 percent from 1980 to 1992, and infectious diseases currently kill 33 percent of persons over 65 years old—primarily due to the rise of antibiotic-resistant bacteria. The annual cost of treating patients infected with antibiotic-resistant strains of microorganisms in the United States alone is more than $30 billion.

Belgian researchers found that antibiotic use dropped by almost 12 percent during a flulike outbreak that occurred after two three-month public awareness campaigns, which took place in 2000–01 and 2001–02 and which stressed the proper use of antibacterials.

According to IMS Health Incorporated, betalactam antibacterials were the most commonly prescribed antibacterials in the world based on 2002 sales. Based on sales figures reported by pharmaceutical companies, worldwide carbapenem (a class of beta-lactam antibacterials) sales increased 13.8 percent to more than $1 billion in 2003 compared to 2002.

The RxList of Top 300 Prescriptions for 2004 (retail and mail order, excluding Wal-Mart) included several antibacterials; among them: amoxicillin, 41,393,538; Zithromax, 37,171,754; cephalexin, 23,665,172.

In 2010, according to IMS Institute for Healthcare Informatics (the public reporting arm of IMS), penicillins were the 17th most prescribed drug class (76.1 million prescriptions dispensed), followed by macrolides "and similar types," with 73.9 million prescriptions. On their ranking of specific drugs, azithromycin ranked seventh, with 52.6 million prescriptions, and amoxicillin eighth, with 52.3 million prescriptions.

Demographics and Cultural Groups

Children are of particular concern for antibiotic resistance because they have the highest rates of antibiotic use. They also have the highest rate of infections caused by antibiotic-resistant pathogens.

In a review of pediatric drug trend data over the previous five years, the Medco Health Solutions 2002 Drug Trend Report revealed that spending on antibacterials for children increased by 42 percent. However, more recent studies have shown that physician prescribing in this category is on the decline.

Development History

Antibacterials are not as new as their development history indicates. The Chinese used moldy curd of soybeans to treat boils and infections 2,500 years ago. In modern medicine, their actions were probably first observed by the French chemist Louis Pasteur in 1877, who discovered that certain bacteria from fungi (molds) can kill anthrax germs. Around the year 1900, the German bacteriologist Rudolf von Emmerich isolated a substance called pyocyanase, which can kill the germs of cholera and diphtheria in the test tube. It was not useful, however, in curing disease.

It was not until the second quarter of the 20th century that the antibacterial era had its real beginnings when penicillin, the first antibacterial, which had been discovered by Alexander Fleming from a mold culture in 1928, was first tested on humans during the winter of 1940–41. Fleming had shown penicillin's effectiveness in laboratory cultures against many disease-producing bacteria, such as those that cause gonorrhea and certain types of meningitis and bacteremia (blood poisoning). However, he performed no experiments on animals or humans. Because the organism that produced the substance that killed the bacteria was a species of *Penicillium*, Fleming named the substance penicillin.

The parent compound of sulfonamides—para-aminobenzenesulfonamide—was synthesized in 1908 by Paul Gelmo, an Austrian industrial chemist. In 1932, the German chemist Gerhard Domagk discovered that the red azo dye Prontosil had antagonistic properties against a wide range of bacteria. Then in 1935, the English medical researcher Leonard Colebrook found that the sulfanilamide portion of the Prontosil molecule was responsible for its antibacterial effect. He introduced sulfamidochrysoidine (trade name Prontosil), the first sulfonamide drug and the first synthetic antibacterial, as a cure for puerperal (childbed) fever, a condition resulting from infection after childbirth or abortion.

The first natural antibacterial to be used in the treatment of human diseases was gramicidin, which was isolated from certain soil bacteria by the American bacteriologist Rene Jules Dubos in 1939. This substance was too toxic for general use, but became useful as a powerful topical antimicrobial agent. Along with Fleming's discovery of penicillin, this finding led the way into the modern era of antibacterial treatment, in which soil organisms played a dominant role.

Beginning in 1939, resources were concentrated on investigating and purifying penicillin, and a team led by the British scientists Howard Walter Florey and Earnest Chain succeeded in producing usable quantities of the purified active ingredient, which were tested on clinical cases—its first use on humans. Results were dramatic, and physicians were elated with the rapid and complete recovery of patients who received penicillin for conditions that had, until then, been difficult to treat, terrible to endure, and frequently fatal. World War II interfered with the large-scale production of penicillin in Great Britain, so methods for its mass production, purification, and stabilization were instead developed in the United States.

As scientists observed other species of mold and other organisms waging a previously unknown level of chemical warfare against bacteria, a large number of substances that inhibit or kill bacteria were rapidly discovered and came into widespread use. The discovery of antibacterials has been ranked among the most important advances in medicine, along with anesthesia and the adoption of hygienic practices by physicians.

Streptomycin was the first aminoglycoside to be discovered (1943) and was the first antibacterial to treat tuberculosis.

Cephalosporins were first isolated in 1948 from cultures of *Cephalosporium acremonium* taken from a sewer in Sardinia by the Italian scientist Giuseppe Brotzu. Brotzu discovered that a substance produced by these cultures was effective against *Salmonella typhi*, the cause of typhoid. The first commercial cephalosporin, cephalothin (Keflin), was launched in 1964 by Eli Lilly (it is no longer on the market in the United States).

Tetracyclines were first isolated in 1949.

Macrolides were first isolated in the 1950s. Erythromycin was derived in 1952 from a strain of *Streptomyces erythreus* from soil in the Philippines.

Carbapenems were introduced in the late 1980s.

Fluoroquinolones were first introduced in 1986.

In 1999, quinupristin-dalfopristin was the first semisynthetic streptogramin to be approved for clinical use in the United States.

In 2000, the FDA approved linezolid, the first entirely new type of antibiotic developed in more than 30 years.

The compound for daptomycin, the first cyclic lipopeptide, was discovered by Eli Lilly researchers in the 1980s, with rights to it bought by Cubist Pharmaceuticals in 1997. They brought it to market following its FDA approval on September 12, 2003.

Telithromycin, the first ketolide, was approved by the European Commission in July 2001 and gained FDA approval on April 1, 2004.

In June 2005, the FDA approved tigecycline as the first in the new glycylcyclines class of antibacterials.

Future Drugs

When announcing the FDA approval of their new antibacterial Tygacil, Wyeth noted that few broad-spectrum antibacterial agents are currently in development. "Antibiotic development has slowed to the point that the FDA has had few opportunities to approve new agents. In fact, development and approvals of new antibacterial agents have decreased by 56 percent over the past 20 years (1998–2002 vs. 1983–87). New classes of antibacterials are needed to address increasing antibiotic resistance among common pathogens."

Dell'Acqua and Balaban explained several obstacles to antibacterial drug development:

- The limited life span of new antibacterials due to a number of factors, including the largely indiscriminate and pervasive use of such drugs (leading to antibiotic resistance), and the fact that newly introduced antibacterials are merely modifications of existing ones. This short life span has also caused Big Pharma to lose interest in new antimicrobials. The total cost to develop and bring a new drug to market is $800 million and requires up to eight years from early testing in animals to product launch. While this investment would produce a favorable return for drugs to treat chronic diseases such as cancer and neurologic and musculoskeletal conditions, the return is not as favorable for antibacterials.

- The increased regulatory requirements for antibacterials. In the early 1990s, the FDA introduced guidelines that resulted in new and costly demands for the development of antibacterials. In an era when hospital- and community-acquired infections are increasingly drug resistant, the efficacy of new antibacterials is benchmarked against susceptible strains, such as methicillin-susceptible *Staphylococcus aureus*.

- New antimicrobials would be more likely to make it to market if the FDA introduced new references, such as drug-resistant strains of bacteria, and used new pathogenic targets to evaluate efficacy, such as the inhibition of toxins or prevention of biofilms. A biofilm is essentially a carpet of bacteria that forms after an organism has entered a host. Within the biofilm, bacteria are encased in a glyco-calix matrix and are protected from the environment. The host's immune defenses and antibiotics are relatively ineffective at eliminating bacteria within a biofilm.

A promising new ketolide is cethromycin, for the treatment of community-acquired pneumonia and other respiratory tract infections. A new drug application was submitted to the FDA in 2008.

Artsimovitch, Irina, et al. "Allosteric Modulation of the RNA Polymerase Catalytic Reaction Is an Essential Component of Transcription Control by Rifamycins." *Cell* 122, no. 3 (August 12, 2005): 351–363.

Bar-Oz, B., et al. "Use of Antibiotic and Analgesic Drugs During Lactation." *Drug Safety* 26, no. 13 (2003): 925–935.

Bauraind, I., et al. "Association Between Antibiotic Sales and Public Campaigns for Their Appropriate Use." *Journal of the American Medical Association* 292, no. 20 (November 24, 2004): 2,468–2,470.

Dell'Acqua, Giorgio, and Naomi Balaban. "Barriers on the Road to New Antibiotics." *The Scientist* 19, no. 5 (March 14, 2005): 42.

Spencer, Jane. "The Risks of Mixing Drugs and Herbs." *Wall Street Journal*, June 22, 2004; D1.

Velicer, Christine, et al. "Antibiotic Use in Relation to the Risk of Breast Cancer." *Journal of the American Medical Association* 291, no. 7 (February 18, 2004): 827–835.

anticoagulants Also called blood thinners, anticoagulants prevent or slow the blood from excessive clotting in the arteries or veins, which blocks blood flow. The body's ability to form blood clots is vital to control bleeding (hemostasis) following tissue injury, such as puncture wounds. However, too much clotting increases the risk of a heart attack, stroke, or pulmonary embolism (PE) (a blood clot blocking an artery of the lungs).

Thrombosis, the abnormal formation of a clot within a blood vessel, is a common cause of death in the United States, with approximately 2 million Americans dying each year from an arterial or venous thrombosis or its consequences. The most common form of thrombosis is deep-vein thrombosis (DVT) in the leg. This type of clot can break apart, travel up the leg and through the heart, lodging in the lungs and causing PE. A study published in 2005 found that more than 900,000 Americans each year suffer from either DVT or PE or both. Almost 300,000 die each year from DVT/PE, usually without forewarning.

Anticoagulants are used to reduce the chance of blood clots forming during open-heart or bypass surgery. They are also used following various other types of surgery, such as orthopedic, abdominal, gynecological-obstetrical, urological, and neurological, to prevent DVT and/or PE. Anticoagulants are also used in people with artificial heart valves, irregular heart rhythms (i.e., atrial fibrillation, atrial flutter), and blood-clotting disorders. People who are at risk for excessive clot formation, such as those who are bedridden, may take anticoagulants in order to maintain normal blood flow. About 4 million Americans take anticoagulants.

The term *antithrombotics* includes anticoagulants, ANTIPLATELETS, and THROMBOLYTICS.

Classes

Anticoagulants are divided into several classes according to their chemical makeup.

- *coumarins* Synthetic anticoagulants. *Example:* warfarin (Coumadin, Jantoven).
- *heparin* (also known as *unfractionated heparin*) A natural anticoagulant derived from

pig intestine. It is one of the oldest anticoagulants available.

- *low molecular weight heparins* (LMWHs) A modified type of heparin. *Examples:* dalteparin (Fragmin), enoxaparin (Lovenox), tinzaparin (Innohep).
- *direct thrombin inhibitors Examples:* argatroban, bivalirudin (Angiomax), dabigatran (Padraxa), lepirudin (Refludan).
- *factor Xa inhibitors Example:* fondaparinux (Arixtra).

How They Work

Anticoagulants do not really *thin* the blood; they inhibit the action of blood proteins called clotting factors. Clotting factors are produced by the liver and interact to form a blood clot. In order for the liver to produce certain clotting factors (specifically, factors II, VII, IX, and X), sufficient amounts of vitamin K must be available. Warfarin decreases the levels of vitamin K within the liver, limiting the production of these clotting factors. As a result, the clotting mechanism is impaired, causing it to take longer for the blood to clot.

Heparin slows down the formation of clots by blocking the action of thrombin (clotting factor IIa), an enzyme produced by the body that plays a pivotal role in the clotting process. It also inhibits clotting factors IX, X, XI, and XII. It does this by binding to and activating one of the body's own anticlotting proteins, antithrombin III. Antithrombin III is then able to bind to thrombin, thereby blocking the activity of thrombin and interfering with the clotting process. By increasing heparin levels in the blood, the time taken for a clot to form is increased.

LMWHs also bind to antithrombin III; however, because they contain far fewer of the large polymers needed for thrombin inactivation, they cause antithrombin III to primarily bind to factor Xa. (LMWHs also have an effect on thrombin [factor IIa], but their primary effect is on factor Xa.) With factor Xa tightly bound to antithrombin III, it cannot interact with prothrombin.

This inhibits the conversion of prothrombin to thrombin and prevents blood clots from forming and getting larger. Unlike standard heparins, LMWHs are less susceptible to interacting with plasma proteins and therefore have a more predictable anticoagulant effect.

Direct thrombin inhibitors interrupt the positive feedback loop responsible for amplifying thrombin generation. The drug maker AstraZeneca explains, "Unlike heparin and LMWH, which inhibit thrombin via potentiation of the effect of antithrombin III, direct thrombin inhibitors bind directly to the thrombin molecule without the need for any additional cofactors, and are active against free circulating thrombin as well as thrombin entrapped in, or bound to, fibrin in a thrombus (clot-bound thrombin)."

Unlike other anticoagulants, which act on multiple sites, factor Xa inhibitors are more specific. These drugs bind to antithrombin III, which then inhibits the activity of factor Xa.

Approved Uses

Warfarin is used to prevent and treat venous thrombosis and PE, as well as thromboembolic complications associated with atrial fibrillation and/or cardiac valve replacement. It is also used to reduce the risk of death, recurrent myocardial infarction (MI), and thromboembolic events such as stroke or systemic embolization after MI.

Heparin is used to prevent and treat venous thrombosis, PE, and peripheral arterial embolism. It is also used to prevent DVT and PE following surgery, to prevent the formation of clots in people with atrial fibrillation, and for patients otherwise at risk of developing thromboembolic disease (blood vessel obstructed by a clot carried in the bloodstream from the site of formation). Heparin is also used to prevent clotting during cardiac and vascular surgery and as an anticoagulant in blood transfusions, extracorporeal circulation (when the blood circulates outside the body, e.g., through a heart-lung machine or artificial kidney), dialysis procedures, and blood samples for laboratory purposes.

Dalteparin is used to prevent DVT (which may lead to PE) in patients undergoing hip replacement or abdominal surgery or in immobile medical patients who are acutely ill and at risk for blood clot complications. Dalteparin can also be used for the treatment of unstable angina or a certain type of heart attack.

Enoxaparin is used to prevent DVT (which may lead to PE) in patients undergoing hip replacement, knee replacement, or abdominal surgery or in immobile medical patients who are acutely ill and at risk for blood clot complications. Enoxaparin is also used along with warfarin for treatment of acute DVT, with or without PE. Enoxaparin can also be used for the treatment of unstable angina or a certain type of heart attack.

Tinzaparin is used along with warfarin for treatment of acute DVT, with or without PE.

Argatroban and lepirudin are used to treat and reduce the risk of blood clots in patients who have had a reaction to heparin that resulted in reduced platelets and associated blood clots (heparin-induced thrombocytopenia, or HIT). Bivalirudin is approved to reduce the risk of blood clotting in adults who are undergoing a procedure to open blocked arteries in the heart (percutaneous coronary intervention, or PCI). Both argatroban and bivalirudin are also approved to reduce the risk of blood clotting in patients undergoing PCI who are at risk or have HIT. Dabigatran is used to help prevent strokes or serious blood clots in people who have atrial fibrillation (irregular heartbeat).

Fondaparinux is used to reduce the risk of DVT, which may lead to PE, in patients undergoing abdominal surgery (specifically for those at risk of blood clot complications), hip fracture surgery, hip replacement surgery, or knee replacement surgery. Fondaparinux is also approved for the treatment of DVT and PE.

Off-Label Uses

Warfarin has been used to prevent recurrent transient ischemic attack (TIA) (caused by the temporary disturbance of blood supply to a restricted area of the brain; sometimes called a ministroke) and to treat antiphospholipid syndrome, an autoimmune disorder characterized by excessive clotting of blood.

Heparin is used to prevent left ventricular blood clots and strokes following MI. Heparin is also used along with warfarin to treat valve thrombosis and to reduce the incidence of stroke in patients with heart valve replacement.

Companion Drugs

Heparin (as well as LMWHs) and warfarin may be given at the same time. Both heparin and LMWHs act quickly. Warfarin takes two to three days before it starts to work. Once the warfarin starts to work, the heparin or LMWH is stopped.

Fondaparinux is used along with warfarin to treat blood clots in the veins and blood clots that have broken off and traveled to the lungs (PE) when the patient is first treated in the hospital. Once the warfarin starts to work, the fondaparinux is stopped.

Administration

Warfarin is the only orally available anticoagulant currently approved for use in the United States. In addition to the tablet form, an intravenous injection is available for patients who cannot take drugs orally.

Heparin is administered via intravenous injection or subcutaneously (under the skin). Intramuscular injections are avoided because of the potential for forming hematomas. Because of its short biologic half-life of approximately one hour, heparin must be given frequently or as a continuous infusion when administered intravenously.

LMWHs are administered by subcutaneous injection and should not be injected directly into the vein or muscle. Because they do not require as much monitoring as heparin, they can often be given to patients at home.

Most direct thrombin inhibitors are administered via intravenous injection. Dabigatran comes as a capsule to take by mouth.

Fondaparinux is administered by subcutaneous injection.

Cautions and Concerns

Patients receiving anticoagulant therapy need to take care to prevent cuts and other accidents because anticoagulants increase the risk of bleeding. Anticoagulants generally should be used with caution in people with conditions that increase the risk of bleeding, such as inflammation of the heart and/or the tissue surrounding the heart; severe uncontrolled high blood pressure; bleeding disorders, including liver failure and certain protein deposits (amyloidosis); active ulcerative colitis and other disorders in the stomach and intestines; bleeding into the brain (hemorrhagic stroke); gastrointestinal bleeding; low platelets (thrombocytopenia); and recent brain, spinal, or eye surgery.

Warfarin therapy is highly individualized and can be affected by numerous factors, including travel, environment, health, diet, medications, and herbals (see *Interactions*). Thus, periodic coagulation testing is essential. During the course of therapy with warfarin, patients will need to have periodic blood tests performed not only to monitor the blood-thinning effects of the drug but also to make sure they are not experiencing adverse bleeding effects.

Periodic monitoring of the blood for platelet counts, hemoglobin, hematocrit (the volume percentage of red blood cells), and occult blood (cannot be seen by the naked eye) in the stool is necessary during anticoagulant therapy.

LMWHs may need to be administered in lower doses in people with kidney disease. Multiple-dose vials of dalteparin and tinzaparin contain benzyl alcohol as a preservative, which has been associated with "gasping syndrome" in premature infants. Tinzaparin contains a sulfite that may cause a severe allergic reaction including life-threatening asthma in patients sensitive to sulfites.

The dose of lepirudin or bivalirudin should be decreased in patients who have kidney disease, while the dose of argatroban should be reduced in patients with liver disease. Dabigatran may cause stomach bleeding. Because daily use of alcohol while using this medicine may increase risk for stomach bleeding, patients should limit or avoid alcoholic beverages.

The most common test used to monitor heparin's effect is the activated partial thromboplastin time (aPTT), which measures the time it takes blood to clot. It is used to determine the most effective dosage for heparin.

Warnings

Hemorrhage can occur at any site in patients receiving anticoagulants. These drugs should be used with extreme caution in patients who have an increased risk of hemorrhage and should be discontinued immediately if hemorrhage occurs.

The most serious risks with warfarin therapy are hemorrhage and, less frequently, necrosis (cell death) and/or gangrene of skin and other tissues. Hemorrhage and necrosis have in some cases resulted in death or permanent disability. About 5 percent of those on warfarin develop serious bleeding problems.

Warfarin may also lead to purple toes syndrome, the sudden appearance of painful purple lesions on the toes and sides of the feet that lose their color with pressure. The syndrome usually develops three to eight weeks after the start of warfarin therapy. Although a rare complication of warfarin therapy, patients need to be monitored for its development.

HIT has occurred in patients receiving heparin with a reported incidence of up to 30 percent. It has been reported to be the most common serious drug reaction in hospitals. Patients on heparin may develop new thrombus formation in association with HIT, resulting from irreversible aggregation of platelets induced by heparin, a condition called white clot syndrome. The process may lead to severe thromboembolic complications such as skin necrosis, gangrene of the extremities (that may lead to amputation), myocardial infarction, pulmonary embolism, stroke, and possibly death.

LMWHs and fondaparinux can cause bleeding into the spine when used in patients who have received epidural or spinal anesthesia or any spinal injection. Bleeding in the spine can cause long-term or permanent paralysis. LMWHs cannot be used interchangeably with other LMWHs.

Dabigatran increases the risk of bleeding and can cause significant and sometimes fatal bleeding. Risk factors for bleeding include the use of drugs that increase the risk of bleeding in general (e.g., antiplatelet agents, heparin, fibrinolytic therapy, and chronic use of NSAIDs) and labor and delivery. Discontinuing anticoagulants, including dabigatran, for active bleeding, elective surgery, or invasive procedures places patients at an increased risk of stroke. Lapses in therapy should be avoided, and if anticoagulation with dabigatran must be temporarily discontinued for any reason, therapy should be restarted as soon as possible.

When Not Advised (Contraindications)

Anticoagulants are contraindicated in patients with a history of major bleeding, aneurysms, severe liver disease, or severe uncontrolled hypertension.

Pregnant women cannot take warfarin, as it passes through the placental barrier and may cause fatal hemorrhage to the fetus. There have been reports of birth defects in children born to mothers who have been treated with warfarin during pregnancy. Also, spontaneous abortion and stillbirth are known to occur, and a higher risk of fetal mortality is associated with the use of warfarin. Low birth weight and growth retardation have also been reported. Warfarin should also not be used in patients with recent or contemplated eye, brain, or spinal cord surgery or any traumatic surgery resulting in large open surfaces.

Heparin should not be used in patients with severe thrombocytopenia, uncontrolled bleeding, or a history of HIT.

LMWHs should not be given to people who are currently experiencing major bleeding or have a history of HIT.

The direct thrombin inhibitors should not be given to individuals who currently have major bleeding.

Fondaparinux should not be given to patients who have severe kidney problems, weigh less than 110 pounds, have active bleeding, have a heart infection (bacterial endocarditis), or have a history of thrombocytopenia due to fondaparinux.

Side Effects

Anticoagulants can cause hemorrhage from any organ or tissue, necrosis (see *Cautions and Concerns* and *Warnings*), and bruising. Complications from hemorrhage may present as paralysis; paresthesia (prickling feeling on the skin); headache, chest, abdomen, joint, muscle, or other pain; dizziness; shortness of breath, difficult breathing or swallowing; unexplained swelling; weakness; abnormally low blood pressure; or unexplained shock.

Patients with hypersensitivity to heparin may experience chills, fever, headache, nausea, or shock. Osteoporosis has been reported following long-term administration of high doses of heparin.

HIT may occur shortly after heparin or an LMWH is given, as well as after a person has been on any of these drugs for a long while.

The most common side effects of LMWHs include irritation and pain at the injection site, easy bruising and bleeding, fever, and allergic reactions.

In addition to bleeding, other side effects of argatroban may include shortness of breath, low blood pressure, fever, and diarrhea. Other side effects of bivalirudin include back pain, nausea, very low or very high blood pressure, headache, injection site pain, insomnia, pelvic pain, anxiety, vomiting, slow heart rate, abdominal pain, and fever. Other side effects of dabigatran include gastrointestinal symptoms (an uncomfortable feeling in the stomach [dyspepsia]), stomach pain, nausea, heartburn, and bloating. Other side effects of lepirudin include abnormal liver function, fever, and allergic skin reactions.

Bleeding is the most common side effect of fondaparinux. Other side effects include fever, injection site reactions, nausea, vomiting, constipation, rash, insomnia, or thrombocytopenia.

Interactions

A variety of foods and herbals should be avoided in patients who are receiving anticoagulant therapy as they may increase the risk of bleeding. Examples of these substances include alfalfa, cranberries, dong quai (angelica), feverfew, garlic, ginger, ginkgo biloba, ginseng, grapefruit, green tea, horseradish, licorice, parsley, red clover, and sweet clover.

Vitamin K produces blood-clotting substances and may reduce the effectiveness of warfarin. Thus, patients on warfarin therapy should not take vitamin K supplements and should maintain a consistent intake of vitamin K–containing foods (such as broccoli, brussels sprouts, cauliflower, kale, spinach, and turnip greens). Significant fluctuations (increase or decrease) in the intake of these foods can lead to variable effectiveness of the warfarin.

Many drugs, both prescription and over-the-counter (OTC), can affect the action of anticoagulants. The use of aspirin, nonsteroidal anti-inflammatory drugs (NSAIDS) (e.g., ibuprofen), clopidogrel, ticlopidine, thrombolytics, or dipyridamole may enhance the action of all anticoagulants (warfarin, heparin, and LMWHs) and lead to an increased risk of bleeding. There are a number of drugs that may also specifically interact with warfarin that could lead to an increased risk of bleeding. Examples of such drugs include acetaminophen, amiodarone, cimetidine, antibacterials, azole antifungals, selective serotonin reuptake inhibitors, statins, thyroid hormones, and vitamin E (400 IU or more).

Some medications may decrease the action of warfarin, which could increase the risk of clot formation. Examples of such drugs include oral contraceptives containing estrogen, barbiturates, and rifampin. Because so many drugs interact with warfarin, it is important for patients on warfarin therapy to alert all of their doctors and

pharmacists of any medications they are currently taking and to consult their medical providers before taking any additional OTC drugs. It is also advisable for patients on warfarin therapy to carry identification to alert emergency personnel that they are taking this drug.

Acute alcohol consumption increases blood levels of warfarin, which may increase the patient's risk for bleeding. Chronic alcohol consumption decreases blood levels of warfarin, which may increase the risk of clot formation.

Concomitant use of dabigatran and strong P-gp inducers (e.g., rifampin, Saint-John's-wort) results in significant reductions in dabigatran exposure and should generally be avoided. Caution is advised in coadministering dabigatran and P-gp inhibitors (e.g., amiodarone, dronedarone, ketoconazole, quinidine, and verapamil), as increased dabigatran exposure may occur.

Sales/Statistics

The annual global market for anticoagulant therapies in 2000 was approximately $6 billion. In 2005, 22.6 million prescriptions for warfarin were dispensed in the United States, with sales totaling $538,671,000.

In 2000, worldwide sales of all heparin products, which includes LMWHs, were estimated to be more than $4 billion, with a 15 percent yearly growth rate. One-third of hospitalized patients in the United States, approximately 12 million in total, receive heparin/LMWH.

U.S. sales of factor Xa inhibitors totaled $1.35 billion in 2003. U.S. sales of direct thrombin inhibitors in 1999 totaled only approximately $15 million but were reported to have the potential to increase significantly in the future.

The IMS Institute for Healthcare Informatics (the public reporting arm of IMS, a pharmaceutical market intelligence firm) reported that warfarin was the 20th most prescribed drug in 2010, with 32 million prescriptions dispensed.

Demographics and Cultural Groups

Warfarin dose requirements vary across ethnic groups. Greaves notes that population studies have suggested "a genetic component to coumarin sensitivity; for example, people of Chinese origin are more sensitive, and African Americans less sensitive, than those of European ancestry."

In a study supported by the Agency for Healthcare Research and Quality, Christian et al. identified 19,051 nursing home residents who had been hospitalized for ischemic stroke in five states over a four-year period. They found that Asian/Pacific Islander, black, and Hispanic residents eligible for anticoagulant therapy received warfarin less often than white residents.

Development History

The development of warfarin can be traced directly to an epidemic of cattle deaths in North Dakota and Canada during the early 1920s. Cattle were dying from uncontrollable bleeding from very minor injuries or sometimes dropped dead from internal hemorrhage. In 1922, Frank W. Schofield, a Canadian veterinarian, traced these deaths to moldy silage containing spoiled sweet clover, which functioned as a potent anticoagulant. Mixing alfalfa, a food rich in vitamin K, into the silage prevented the disease.

However, the identity of the anticoagulant substance in spoiled sweet clover remained a mystery. In 1931, a North Dakota veterinarian, L. M. Roderick, found that the hemorrhaging was caused by the reduced activity of prothrombin, a clotting factor in blood. Isolating prothrombin was finally accomplished in 1939 by Karl Link and H. A. Campbell, working at the University of Wisconsin agricultural college. The chemists determined that the anticoagulant substance was the coumarin derivative 4-hydroxycoumarin. Over the next few years, numerous similar chemicals were found to have the same anticoagulant properties. The first of these to be widely commercialized was dicumarol, patented in 1941. During the 1940s, dicumarol was widely used in the United States to treat postoperative thrombosis. Link continued working on developing more potent coumarin-based anticoagulants for use as rodent poisons, resulting in warfarin in 1948, which was first registered for use as a rodenticide.

Because of its apparent toxicity, the medical community hesitated to use warfarin on human patients. Then, in 1951, a naval recruit unsuccessfully attempted suicide with large amounts of warfarin and recovered fully. Soon studies began with the use of warfarin as a therapeutic anticoagulant. It was found to be generally superior to dicumarol and in 1954 was approved for medical use in humans.

Heparin is one of the oldest drugs currently still in widespread clinical use. It was originally isolated from liver cells, thus its name (hepar is Greek for liver). William Henry Howell, the first professor of physiology at the Johns Hopkins Medical School, had been searching for years for an anticoagulant that could work safely in humans. His student Jay McLean in 1916 found a compound extracted from dog liver that acted as an anticoagulant. After McLean left Johns Hopkins, Howell continued working on the liver extract; however, he was unable to obtain a product pure enough for human use.

In the early 1930s, University of Toronto researchers successfully prepared a pure product, first from beef liver and later from beef lung, and developed practical methods for standardizing the drug. The Canadian surgeon Gordon Murray was chosen to evaluate the potential of the new drug. After his animal experiments demonstrated that heparin made operations on blood vessels possible, Murray began treating human patients with heparin in 1935.

Dissatisfaction linked with the limitations of these older drugs prompted the search for and study of new anticoagulants. Nenci wrote, "While the old anticoagulants were discovered by chance, most of the new molecules have been developed following a rational design aimed at overcoming the drawbacks as well as potentiating the benefits of already existing agents. Only a few of the more recent drugs are extracted from the animal world (e.g., leeches, worms, ticks); indeed, most of them are synthetic even if some reproduce or mimic the active part of naturally occurring anticoagulants."

The development of LMWHs began in the early 1970s, when Canadian researchers led by the anticoagulant expert Jack Hirsh, M.D., were studying the optimal way to deliver heparin in an experimental rabbit model. According to Dr. Hirsh, "By chance we noted that a fragment of heparin about a third of the size of standard heparin produced less bleeding for an equivalent anti-clotting effect. This was followed by ten years of experimental work." Enoxaparin was the first LMWH approved for use in the United States, in 1993.

The first direct thrombin inhibitor to be approved by the FDA (1998) was lepirudin, a synthetic hirudin, which is a natural substance derived from the saliva of the medicinal leech *Hirudo medicinalis.* Approval of argatroban and bivalirudin followed in 2000, and dabigatran was approved in 2010.

Bauer noted that "breakthroughs in polysaccharide chemistry made possible the synthesis of a new class of antithrombotic compounds, the synthetic oligosaccharides." Fondaparinux, the first of this new class, a selective inhibitor of factor Xa, received FDA approval in 2001.

Future Drugs

Decision Resources, Inc., a market research firm, predicted in September 2005 that the launch of new drugs would generate 12 percent annual growth in the anticoagulant drug market over the next 10 years. The firm specifically mentioned the forthcoming oral factor Xa inhibitor rivaroxaban (Bayer), which was submitted to the FDA in January 2011 for approval for the prevention of stroke and systemic embolism in patients with nonvalvular atrial fibrillation. Myriad Genetics, Inc. announced in October 2005 that it was nearing completion of the preclinical data package on MPC-0920, its oral direct thrombin inhibitor drug candidate, for submission to the FDA prior to beginning human clinical trials. Bristol-Myers Squibb is also developing an oral factor Xa inhibitor, razaxaban, which is currently in Phase IIb clinical trials.

Bauer, Kenneth A. "New Pentasaccharides for Prophylaxis of Deep Vein Thrombosis: Pharmacology." *Chest* 124, no. 6 Suppl. (December 2003): 364A-370S.

Christian, Jennifer B., Kate L. Lapane, and Rebecca S. Toppa. "Racial Disparities in Receipt of Secondary Stroke Prevention Agents among U.S. Nursing Home Residents." *Stroke* 34, no. 11 (November 2003): 2,693–2,697.

Greaves, Mike. "Pharmacogenetics in the Management of Coumarin Anticoagulant Therapy: The Way Forward or an Expensive Diversion?" *PLoS Medicine* 2, no. 10 (October 2005). Available online. URL: http://medicine.plosjournals.org/perlserv?request=get-document&doi=10.1371/journal.pmed.0020342.

Hirsh, Jack. "Anticoagulants." Canadians for Health Research. Available online. URL: http://www.chrcrm.org/main/modules/pageworks/index.php?page=011&id=195. Downloaded on May 26, 2006.

Nenci, Giuseppe G. "Novel Factor Xa– and Thrombin-Inhibitors." *Current Pharmaceutical Design* 11, no. 30 (November 2005): 3,853.

anticonvulsants Also called antiepileptics or antiseizure medications, anticonvulsants include a diverse group of drugs used to relieve or prevent the occurrence of epileptic seizures or convulsions. Epilepsy is a brain disorder in which clusters of nerve cells, or neurons, in the brain sometimes signal abnormally. Neurons normally generate electrochemical impulses that act on other neurons, glands, and muscles to produce human thoughts, feelings, and actions. In epilepsy, the normal pattern of neuronal activity becomes disturbed, causing strange sensations, emotions, and behavior or sometimes convulsions, muscle spasms, and loss of consciousness. Seizures are called simple if there is no loss of consciousness and complex if there is a loss of consciousness. During a seizure, neurons may fire as many as 500 times a second, much faster than the normal rate of about 80 times a second. In some people, this happens only occasionally; for others, it may happen up to hundreds of times a day. More than 2 million people in the United States—about one in 100—have experienced an unprovoked seizure or been diagnosed with epilepsy. However, having a seizure does not by itself mean a person has epilepsy. First-time seizures (often occurring in reaction to anesthesia or a strong drug but sometimes without any obvious triggering factor), febrile seizures (childhood seizures during the course of an illness with a high fever), nonepileptic events (resemble seizures, but the brain shows no seizure activity), and eclampsia (a life-threatening condition that can develop in pregnant women) are examples of seizures that may not be associated with epilepsy.

Classes

Anticonvulsants are grouped into classes according to how they work in the brain.

- *Barbiturates* have been used as anticonvulsants for nearly 100 years. *Examples:* Phenobarbital is the oldest epilepsy drug still in use. Although all barbiturates exhibit anticonvulsant actions, only phenobarbital is commonly used today for treatment of seizures. Pentobarbital (Nembutal) is sometimes used to treat seizures; mephobarbital (Mebaral) is more rarely used. Today barbiturates are used less often for treating seizures because of their sedative effects and addiction potential. (See also ANTIANXIETY AGENTS.)

- *Benzodiazepines* are not used for chronic therapy to prevent seizures from recurring, but they are used in the treatment of status epilepticus. While occasional use can be helpful, most patients do not respond well to them over long periods of time due to a diminution of their pharmacological effects. *Examples:* Clonazepam (Klonopin), clorazepate (Tranxene), diazepam (Valium), and lorazepam (Ativan). (See also ANTIANXIETY AGENTS.)

- *Hydantoins* have a slow onset of action. *Examples:* fosphenytoin (Cerebyx), phenytoin (Dilantin).

- *Oxazolidinediones.* Trimethadione (Tridione) is the only oxazolidinedione that is currently available, and it is not often used.

- *Succinimides* are generally used to control absence (formerly called petit mal) seizures. *Examples:* ethosuximide (Zarontin), methsuximide (Celontin).

- *Miscellaneous unique drugs* that do not fall into the above classes. These are adjuncts to the more widely used anticonvulsants and are used in patients who do not respond adequately to the other anticonvulsants. *Examples:* acetazolamide (Diamox), carbamazepine (Carbatrol, Tegretol, Epitol), felbamate (Felbatol), gabapentin (Neurontin), lamotrigine (Lamictal), levetiracetam (Keppra), oxcarbazepine (Trileptal), pregabalin (Lyrica), primidone (Mysoline), tiagabine (Gabitril), topiramate (Topamax), valproic acid (Depakene, Depakote), zonisamide (Zonegran).

How They Work

Anticonvulsant drugs generally inhibit seizure activity by depressing the abnormal neural discharges in the central nervous system (CNS). Roach and Scherer explain, "Generally, anticonvulsants reduce the excitability of the neurons (nerve cells) of the brain. When neuron excitability is decreased, seizures are theoretically reduced in intensity and frequency of occurrence or, in some instances, are virtually eliminated." Some anticonvulsants try to influence the action of gamma-amino butyric acid (GABA), a neurotransmitter that carries messages between brain nerve cells. GABA inhibits the transmission of nerve signals, thereby reducing nervous excitation. Other anticonvulsants limit the spread of impulses from one nerve to another inside the brain. When a patient does not respond well to one anticonvulsant, the physician will prescribe a different one or a combination of drugs until the appropriate treatment regimen is determined. During early treatment, dosages may need to be increased or decreased until the correct dosage for that person is determined.

Barbiturates and primidone (metabolized into phenobarbital) work similarly and elevate the seizure threshold by decreasing the excitability of the neurons in the brain.

Benzodiazepines prevent or stop seizures by slowing down the CNS, thereby making abnormal electrical activity less likely.

The precise mechanism by which hydantoins work is not known, but they are thought to reduce the flow of sodium into and out of nerve cells, making the cells less likely to send out spontaneous impulses and begin seizures.

Succinimides elevate the seizure threshold, making it more difficult for a nerve impulse to spread from one nerve to another.

The mechanism by which acetazolamide works against seizures is unclear, but it appears to reduce the firing of neurons in the brain. It is not used often because most people tend to build up a resistance to it.

The mechanism of action of carbamazepine and its derivatives (e.g., oxcarbazepine) is not well understood, but they appear to prevent seizures by reducing the influx of sodium into nerve cells.

It is not known exactly how felbamate prevents seizures; however, it is thought that it prevents seizures by blocking the effects of some of the brain chemicals that stimulate the CNS.

The precise mechanism by which gabapentin and levetiracetam prevent seizures is not clear. However, it is thought that gabapentin may inhibit calcium channels.

Lamotrigine primarily works by inhibiting the release of glutamate (an excitatory hormone) and by inhibiting sodium and calcium channels.

Pregabalin works by blocking a receptor on over-firing neurons, which is believed to help reduce the excessive activity that can cause seizures.

Tiagabine and topiramate are believed to work, in part, by enhancing the actions of GABA. Topiramate is also thought to inhibit sodium channels.

Valproic acid is believed to increase the availability, enhance the actions, or mimic the effects of GABA.

While the mechanism by which zonisamide prevents seizures is unclear, it is thought to work by inhibiting sodium and calcium channels.

Approved Uses

Most anticonvulsants are used to treat specific types of seizures. Roach and Scherer note, "Drugs that control generalized tonic-clonic seizures are not effective for absence seizures." (*Tonic-clonic* is the newer term for grand mal or major motor seizure, characterized by loss of consciousness, falling, stiffening, and jerking.) Some anticonvulsants also have other medical uses, such as relieving certain types of pain.

Phenobarbital is used for controlling simple and complex partial seizures (formerly called psychomotor seizures or temporal lobe epilepsy) and generalized tonic-clonic seizures in patients of all ages. It is also used for emergency treatment of acute convulsive episodes, such as those associated with status epilepticus, eclampsia (coma and convulsions during or immediately after pregnancy), tetanus, or toxic reactions to strychnine or local anesthetics. Although phenobarbital is sometimes used alone, it is more commonly used in combination with other anticonvulsants.

Pentobarbital is used to treat acute convulsive episodes or to place patients with head injuries in a drug-induced coma.

Benzodiazepines stop seizures quickly. Diazepam and lorazepam are often used to treat prolonged seizures or status epilepticus. Diazepam may be used during short periods of increased, repeated, or prolonged seizures (acute repetitive seizures or clusters) in people who are taking other antiseizure drugs for long-term treatment.

Phenytoin is used to control generalized tonic-clonic and complex partial seizures as well as to prevent and treat seizures that occur during or following neurosurgery. Fosphenytoin is approved for the short-term (five days or less) treatment of seizures when the usual means of phenytoin administration are not possible or are ill-advised. Fosphenytoin is also used for the treatment of generalized convulsive status epilepticus as well as to prevent and treat seizures that occur during or following neurosurgery.

Trimethadione is used to control absence seizures. Trimethadione and methsuximide are used when these seizures are resistant to other drugs.

Although succinimides can be used to control and prevent absence seizures, they are most often used in conjunction with other anticonvulsants to control other types of seizures, such as other generalized seizures (e.g., tonic-clonic).

Acetazolamide is used to treat glaucoma, epileptic seizures, edema, and high-altitude sickness in mountain climbers. In epilepsy, its main use is in absence seizures, particularly in children, with some benefit in other seizure syndromes.

Carbamazepine is used to treat simple and complex partial seizures and in generalized tonic-clonic seizures. It is used to treat a painful nerve condition of the face called trigeminal neuralgia. Oxcarbazepine is used alone and with other drugs to treat partial seizures in adults and children as young as four years of age.

Because of the potential serious side effects that may exceed those of primary anticonvulsants, felbamate is recommended for use only in certain patient populations with partial seizures who have responded inadequately to other treatments.

Gabapentin is used in combination with other anticonvulsants to treat partial seizures. It is also approved to manage postherpetic neuralgia in adults.

Lamotrigine is used to treat partial seizures and generalized seizures associated with Lennox-Gastaut syndrome (LGS), a severe form of epilepsy that typically develops before age four and is associated with developmental delays. In 2003, lamotrigine was also approved by the Food and Drug Administration (FDA) for use as a maintenance treatment for people with bipolar disorder.

Levetiracetam is used as an adjunct treatment for partial-onset seizures in adults and children.

Pregabalin was approved on June 10, 2005, as a treatment for partial onset seizures in adults. It had originally been approved on December 21, 2004, for the management of neuropathic pain associated with diabetic peripheral neuropathy and postherpetic neuralgia.

Primidone is used either alone or in conjunction with other anticonvulsants to control tonic-clonic, partial, or focal seizures.

Tiagabine is used in combination with other anticonvulsants to treat partial seizures in adults and children at least 12 years of age.

Topiramate is used either alone or in combination with other anticonvulsants to treat partial or primary generalized tonic-clonic seizures in adults and children. It can also be used in combination with other anticonvulsants to treat seizures associated with LGS in adults and children. Topiramate is also approved for prevention of migraine headaches in adults. Its usefulness in the acute treatment of migraine headaches has not been studied.

Valproic acid is used either alone or in conjunction with other anticonvulsants in the treatment of complex partial seizures. It is also used alone or with other anticonvulsants in the treatment of simple and complex absence seizures and along with other anticonvulsants in patients with multiple seizure types that include absence seizures. Also, valproic acid is approved for the treatment of manic episodes associated with bipolar disorder and for the prevention of migraine headaches in adults.

Zonisamide is used along with other anticonvulsants to manage partial seizures in adults.

Off-Label Uses

A three-part investigative series by Knight Ridder Newspapers in 2003 found that three-quarters of antiseizure medications are prescribed off-label for such things as depression and hot flashes and to help people lose weight.

Hydantoins have been shown to be helpful in treating trigeminal neuralgia (shooting pains in the facial area). Phenytoin has also been used to treat ventricular arrhythmias, especially those associated with digoxin toxicity.

Carbamazepine has been used for relief of pain due to diabetic neuropathy, relief of pain and control of paroxysmal symptoms of multiple sclerosis, augmenting treatment of schizo-phrenia and bipolar disorder, and management of alcohol withdrawal, restless leg syndrome, postherpetic neuralgia, and intermittent explosive disorder and other rage disorders.

According to Knight-Ridder researchers, 90 percent of gabapentin prescriptions are written for off-label use, with annual off-label sales of $1.8 billion. Its off-label uses include treatment of migraines, social anxiety, bipolar disorder, chronic pain, multiple sclerosis, and restless leg syndrome.

Oxcarbazepine, tiagabine, and zonisamide can be used as an alternative treatment for bipolar disorder.

Pregabalin is used for treating anxiety as well as mood and sleep disorders.

Primidone has been found to be effective in treating essential tremor.

Common off-label uses of topiramate include the prevention of migraine headaches and treatment of bipolar disorder, infantile spasms, alcohol dependence, and bulimia nervosa.

Valproic acid has been used to treat agitation and aggressive behavior in patients with dementia.

Companion Drugs
Many anticonvulsants (e.g., carbamazepine, gabapentin, lamotrigine, topiramate, and valproic acid) are also used along with antidepressants and/or antipsychotics as mood stabilizers for treatment of bipolar disorder and as sedating agents for anxiety.

Administration
Phenobarbital is available in various forms: tablets, capsules, liquid, and injection. Intravenous (IV) injection is used only in emergencies, when taking the medication by mouth is impossible or impractical.

Benzodiazepines are commonly used IV and occasionally rectally to treat status epilepticus. Clonazepam is available in tablet form. Diazepam and lorazepam are available in an IV form for the treatment of prolonged seizures or status epilepticus. Diazepam is also available in a gel form for rectal administration.

Phenytoin is available in oral and injectable forms. Orally, phenytoin is available in the form of tablets, capsules, or oral suspension. Fosphenytoin is available only as an injectable.

Succinimides are available in capsule form, and ethosuximide also is available as a syrup.

Acetazolamide is available in tablets, extended-release capsules, and IV injection.

Carbamazepine is available in several oral forms: conventional and chewable tablets, extended-release capsules and tablets, and suspension.

Felbamate and oxcarbazepine are available in tablets and as an oral suspension.

Gabapentin is available in tablets and capsules as well as an oral solution.

Lamotrigine is available as conventional and chewable tablets.

Levetiracetam is available in tablets and as an oral solution.

Pregabalin and zonisamide are available in capsules.

Primidone and tiagabine are available in tablets.

Topiramate is available in tablets or sprinkle capsules.

Valproic acid is available in a number of oral forms (capsules, delayed-release tablets, extended-release tablets, sprinkle capsules, and syrup) as well as IV injection.

Cautions and Concerns
Anticonvulsants have sleep-inducing effects, which make driving or operating dangerous machinery potentially hazardous. Thus, patients are advised to temporarily cease driving during the time of anticonvulsant medication initiation, withdrawal, or dosage change. If there is significant risk of recurrent seizure during medication withdrawal or change, the patient should cease driving during this time and for at least three months thereafter.

Although most pregnant women who take anticonvulsants deliver normal babies, there have been reports of increased birth defects when these medicines were used during pregnancy. Phenobarbital, valproic acid, and hydantoins have been associated with significantly increased risks for birth defects. In addition, hydantoins may cause a bleeding problem in the mother during delivery and in the newborn. Also, pregnancy may cause a change in the way anticonvulsants are absorbed in the body, leading to more seizures even when the medicine is taken regularly. For this reason, using as few medications as possible and at the lowest dose needed to control seizures is the goal of treatment during pregnancy.

Because anticonvulsants interact with many other drugs, they may cause special problems in older patients who use multiple medications for other health problems. Elderly patients, in particular, should have liver and kidney function tests performed before starting anticonvulsant therapy.

Carbamazepine has been associated with increased frequency of generalized convulsions in patients with a mixed seizure disorder that includes atypical absence seizures. Also, hepatic effects, ranging from slight elevations in liver enzymes to rare cases of hepatic failure, have been reported. In some cases, hepatic effects may progress despite discontinuation of the drug. Loss of red blood cells, white blood cells, and platelets have been reported with the use of carbamazepine. These side effects can be life-threatening if unnoticed, so complete blood counts are required for the first few months followed by three or four a year to detect these abnormalities.

Because photosensitization may occur when taking felbamate, patients need to take protective measures against exposure to ultraviolet light or sunlight until their tolerance is determined.

Because primidone therapy generally extends over prolonged periods, complete blood counts, electrolytes, and liver function tests should be monitored every six months.

Serious risks associated with topiramate include decreased sweating, increased body temperature, kidney stones, sleepiness, dizziness, confusion, and difficulty concentrating.

Warnings

Discontinuing anticonvulsant medications should be done only with a doctor's approval and supervision. Discontinuing anticonvulsants without a doctor's advice is a primary cause of people who have been seizure-free to begin having new seizures. Seizures that result from suddenly stopping medication can be very serious and can lead to status epilepticus.

Because severe, even fatal, blood disorders (aplastic anemia) and liver problems have occurred with usage of felbamate, it should be used only in people with severe epilepsy and only after careful consideration. Aplastic anemia may occur even after the drug has been stopped.

In rare cases, lamotrigine has been known to cause the development of serious rashes, including the life-threatening Stevens-Johnson syndrome. Although nearly all cases of life-threatening rashes associated with lamotrigine have occurred within two to eight weeks of beginning treatment, isolated cases have been reported after more prolonged use.

Evidence shows that in mothers treated with primidone who breast-feed, the drug appears in the milk in substantial quantities. Spencer et al. write, "Although anticonvulsants are excreted into breast milk, most mothers who require the use of these drugs can safely breast-feed their infants. During breast-feeding, anticonvulsants other than phenobarbital and primidone are preferred because the slow rate of barbiturate metabolism by the infant may cause sedation. Infant serum levels may be helpful in monitoring toxicity."

Off-label use of tiagabine is strongly discouraged, as its use has been associated with the occurrence of seizures in patients without epilepsy. In February 2005, the FDA announced that a bolded Warning would be added to the labeling for tiagabine to warn health-care professionals and patients of this risk.

An FDA alert to physicians and patients warned that regular use of topiramate may cause temporary or permanent loss of vision. Symptoms, which typically begin in the first month of use, include blurred vision and eye pain. Early discontinuation of topiramate may halt any eye damage and reverse any loss of vision.

Valproic acid can cause serious damage to the liver, especially in children under two years of age, and can also cause life-threatening inflammation of the pancreas.

Zonisamide has been known to cause the development of serious rashes, including the life-threatening Stevens-Johnson syndrome and toxic epidermal necrolysis. Most cases of these skin reactions occur within two to 16 weeks of beginning treatment. Additionally, zonisamide has been associated with decreased sweating and increased body temperature in children. Because the safety and effectiveness of zonisamide has not been demonstrated in children, its use should be reserved for adults.

When Not Advised (Contraindications)

Because many anticonvulsants are potentially teratogenic (causing malformations of an embryo or fetus), they should be considered for women of childbearing potential only after the risk has been thoroughly discussed with the patient and weighed against the potential benefits of treatment. Specifically, according to Julian Robinson, M.D., valproate and carbamazepine are associated with neural tube defects (NTDs), and phenytoin and phenobarbital are linked to coronary heart disease and cleft lip and palate. Also, therapy using multiple anticonvulsants carries a higher risk for birth defects than monotherapy. Robinson adds, "The newer anticonvulsants—gabapentin, lamotrigine, levetiracetam, oxcarbazepine, tiagabine, topiramate, and zonisamide—may be safer than the older anticonvulsants to control seizure activity in women of childbearing age."

Barbiturates are not advised in patients with a history of severe liver dysfunction or porphyria, a disorder in which porphyrins build up in the blood and urine.

Because of their effect on conduction, intravenous phenytoin and fosphenytoin should not be used in patients with sinus bradycardia or heart block.

Acetazolamide should not be taken by individuals who are allergic to sulfa medications or have liver or kidney disease.

Carbamazepine should not be used in patients with a history of previous bone marrow depression or known sensitivity to any of the tricyclic antidepressants. Likewise, its use with monoamine oxidase (MAO) inhibitors is not recommended. Before administration of carbamazepine, MAO inhibitors should be discontinued for a minimum of 14 days.

Felbamate should not be used in patients with a history of any blood disease or liver dysfunction.

People who have had porphyria should not take primidone. Those who are sensitive to phenobarbital also are advised to avoid primidone, because the body produces phenobarbital when it processes primidone.

Valproic acid should not be used in patients with liver dysfunction (see *Warnings*).

Zonisamide should not be taken by individuals who are allergic to sulfa medications.

Side Effects

Because anticonvulsants can cause numerous side effects, particularly as their dosage is increased, patients may stop taking their medication. (See *Warnings*.) However, many side effects are mild and either disappear or occur less frequently as the body adjusts to the drug. Because of the troublesome side effects, physicians frequently have to start patients' prescriptions at subtherapeutic levels. Most anticonvulsants cause some drowsiness and stomach upset.

Barbiturates may cause dizziness, lightheadedness, faintness, clumsiness, impaired judgment, sedation, skin rashes, or constipation. They also may promote or enhance depression.

The most common side effects of benzodiazepines include drowsiness or sedation, fatigue, headache, dizziness, blurred vision, loss of muscle coordination, behavior changes (nervousness, anxiety, confusion, aggression, hallucinations, and agitation), slowed breathing, slowed heart rate, increased or decreased appetite, or rash and itching.

Hydantoins can cause gingival hyperplasia (enlargement of the gums) and hirsutism (excessive facial and body hair). Some side effects, especially bleeding, tender or enlarged gums, and enlarged facial features, are more likely to occur in children and young adults. Excessive hair growth is more noticeable in young girls. In addition, some children may not do as well in school after using high doses of hydantoins for an extended period of time. Hydantoins can also cause confusion, dizziness, severe skin reactions, stuttering, and trembling. Phenytoin has a number of side effects that may be hazardous to the elderly, including muscle incoordination, sedation, and osteomalacia (a softening of the bones).

Succinimides can cause dizziness and loss of balance, severe skin reactions, depression, headache, or aggressive behavior.

Common side effects of acetazolamide include numbness and tingling in the fingers and toes and taste alterations, both usually due to low potassium levels. Some may also experience blurred vision, but this usually disappears shortly after stopping the medication. More frequent urination is common. Other reported side effects include lethargy, loss of appetite, nausea, and, occasionally, kidney stones.

Common side effects of carbamazepine include drowsiness, dizziness, blurry or doubled vision, motor-coordination impairment, and upset stomach.

Felbamate side effects include nausea, vomiting, loss of appetite, constipation, drowsiness, dizziness, difficulty sleeping, headache, and itching.

The most common side effects of gabapentin are drowsiness, dizziness, unsteady gait, fatigue, tremor, nausea, vomiting, diarrhea, and eye twitching.

Common side effects of lamotrigine include headache, dizziness, unsteady gait, drowsiness, nausea, blurred vision, and rash.

Common side effects of levetiracetam include behavioral problems, drowsiness, dizziness, headache, diarrhea, vomiting, loss of appetite, and muscle weakness.

Oxcarbazepine occasionally causes fatigue, nausea, vomiting, headache, dizziness, drowsiness, abdominal pain, tremor, indigestion, abnormal gait, and blurred or double vision. It can cause hyponatremia (a deficiency of sodium in the blood), so blood sodium levels are tested in patients who complain of severe fatigue.

Some of the most common side effects reported in clinical trials of pregabalin were dizziness, drowsiness, tremor, dry mouth, swelling of hands and feet, blurred vision, and weight gain.

Primidone may be associated with drowsiness, dizziness, unsteady gait, fatigue, vertigo, nausea, vomiting, sexual impotency, double vision, twitching eyes, and decreased appetite.

Tiagabine may cause a serious and life-threatening rash. Other side effects include dizziness, lightheadedness, low energy, nausea, nervousness, irritability, tremors, stomach pain, impaired concentration, speech or language problems, confusion, drowsiness, and fatigue.

Common side effects of topiramate are tingling in arms and legs, loss of appetite, nausea, diarrhea, taste change, and weight loss.

Valproic acid can cause nausea, vomiting, diarrhea, headache, drowsiness, dizziness, insomnia, weight gain or loss, hair loss, decreased platelets, tremor, blurred or double vision, or menstrual bleeding changes.

The most common side effects of zonisamide are drowsiness, loss of appetite, dizziness, headache, nausea, and agitation/irritability.

Interactions

Because many anticonvulsants can potentially decrease the effectiveness of hormonal contraceptives (oral, progesterone implants, and progesterone injections), an alternative method of contraception should be used.

Many drugs are capable of lowering seizure threshold and may decrease the effectiveness of anticonvulsants, including tricyclic antidepressants and phenothiazines.

Barbiturates stimulate the metabolism of many drugs that are metabolized by the liver, decreasing their effectiveness.

Acute alcohol consumption increases the availability (the amount of the drug that is active in the body) of phenytoin and the risk of drug-related side effects. Chronic drinking may decrease phenytoin availability, significantly reducing the patient's protection against epileptic seizures, even during a period of abstinence. Also, phenytoin and warfarin affect the metabolism of each other, making it difficult to use these two drugs simultaneously in a patient.

The use of succinamides with benzodiazepines, phenobarbital, or narcotic agents may increase its sedative effects. A number of drugs such as erythromycin, ketoconazole, itraconazole, calcium channel blockers, and protease inhibitors may increase the blood levels of succinamides.

Acetazolamide may enhance the effect of amphetamines, phenytoin, and quinidine, may elevate cyclosporine levels, and may decrease lithium levels.

Carbamazepine interacts with many different drugs; therefore, it is important that the patient's physician and pharmacist are made aware of all prescription and over-the-counter medicines being taken. Also, grapefruit juice increases the blood levels of carbamazepine, thereby increasing the risk for side effects.

Felbamate interacts with other anticonvulsants; for example, felbamate increases blood levels of phenytoin, phenobarbital, and valproic acid, yet decreases blood levels of carbamazepine. The effects of felbamate may be increased with the use of fluconazole, ketoconazole, itraconazole, clarithromycin, erythromycin, nefazodone, protease inhibitors, quinidine, and verapamil. The use of carbamazepine, phenobarbital, phenytoin, or rifampin may decrease the effects of felbamate.

Antacids reduce the effectiveness of gabapentin; therefore, gabapentin should be taken at least two hours following antacid administration. Studies have shown hydrocodone and morphine to increase blood levels of gabapentin.

Acetaminophen (chronic use), carbamazepine, estrogen, primidone, phenobarbital, phenytoin, and rifampin may lower blood levels of lamotrigine. Valproic acid may increase blood levels of lamotrigine.

Oxcarbazepine may increase blood levels of phenobarbital and phenytoin. Valproic acid, carbamazepine, phenobarbital, phenytoin, and verapamil may reduce the effectiveness of oxcarbazepine. Oxcarbazepine may also reduce the effectiveness of calcium channel blockers and hormonal contraceptives.

Patients taking certain diabetes medications called glitazones (e.g., pioglitazone, rosiglitazone) along with pregabalin may have a higher chance of developing swelling or gaining weight.

Primidone may heighten the effects of CNS depressants such as alcohol and barbiturates, but it may decrease the effects of a number of drugs, some of which include beta-blockers, calcium channel blockers, carbamazepine, citalopram, cyclosporine, fluoxetine, hormonal contraceptives, methadone, phenytoin, protease inhibitors, rifampin, sulfonamides, quinidine, tacrolimus, theophylline, and warfarin. Taking primidone within two weeks of taking monoamine oxidase (MAO) inhibitors may prolong the effects of primidone.

Carbamazepine, phenytoin, primidone, and phenobarbital lower blood levels of tiagabine by inducing its metabolism and may decrease its effectiveness.

Topiramate may increase the blood levels of phenytoin and may decrease blood levels of digoxin and hormonal contraceptives. Carbamazepine and phenytoin may decrease the effectiveness of topiramate. The use of topiramate and valproic acid together may increase the risk of developing increased ammonia levels in the blood, which could lead to encephalopathy. Alcohol consumption while taking topiramate may cause increased sedation or drowsiness.

Valproic acid may increase, decrease, or have no effect on blood levels of carbamazepine and phenytoin. Valproic acid may increase blood levels of lamotrigine, phenobarbital, tricyclic antidepressants, warfarin, and zidovudine. Clarithromycin, erythromycin, felbamate, and isoniazid may increase blood levels of valproic acid.

The effects of zonisamide may be increased by ketoconazole, clarithromycin, erythromycin, fluconazole, protease inhibitors, quinidine, and verapamil, while its effects may be decreased by carbamazepine, phenobarbital, phenytoin, and rifampin. Alcohol consumption while taking zonisamide may cause increased sedation or drowsiness

Sales/Statistics

Spending on anticonvulsants grew by 21.9 percent in 2004, which was down from the 28.9 percent increase in 2003, according to a survey by Express Scripts Inc., a St. Louis pharmacy-benefit management company. The smaller increase in spending was mainly attributed to a decrease in utilization of these drugs. Utilization growth slowed to 8.7 percent in 2004, down from 13.3 percent in 2003. The introduction of the first generic versions of gabapentin, with their lower costs, also played a role in the smaller spending increase, according to the report. Utilization of anticonvulsants is expected to grow as their off-label use for pain relief becomes more widespread and acceptable. Drug inflation among anticonvulsants was 9.7 percent in 2004, the second highest of the top 25 therapy classes in this report.

Examining trends from 1994 to 2003 in the use of anticonvulsants by enrollees aged five to 17 years of Kaiser Permanente in northern California, Hunkeler et al. found that the use of anticonvulsants nearly doubled, from 3.5 per 1,000 enrollees to 6.9 per 1,000 enrollees. An increasing percentage of anticonvulsant users had a diagnosis of bipolar disorder.

According to Pharmacor, an advisory service that analyzes and forecasts the commercial outlook for drugs in research and development,

dollar sales of anticonvulsants were expected to begin a steady decline after 2008 as they lose patent protection. In 2010, according to IMS Institute for Healthcare Informatics, anticonvulsants ranked 16th in U.S. drug spending, with $5.6 billion in sales, and 10th in prescriptions (121.7 million prescriptions dispensed).

Demographics and Cultural Groups

According to the Epilepsy Foundation, males are slightly more likely to develop epilepsy than females. The incidence of epilepsy is greater in black and socially disadvantaged populations. The trend shows decreased incidence in children and increased incidence in the elderly. The prevalence of active epilepsy is higher among racial minorities than among whites.

Development History

Although Hippocrates recognized epilepsy as a brain disorder in 400 B.C., it was not until 1912 that scientists learned the recently introduced phenobarbital could be effective against seizures. LeWinn explains, "It was discovered that phenobarbital not only has a calming effect and causes sleep, depending on the size of the dose, but that, to a degree much greater than that of other barbiturates, it also suppresses seizures. Efforts were then begun to modify the chemical structure of phenobarbital so as to eliminate its sedative effect and enhance its anticonvulsant capability."

In 1939, the discovery and clinical testing of phenytoin introduced both a major new non-sedating anticonvulsant and an animal model of epilepsy. Phenytoin was first synthesized by a German physician named Heinrich Biltz in 1908. Biltz sold his discovery to Parke-Davis, which did not find an immediate use for it. In 1938, outside scientists discovered phenytoin's usefulness for controlling seizures without the sedation effects associated with phenobarbital.

Many antiepileptic drugs were discovered by testing their ability to prevent seizures in experimental animals after electrical stimulation of the brain or after the administration of convulsant drugs such as strychnine or pentylenetetrazol. Others, such as phenytoin, were discovered as a result of persistent testing of a series of drugs.

Beginning in the 1950s, a number of drugs were introduced and approved over the next 20 years to treat seizures, including carbamazepine, ethosuximide, and sodium valproate.

Since 1975, the Epilepsy Branch of the National Institute of Neurological Disorders and Stroke, National Institutes of Health, through its Antiepileptic Drug Development (ADD) Program, has collaborated with the pharmaceutical industry in developing new therapeutic agents for the treatment of seizure disorders. In 1993, felbamate, the first new drug in nearly two decades, was approved for sale in the United States. Felbamate's development was a collaborative effort of both the pharmaceutical sponsor and ADD Program. Several other drugs are now in early clinical development.

Future Drugs

A handful of new anticonvulsant drugs are under development. Although they have unique mechanisms of action for the treatment of epilepsy and other seizure disorders, they probably will gain initial approval for use as adjunctive therapy for patients who are not adequately controlled with current therapy. Although a key patent for lamotrigine did not expire until 2009, its manufacturer made an agreement that allowed generics to enter the market before its scheduled patent-expiration date.

Agents known as AMPA receptor antagonists have antiseizure properties and are under investigation. Talampanel is one such potentially effective anticonvulsive and is currently in early trials. Other antiseizure agents being investigated include carabersat, fluorofelbamate, harkoseride, safinamide, and valrocemid.

Ezogabine (Potiga, Valeant Pharmaceuticals and GlaxoSmithKline [GSK]) was nearing final FDA approval in mid-June 2011 as an add-on medication to treat seizures associated with epilepsy in adults. In their announcement release, GSK noted, "FDA has recommended that ezo-gabine be scheduled as a controlled substance under the Controlled Substances Act. Final classification is still under review by the U.S. Drug Enforcement Administration (DEA) and ezogabine will not be available until this process is complete." Ezogabine's approval was for the treatment of "partial seizures and is the first in its class as an activator of voltage-gated potassium channels in the brain developed for the treatment of epilepsy. The exact mechanism of action is unknown, but ezogabine may act as an anticonvulsant by reducing excitability through the stabilization of neuronal potassium channels in an 'open' position," according to Medscape Medical News on June 13, 2011.

Hunkeler, Enid M., et al. "Trends in Use of Antidepressants, Lithium, and Anticonvulsants in Kaiser Permanente-Insured Youths, 1994–2003." *Journal of Child and Adolescent Psychopharmacology* 15, no. 1 (February 2005): 26–37.
LeWinn, Edward B. "A Bill of Particulars on Seizures and on Discontinuing Anticonvulsant Drugs." The Institutes for the Achievement of Human Potential. Available online. URL: http://www.iahp.org/A_Bill_of_Particulars.303.0.html. Downloaded on November 27, 2005.
Roach, Sally S., and Jeanne C. Scherer. *Introductory Clinical Pharmacology.* Philadelphia: Lippincott Williams & Wilkins, 2003.
Robinson, Julian N. "Gynecologic and Obstetric Management of Women on Anticonvulsant Drugs." *The Female Patient Supplement,* July 2004. Available online. URL: http://www.femalepaticnt.com/pdf/sup0704_4.pdf.
Spencer, Jeanine P., Luis S. Gonzalez III, and Donna J. Barnhart. "Medications in the Breast-Feeding Mother." *American Family Physician* 64, no. 1 (July 1, 2001): 119–126.

antidepressants Medications that relieve the symptoms of depression, the most commonly diagnosed mental health disorder. In the United States, around 19 million adults suffer from some type of depression each year. Major depressive disorder, also known as clinical or unipolar depression, is the leading cause of disability in the United States, affecting 5 percent of the American population (around 15 million), with women being affected more than two times as often as men. Studies have estimated that as many as 12 percent of men and 25 percent of women will experience a depressive episode serious enough to seek treatment at least once in their lifetimes. Estimates are that as many as 340 million people worldwide suffer from major depression. Modern treatment of depression began with the introduction of the early antidepressants in the late 1950s, and by December 1998, 1,175 antidepressant drug products (including all dosage forms and strengths) were on the market in the United States.

Classes

Antidepressants are separated into classes according to their chemical structure and action on the brain.

- *Tricyclic antidepressants* (TCAs) First-generation antidepressants. They block the reuptake of norepinephrine, serotonin, or both. *Examples:* amitriptyline, clomipramine (Anafranil), desipramine (Norpramin, Pertofrane), doxepin (Sinequan), imipramine (Tofranil), nortriptyline (Pamelor), protriptyline (Vivactil), and trimipramine (Surmontil).

- *Monoamine oxidase inhibitors* (MAOIs) Also first-generation antidepressants. They block monoamine oxidase, which breaks down norepinephrine, serotonin, and dopamine. *Examples:* isocarboxazid (Marplan), phenelzine (Nardil), selegiline (Emsam), and tranylcypromine (Parnate).

- *Selective serotonin reuptake inhibitors* (SSRIs) Second-generation antidepressants, and currently the most widely prescribed because they tend to have fewer side effects than the first-generation antidepressants. They primarily block the reuptake of serotonin, making more of it available in the brain. *Examples:* citalopram (Celexa), escitalopram (Lexapro), fluoxetine (Prozac), fluvoxamine (Luvox), paroxetine (Paxil), and sertraline (Zoloft).

- *Serotonin-norepinephrine reuptake inhibitors* (SNRIs) Also second-generation antidepressants, they are potent inhibitors of the reuptake of serotonin and norepinephrine and are weak inhibitors of the reuptake of dopamine. *Examples:* duloxetine (Cymbalta) and venlafaxine (Effexor).

- *Miscellaneous antidepressants* Not chemically structured like the other classes, plus each drug in this category affects one or more of the brain chemicals in different ways. *Examples:* bupropion (Wellbutrin)—a relatively weak inhibitor of the reuptake of serotonin, norepinephrine, and dopamine (its mechanism of action is not fully understood); maprotiline (Ludiomil)—a strong norepinephrine reuptake inhibitor with only weak effects on serotonin and dopamine reuptake; mirtazapine (Remeron)—affects serotonin and norepinephrine; nefazodone (Serzone)—acts mostly on serotonin reuptake; and trazodone (Desyrel)—a serotonin reuptake inhibitor and 5-HT$_2$ receptor antagonist.

How They Work

Because scientists cannot "model" major depression in animals, they have not been able to determine exactly how antidepressants achieve their therapeutic results. Although the effects of antidepressants on the brain are not fully understood, there is substantial evidence that they somehow restore the brain's chemical balance. Brain-imaging research has revealed that in depression, neural circuits responsible for moods, thinking, sleep, appetite, and behavior fail to function properly and that the regulation of critical neurotransmitters—specifically, norepinephrine (called noradrenalin in the United Kingdom), serotonin, and dopamine—is impaired. Neurotransmitters are the chemicals that transmit signals between the cells in our brains. Existing antidepressants influence the functioning of one or all of those neurotransmitters by either raising their levels (increasing their activity) or by preventing them from becoming inactive.

Antidepressants usually can control depressive symptoms in four to eight weeks; two-thirds of the people who use them improve within three weeks. Duloxetine, introduced in 2004, became effective in one week during trials. Antidepressants are typically taken for at least four to six months, with many patients continuing to take them for six months to a year following a major depressive episode to avoid relapse. Any given antidepressant may fail to work in 10–30 percent of people who take it, so it may take several months to find the right medication and dose.

Studies have found that after three months of antidepressant treatment, between 50 percent and 65 percent of the people who take them will be much improved. This compares with 25 to 30 percent of people who benefit due to the placebo effect. The placebo effect can be so substantial that drug companies often face challenges in proving the effectiveness of their antidepressant drugs.

Antidepressants do not cure depression; they alleviate the symptoms. In some cases they can help the person get on with life by lifting the dark moods of depression, which then allows psychotherapy treatment to be more effective.

Approved Uses

The TCAs are approved to treat depression, except for clomipramine, which is approved only for treatment of obsessive-compulsive disorder (OCD). Doxepin is used to treat psychoneurotic patients with depression or anxiety and to treat depression or anxiety associated with alcoholism, organic disease, or psychotic depressive disorders. Imipramine is also used to treat bed-wetting in children at least six years of age.

The MAOIs are used to treat patients with atypical depression and patients unresponsive to other antidepressants.

The SSRIs are approved to treat depression, except for fluvoxamine, which is only approved for the treatment of OCD. The Food and Drug Administration (FDA) has approved escitalopram to also treat generalized anxiety disorder (GAD). Fluoxetine is approved to also treat panic disorder, premenstrual dysphoric disorder (PMDD), OCD, and bulimia nervosa. Among antidepressants, only fluoxetine is approved for the treatment of pediatric major depressive disorder. Fluoxetine, fluvoxamine, and sertraline are approved for pediatric OCD. Paroxetine has been approved also for OCD, panic disorder, GAD, social anxiety disorder, PMDD, and post-traumatic stress disorder (PTSD). Sertraline has also been approved for social anxiety disorder, OCD, panic disorder, PTSD, and PMDD.

The SNRIs are approved to treat major depression. In addition, duloxetine is used in the management of neuropathic pain associated with diabetic peripheral neuropathy. Venlafaxine is approved for the treatment of GAD, social anxiety disorder, and panic disorder.

The miscellaneous antidepressants are all approved to treat depression. In addition, bupropion is approved as an aid to smoking cessation treatment under the brand name Zyban. Maprotiline is also used for the relief of anxiety associated with depression.

Off-Label Uses

A survey of more than 1,000 patients receiving antidepressants found that a majority of usage (56 percent) was for conditions other than those for which the FDA had approved the drugs. Doctors have prescribed antidepressants off-label for years to manage chronic pain, such as from migraine and chronic tension headaches, cancer, and arthritis. Although the evidence is fairly strong that these drugs are helpful in the management of chronic pain, it is not definitive.

An FDA review of prescribing data for children younger than 12 years of age indicated that 18 percent of the antidepressant prescriptions were for patients who had attention-deficit disorder, or the related attention-deficit/hyperactivity disorder (ADHD). None of the antidepressant drugs are approved to treat attention-deficit disorders.

Because antidepressants sometimes cause delayed ejaculation in men, some doctors have prescribed them in cases of premature ejaculation.

Among the TCAs, amitriptyline, desipramine, and imipramine are used off-label to treat bulimia nervosa; clomipramine, desipramine, and nortriptyline are used to treat premenstrual symptoms; desipramine and imipramine are used to treat cocaine withdrawal; doxepin and protriptyline are used to treat sleep apnea; and trimipramine is used to treat peptic ulcer disease.

The MAOIs have been used off-label to treat bulimia nervosa. Phenelzine has been used to treat cocaine addiction, and small studies have shown it effective for night terrors and PTSD. Phenelzine and tranylcypromine are used for some migraines resistant to other therapies and for panic disorder with associated agoraphobia.

Among the SSRIs, citalopram is used off-label to treat GAD, OCD, panic disorder, PMDD, and PTSD. Escitalopram is used to treat panic disorder. Fluoxetine is used to treat GAD, PTSD, Raynaud's syndrome, and hot flashes and to prevent migraines. Fluvoxamine is used to treat bulimia nervosa, depression, panic disorder, and social anxiety disorder. Paroxetine is used to treat hot flashes and diabetic neuropathy.

Among the SNRIs, duloxetine has been used off-label to treat panic disorder, anxiety, bipolar depression, fibromyalgia, urinary incontinence, interstitial cystitis, and irritable bowel syndrome. Some clinicians have found venlafaxine to be helpful in treating OCD, premenstrual dysphoria, borderline personality, fibromyalgia, hot flashes, and ADHD, but the data is preliminary.

Bupropion has been used off-label to treat neuropathic pain and ADHD and to enhance weight loss.

Trazodone has been used off-label to treat aggressive behavior, cravings for alcohol, panic disorder, agoraphobia with panic attacks, and cocaine withdrawal. Low doses of trazadone along with an SSRI are used to treat insomnia.

Administration

Antidepressants are available only with a doctor's prescription. Tricyclic antidepressants are available in tablet, capsule, or oral solution form, depending on the particular medicine. MAO inhibitors are available in tablet form, except for selegiline, which is a skin (transdermal) patch. SSRIs are available in tablet, capsule, or oral solution form, and all have dosage forms that can be administered once daily, with fluoxetine and fluvoxamine prescribed twice daily when larger doses are used. SNRIs are available in tablets and capsules: Duloxetine comes in a capsule and can be taken once a day. Venlafaxine is available as tablets and extended-release capsules. Bupropion is available as tablets, 12-hour sustained-release tablets, and 24-hour extended-release tablets. Maprotiline, mirtazapine, nefazodone, and trazodone are available as tablets. Antidepressants can be taken with or without food.

Cautions and Concerns

Although antidepressants are not addictive, they sometimes cause withdrawal symptoms. Care is needed when antidepressants are discontinued, because quickly stopping certain antidepressants can be linked to side effects ranging from flulike symptoms to sensory disturbances. As a result, new labeling, as specified by the FDA, recommends that patients taper off these medications slowly. If a person encounters problems going off a drug, he or she is advised to consult a physician rather than reduce dosage without supervision.

In September 2005, the FDA notified healthcare professionals that an epidemiologic study of major congenital malformations in infants born to women taking antidepressants during the first trimester of pregnancy had shown a greater risk for birth defects for paroxetine compared to other antidepressants.

In October 2005, the FDA notified healthcare professionals that patients with preexisting liver disease who take duloxetine may have an increased risk for further liver disease. Although the effects of heat on the selegiline patch are not known, the drug labeling advises health-care professionals and patients about the possible effects of direct heat applied to the patch. Direct heat may result in an increased amount of the drug absorbed from the patch. Patients should avoid exposing the patch to heating pads, electric blankets, heat lamps, saunas, hot tubs, or prolonged sunlight.

Warnings

Nefazodone carries an FDA black-box warning on the label about rare cases of liver failure.

On March 22, 2004, the FDA requested that manufacturers include a Warning Statement in the labeling for 10 antidepressants (Prozac, Zoloft, Paxil, Luvox, Celexa, Lexapro, Wellbutrin, Effexor, Serzone, and Remeron) to encourage close observation of adult and pediatric patients treated with these drugs for worsening depression or the emergence of suicidal thoughts. The FDA noted there was no evidence that the drugs cause suicidal behavior in children, but it was reevaluating drug-company studies to see if a credible link might be established. The FDA concerns did cause increased vigilance among physicians, but this greater caution has not led to a decline in prescribing of SSRI or SNRI antidepressants for children or adolescents. The majority of physicians believe that the benefits of antidepressants outweigh the risks, with parents seeming to agree with this view and not pressuring doctors to remove their children from these drugs.

When Not Advised (Contraindications)

Patients recovering from myocardial infarction (MI) are generally advised not to take any TCAs because they have been known to complicate some heart problems. Specifically, they may affect a person's blood pressure and heart rate. Also, patients who have narrow-angle glaucoma or who tend to have urinary retention should not take doxepin.

MAOIs are not advised for patients with chronic heart failure, history of liver disease, severe kidney impairment, hypertension, or history of headaches.

In clinical trials, duloxetine use was associated with an increased risk of mydriasis (an excessive dilation of the pupil of the eye). Therefore, its use should be avoided in patients with uncontrolled narrow-angle glaucoma.

Bupropion is not recommended for patients with a history of seizure disorder, anorexia, or bulimia. It is also not recommended for patients undergoing abrupt discontinuation of alcohol or sedatives.

Side Effects

Not all antidepressants produce the same side effects in every person. Some side effects disappear quickly; others may remain for the length of treatment.

The older TCAs have unpleasant and sometimes dangerous side effects, such as dry mouth, blurred vision, slight tremor, heart palpitations, constipation, sleepiness, and weight gain. Particularly in older people, they may cause confusion, slowness in starting and stopping when urinating, low blood pressure, lightheadedness, and falls. Men may experience difficulty in getting or keeping an erection or delayed ejaculation. An overdose of a TCA is dangerous and potentially lethal. Symptoms of an overdose develop within an hour and may begin with rapid heartbeat, dilated pupils, flushed face, and agitation. Any of these may then progress to confusion, unconsciousness, seizures, irregular heartbeat, and even death.

The more common MAOI side effects include hypotension, fainting, palpitations, tachycardia, dizziness, headache, tremors, confusion, memory impairment, sleep disturbances, constipation, nausea, diarrhea, abdominal pain, dry mouth, weight gain, blurred vision, impotence, and chills. Side effects of selegiline detected in trials included a mild skin reaction where the patch is placed, lightheadedness related to a drop in blood pressure, headache, diarrhea, insomnia, and dry mouth.

During the first couple of weeks of taking SSRIs, the patient may experience nausea or headache and feel jittery or agitated. Some of these can produce indigestion, which can usually be avoided by taking them with food. They may interfere with sexual function. There have also been reports of episodes of aggression, although these are rare.

In duloxetine clinical trials, people reported side effects such as nausea, dry mouth, constipation, low appetite, sleepiness, and increased sweating.

Common side effects of venlafaxine include headache, nausea, dizziness, sleepiness, insomnia, vertigo, dry mouth, anorexia, constipation, sexual dysfunction, sweating, vivid dreams, and increased blood pressure.

Common side effects of bupropion include dry mouth, tremors, nausea, anxiety, loss of appetite, agitation, dizziness, headache, excessive sweating, increased risk of seizure, and insomnia.

The most common side effects of maprotiline include dizziness, drowsiness, fatigue, dry mouth, insomnia, anxiety, headache, constipation, nausea, tremor, blurred vision, and agitation.

Side effects of mirtazapine may include drowsiness, dizziness, anxiousness, confusion, increased weight and appetite, dry mouth, constipation, increased cholesterol, and vivid and unusual dreams or nightmares.

Nefazodone may cause dry mouth, nausea, headache, dizziness, constipation, agitation, and drowsiness.

Trazodone's most common side effects are drowsiness, fatigue, insomnia, nausea, vomiting, headache, dizziness, blurred vision, and dry mouth.

Interactions

Alcoholism and depression are frequently associated, leading to a high potential for alcohol-antidepressant interactions. Alcohol increases the sedative effect of TCAs, impairing mental skills required for driving. Acute alcohol consumption increases the availability of (or activity of) some TCAs, potentially increasing their sedative effects; chronic alcohol consumption appears to increase the availability of some TCAs and to decrease the availability of others. The significance of these interactions is unclear. These chronic effects persist in recovering alcoholics.

Taking a TCA concurrently with an MAO inhibitor has caused high fever crises, increased blood pressure and heart rate, severe convulsions, and fatalities. In addition, patients who had been taking an MAO inhibitor have been advised to have discontinued the MAOI use for at least two weeks before beginning treatment with any TCA.

MAO inhibitors have many dietary restrictions, and people taking them need to follow the dietary guidelines and physician's instructions very carefully. A rapid, potentially fatal increase in blood pressure can occur if foods or alcoholic beverages containing the chemical tyramine are consumed while taking MAO inhibitors. As little as one standard alcoholic drink may lead to the development of this interaction. The FDA cautions that the following beverages must be avoided: beer, red wine, and malted beverages. In addition, the following foods that are high in tyramine should be avoided in patients taking an MAO inhibitor: American processed, cheddar, blue, brie, mozzarella, and Parmesan cheese; yogurt and sour cream; beef or chicken liver; cured meats such as sausage and salami; game meat; caviar; dried fish; avocados, bananas, yeast extracts, raisins, sauerkraut, soy sauce, and miso soup; broad (fava) beans, ginseng, and caffeine-containing products (colas, chocolate, coffee, and tea). The lowest dose of the MAOI patch, which delivers 6 milligrams (mg) of the medication over a 24-hour period, can be used without such dietary restrictions. However, avoiding tyramine-containing foods is necessary with the 9 mg/24 hr patch and the 12 mg/24 hr patch.

Antidepressants can have an effect on many other medicines. Thus, it is important for patients to inform their doctors of every medication they are currently taking prior to starting any antidepressant. Taking an MAOI antidepressant at the same time as any other antidepressants or certain over-the-counter medicines for colds and flu can cause a dangerous reaction.

The herb Saint-John's-wort may interact with antidepressants because it is believed to act similarly to the way in which SSRIs work. Thus, using Saint-John's-wort with SSRIs in particular can lead to exacerbation of side effects including headache, dizziness, nausea, agitation, anxiety, lethargy, and confusion. Clinicians have reported cases of clinically diagnosed serotonin syndrome among elderly patients who combined prescription antidepressants with Saint-John's-wort.

Duloxetine should not be used along with any MAO inhibitor; it also should not be taken along with thioridazine.

People who take an antidepressant such as trazodone as a sleeping pill plus another antidepressant for depression have been known to develop serotonin syndrome (see How Drugs Work in the Body, p. xxi). Serotonin syndrome can occur if the patient uses any two antidepressants that increase serotonin levels.

Sales/Statistics

Antidepressants reached more than $17 billion in sales worldwide in 2003 and were the third-largest therapeutic group of drugs by sales. Although the global antidepressant market saw extraordinary growth between 1993 and 2003, with few new entrants and a flood of patents expiring by 2014, the dynamics of the antidepressant market have changed. With seven of the eight leading brands losing U.S. patents, dollar sales for antidepressants have decreased as physicians have encouraged patients to use cheaper generics.

In 2010, according to IMS Institute for Healthcare Informatics (the public reporting arm of IMS), antidepressants were the seventh-largest U.S. drug class, with $11.6 billion in sales. However, they ranked second in prescriptions dispensed (253.6 million). Cymbalta was the top-selling antidepressant ($3.2 billion) and the 13th top-selling drug overall; Lexapro ranked 19th overall, with $2.8 billion in sales. The generic sertraline was the 17th most prescribed drug in the United States in 2010, with 35.7 million prescriptions dispensed. Citalopram ranked 19th, with 32.1 million prescriptions.

Demographic and Cultural Groups

The use of antidepressant drugs in children is growing by 10 percent a year, with the fastest-growing user group being preschoolers. This growth has occurred while evidence for their effectiveness and safety in children and adolescents has been scant and widely debated. The increased pediatric usage has occurred particularly among SSRIs, according to researchers, who found a 4.5-fold increase in the rate of prescriptions for SSRIs for children between 2000 and 2002.

Although depression is common among the elderly, a Duke University study published in 2000 suggests that its symptoms are being overlooked in many older black people. This study found that elderly white people are more than three times as likely to be prescribed antidepressant drugs as elderly blacks. Part of the problem, researchers say, may be reluctance on the part of black patients to take antidepressants. One large study showed that of those who did receive antidepressant medications, blacks were less likely to receive the newer SSRI medications than were the white patients. Other studies have shown that black women may be more sensitive to certain antidepressants and may require smaller dosages than traditional treatment advises. Black patients have also been found to metabolize antidepressants more slowly than white patients and may experience serious side effects from inappropriate dosages.

An earlier study by Washington State University researchers had similar findings regarding African Americans being underprescribed antidepressants and also found that Hispanic patients diagnosed with depression are prescribed antidepressants less frequently than similarly diagnosed non-Hispanic white patients. In a separate study, the same authors reviewed data from more than 18 million physician office visits from the 1995 National Ambulatory Medical Care Survey and found that physicians were more likely to prescribe antidepressants to patients who were younger (18 to 49 years old), female, and who self-reported depression as their reason for scheduling an office visit.

Some research suggests that Asian Americans metabolize antidepressants more slowly than white patients do. Therefore, Asian Americans may suffer from increased side effects and may be less medication adherent than white patients.

Development History

The treatment of depression was revolutionized in the 1950s, when two classes of drugs were discovered—entirely by serendipity—to be effective antidepressants: the TCAs and the MAO inhibitors. The TCAs, the first of which was imipramine, arose from antihistamine research, whereas the early MAO inhibitors, the first of which was iproniazid, were derived from treating tuberculosis.

Clinicians observed in 1953 that iproniazid improved tuberculosis patients' mood and gave them boundless energy. Nathan Kline first investigated its psychological effects and suggested it might prove useful in treating depression. In 1957, following initial success in trials, more than 400,000 prescriptions of iproniazid were issued within a year. However, after a number of people treated with this drug developed jaundice, the manufacturer withdrew the drug from the market.

About this same time, imipramine was found through clinical observation to have unexpected antidepressant effects. Imipramine was the first commercially available antidepressant, being launched in 1958. The clinical success of this drug led to the development of a successful series of other tricyclic and nontricyclic antidepressants.

It took almost 30 years for researchers to unravel enough of the brain's functioning to understand how MAOIs and TCAs worked to increase levels of the brain chemicals serotonin and norepinephrine simultaneously. Their disadvantage was that they could be difficult to tolerate because of significant side effects. Thus, the search began for medications that could selectively increase one of the chemicals responsible for improved mood, but not all of the chemicals at the same time—resulting in the second generation of antidepressants: SSRIs and, later, SNRIs. The first SSRI to be approved by the FDA was fluoxetine, in 1987.

The introduction of duloxetine in 2004 raised hope that another corner had been turned in treating depression due to its ability to treat physical pain associated with depression.

Future Drugs

Stahl and Grady noted that all classes of antidepressants currently available in the United States affect serotonin, norepinephrine, and/or dopamine neurotransmission. "New agents in development also affect neurotransmission of such monoamines and include serotonin-norepinephrine reuptake inhibitors, serotonin-selective agents, selective monoamine oxidase inhibitors, and selective norepinephrine reuptake inhibitors. Treatments with entirely new mechanisms of action are also being studied, including hormone-linked treatments such as estrogen replacement therapy and the steroid antagonist mifepristone (RU-486 or C-1073); novel antagonist peptides such as corticotropin-releasing factor, neurokinins, and injectable pentapeptides; and agents that affect glutamate neurotransmission. The introduction of antidepressants with novel mechanisms of action could potentially revolutionize the treatment of depression."

In September 2005, pharmaceutical companies had 28 new depression drugs under development, according to the trade group Pharmaceutical Research and Manufacturers of America.

Stahl, S. M., and M. M. Grady. "Differences in Mechanism of Action between Current and Future Antidepressants." *Journal of Clinical Psychiatry* 64, Suppl. 13 (2003): 13–17.

antidiabetic agents Drugs used to treat diabetes mellitus, a group of diseases marked by high levels of blood glucose (sugar), a condition known as hyperglycemia, resulting from defects in insulin production, insulin action, or both. Type 1 diabetes is an autoimmune disease in which the immune system attacks and destroys the insulin-producing beta cells in the pancreas. The pancreas then produces little or no insulin. Because Type 1 diabetes develops most often in children and young adults, it used to be called juvenile diabetes. A person who has Type 1 diabetes must take insulin daily to live; for this reason, this condition was also formerly called insulin-dependent diabetes. When Type 2 diabetes is diagnosed, the pancreas is usually producing enough insulin, but for unknown reasons, the body cannot use the insulin effectively, a condition called insulin resistance. After several years, insulin production decreases. The result is the same as for Type 1 diabetes—glucose builds up in the blood, and the body cannot make efficient use of its main source of fuel. Many people with Type 2 diabetes require oral medication, insulin, or both to control their blood glucose levels. Type 2 diabetes was formerly called adult-onset or non–insulin-dependent diabetes. A third type of diabetes, gestational diabetes, develops in some women late in pregnancy, caused by the hormones of pregnancy or a shortage of insulin. Although this form of diabetes usually disappears after the birth of the baby, women who have had gestational diabetes have a 20 to 50 percent chance of developing Type 2 diabetes within five to 10 years. Treatment for gestational diabetes may include insulin. Diabetes can lead to serious complications and premature death unless steps are taken to control the disease and lower the risk of complications.

In 2005, the National Diabetes Information Clearinghouse (NDIC), a service of the National Institute of Diabetes and Digestive and Kidney Diseases (NIDDK), reported that 20.8 million Americans—7 percent of the U.S. population—have diabetes. Of those, 14.6 million have been diagnosed; 6.2 are undiagnosed. About 90 to 95 percent of people with diabetes have Type 2 diabetes, which is most often associated with older age, obesity, family history of diabetes, previous history of gestational diabetes, physical inactivity, and certain ethnicities. About 80 percent of people with Type 2 diabetes are overweight. According to 2006 estimates from the Centers

for Disease Control and Prevention (CDC), diabetes will affect one in three people born in 2000 in the United States. The CDC also projects the prevalence of diagnosed diabetes in the United States will increase by 165 percent by 2050.

Classes
Antidiabetic drugs are divided into eight classes.

- *Insulin* Most synthetic insulins are now produced by recombinant DNA techniques and are chemically identical to natural human insulin, the hormone responsible for glucose utilization. Insulin is further subdivided into four main types according to their speed and duration of action: A.) Rapid-acting insulin, which begins to work within five to 15 minutes and lasts three to five hours. *Examples:* insulin aspart (NovoLog), insulin lispro (Humalog), insulin glulisine (Apidra). B.) Short-acting insulin, which starts working within 30 minutes and lasts five to eight hours. *Examples:* insulin regular (Humulin R, Novolin R). C.) Intermediate-acting insulin, which starts working in one to three hours and lasts six to 12 hours. *Examples:* NPH insulin suspension (Humulin N, Novolin N). D.) Long-acting insulin, which starts working in one to two hours and lasts 24 hours. *Example:* insulin detemir (Levemir), insulin glargine (Lantus). In addition, a variety of insulin mixture products are available.

- *Sulfonylureas* Stimulate the pancreas to make more insulin and help the body use the insulin it makes to better lower blood glucose. *Examples:* First generation: acetohexamide (Dymelor), chlorpropamide (Diabinese), tolazamide (Tolinase), and tolbutamide (Orinase). Second generation: glimepiride (Amaryl), glipizide (Glucotrol), and glyburide (DiaBeta, Glynase PresTab, Micronase).

- *Alpha-glucosidase inhibitors* Slow the absorption of starches, which causes a slower and lower rise of blood glucose through the day, particularly right after meals. *Examples:* acarbose (Precose) and miglitol (Glyset).

- *Biguanides* Decrease the amount of glucose made by the liver and increase insulin sensitivity. *Example:* metformin (Fortamet, Glucophage, Glumetza, Riomet).

- *Meglitinides* Stimulate the pancreas to make more insulin immediately following meals, which lowers blood glucose. *Examples:* nateglinide (Starlix) and repaglinide (Prandin).

- *Thiazolidinediones* (also called glitazones) Increase insulin sensitivity. *Examples:* pioglitazone (Actos) and rosiglitazone (Avandia).

- *Incretin mimetics* (also called glucagon-like peptide-1 [GLP-1] analogs or GLP-1 receptor agonists) Stimulate the pancreas to make more insulin (especially in the presence of elevated glucose levels) and slow gastric emptying. *Examples:* exenatide (Byetta) and liraglutide (Victoza).

- *Dipeptidyl peptidase-4 (DPP-4) inhibitors* Decrease the inactivation of and increase levels of incretin hormones, such as GLP-1, to lower blood glucose. *Examples:* saxagliptin (Onglyza) and sitagliptin (Januvia).

How They Work

Insulin is a hormone in the body that lowers blood glucose by moving glucose from the blood into the body's cells. Once inside the cells, glucose provides energy. Insulin also helps the body process the carbohydrates, fats, and proteins taken in as food and drink. When insufficient insulin is produced by the body to meet its needs, artificial insulin works to keep blood glucose levels within an acceptable range. Some people take the same amount of insulin every day to accomplish this; others need to adjust the dosage depending on their exercise, diet, and blood sugar patterns.

Sulfonylureas increase insulin release from the beta cells in the pancreas. Evidence also points to their sensitizing the beta cells to glucose, limiting glucose production in the liver, decreasing the breakdown of fatty acids, and decreasing clearance of insulin by the liver.

Alpha-glucosidase inhibitors block the enzymes that break down (digest) complex carbohydrates (starches) from food into glucose.

Delaying the digestion of dietary carbohydrates reduces blood glucose levels.

Biguanides help lower blood glucose by making sure the liver does not make too much glucose. They also tend to make the cells of the body more willing to absorb glucose already present in the bloodstream, thereby further reducing blood glucose.

Meglitinides block the potassium channels in beta cells, which opens the cells' calcium channels. The resulting calcium influx causes the cells to secrete insulin.

Thiazolidinediones help make the body's fat, liver, and muscle cells more sensitive to insulin, making it easier for the insulin to move glucose from the blood into these cells for energy. They act by binding to PPARs (peroxisome proliferator-activated receptors), a group of receptor molecules inside the cell nucleus. The normal molecules for these receptors are free fatty acids (FFAs) and eicosanoids. When activated, the receptor migrates to the DNA, activating transcription of a number of specific genes, resulting in decreased insulin resistance.

Incretin mimetics work by signaling the pancreas to make the right amount of insulin when blood sugar levels are high by stopping the liver from overproducing glucose when it is unneeded and by helping slow down the speed of food and glucose leaving the stomach, which also prevents hyperglycemia. These drugs mimic the effects of incretin hormones, such as GLP-1, which helps to lower blood glucose levels by increasing the ability of the beta cells to secrete insulin only when needed.

DPP-4 inhibitors work by increasing the level of incretins, which are hormones secreted by the gut. The most prominent incretin they enhance is GLP-1.

Approved Uses

Insulin is approved for use in all types of diabetes. All patients with Type 1 diabetes need insulin treatment permanently, unless they receive a pancreas transplant. Insulin is prescribed for Type 2 diabetes when diet, weight reduction, exercise, and oral antidiabetic agents do not sufficiently control blood glucose. Many patients with Type 2 diabetes will require insulin as their beta cell function declines over time.

Sulfonylureas are used to lower blood glucose levels in patients with Type 2 diabetes whose hyperglycemia cannot be controlled by diet and exercise alone. Many patients need combination therapy with several oral antidiabetic agents.

Alpha-glucosidase inhibitors are used along with diet to lower blood glucose in patients with Type 2 diabetes whose hyperglycemia cannot be managed on diet alone.

Metformin is used along with diet and exercise to improve glycemic control in patients with Type 2 diabetes.

Repaglinide is used along with diet and exercise to lower the blood glucose in patients with Type 2 diabetes whose hyperglycemia cannot be controlled satisfactorily by diet and exercise alone. Nateglinide is used to lower blood glucose in patients with Type 2 diabetes whose glycemia cannot be adequately controlled by diet and exercise and who have not been chronically treated with other antidiabetic agents.

Thiazolidinediones are used along with diet and exercise to improve glycemic control in patients with Type 2 diabetes.

Exenatide is used to lower blood sugar in patients with Type 2 diabetes when oral agents are no longer sufficiently effective by themselves. It is specifically for patients receiving metformin, a sulfonyolurea, a glitazone, or a combination of these agents.

Liraglutide is intended to help lower blood sugar levels in addition to diet, exercise, and selected other diabetes medicines.

Saxagliptin and sitagliptin are used along with diet and exercise to improve glycemic control in patients with Type 2 diabetes.

Off-Label Uses

Chlorpropamide has been used in the treatment of diabetes insipidus, a disease characterized by intense thirst and excessive urination, which cannot be reduced when fluid intake is decreased.

Exenatide is often prescribed off-label with insulin and is being studied for this usage. However, when this combination is used, the patients need to be counseled on the fact that it is not FDA-indicated, that there is a higher risk for hypoglycemia (low blood sugar) in that combination, and that they need to be monitoring their blood sugars carefully.

Companion Drugs

If one type of antidiabetic agent does not control a patient's blood glucose, the patient may be prescribed two kinds of pills or insulin and a pill. Pills used together:

- a sulfonylurea and metformin
- a sulfonylurea and acarbose
- metformin and acarbose
- repaglinide and metformin
- nateglinide and metformin
- pioglitazone and a sulfonylurea
- pioglitazone and metformin
- rosiglitazone and metformin
- rosiglitazone and a sulfonylurea

Drugs with similar mechanisms of action, such as meglitinides and sulfonylureas, should not be used in combination.

Several fixed-combination pills are also available. Although they offer less flexibility (if the dose of one ingredient needs to be adjusted, both would end up being adjusted), the benefits of an easier routine may help patient compliance. *Examples:* glyburide plus metformin (GlucoVance), glipizide plus metformin (Metaglip), rosiglitazone plus metformin (Avandamet), rosiglitazone plus glimepiride (Avandaryl), pioglitazone plus metformin (Actoplus Met), pioglitazone plus glimepiride (Duetact), and metformin plus sitagliptin (Janumet).

Insulin may be taken along with one of these diabetes pills: a sulfonylurea, metformin, or pioglitazone.

Administration

Insulin is administered via injection just under the skin with a small, short needle. Several devices for taking insulin are available. One is the insulin pen, which provides the convenience of carrying insulin in a discreet way. An insulin pen looks like a pen with a cartridge. Some of these devices use replaceable cartridges of insulin; other pen models are totally disposable. A short, fine needle, similar to the needle on an insulin syringe, is on the tip of the pen. Users turn a dial to select the desired dose of insulin and press a plunger on the end to deliver the insulin just under the skin. Insulin jet injectors send a fine spray of insulin through the skin by a high-pressure air mechanism instead of needles.

With subcutaneous infusion sets, also called insulin infusers, a catheter (flexible hollow tube) is inserted into the tissue just beneath the skin and remains in place for several days. Insulin is then injected into the infuser instead of through the skin. External insulin pumps deliver insulin through narrow, flexible plastic tubing that ends with a needle inserted just under the skin near the abdomen. The insulin pump is about the size of a deck of cards, weighs about 3 ounces, and can be worn on a belt or carried in a pocket. Users set the pump to give a steady trickle or "basal" amount of insulin continuously throughout the day. Pumps release "bolus" doses of insulin (several units at a time) at meals and at times when blood glucose is too high based on the programming set entered by the user. They also can be programmed to release smaller amounts of insulin throughout the day. Frequent blood glucose monitoring is essential to determine insulin dosages and to ensure that insulin is delivered.

If an entire vial of insulin will be used within 30 days, that vial may be kept at room temperature. After 30 days, these vials must be discarded. Vials of insulin that will not be used up within 30 days should be stored in the refrigerator all the time. If insulin gets too hot or too cold, it breaks down and does not work. Thus, insulin should not be kept in very cold places such as a freezer, or in hot places, such as by a window or in a car's glove compartment during warm weather.

Exenatide is an injectable drug, administered subcutaneously twice a day prior to the two biggest meals. It needs to be refrigerated before first use, and then it can be kept at room temperature not to exceed 77 degrees. Liaglutide is an injectable medication taken once a day via an injection pen.

All other antidiabetic agents are taken orally in tablet form.

Cautions and Concerns

In rare instances, insulin resistance may occur, meaning the muscle, fat, and liver cells do not use insulin properly. The pancreas tries to keep up with the demand for insulin by producing more. Eventually, the pancreas cannot keep up with the body's need for insulin, and excess glucose builds up in the bloodstream. Many people with insulin resistance have high levels of blood glucose and high levels of insulin circulating in their blood at the same time.

Insulin, sulfonylureas, meglitinides, and combination medicines can make blood glucose go too low. Hypoglycemia can result from delaying or skipping a meal, eating too little food at a meal, getting more exercise than usual, taking too much diabetes medicine, or drinking alcohol.

Insulin omission may lead to diabetic ketoacidosis (DKA), an emergency condition in which extremely high blood glucose levels result in the breakdown of body fat for energy and an accumulation of ketones in the blood and urine. Signs of DKA are nausea and vomiting, stomach pain, fruity breath odor, and rapid breathing. Untreated DKA can lead to coma and death. Diabetic ketoacidosis may also develop slowly after a long period of poor insulin control.

Lipoatrophy, the loss of fat under the skin resulting in small dents, may be caused by repeated injections of insulin in the same spot. Lipoatrophy may delay insulin absorption. Lipohypertrophy, the buildup of fat below the surface of the skin, causing lumps, may also be caused by repeated injections of insulin in the same spot. Lipohypertrophy may interfere with insulin absorption from the site. To minimize the occurrence of either of these conditions, the injection site should be rotated.

Patients taking insulin must follow a prescribed diet and exercise regimen regularly, including the set timing of insulin administration and meals.

Patients with hyperthyroidism may need more insulin to control their diabetes; those with hypothyroidism may require less insulin.

A patient who is stabilized on any oral diabetic regimen and experiences fever, trauma, infection, or surgery may lose glucose control and may need to discontinue the oral drug and take insulin.

All sulfonylureas may produce severe hypoglycemia. Thus, proper usage is important to avoid hypoglycemic episodes. Chlorpropamide remains active for up to 60 hours, requiring special caution with elderly patients or patients with liver or kidney impairment. A sulfonylurea-induced facial flushing may occur when chlorpropamide is administered with alcohol. Controlling blood glucose in Type 2 diabetes with sulfonylureas has not been established to definitely prevent long-term cardiovascular or neurologic complications of diabetes.

Metformin use should be temporarily suspended for surgical procedures restricting intake of food and fluids and should not be restarted until the patient's oral intake has resumed and kidney function is normal. Metformin should also be temporarily discontinued in patients who undergo procedures requiring contrast dye (e.g., cardiac catheterization, CT scans) because of the risk of renal failure.

All patients treated with thiazolidinediones should have liver enzyme monitoring prior to initial use and periodically thereafter (see *Warnings*).

Patients receiving exenatide should be observed for signs and symptoms of hypersensitivity reactions. There have also been postmarketing reports of pancreatitis associated with exenatide. The use of exenatide with a sulfo-nylurea may lead to hypoglycemia. The dose of the sulfonylurea may need to be reduced while taking exenatide.

Pancreatitis, seen with the first marketed incretin mimetic (exenatide), was also observed with liraglutide in several patients in clinical trials. When liraglutide is combined with other antidiabetic agents, the risk of hypoglycemia increases.

When saxagliptin is used with certain other diabetes medicines, such as a sulfonylurea, to treat high blood sugar, hypoglycemia may occur. When saxagliptin is used with a thiazolidinedione (TZD), such as pioglitazone or rosiglitazone, to treat high blood sugar, peripheral edema (fluid retention) may become worse.

A sitagliptin dosage adjustment is recommended in patients with moderate or severe kidney insufficiency. When sitagliptin is used with a sulfonylurea, hypoglycemia can occur.

Warnings

Types or brands of insulin should be changed only under medical supervision, as changes in purity, strength, manufacturer, or type may require dosage adjustment. Also, when changing insulin types or brands, any oral antidiabetic drugs being taken may need to be adjusted.

Hypersensitivity reactions to insulin may occur. Local allergy, with the patient occasionally experiencing redness, swelling, and itching at the site of injection of insulin, usually clears up in a few days to a few weeks. In some instances, this condition may be related to factors other than insulin, such as irritants in a skin cleansing agent or poor injection technique. Systemic allergy, which is less common but potentially more serious than local allergy, is considered a generalized allergy to insulin. It may cause rash over the whole body, shortness of breath, wheezing, reduction in blood pressure, fast pulse, or sweating. Severe cases of generalized allergic reaction may be life threatening. Any suspected generalized allergic reaction to insulin must be reported to a doctor immediately.

Careful glucose monitoring and dose adjustments of insulin may be necessary in patients with kidney or liver function impairment.

The administration of sulfonylureas has been associated with increased cardiovascular mortality as compared with treatment with diet alone or diet plus insulin. Although some controversy has surrounded the interpretation of these findings, patients should be informed of potential risks, advantages, and alternative treatment options. Sulfonylureas should be used with caution in Type 2 diabetes patients with impaired kidney or liver function and only with frequent monitoring of these organ functions. Dosing of sulfonylureas in the elderly should be conservative to avoid hypoglycemic reactions.

Gastrointestinal problems are the most common reactions to alpha-glucosidase inhibitors (see *Side Effects*), but the incidence of diarrhea and abdominal pain tend to diminish considerably with continued treatment.

Lactic acidosis is a rare but serious metabolic complication that can occur because of metformin accumulation during treatment; when it occurs, it is fatal in about half the cases. The few reported instances of metformin-associated lactic acidosis have occurred primarily in diabetic patients with impaired liver and/or kidney function. The risk of metformin accumulation and lactic acidosis increases with the degree of kidney function impairment. Because aging is associated with reduced kidney function, metformin should be used with caution as age increases. Patients with heart failure may also be predisposed to lactic acidosis.

Patients with impaired liver function may be exposed to higher concentrations of meglitinides than would patients with normal liver function receiving usual doses. Therefore, these drugs should be used cautiously in patients with impaired liver function.

Liver enzymes should be monitored regularly during the first year of treatment with thiazolidinediones to ascertain that no liver damage is occurring and periodically thereafter. If jaundice is observed, therapy should be discontinued.

Thiazolidinediones, alone or in combination with other antidiabetic agents, can cause fluid retention, which may exacerbate or lead to edema or heart failure. (This is especially the case when used with insulin.) Therefore, thiazolidinediones should not be used in patients with symptomatic heart failure and should be discontinued if any signs or symptoms of heart failure develop (e.g., excessive, rapid weight gain, shortness of breath, edema). In June 2011, the FDA announced that the use of pioglitazone for more than one year might increase the risk of bladder cancer.

Rosiglitazone may be associated with an increased risk of myocardial ischemia in some patients. In premenopausal women on birth control pills, thiazolidinediones may result in resumption of ovulation, putting these patients at risk for pregnancy. Thiazolidinediones are not recommended for use with insulin because of the risk of edema and heart failure. In 2006, the FDA notified health-care professionals regarding very rare postmarketing reports of new onset or worsening macular edema in patients receiving rosiglitazone. A number of studies have also demonstrated thiazolidinedione-induced bone loss in postmenopausal women, which is consistent with reports that thiazolidinediones may be associated with an increased fracture risk in women.

In animal studies, liraglutide caused tumors of the thyroid gland in rats and mice. Some of these tumors were cancers, which were significantly increased in rats who received excessive doses that were eight times higher than what humans would receive. It is not known if liraglutide could cause thyroid tumors or a very rare type of thyroid cancer called medullary thyroid cancer in people. For this reason, liraglutide should not be used as the first-line treatment for diabetes until additional studies are completed that support expanded use.

When Not Advised (Contraindications)

Antidiabetic agents are contraindicated during episodes of hypoglycemia.

Oral antidiabetic agents should not be used in patients with diabetic ketoacidosis (increased ketones in the blood or urine) or Type 1 diabetes.

Sulfonylureas should not be used when diabetes is complicated by ketoacidosis.

Safety during pregnancy for oral antidiabetic agents has not been adequately studied in humans; thus, these drugs should not be used during pregnancy unless the benefit outweighs the risk.

Alpha-glucosidase inhibitors should be avoided entirely in patients with inflammatory or obstructive bowel disease, diabetic ketoacidosis or cirrhosis, or digestion disorders. They are not recommended for patients with kidney dysfunction.

Metformin is contraindicated in patients with kidney or liver dysfunction, symptomatic congestive heart failure, sepsis, or diabetic ketoacidosis. It should not be used during acute illness requiring hospitalization or within 48 hours of radiologic studies involving the use of iodinated contrast materials.

Initiation of rosiglitazone or pioglitazone is contraindicated in patients with New York Heart Association class III or IV heart failure. Pioglitazone should not be used in patients with active bladder cancer, and the FDA has urged caution in using pioglitazone in patients with a history of bladder cancer

Liraglutide should not be used in people already at risk for medullary thyroid cancer, such as those who have medullary thyroid cancer in the family or those with a rare genetic condition known as multiple endocrine neoplasia syndrome type 2.

Side Effects

Hypoglycemia is a common side effect of diabetes treatment. Antidiabetic drugs that generally can lead to hypoglycemia include insulins, sulfonylureas, and meglitinides. For people taking these medications, blood sugar can fall too low for a number of reasons: meals or snacks that are too small, delayed, or skipped; excessive doses of these drugs; increased activity or exercise; or excessive drinking of alcohol. Patients should always take these drugs in the recommended doses and at the recommended times.

The NDIC recommends that patients who think their blood glucose is too low should use a blood glucose meter to check their level. If it is 70 mg/dL or below, the patient should have one of the following "quick fix" foods right away to raise his or her blood glucose:

- 2 or 3 glucose tablets
- 1/2 cup (4 ounces) of any fruit juice
- 1/2 cup (4 ounces) of a regular (not diet) soft drink
- 1 cup (8 ounces) of milk
- 5 or 6 pieces of hard candy
- 1 or 2 teaspoons of sugar or honey

After 15 minutes, the patient should check blood glucose again to make sure that it is no longer too low. If it is still too low, the patient should have another serving, then repeat these steps until the blood glucose is at least 70 mg/dl. Then, if it will be an hour or more before the next meal, he or she should have a snack.

Patients who take any of these drugs that can cause hypoglycemia should always carry one of the quick-fix foods with them. Wearing a medical identification bracelet or necklace is also a good idea. When used alone, certain drugs do not generally cause hypoglycemia (e.g., metformin, thiazolidinediones, exenatide, sitagliptin).

Hypokalemia (an abnormally low level of potassium, which can lead to weakness and heart abnormalities) is a potential side effect of all insulins. Allergic reactions (swelling, itching, or redness at the injection site; fast pulse, low blood pressure, perspiration, rash over the entire body, shortness of breath, shallow breathing, or wheezing) may also occur. Insulin may also lead to weight gain.

Sulfonylureas may induce upset stomach, headache, skin rash or itching, or weight gain. Because of a risk of photosensitivity reactions with these drugs, patients need to wear sunscreen when out in the sun.

The most frequent side effects of alpha-glucosidase inhibitors are gastrointestinal in nature and may include gas, bloating, abdominal pain, and diarrhea.

The most common side effects of metformin include diarrhea, nausea, gas, weakness, tiredness, dizziness, metallic taste, and flu symptoms.

The most common side effects of meglitinides include weight gain, upper respiratory tract infection, chest pain, and headache.

The main side effect of thiazolidinediones is fluid retention, leading to edema, weight gain, and potentially aggravating heart failure. Thiazolidinediones also have a potential for liver dysfunction (see *Warnings*). Other common side effects include headache, anemia, myalgia, flulike symptoms, and upper respiratory tract infection.

Mild to moderate nausea is the most common side effect of exenatide, usually occurring early in treatment and tending to go away as treatment continues. Other less common side effects with exenatide include diarrhea, dizziness, headache, and feeling jittery.

The most common side effects observed with liraglutide have been headache, nausea, and diarrhea. Other side effects included allergiclike reactions such as hives.

The most common side effects reported with saxagliptin were upper respiratory tract infection, urinary tract infection, and headache. Hypersensitivity-related events (e.g., urticaria, facial edema) were reported more commonly in patients treated with saxagliptin than in patients treated with placebo.

Although clinical trials showed sitagliptin to be free of side effects, postmarketing reports have revealed some nasopharyngitis, headache, and upper respiratory tract infections.

Interactions

Several drugs increase the action of insulin and may lower blood glucose to a dangerous level. Monoamine oxidase (MAO) inhibitors, angiotensin-converting enzyme (ACE) inhibitors, beta-blockers, NSAIDs, probenecid, salicylates (including aspirin), alcohol, anabolic steroids, tetracyclines, and sulfonamides may cause hypoglycemia in combination with antidiabetic agents, so blood glucose levels should be closely monitored when one of these drugs is initiated or discontinued. To prevent hypoglycemia when these drugs are used, the dosage of the antidiabetic agent may need to be reduced.

Certain drugs may decrease the effect of antidiabetic agents and cause worsening hyperglycemia. These include antiretrovirals, albuterol, calcium channel blockers, corticosteroids, danazol, diuretics, estrogens, isoniazid, niacin, nicotine, oral contraceptives, phenothiazines, phenytoin, sympathomimetics, and thyroid supplements. Blood glucose levels should be closely monitored when one of these drugs is added or discontinued during antidiabetic drug therapy.

Drugs that may increase the effectiveness of sulfonylureas include androgens, warfarin, azole antifungals, beta-blockers, chloramphenicol, fluoroquinolones, fluconazole, gemfibrozil, and H_2 antagonists.

Drugs that may decrease the effectiveness of sulfonylureas include cholestyramine, carbamazepine, phenytoin, and rifampin. Absorption of glipizide is delayed by about 40 minutes when taken with food. Other sulfonylureas may be taken with or without food.

Alpha-glucosidase inhibitors may reduce serum digoxin concentrations, decreasing the therapeutic effects. Digestive enzymes and intestinal adsorbents, such as charcoal, will decrease the effect of alpha-glucosidase inhibitors. Miglitol decreases the bioavailability of propranolol and ranitidine.

Acute or chronic alcohol use while taking metformin increases the risk for lactic acidosis. Nifedipine may enhance metformin absorption. Cationic drugs (e.g., amiloride, cimetidine, cotrimoxazole, digoxin, dofetilide, morphine, procainamide, quinidine, quinine, ranitidine, triamterene, and vancomycin) theoretically increase the risk for lactic acidosis by interfering with the renal tubular transport of metformin.

Azole antifungals, gemfibrozil, erythromycin, and clarithromycin may interfere with the metabolism of repaglinide, resulting in hypoglycemia. Gemfibrozil and repaglinide in particular should not be used together. Rifampin may decrease the effectiveness of repaglinide, resulting in hyperglycemia.

When thiazolidinediones are used with other antidiabetic agents, dosage of the other agents may need to be reduced. Gemfibrozil may increase rosiglitazone and pioglitazone concentrations. Rifampin may lower rosiglitazone and pioglitazone concentrations. Pioglitazone may decrease effectiveness of oral contraceptives. Thiazolidinediones should not be used with insulin because of the risk of edema, heart failure, and myocardial ischemia. Taking rosiglitazone with nitrates may increase the risk of myocardial ischemia.

Incretin mimetics can slow gastric emptying, which may have an effect on drugs being absorbed. It is recommended that orally administered drugs be taken at least one hour before exenatide. In clinical pharmacology trials, liraglutide did not affect the absorption of the tested orally administered medications to any clinically relevant degree. Nonetheless, caution should be exercised when oral medications are concomitantly administered with liraglutide.

Because ketoconazole, a strong CYP 3A4/5 inhibitor, increased saxagliptin exposure, the dose of saxagliptin should be limited to 2.5 mg when coadministered with a strong CYP 3A4/5 inhibitor (e.g., atazanavir, clarithromycin, indinavir, itraconazole, ketoconazole, nefazodone, nelfinavir, ritonavir, saquinavir, and telithromycin).

Taking sitagliptin and digoxin together can slightly increase the level of digoxin in the blood. The risk of hypoglycemia with both exenatide and sitagliptin significantly increases when used with a sulfonylurea.

Sales/Statistics

According to the 2007–2009 National Health Interview Survey (National Institute of Diabetes and Digestive and Kidney Diseases), among adults with diagnosed diabetes, 12 percent take insulin only, 14 percent take both insulin and oral medication, 58 percent take oral medication only, and 16 percent do not take either insulin or oral medications.

Espicom Business Intelligence, which monitors the pharmaceuticals market, estimated the global market for antidiabetic drugs in 2005 to be $11.8 billion, an increase of 12 percent over the previous year. Oral antidiabetic agents accounted for more than 60 percent of sales ($7 billion) versus insulin ($4.6 billion).

In the United States, *Drug Topics* magazine ranked three antidiabetic agents among the top 50 brand-name drugs in retail dollars in 2006: Actos ranked 14th ($1,926,293,000), Avandia ranked 17th ($1,664,459,000), and Lantus ranked 38th ($1,057,914,000). Avandia ranked 28th in units sold (11,331,000), Actos 29th (11,329,000 units), and Lantus 39th (9,519,000). Three other antidiabetics made one or both of the top 200 lists—Byetta, Humalog, Novolin 70/30, and NovoLog Mix 70/30. Within the first two years of its launching, 600,000 patients had been treated with Byetta.

Drug Topics ranked metformin #11 among the top 50 generic drugs in retail dollars ($670,167,000) and #10 in generic units sold (34,815,000). Other generic antidiabetics on the top 200 lists were glyburide, glipizide, and glimepiride.

In 2010, according to the IMS Institute for Healthcare Informatics, antidiabetic agents ranked fourth in U.S. drug spending, with $16.9 billion in sales, and sixth in prescriptions dispensed (165 million). Actos ranked ninth in sales ($3.5 billion) and generic metformin ninth in prescriptions dispensed (48.3 million).

Demographics and Cultural Groups

Type 1 diabetes occurs equally among males and females but is more common in whites than in nonwhites. Data from the World Health Organization's Multinational Project for Childhood Diabetes indicate that Type 1 diabetes is rare in most African, American Indian, and Asian populations. However, some northern European countries, including Finland and Sweden, have high rates of Type 1 diabetes. The reasons for these differences are unknown. Type 1 diabetes develops most often in children but can occur at any age.

Type 2 diabetes is more common in older people, especially in people who are overweight, and occurs more often in African Americans, American Indians, some Asian Americans, Native Hawaiians and other Pacific Islander Americans, and Hispanics/Latinos. On average, non-Hispanic African Americans are 1.8 times as likely to have diabetes as non-Hispanic whites of the same age. Mexican Americans are 1.7 times as likely to have diabetes as non-Hispanic whites of similar age. (Data are not available for estimation of diabetes rates in other Hispanic/Latino groups.) American Indians have one of the highest rates of diabetes in the world. On average, American Indians and Alaska Natives are 2.2 times as likely to have diabetes as non-Hispanic whites of similar age. Although prevalence data for diabetes among Asian Americans and Pacific Islanders are limited, some groups, such as Native Hawaiians, Asians, and other Pacific Islanders residing in Hawaii (aged 20 or older) are more than twice as likely to have diabetes as white residents of Hawaii of similar age.

Development History

The treatment of Type 1 diabetes was revolutionized during the summer of 1921 with the discovery of insulin by a group of researchers at the University of Toronto. Frederic Banting, Charles Best, J. B. Collip, and J. J. R. Macleod all played a role in making a pancreatic extract with antidiabetic characteristics. Banting and Macleod received the Nobel Prize for the discovery of insulin in 1923. The first successful use of insulin was in treating a diabetic dog. In 1922, the first diabetes patient was successfully treated with insulin.

In 1944, a standard insulin syringe was developed, helping to make diabetes management more uniform. This was followed in 1948 by the development of delayed action insulin, which reduced the number of daily insulin injections. In 1977, the insulin pump was introduced, allowing continuous delivery of insulin. Then in 1983, the first biosynthetic human insulin, Humulin, was introduced by Eli Lilly. Humulin was the first medication produced using modern genetic engineering techniques, in which actual human DNA is inserted into a host cell (*E. coli* in this case). The host cells are then allowed to grow and reproduce normally, and due to the inserted human DNA, they produce actual human insulin.

Sulfonylureas were discovered during World War II by the French university pharmacologist Marcel Janbon, who was studying sulfonamide antibiotics in an attempt to find an effective treatment for typhoid. While testing sulfonylurea in animals, he discovered that the drug induced hypoglycemia in the animals. Janbon convinced a medical colleague, August Loubatieres, to try it on his diabetic patients. After the drug triggered a fall in these patients' blood sugars, follow-up experiments revealed that the sulfonylurea stimulated pancreas cells to release insulin. In 1957, tolbutamide, the first of four sulfonylureas, debuted as the first class of oral antidiabetic agents. The other first-generation sulfonylureas gained approval in 1959 (chlorpropamide), 1964 (acetohexamide), and 1966 (tolazamide). Glipizide and glyburide, the first two second-generation sulfonylureas, gained FDA approval in 1964; glimepiride followed in 1995.

The biguanides class originates from the French lilac or goat's rue, a plant known since medieval times to improve the symptoms of diabetes mellitus. Researchers had tried over the years to use one of the plant's compounds, guanidine, to treat diabetes; however, its side effects proved too dangerous. Patlak writes, "A number of researchers tried to synthesize less toxic versions of guanidine that still lowered blood sugar levels. One of those versions, called a biguanide because it was comprised of two molecules of guanidine linked together, was first synthesized in 1922 by two English chemists. Dogged by toxic reactions, many researchers abandoned their efforts to develop biguanides into anti-diabetes drugs once insulin became available. The torch wasn't taken up again until the 1940s, when doctors tried using biguanides to treat people afflicted with malaria or influenza because there were no other treatments available for these often-fatal diseases. A side effect of the drug—the lowering of blood sugar—sparked the interest of the French doctor Jean Sterne, who decided to study one of the biguanides called metformin."

Once Sterne confirmed the blood sugar–lowering property of metformin and also showed that the drug had none of the serious side effects plagued by the other guanidines and biguanides, metformin made its debut in France in 1959. Soon it was being used in many European countries. However, the FDA continued to express concern about its potential toxicity and did not approve metformin for use in the United States until December 1994, following additional testing.

Acarbose received FDA approval in 1995 and miglitol in 1996.

Precursor drugs to repaglinide were invented in late 1983 by scientists at a German drug manufacturer. The drug that became repaglinide was later licensed to Novo Nordisk, which filed an Investigational New Drug application for the compound with the FDA in April 1992. Novo Nordisk filed its New Drug Application for Prandin in July 1997, and it was quickly approved, gaining FDA approval in December 1997. The drug was the first of the meglitinide class. It was branded Prandin because its quick onset and short duration of action concentrates its effect around meal time (the prandium was the Roman meal comparable to the modern lunch). The FDA approval of Starlix followed in 2000.

Scientists at several drug companies had created more potent antidiabetic drugs known as thiazolidinediones, but no one knew how they worked. Patlak writes, "That riddle was solved by molecular biologists at the Glaxo Research Institute in North Carolina, who were trying to figure out what causes fat cells to mature. Other scientists had shown that PPAR gamma was produced in large amounts by mature fat cells. In addition, researchers had reported that glitazones induced precursor fat cells (pre-adipocytes) to mature into fat cells. Putting two and two together, Steven Kliewer (University of Texas molecular biologist) and his colleagues used some clever laboratory manipulations to show, in 1995, that glitazones activated PPAR gamma. This discovery gave researchers a major new target for antidiabetes drugs—compounds that could activate PPAR gamma. Two such drugs, rosiglitazone (Avandia) and pioglitazone (Actos), came on the market in 1999."

Although John Eng, M.D., an endocrinologist at the Bronx Veterans Affairs Medical Center in New York City, discovered the unique ability of a salivary tissue protein from the Gila monster to lower blood sugar, the resultant exenatide drug is not derived specifically from the Gila monster, but rather is a synthetic. The exenatide protein was patented in 1993, with FDA approval in April 2005.

In the late 1970s, the Harvard Medical School professor Joel Habener was studying diabetes hormones in monkfish when he discovered the GLP-1 hormone, which scientists eventually realized lowers blood sugar only when it gets too high. However, making a pill form of GLP-1 proved challenging. The Merck researchers Nancy Thornberry and Ann Weber later identified the molecule that would become sitagliptin, with FDA approval for this drug being achieved in 2006.

Saxagliptin was approved on July 31, 2009, and liraglutide on January 25, 2010.

Fixed-combination pill FDA approvals: Gluco-Vance on July 31, 2000; Avandamet on October 10, 2002; Metaglip on October 22, 2002; Acto-plus Met on August 30, 2005; Avandaryl on November 23, 2005; Duetact on July 28, 2006; Janumet on April 2, 2007.

Future Drugs

Vildagliptin (Galvus), which was being developed by Novartis, is an oral DPP-4 inhibitor drug, similar to sitigliptin, that is administered once daily. When Novartis received a request from the FDA for additional information, the company withdrew its intent to submit vildagliptin to the FDA as of July 2008. The drug is already approved and available in Mexico, Brazil, and the European Union and in Australia with certain restrictions.

Dapagliflozin, being developed by AstraZeneca and Brsitol-Myers Squibb, has a novel mechanism of action that is called an SGLT2 inhibitor, or sodium glucose cotransporter 2. Although glucose is normally filtered by the kidney, nearly all of it is reabsorbed in the proximal tubule by SGLT2. For patients with diabetes, retention of excess glucose by this pathway contributes to persistent high blood glucose levels. Research in animal models indicates that modifying this glucose absorption with SGLT2 inhibition reduces blood glucose independent of insulin secretion or action. Dapagliflozin allows the kidney to excrete glucose specifically, so it comes out in the urine and does not get reabsorbed in the blood. It is being studied as a once-daily oral agent. The FDA accepted for review a New Drug Application for dapagliflozin in March 2011.

Herper, Matthew. "Merck Starts Diabetes Race." Forbes.com. Available online. URL: http://www.forbes.com/2006/10/17/merck-diabetes-drug-januvia-biz-cz_mh_1017merck.html. Posted on October 17, 2006.

Patlak, Margie. "New Weapons to Combat an Ancient Disease: Treating Diabetes." *The FASEB Journal* 16, no. 14 (December 2002): 1,853E.

antidiarrheals Drugs used to prevent or treat diarrhea—loose, watery stools occurring more than three times in one day—and some of its symptoms. Symptoms of diarrhea may include cramping abdominal pain, bloating, nausea, or an urgent need to use the bathroom. Depending on the cause, a person may have a fever or bloody stools. Stool is what is left after the digestive system (stomach, small intestine, and colon) absorbs nutrients and fluids from what one eats and drinks. Stool passes out of the body through the rectum. If fluids are not absorbed, or if the digestive system produces extra fluids, stools will be loose and watery. Diarrhea is not a disease itself, but rather a symptom of some other problem or disease. Diarrhea may be caused by a temporary problem, such as food intolerance or an infection, or a chronic problem, such as an intestinal disease.

Classes

Antidiarrheal drugs are divided into two types according to how they work—adsorbents and intestinal muscle relaxants.

- Adsorbents adhere to chemicals, toxins, and some infectious organisms in the gastrointestinal tract. Some adsorbents can also help firm up the stool. Adsorbents are available over the counter (OTC). *Examples:* bismuth subsalicylate (Kaodene Non-Narcotic, Kaopectate, Pepto-Bismol).

- Intestinal muscle relaxants, or antispasmodics, slow spasms of the bowel muscles so that the contents are propelled more slowly. They are more potent than adsorbents. *Examples:* difenoxin and atropine (Motofen), diphenoxylate and atropine (Lomotil, Lonox), and loperamide (Imodium). Difenoxin/atropine, diphenoxylate/atropine, and loperamide capsules are available only by prescription. Loperamide tablets and liquid are available OTC.

How They Work

By adsorbing (binding or attaching to) toxins (poisons) or bacteria that are causing the problem in the intestine, bismuth neutralizes the toxins so that they are not harmful. Bismuth also decreases the amount of liquid in the intestine. Bismuth subsalicylate also displays anti-inflammatory action (due to salicylate) and also acts as an antacid and mild antibiotic.

Intestinal muscle relaxants relax the muscles of the large intestine, causing the stools to move more slowly through. As a result, feces remain for an extended period of time in the intestine. This produces less stool volume, increased stool viscosity, and decreased fluid loss.

Difenoxin and atropine is a combination of an antidiarrheal (difenoxin) and an anticholinergic (atropine). Difenoxin is the principal active metabolite of diphenoxylate and is effective at one-fifth the dosage of diphenoxylate. Because difenoxin is chemically related to meperidine, a narcotic, it may be habit-forming if taken in doses that are larger than prescribed. To help prevent possible abuse, atropine has been added. If higher than normal doses of the combination are taken, the atropine will cause unpleasant effects, making it unlikely that such doses will be taken again. Similarly, diphenoxylate is available commercially only in combination with atropine sulfate in low quantity to discourage intentional abuse.

Approved Uses

Bismuth subsalicylate is used to treat indigestion and nausea, to relieve abdominal cramps, and to control diarrhea, including traveler's diarrhea, within 24 hours. Traveler's diarrhea affects an estimated 10 million international travelers each year who eat or drink contaminated food or water. High-risk destinations are the developing countries of Latin America, Africa, the Middle East, and Asia.

Diphenoxylate/atropine is used to treat acute diarrhea (diarrhea of limited duration). It may be useful in the treatment of mild or uncomplicated traveler's diarrhea.

Difenoxin/atropine is used as adjunctive therapy in the management of acute nonspecific diarrhea and acute exacerbations of chronic functional diarrhea.

Prescription loperamide is effective against diarrhea resulting from gastroenteritis or inflammatory bowel disease. Lembo and Rink write, "Loperamide appears to enhance the resting internal anal sphincter tone, which helps to improve stool leakage in irritable bowel syndrome (IBS), especially at night. It does not,

however, have any effect on abdominal pain or distention." OTC loperamide is used to control the symptoms of diarrhea, including traveler's diarrhea.

Off-Label Uses

Bismuth subsalicylate has been used in larger doses to prevent traveler's diarrhea in up to 65 percent of patients. It has also been used to treat chronic diarrhea in infants but should not be used in children under three years of age without a physician's approval.

Loperamide has been used to treat chronic diarrhea caused by bowel resection or organic lesions.

Administration

Antidiarrheals are taken by mouth, either as a tablet, caplet, chewable, or liquid. Bismuth subsalicylate liquid must be shaken well before using.

Because diarrhea helps rid the body of infection, patients should avoid using antidiarrheals for the first 24 hours, and after that use only if cramping and pain continue with no other signs of illness, such as fever.

Because taking too much diarrhea medicine can cause constipation, it should not be taken for longer than two days in a row even if the stool has not become less watery.

Cautions and Concerns

Antidiarrheals are not recommended for people whose diarrhea is caused by a bacterial infection or parasite: Stopping the diarrhea traps the organism in the intestines, prolonging the problem. Instead, doctors usually prescribe antibiotics in these instances.

Because adsorbents also adsorb the bacteria needed for digestion, they are not advised for long-term use.

Because bismuth subsalicylate may cause salicylate absorption, patients with bleeding disorders need to be watched closely. It may also cause impaction (bowel obstruction) in infants and weakened patients.

Warnings

Hepatic coma has been reported in patients with cirrhosis who have taken diphenoxylate/atropine and difenoxin/atropine. Extreme caution should be taken when using these drugs in patients with cirrhosis, advanced hepatorenal disease, or abnormal liver function.

When Not Advised (Contraindications)

Antidiarrheals can worsen colitis and dysentery. When there is a possibility that a patient may have infectious diarrhea (such as *Clostridium dificile* or other bacteria), and that patient is given one of these agents that slows intestinal motility, there is a potential that the toxins may accumulate in the intestine and cause damage.

Bismuth subsalicylate should not be used in patients who have a history of gastrointestinal bleeding.

Children and teenagers who have or are recovering from chicken pox or flulike symptoms should not take bismuth subsalicylate. Changes in behavior with nausea or vomiting when taking it could be an early sign of Reye's syndrome, a rare but serious illness.

Diphenoxylate/atropine is not recommended for children under two years of age because of a narrow therapeutic range between the beneficial dose and an at-risk dosage in this age group.

Loperamide is not recommended for children under two years of age unless a pediatrician advises otherwise. It is also not recommended for patients who could suffer detrimental effects from rebound constipation.

Side Effects

Bismuth subsalicylate has a normal side effect of turning the stool and tongue black. This occurs when bismuth combines with trace amounts of sulfur in the saliva and gastrointestinal tract, causing a black-colored substance (bismuth sulfide) to form. Temporary and harmless, this discoloration can last several days after a person stops taking bismuth subsalicylate. This discoloration is different from blackened stools caused from internal bleeding. Rarely, bismuth subsalicylate may cause ringing in the ears.

Diphenoxylate/atropine and difenoxin/atropine may cause dry mouth, dry skin, headache, constipation, and blurred vision. Because they also may cause drowsiness or dizziness, caution should be taken when driving or operating hazardous machinery.

The most common side effects of loperamide include constipation, abdominal pain or discomfort, nausea, drowsiness, and dizziness. Any of these are more likely to occur when treating chronic diarrhea. Children may be more susceptible to feeling drowsy or dizzy while taking loperamide.

Interactions

Antidiarrheals can prolong side effects caused by antibiotics such as cephalosporin, erythromycin, and tetracycline.

Antidiarrheals can worsen the constipation caused by opiate ANALGESICS such as oxycodone, hydrocodone, morphine, and codeine.

Bismuth subsalicylate should not be taken with aspirin or any other drugs containing salicylates. It may also interact with blood thinners and drugs used to treat diabetes, gout, and arthritis.

Diphenoxylate/atropine taken along with monoamine oxidase inhibitors can cause severe high blood pressure with the possibility of a stroke. When taken along with barbiturates, tranquilizers, and alcohol, diphenoxylate/atropine may increase central nervous system depression.

Sales/Statistics

According to the Consumer Healthcare Products Association, OTC antidiarrheal sales in 2004 amounted to $180 million (sold in groceries, drug stores, and mass merchandisers, but not Wal-Mart).

Development History

According to Procter & Gamble, the current marketers of Pepto-Bismol, this antidiarrheal was originally developed early in the 20th century as a treatment for "cholera infantum," a sometimes fatal disease that was striking infants suddenly. Infants with the disease suffered from diarrhea and vomiting. "A doctor concocted a formula in his home that proved effective against these symptoms. The formula was made from pepsin, bismuth salicylate, zinc salts, salol, and oil of wintergreen, along with a colorant to make it pink, and he called it Mixture Cholera Infantum."

Although it was later discovered that cholera infantum was caused by a bacterial infection treatable with antibiotics, the pink mixture had proven so successful at treating the disease's symptoms that demand continued for it. Unable to meet the demand from home, the inventor took the formula to Norwich Pharmacal Company, which increased production by making it in 20-gallon tubs and sold it to medical professionals. Eventually, researchers discovered that bismuth subsalicylate was the active ingredient. A name change to Pepto-Bismol in 1919 made it marketable to adults as well as children.

Diphenoxylate/atropine was approved by the FDA on September 15, 1960.

Loperamide received its first approval on December 28, 1976.

Difenoxin/atropine was approved on July 14, 1978.

Future Drugs

In April 2005, Genzyme Corporation announced the first Phase III clinical study for tolevamer, an investigational therapy for patients with *Clostridium difficile*–associated diarrhea (CDAD), a form of infectious diarrhea caused by the bacterium *C. difficile*. According to the company's news release, "Tolevamer is being developed as a new, non-absorbed therapy that could be the first non-antibiotic treatment approved for CDAD. Tolevamer is designed to bind and remove from the body toxins released by *C. difficile* that damage the intestine."

Lembo, Tony, and Rebecca Rink. "Current Pharmacologic Treatments of Irritable Bowel Syndrome." *Participate*, IFFGD 11, no. 2 (Summer 2002). Available online. URL: http://www.aboutibs.org/Publications/Pharma.html.

antiemetics Drugs that are effective against nausea and vomiting (emesis). Antiemetics are typically used to treat motion sickness, gastroenteritis, morning sickness, and the side effects of narcotic analgesics, chemotherapy, radiation, or surgery. Certain antiemetics are also used to treat the effects of vertigo, the sensation of spinning produced by an illusion of movement. Chronic vomiting can result in dehydration, which can become a serious and potentially life-threatening condition when the body contains an insufficient volume of water for normal functioning. Flake et al. note that "pregnancy-induced nausea alone has been estimated to cause 8.5 million lost working days annually. Postoperative nausea and vomiting have been shown to increase hospitalization costs by $415 per patient. Nausea affects an estimated 30 percent of patients within 24 hours of surgery." According to the National Cancer Institute, more than 500,000 Americans received chemotherapy in 2004. An estimated 75 percent suffer from nausea or vomiting within 24 hours of treatment, and about 90 percent of all patients suffer from chemotherapy-induced nausea or vomiting two to five days after treatment. Most antiemetics require a prescription, but several are available over-the-counter (OTC).

Classes

Antiemetics are divided into several classes according to their primary action; some agents affect multiple receptors.

- Antidopaminergics (commonly called dopamine antagonists) block dopamine receptors. *Examples:* Phenothiazines (see ANTIPSYCHOTICS)—chlorpromazine (Thorazine), perphenazine (Trilafon), prochlorperazine (Compazine), and promethazine (Phenergan). Others—metoclopramide (Reglan) and droperidol (Inapsine).

- Antihistamines act on histamine receptors. *Examples:* cyclizine (Marezine), dimenhydrinate (Dramamine), diphenhydramine (Benadryl), hydroxyzine (Atarax, Vistaril), and meclizine (Antivert, Bonine, Dramamine).

- Anticholinergics block acetylcholine receptors. *Examples:* scopolamine (Transderm Scop, Scopace, Maldemar) and trimethobenzamide (Tigan).
- Selective 5-HT$_3$ receptor antagonists (also called selective serotonin antagonists) block peripheral serotonin receptors. *Examples:* dolasetron (Anzemet), granisetron (Kytril), ondansetron (Zofran), and palonosetron (Aloxi).
- Substance P/Neurokinin 1 receptor antagonists block the action of neurokinin. *Examples:* aprepitant (Emend) and fosaprepitant (Emend for Injection).
- Cannabinoids work on cannabinoid receptors in the brain. *Examples:* dronabinol (Marinol) and nabilone (Cesamet).
- Corticosteroids are believed to affect prostaglandin activity in the brain. *Examples:* dexamethasone (Decadron) and methylprednisolone (Solu-Medrol).
- Benzodiazepines modulate the gamma-amino butyric acid (GABA) receptor within the brain. *Example:* lorazepam (Ativan).

How They Work

Both nausea and vomiting are controlled or mediated by the central nervous system but by different mechanisms. Nausea is controlled by a part of the central nervous system that controls involuntary bodily functions. Vomiting is a reflex coordinated in the base of the brain (brainstem) in a location called the vomiting center. Several neurotransmitter receptor sites along the pathways that send information to this vomiting center participate in the process. For example, the chemoreceptor trigger zone (CTZ), which stimulates the brain's vomiting center, has numerous dopamine type 2 (D$_2$) receptors, serotonin (5-HT$_3$) receptors, opioid receptors, acetylcholine receptors, histamine receptors, and receptors for neurokinin. Chemoreceptors in the upper gastrointestinal (GI) tract and mechanoreceptors in the wall of the GI tract also play a part in the process. Because activation of the various receptors leads to nausea and/or vomiting, most antiemetic agents target one or more of these receptor sites.

Dopamine antagonists block dopamine in the intestines and CTZ, which is stimulated primarily through D$_2$ receptors.

Antihistamines work by blocking the effects of histamine, a chemical in the body that stimulates gastric secretion.

Anticholinergics antagonize the action of the neurotransmitter acetylcholine, which is released at some (cholinergic) nerve endings, passing on a nerve impulse to the next nerve.

Antihistamines and anticholinergics also have the ability to block the transmission of information from the vestibular apparatus (the part of the middle ear that is involved in balance) to the vomiting center in the brain.

Selective 5-HT$_3$ receptor antagonists block serotonin binding in the GI tract. This, in turn, prevents stimulation from the gut to the CTZ in the brain.

Substance P/Neurokinin 1 receptor antagonists block the actions of substance P, a neurotransmitter in the brain that activates the neurokinin-1 pathway, which has been implicated in the development of nausea and vomiting.

Cannabinoids activate the cannabinoid CB$_1$ receptors in higher cortical areas, which suppresses the stimulatory nerve signals to the brainstem vomiting center, thereby reducing the vomiting reflex.

It is not known exactly how corticosteroids work to control nausea and vomiting. Because they improve the antiemetic characteristics of other medications, they are frequently used along with other antiemetic drugs.

Benzodiazepines work by acting on GABA receptors in the brain, which causes the release of the GABA neurotransmitter. GABA acts as a natural nerve-calming agent. Benzodiazepines are not very effective for controlling vomiting when used alone; therefore, they are frequently combined with other antiemetic medicines such as 5:HT$_3$ antagonists to increase their effectiveness.

Approved Uses

Chlorpromazine is approved to control nausea and vomiting and for relief of intractable hiccups (see also ANTIPSYCHOTICS). Perphenazine is used to control severe nausea and vomiting in adults. Prochlorperazine is used to control severe nausea and vomiting. Promethazine is approved to prevent and treat active motion sickness, to prevent and control nausea and vomiting associated with anesthesia and surgery, and as an antiemetic in postoperative patients. Metoclopramide is used to prevent nausea and vomiting associated with cancer chemotherapy, to treat gastroesophageal reflux (GERD), and to relieve symptoms associated with acute and recurrent diabetic gastric stasis. Droperidol is approved to reduce nausea and vomiting associated with surgical and diagnostic procedures.

Antihistamines are approved to prevent and treat nausea, vomiting, and the dizziness of motion sickness. Dimenhydrinate is also used to prevent and treat vertigo of motion sickness. (Dizziness of motion sickness refers to the feeling of lightheadedness or loss of balance. Vertigo of motion sickness refers to feeling that the room is spinning.)

Scopolamine is used to prevent nausea and vomiting associated with motion sickness, anesthesia, or surgery as well as an antispasmodic to reduce smooth muscle contractions. Trimethobenzamide is used to treat nausea and vomiting following surgery and for nausea associated with gastroenteritis (flu).

Dolasetron is used to prevent nausea and vomiting following cancer chemotherapy and to prevent and treat postoperative nausea and vomiting. Granisetron and ondansetron are used to prevent nausea and vomiting associated with cancer chemotherapy or radiation as well as to prevent and treat postoperative nausea and vomiting. Palonosetron is used to prevent acute and delayed nausea and vomiting associated with cancer chemotherapy.

Aprepitant and fosaprepitant are used in the prevention of acute and delayed chemotherapy-induced nausea and vomiting and in the prevention of postoperative nausea and vomiting.

Dronabinol and nabilone are used to treat nausea and vomiting associated with chemotherapy in patients not responding adequately to standard antiemetic treatment regimens. Dronabinol is also approved to treat anorexia associated with weight loss in patients with acquired immune deficiency syndrome (AIDS).

Off-Label Uses

Chlorpromazine is occasionally used off-label for treatment of severe migraine.

Metoclopramide has been used off-label to treat nausea and vomiting during pregnancy and labor.

All 5-HT$_3$ antagonists are used off-label to treat nausea and vomiting during pregnancy, to reduce bulimic episodes in patients with bulimia nervosa, and to treat intense itching resulting from spinal or epidural morphine. Dolasetron is used off-label to treat radiation-induced nausea and vomiting and to treat hyperemesis gravidarum, a severe form of nausea and vomiting in pregnancy. Granisetron is used off-label in the prevention of anesthetic-induced shivering.

Corticosteroids are used off-label to augment the antiemetic effect of 5-HT$_3$ receptor antagonists. (See also ANTIGOUT AGENTS and CORTICOSTEROIDS).

Lorazepam is used off-label to prevent nausea and vomiting following chemotherapy. (See also ANTIANXIETY AGENTS.)

Administration

Chlorpromazine is available as tablets and an injection (intravenous or intramuscular). Prochlorperazine is available as tablets, suppositories, and an injection (intravenous or intramuscular). Perphenazine is available only as tablets. Promethazine is available as tablets, suppositories, syrup, or injection (intravenous or intramuscular). Metoclopramide is available as tablets, syrup, or injection (intravenous or intramuscular). Droperidol can be administered via intramuscular or intravenous injection.

Antihistamines are available in many different formulations. See ANTIHISTAMINES.

Scopolamine is administered orally via tablets as well as via a skin patch placed behind the ear. Trimethobenzamide is administered via capsules or intramuscular injection.

All selective 5-HT$_3$ receptor antagonists can be administered via intravenous injection; ondansetron can also be administered intramuscularly. Dolasetron, granisetron, and ondansetron are also administered orally as tablets. Ondansetron is also available as orally disintegrating tablets that rapidly dissolve when placed on the tongue. Granisetron and ondansetron are also available as a liquid.

Aprepitant and cannabinoids are administered orally via capsules.

Fosaprepitant is given slowly through an IV infusion, which can take 15 to 30 minutes to complete. The first dose of fosaprepitant is usually given 30 minutes prior to chemotherapy treatment. Fosaprepitant is administered together with other drugs, such as aprepitant, a corticosteroid, and a 5-HT$_3$ antagonist.

Corticosteroids and lorazepam are administered orally via tablets or liquid or by intramuscular or intravenous injection.

Cautions and Concerns

Antiemetics can cause sleepiness, disorientation, and lack of concentration; thus, patients should avoid driving, operating machinery, or performing other tasks that require alertness.

For cautions with phenothiazines, see ANTIPSYCHOTICS; for cautions with promethazine and antihistamines, see ANTIHISTAMINES.

Dopamine antagonists should be used with caution in Parkinson's disease as they may worsen symptoms. Caution should be exercised when metoclopramide is used in patients with hypertension. The initial dose of droperidol should be appropriately reduced in elderly, debilitated, and other poor-risk patients. Droperidol should be administered with caution to patients with liver and kidney dysfunction.

After applying or removing a scopolamine patch, hands should be washed thoroughly with soap and water immediately to prevent any transfer of the drug to other parts of the body, especially the eyes. Scopolamine should be used with caution in the elderly and in individuals with kidney or liver dysfunction. Patients using the scopolamine patch longer than three days have reported dizziness, nausea, vomiting, and headache after discontinuing its use.

Central nervous system (CNS) reactions such as spasms, convulsions, coma, and extrapyramidal symptoms have occurred with use of trimethobenzamide, especially in children, the elderly, and the debilitated who have concurrent acute febrile illness, encephalitis, gastroenteritis, dehydration, or electrolyte imbalance. In such disorders, trimethobenzamide should be used with caution in patients who have recently received other CNS-acting agents (phenothiazines, barbiturates, belladonna derivatives).

Dolasetron and palonosetron should be administered with caution in patients who have or may be at risk for developing a prolonged QT interval (length of the heart's electrical cycle). The use of ondansetron or granisetron in patients following abdominal surgery or in patients with chemotherapy-induced nausea and vomiting may mask a progressive ileus and/or gastric distention.

Aprepitant and fosaprepitant should be used with caution in patients taking drugs that are metabolized by the CYP3A4 enzyme, as aprepitant and fosaprepitant could affect the blood levels of these drugs. Chronic continuous use of aprepitant or fosaprepitant for prevention of nausea and vomiting is not recommended because these drugs have not been studied and because the drug interaction profile may change during chronic continuous use. Aprepitant and fosaprepitant should also be used with caution in patients with severe liver disease.

Dronabinol should be used with caution in patients with a history of seizure disorder, as it may lower the seizure threshold. Both dronabinol and nabilone should be used with caution in patients with cardiac disorders because these drugs may increase or decrease blood pressure or cause fainting or tachycardia (abnormally rapid heart rate). Because they are highly abusable, these drugs should be used with caution in patients with a history of substance abuse. Dronabinol and nabilone should be used with caution and careful psychiatric monitoring in patients with mania, depression, or schizophrenia, as they may worsen these conditions. Both of these drugs should also be used with caution in the elderly, as these patients may be at increased risk for side effects.

For cautions with dexamethasone and methylprednisolone, see CORTICOSTEROIDS.

Lorazepam should be used with caution in patients with severe liver, kidney, or lung impairment. Because abruptly stopping lorazepam can cause anxiety, dizziness, nausea and vomiting, and tiredness, it should be gradually stopped. (See *Warnings*.)

Warnings

Antiemetics should be used only under close medical supervision in children with chickenpox, CNS infections, measles, gastroenteritis, or dehydration, as these patients appear to be more susceptible to neuromuscular reactions.

For warnings with phenothiazines, see ANTIPSYCHOTICS; for warnings with promethazine and antihistamines, see ANTIHISTAMINES.

Because metoclopramide can cause depression, patients with a history of severe depression should take this drug only if absolutely necessary. In addition, metoclopramide should be used with caution in patients with Parkinson's disease, as it may worsen the symptoms of their condition.

When administering droperidol, fluids and other countermeasures to manage hypotension should be readily available. Very rare reports of neuroleptic malignant syndrome (altered consciousness, muscle rigidity, and autonomic instability) have occurred in patients who have received droperidol. Droperidol carries an FDA-required black-box warning citing concerns of QT prolongation and torsades de pointes. Some cases have occurred in patients with no known risk factors, and some cases have been fatal. Droperidol should be used with extreme caution in patients who may be at risk for developing QT interval prolongation, including those with bradycardia (abnormally slow heart rate), heart disease, or electrolyte disorders such as hypokalemia (low potassium levels) or hypomagnesemia (low magnesium levels).

Because scopolamine may cause an increase in pressure inside the eye, glaucoma therapy in patients with chronic open-angle (wide-angle) glaucoma needs to be monitored and may need to be adjusted during scopolamine use.

Trimethobenzamide should be used with caution in children who have a viral illness, as it may mask or mimic the symptoms of Reye's syndrome.

Isolated reports of immediate hypersensitivity reactions, including flushing, erythema, and dyspnea, have occurred during infusion of fosaprepitant. These hypersensitivity reactions have generally responded to discontinuation of the infusion and administration of appropriate therapy. It is not recommended to reinitiate the infusion in patients who experience hypersensitivity reactions.

Both psychological and physiological dependence have been noted in healthy individuals receiving dronabinol after prolonged high-dose administration.

For warnings with dexamethasone and methylprednisolone, see CORTICOSTEROIDS.

Benzodiazepines can cause psychological and/or physical dependence. Withdrawal symptoms similar in character to those of alcohol and barbiturates have been observed after abrupt discontinuation; therefore, a gradual taper is recommended over a period of weeks or even months, depending on the length of time the drug was used and the dosage taken.

When Not Advised (Contraindications)

Antiemetics are not recommended for treatment of uncomplicated vomiting in children; their use should be limited to prolonged vomiting of known cause.

For contraindications with phenothiazines, see ANTIPSYCHOTICS; for contraindications with promethazine and antihistamines, see ANTIHISTAMINES.

Patients with a history of seizures should not take metoclopramide, as it may increase the frequency and severity of the seizures. Metoclopramide should also not be used in patients with intestinal problems such as bleeding, tears, or blockages.

Because of the risk of torsades de pointes, droperidol should be not be used in patients with QT interval prolongation or who are receiving monoamine oxidase inhibitors (MAOIs), antiarrhythmics, or other drugs that may prolong the QT interval.

Anticholinergics should not be used in patients with narrow-angle glaucoma, severe hemorrhage, tachycardia, or myasthenia gravis. The scopolamine skin patch should not be used on children.

Aprepitant or fosaprepitant should not be used in patients receiving pimozide or cisapride because of the potential for causing a life-threatening reaction.

Dronabinol should not be used in patients with hypersensitivity to sesame oil.

For contraindications with dexamethasone and methylprednisolone, see CORTICOSTEROIDS.

Lorazepam is not recommended for use in patients with a primary depressive disorder or psychosis. It is also contraindicated in patients with acute narrow-angle glaucoma.

Side Effects

Side effects of antiemetics that may impair driving performance include sedation, blurred vision, headache, confusion, and involuntary muscle contractions. Significant impairment may be present even in the absence of these symptoms. (See *Cautions and Concerns*.)

For specific side effects of phenothiazines, see ANTIPSYCHOTICS; for side effects of promethazine and antihistamines, see ANTIHISTAMINES.

Common side effects associated with metoclopramide include restlessness, drowsiness, dizziness, fatigue, headache, nausea, and diarrhea. The most common side effects with droperidol are hypotension (abnormally low blood pressure), tachycardia, QT interval prolongation, drowsiness, restlessness, hyperactivity, and anxiety. Both metoclopramide and droperidol can cause extrapyramidal side effects such as restlessness, tongue protrusion, and involuntary movements.

The most common side effects of scopolamine are dry mouth, drowsiness, and blurred vision. Memory disturbances; restlessness; confusion; dizziness; difficulty urinating; skin rash; dry, red, itchy eyes; and acute narrow angle glaucoma may also occur. Side effects of trimethobenzamide may include allergic reactions (hives, difficulty breathing, facial swelling), jaundice (yellowing of the skin), convulsions, easy bruising or bleeding, weakness, uncontrolled shaking, muscle cramps, drowsiness, dizziness, headache, and blurred vision.

Headache, hypertension, dizziness, chills, abdominal pain, diarrhea, and constipation are the most commonly reported side effects associated with selective 5-HT$_3$ receptor antagonists.

Common side effects of aprepitant include headache, dizziness, fatigue, weakness, loss of appetite, constipation, diarrhea, nausea, vomiting, heartburn, hypotension, bradycardia, and hiccups.

Because fosaprepitant is converted to aprepitant, those side effects associated with aprepitant might also be expected to occur with fosaprepitant. In addition, side effects observed in patients receiving fosaprepitant and not reported for aprepitant include infusion site redness, itching, and pain (see *Warnings*) as well as increased blood pressure and thrombophlebitis.

Common side effects of dronabinol include euphoria, paranoia, drowsiness, dizziness, abdominal pain, nausea, and vomiting. Common side effects of nabilone include dizziness, hypotension, loss of strength and muscle coordination, concentration difficulties, drowsiness, sleep disturbance, headache, vertigo, dry mouth, visual disturbance, depression, euphoria, loss of appetite, nausea, and weakness.

For side effects with dexamethasone and methylprednisolone, see CORTICOSTEROIDS.

The most common side effects of lorazepam are dizziness, drowsiness, and lethargy. Other side effects may include headache, mental depression, blurred vision, hypotension, nausea, and skin rashes.

Interactions

Antiemetics may enhance patients' response to alcohol; similarly, added sedative effects can occur when antiemetics are given along with barbiturates, hypnotics, narcotics, or tranquilizers.

For interactions with phenothiazines, see ANTIPSYCHOTICS; for interactions with promethazine and antihistamines, see ANTIHISTAMINES.

Metoclopramide should be used cautiously, if at all, in patients receiving MAOIs. Absorption of drugs from the stomach (e.g., digoxin) may be decreased by metoclopramide, while the absorption of drugs from the small bowel (e.g., acetaminophen, tetracycline, levodopa, ethanol, cyclosporine) may be increased. The use of droperidol should be avoided in patients receiving medications that prolong the QT interval (e.g., antiarrhythmics, antidepressants, fluoroquinolones). Droperidol should also be used with caution in patients receiving diuretics because the hypokalemia or hypomagnesemia that may result from diuretic therapy may predispose the patient to torsade de pointes. When patients have received CNS depressants, the dose of droperidol required will be less than usual.

The absorption of oral medications may be decreased during the concurrent use of scopolamine because of decreased gastric motility and delayed gastric emptying. Scopolamine interferes with the absorption of ketoconazole; it may also interact with other anticholinergic drugs, antidepressants, and antihistamines.

Blood levels of hydrodolasetron (dolasetron's active metabolite) may increase when dolasetron is coadministered with cimetidine and may decrease when used with rifampin. Dolasetron and palonosetron should be used cautiously, if at all, in patients receiving drugs that prolong the QT interval. The use of rifampin, phenytoin, or carbamazepine may reduce the antiemetic effect of ondansetron.

Concurrent use of aprepitant with other medications that are metabolized by CYP3A4 may result in altered blood levels of these agents. The use of aprepitant with the following chemotherapy agents that are metabolized by CYP3A4 could result in increased toxicity from these agents: docetaxel, paclitaxel, etoposide, irinotecan, ifosfamide, imatinib, vinorelbine, vinblastine, and vincristine. Aprepitant may also increase blood levels of benzodiazepines and corticosteroids. Aprepitant may also decrease the effects of warfarin, oral contraceptives, and tolbutamide. Concurrent use of aprepitant with CYP3A4 inhibitors (e.g., ketoconazole, itraconazole, nefazodone, clarithromycin, ritonavir, nelfinavir, and diltiazem) may increase the blood levels and effects of aprepitant. Concurrent use of aprepitant with CYP3A4 inducers (e.g., rifampin, carbamazepine, and phenytoin) may decrease the blood levels and effects of aprepitant. Drug interactions following administration of fosaprepitant are likely to occur with drugs that interact with oral aprepitant.

Cannabinoids may increase the effects of other drugs that cause drowsiness, including antidepressants, alcohol, antihistamines, sedatives, pain relievers, anxiety medicines, seizure medicines, and muscle relaxants.

For interactions with dexamethasone and methylprednisolone, see CORTICOSTEROIDS.

Lorazepam produces increased CNS-depressant effects when administered with other medications and drugs that slow the brain's processes, such as alcohol, barbiturates, narcotics, antipsychotics, anxiolytics, antidepressants, antihistamines, anticonvulsants, and anesthetics.

Sales/Statistics

According to the "Top 200 Generic Drugs by Total Prescriptions in 2010" (*Drug Topics*, June 2011), lorazepam ranked #26 with 23,428,627 prescriptions, and metoclopramide ranked #126 (4,418,452 prescriptions). However, because these drugs are used for multiple indications, not all these prescriptions would be for antiemetic use. Total in retail dollars in 2010 for lorazepam was $302,154,620 (ranking #45 among generic drugs). Zofran had ranked #53 in the "Top 200 Brand-Name Drugs by Retail Dollars in 2006" with $645,411,000 in sales. Antiemetics are often included in the general gastrointestinals category on industry reports. Thus, sales statistics for antiemetic use are not usually available.

Development History

Among the earliest drugs approved as antiemetics were phenothiazines and antihistamines, which were FDA-approved in the 1950s. Promethazine has been available as an antiemetic since 1951. Metoclopramide was approved in 1979, and dronabinol in 1985.

The FDA initially approved the scopolamine patch in December 1979 to prevent nausea and vomiting associated with motion sickness. Following the manufacturer's removal of the product from the marketplace in 1994 due to manufacturing problems, the FDA approved scopolamine again in October 1997 for the additional indication of preventing nausea and vomiting during or after surgery. In June 1997, the FDA approved scopolamine soluble tablets.

The selective 5-HT$_3$ receptor antagonists revolutionized the treatment of chemotherapy-induced nausea and vomiting. Ondansetron was granted FDA approval in January 1991, with oral ondansetron gaining approval in December 1992 and the orally disintegrating formulation gaining approval in January 1999. Granisetron injection was approved in March 1994; oral in March 1995. Dolasetron was approved in September 1997, and palonosetron in 2003.

Aprepitant, the first substance P/Neurokinin 1 receptor antagonist approved to treat chemotherapy-induced nausea and vomiting, was approved by the FDA in March 2003. Fosaprepitant was approved in January 2008.

Tetrahydrocannabinol, also known as THC, the main psychoactive substance found in the cannabis plant, was isolated by Israeli scientists in 1964. In the late 1970s, two National Cancer Institute (NCI) pilot studies were performed with smoked marijuana as well as oral THC. These small studies suggested that the utility of smoked and oral THC varied in part by the type of cancer chemotherapy being administered. As information developed regarding the potential benefit of THC as an antiemetic for patients undergoing chemotherapy, the NCI supported the development of the drug dronabinol—synthetic THC—as an oral antiemetic for such patients. In 1985, the FDA approved dronabinol for treatment of nausea and vomiting associated with cancer chemotherapy in patients who have not responded to conventional antiemetic therapy. The FDA also approved dronabinol in 1992 for use in loss of appetite and weight loss related to AIDS. Nabilone, also a synthetic cannabinoid, was approved in December 1985.

See also BENZODIAZEPINES, CORTICOSTEROIDS.

Future Drugs

Abeille Pharmaceuticals, Inc. has in development a novel transdermal patch for the relief of chemotherapy-induced nausea and vomiting. The patch (code name AB-1001) is designed to deliver a continuous dose of a commercially available 5-HT$_3$ antagonist for up to five days of continuous symptom relief from emetogenic chemotherapy.

In 2006, Hana Biosciences submitted a New Drug Application (NDA) for Zensana, an oral spray formulation of ondansetron. Hana believes Zensana is statistically bioequivalent to ondansetron tablets with faster initial delivery. In March 2007, Hana withdrew its pending NDA following their decision to file a different formulation of Zensana with the FDA after running into manufacturing problems with the therapy.

BioDelivery Sciences International, Inc. is developing Emezine, a buccal tablet formulation of prochlorperazine, for the treatment of severe nausea and vomiting. If approved, it will be the first buccal antiemetic in the United States, avoiding the discomfort of injections and inconvenience of suppositories. However, a non-approvable letter from the FDA in March 2006 caused the company to reevaluate the direction it intended to pursue regarding Emezine. Reckitt Benckiser Healthcare (U.K.) Limited distributes a similar product in the United Kingdom.

GlaxoSmithKline is developing vestipitant, another substance P/Neurokinin 1 receptor antagonist.

Flake, Zachary A., Robert D. Scalley, and Austin G. Bailey. "Practical Selection of Antiemetics." *American Family Physician* 69, no. 5 (March 1, 2004): 1,169–1,174.

antifungals Drugs used to treat fungal infections, the most common of which affect the hair, skin, nails, or mucous membranes. Fungal infections can include but are not limited to athlete's foot, ringworm, and candidiasis (a yeast infection), as well as serious systemic infections such as cryptococcal meningitis. A system-wide fungal infection is called a mycosis. Antifungal drugs destroy or inhibit the growth of fungi.

Visible only through a microscope, fungi survive by attaching themselves to and living off of other cells. Fungi can occur as yeasts, molds, or as a combination of both forms. Filamentous fungi grow as long, multicelled strands (filaments). Fungi particularly thrive in moist, dark places. Some fungal infections are spread by sharing combs or hairbrushes and in public showers, pools, and locker rooms. Taking ANTIBACTERIALS can also cause some people to get fungal infections. While killing intended harmful bacteria, antibacterials sometimes also kill harmless bacteria that normally fight with the fungus or yeast for a place to live. When antibacterials kill these harmless bacteria, the fungus is free to grow. Similarly, fungus infections have become more common with the increasing use of chemotherapeutic agents to fight cancer.

Mycoses may also be caused by opportunistic fungi in patients who are being treated with corticosteroids or immunosupressants as well as in people with weakened immune systems, such as with HIV or AIDS. Babies with low birth weight are also at risk for opportunistic fungal infections.

Adhikari, a pharmaceutical industry analyst, wrote, "Systemic fungal infections are estimated at 335,000 incidences per year worldwide (World Health Organization, 2004). Most common is systemic candidiasis, representing approximately 70 percent of all such infections with a mortality rate of approximately 40 percent."

Classes

Antifungal drugs may be systemic (spread throughout the body) or topical (effective only in a certain area, such as the skin). Systemic antifungals are available by prescription only. Some of the topical antifungals are available over the counter (OTC), while others are available only by prescription. Antifungals are classified according to their mechanism of action, site of action, and chemical make-up.

- *Polyenes* are naturally occurring compounds isolated from the *Streptomyces nodosus* species, an organism found in the soil. *Examples:* amphotericin B (Amphocin, Fungizone)—systemic, amphotericin B lipid-based (Abelcet, AmBisome, Amphotec)—systemic, natamycin (Natacyn)—ophthalmic, and nystatin (Mycostatin, Nilstat, Nystop)—topical.

- *Azoles* are classified into imidazoles and triazoles according to their chemical structure; however, their antifungal activity is due to the same molecular mechanism. *Examples:* imidazoles: butoconazole (Mycelex-3, Gynazole-1)—topical, clotrimazole (Cruex, Mycelex-7)—topical, econazole (Spectazole)—topical, ketoconazole (Nizoral)—systemic and topical, miconazole (Monistat)—topical, oxiconazole (Oxistat)—topical, sulconazole (Exelderm)—topical, and tioconazole (Vagistat-1)—topical; triazoles: fluconazole

(Diflucan)—systemic, itraconazole (Sporanox)—systemic, posaconazole (Noxafil)—systemic, terconazole (Terazol)—topical, and voriconazole (Vfend)—systemic.

- *Allylamines* are synthetic antifungal agents similar to the azoles. *Examples:* butenafine (Lotrimin Ultra, Mentax)—topical, naftifine (Naftin)—topical, and terbinafine (Lamisil)—systemic and topical.

- *Echinocandins* are also known as glucan synthesis inhibitors. *Examples:* anidulafungin (Eraxis)—systemic, caspofungin (Cancidas)—systemic, and micafungin (Mycamine)—systemic.

- *Pyrimidines Example:* flucytosine, also called 5-flurocytosine or 5-FC (Ancobon)—systemic.

- *Miscellaneous* Ciclopirox (Loprox, Penlac)—topical, griseofulvin (Fulvicin, Grifulvin, Gris-PEG)—a systemic antifungal derived from the mold *Penicillium griseofulvum*, and tolnaftate (Tinactin)—topical.

How They Work

The polyene antifungals bind with sterols, particularly ergosterol, in the fungal cell membrane. This binding causes the cell's contents to leak out through the membrane, and the cell eventually dies. The body's cells contain cholesterol instead of ergosterol, so they are much less susceptible to the antifungal agent.

The azole antifungals interrupt the synthesis of ergosterol by inhibiting the fungal enzyme 14-alpha demethylase. This enzyme normally converts lanosterol to ergosterol, and is required in fungal cell wall synthesis. When the cell membrane lacks sufficient amounts of ergosterol, it becomes weak and unable to support further growth. Eventually, the fungal cells die as a result of this deficiency. At higher concentrations, azoles appear to cause direct damage to cell walls. These drugs also block steroid synthesis in humans. Because they inhibit many human enzymes involved in drug metabolism, they are particularly susceptible to interactions with other drugs metabolized through the same pathway.

Like the azoles, allylamines disrupt the production of ergosterol in the fungus cell membrane, leading to the eventual death of the fungus. However, the allylamines block an earlier step in the ergosterol production process by inhibiting the enzyme squalene epoxidase. Also like the azoles, terbinafine, in particular, is susceptible to interactions with other drugs metabolized through the same pathway.

The echinocandins inhibit the enzyme 1,3-beta-D-glucan synthase, which forms glucan polymers in the fungal cell wall. By inhibiting this enzyme, echinocandins prevent more than 90 percent of glucose incorporation into glucan. This results in an abnormally weak fungal cell wall.

Once flucytosine enters into the fungal cell wall, it is converted into 5-fluorouracil by the enzyme cytosine deaminase. At this point, flucytosine has two mechanisms of action. One is that the 5-fluorouracil is converted to 5-fluorouridine triphosphate, which is incorporated into fungal RNA and disturbs the production of certain essential proteins. The other mechanism is that 5-fluorouracil is converted into 5-fluorodeoxyuridylic acid monophosphate, which inhibits fungal DNA-synthesis.

Ciclopirox works by binding to iron and aluminum ions, which inhibits the metal-dependent enzymes that are responsible for the destruction of peroxides in the fungal cell. This results in an accumulation of peroxides, which can be toxic to the fungal cell.

Griseofulvin inhibits fungal cell mitosis (the process by which a cell separates its duplicated genome into two identical halves) by disrupting mitotic spindle formation—a critical step in cellular division.

Tolnaftate works in a manner that is similar to the allylamine antifungal agents.

Approved Uses

Amphotericin B, a broad-spectrum antifungal agent, is the drug of choice in treating life-threatening systemic fungal infections and for most other mycoses. It has been called the gold standard for the treatment of serious fungal infections. Among the fungal infections it is used to treat are aspergillosis, blastomycosis, candidiasis, coccidioidomycosis, cryptococcosis, histoplasmosis, and mucormycosis.

Natamycin, an ophthalmic antifungal, is used to treat fungal keratitis (inflammation of the cornea), fungal blepharitis (inflammation of eyelids and eyelashes), and conjunctivitis (commonly called pinkeye) caused by fungus. It is especially effective against cabdida, aspergillus, and fusarium ophthalmologic infections.

Nystatin is used to treat fungal infections of the skin, mouth, vagina, and intestinal tract caused by *Candida.*

Butoconazole is available by prescription and OTC and is used to treat vaginal yeast infections.

Clotrimazole is used for treating athlete's foot, jock itch, ringworm, topical treatment of mild to moderate candidiasis (vaginal yeast infections or oral thrush), and tinea versicolor. It is also used as a preventive in order to reduce the incidence of oral thrush in patients with neutropenia (low neutrophils in blood).

Econazole is used to treat athlete's foot, jock itch, ringworm, tinea versicolor (skin infection caused by the yeast *Malassezia furfur,* sometimes called "sun fungus"), and cutaneous candidiasis (a skin infection).

Systemic ketoconazole is used to treat fungal infections such as candidiasis, oral thrush, blastomycosis, coccidioidomycosis, histoplasmosis, candiduria, chromomycosis, and paracoccidioidomycosis. Topical ketoconazole is used to treat athlete's foot, ringworm, cutaneous (skin) candidiasis, jock itch, and tinea versicolor. The shampoo formulation is used to reduce scaling due to dandruff.

Both OTC and prescription miconazole are used to treat athlete's foot, jock itch, and ringworm. Prescription miconazole is used to treat tinea versicolor and cutaneous candidiasis. Miconazole OTC is also used internally to treat vaginal yeast infection as well as for relief of itching and irritation associated with vaginal candidiasis.

Oxiconazole and sulconazole are both used to treat athlete's foot, jock itch, and ringworm. Sulconazole can also be used to treat tinea versicolor.

Tioconazole is available OTC and is used to treat vaginal yeast infections.

Fluconazole is used especially to treat fungal infections caused by *Candida*—namely, yeast infections of the vagina, mouth, throat, esophagus, urinary tract, abdomen, lungs, blood, and other organs and cryptococcal meningitis, an infection of the membranes covering the brain and spine. Fluconazole is also used to prevent yeast infections in patients undergoing bone marrow transplantation who receive chemotherapy or radiation therapy.

Itraconazole has a broader spectrum of activity than fluconazole. In particular, it is active against aspergillosis, which fluconazole has no activity against. It is also used to treat blastomycosis, histoplasmosis, and onychomycosis. The oral solution is approved for treatment of mouth and throat candidiasis.

Posaconazole is used to prevent serious fungal infections in people with a weakened ability to fight infection. Posaconazole is also used to treat yeast infections of the mouth and throat, including yeast infections that could not be treated successfully with other medications.

Terconazole, available only by prescription, is used to treat vaginal yeast infections.

Voriconazole is used to treat serious invasive fungal infections that are generally seen in people with weak immune systems, such as patients with cancer or who have received organ or bone marrow transplants. These infections include invasive candidiasis and aspergillosis.

Prescription and OTC butenafine are used to treat athlete's foot, jock itch, and ringworm. The prescription product is also used to treat tinea versicolor.

Naftifine is a prescription topical antifungal used to treat athlete's foot, jock itch, and ringworm.

Oral terbinafine is available by prescription only and is used to treat fungal infections of the fingernails and toenails. Topical terbinafine is available OTC and is used to treat athlete's foot, jock itch, and ringworm.

Anidulafungin has been approved to treat candidemia, the most deadly of the common hospital-acquired bloodstream infections, and potentially life-threatening, as well as other infections caused by the *Candida* fungus, including peritonitis (infection of the abdominal cavity), intra-abdominal abscesses, and esophageal candidiasis.

Caspofungin is used for the treatment of invasive aspergillosis in patients who cannot tolerate or who do not respond to standard treatments for infections caused by *Aspergillus* fungus. It has not been studied as an initial therapy for invasive aspergillosis, and it is not recommended for such use. Caspofungin is also approved for presumed fungal infections in patients who have a fever and neutropenia as well as for *Candida* fungal infections of the blood (candidemia), esophageal candidiasis, and the following *Candida* infections: intra-abdominal abscesses, peritonitis, and pleural space infections.

Micafungin is used to treat esophageal candidiasis and to prevent fungal infections caused by *Candida* in patients who are undergoing a stem cell transplant.

Flucytosine is a systemic antifungal used to treat serious fungal infections caused by *Candida* or *Cryptococcus*. In life-threatening fungal infections, flucytosine is not administered as sole agent due to its relatively weak antifungal effects and fast development of resistance. Rather, it should be used in combination with amphotericin B. Minor infections such as candidal cystitis may be treated with flucytosine alone.

Ciclopirox is available by prescription only in a number of topical formulations. The cream and topical suspension are used to treat athlete's foot, jock itch, ringworm, cutaneous candidiasis, and tinea versicolor. The gel is used to treat athlete's foot, ringworm, and seborrheic dermatitis of the scalp. The nail lacquer is used to treat fungal infections of the fingernails and toenails. The shampoo is used to treat seborrheic dermatitis of the scalp.

Griseofulvin is used to treat fungal skin infections such as jock itch, athlete's foot, and ringworm and fungal infections of the scalp, fingernails, and toenails.

Tolnaftate is available OTC and is used to treat athlete's foot, jock itch, and ringworm.

Off-Label Uses

Amphotericin B is used as a fungal infection preventive in patients with bone marrow transplantation and also as a bladder irrigation for candidal cystitis.

Nystatin is used as a preventive in patients who are at risk for fungal infections, such as certain AIDS patients and patients receiving chemotherapy.

Systemic ketoconazole has been used successfully to treat tinea versicolor, vaginal yeast infections, excessive hair growth in women, and eumycetoma (the fungal form of mycetoma, a disease of the skin and of connective tissue). The decrease in testosterone caused by ketoconazole makes it useful for treating prostate cancer. Because it inhibits adrenal steroidogenesis, ketoconazole has been used in the treatment of Cushing's disease.

Fluconazole has been used as an alternative treatment of blastomycosis as well as to treat deep or recurrent skin fungi such as ringworm, jock itch, and athlete's foot when local treatment was not successful.

Itraconazole oral solution is used as an alternative for long-term prevention of recurrence or relapse of mucocutaneous candidiasis (throat, oral, vaginal) in HIV-infected infants, children, adolescents, and adults. It is also used as alternative treatment for coccidioidomycosis, chromomycosis, cryptococcosis, and sporotrichosis.

Voriconazole has been used in specific clinical settings for the management of presumed fungal infections in febrile neutropenia patients.

Systemic terbinafine is used to treat ringworm of the scalp and body. Topical terbinafine is effective in the treatment of cutaneous candidiasis and tinea versicolor.

Flucytosine is used in conjunction with amphotericin B for treatment of invasive aspergillosis.

Administration

Systemic antifungals are available in tablet, capsule, liquid, vaginal suppository, and injectable forms. Topical antifungals are available as creams, lotions, ointments, gels, lacquers, powders, liquids, aerosol sprays, shampoos, and vaginal suppositories.

Amphotericin B is administered intravenously.

Natamycin is available as an ophthalmic suspension. Natamycin is for topical eye use only and not for injection. Touching the dropper tip to any surface may contaminate the suspension.

Nystatin is available as a tablet and a suspension (liquid) to take by mouth; a tablet and cream to be inserted into the vagina; and in powder, ointment, and cream to be applied to the skin.

Butoconazole is available as a vaginal cream.

Clotrimazole is available as oral lozenges (called troches) as well as for topical use as a cream, solution, and vaginal tablets (suppositories).

Econazole is available only as a topical cream.

Systemic ketoconazole is available in tablet form. Topical ketoconazole is available as a prescription cream, as a prescription shampoo, and in a weaker dosage as an over-the-counter shampoo.

Miconazole is available as a topical spray (liquid and powder), effervescent tablet, tincture, powder, cream, and ointment as well as vaginal suppositories and cream.

Oxiconazole is available as a topical cream and lotion.

Sulconazole is available as a topical cream and solution.

Tioconazole is available as a vaginal ointment.

Fluconazole is administered either orally (tablets or suspension) or by injection.

Itraconazole is available as capsules, as an oral solution, or by an injection.

Posaconazole is available as a suspension to take by mouth.

Terconazole is available as a vaginal cream and suppositories.

Voriconazole is administered orally (tablets or suspension) or by injection.

Butenafine is available only as a topical cream.

Naftifine is available as a topical cream (applied once a day) or gel (applied twice a day).

Systemic terbinafine comes as a tablet to take by mouth. Topical terbinafine is available as a cream or spray.

Anidulafungin, caspofungin, and micafungin are administered by intravenous injection.

Flucytosine is available as capsules.

Ciclopirox is available as a topical cream, gel, shampoo, lacquer, and suspension.

Griseofulvin is available as tablets or a suspension taken by mouth.

Tolnaftate is available as a topical spray (liquid and powder), cream, powder, solution, and swab.

Cautions and Concerns

Because of the high risk of adverse events in patients receiving amphotericin B, kidney and liver function and blood counts need to be closely monitored.

Ketoconazole cream contains sulfites that may cause allergic reactions or asthmatic episodes in susceptible persons.

Fluconazole, ketoconazole, itraconazole, and posaconazone should be administered with caution to patients with potentially proarrhythmic conditions.

Because voriconazole causes some people to have blurred vision or other visual disturbances, especially during the first two weeks of use, using machines, driving motor vehicles, or performing other tasks that could be considered dangerous when vision is impaired are not recommended.

Liver function test abnormalities as well as hepatic dysfunction have been reported in patients receiving anidulafungin.

Micafungin may cause liver inflammation, worsening of liver failure, and abnormal liver function tests; kidney problems, kidney failure, and abnormal kidney function tests; and problems with red blood cells called hemolysis or hemolytic anemia. Patients should be watched closely for worsening liver function, worsening kidney function, and worsening blood disorder.

Blood counts and kidney and liver function tests should be taken frequently during flucytosine therapy. Patients with preexisting bone marrow depression and liver impairment should be treated with caution. Patients with kidney disease should receive flucytosine cautiously and in reduced doses.

Lupus symptoms in patients who have lupus erythematosus (SLE) have worsened when taking griseofulvin. Because of possible photosensitivity reactions, patients taking griseofulvin (particularly those who have SLE) should wear protective clothing and use sunscreen to protect against exposure to sunlight or ultraviolet light.

Warnings

Kidney damage is a major issue with the use of amphotericin B and can be severe and irreversible. Electrolyte imbalances may also occur.

Ketoconazole has been associated with liver damage, including some fatalities. Patients need to be closely monitored.

Fluconazole has been associated with liver toxicity, but less than that with ketoconazole.

Liver function monitoring in patients taking itraconazole, posaconazole, or voriconazole is suggested for all patients, but particularly in those patients with preexisting liver disease.

Itraconazole can cause congestive heart failure (CHF) in patients at risk for CHF, such as those who have a history of heart failure, a heart attack, or serious irregular heart rhythms. Taking dofetilide, pimozide, or quinidine while taking itraconazole can cause potentially serious cardiovascular events, including QT (length of the heart's electrical cycle) prolongation, torsades de pointes, ventricular tachycardia, cardiac arrest, and/or sudden death.

In rare cases, systemic terbinafine has caused severe liver damage, sometimes resulting in liver transplant or death, in individuals with and without preexisting liver disease.

Isolated cases of severe hypersensitivity reactions have been reported in patients receiving micafungin. If these reactions occur, micafungin infusion should be discontinued.

Because of potential fertility and pregnancy problems, men should wait at least six months after completing griseofulvin therapy before fathering a child, and neither pregnant women nor women considering pregnancy should take this drug. Rare cases of conjoined twins have been reported in women who took griseofulvin during the first three months of pregnancy.

When Not Advised (Contraindications)

Any of the antifungals used to treat onychomycosis (a fungal infection of the fingernails or toenails) should not be used during pregnancy or in women contemplating pregnancy, since this is not a condition that requires urgent treatment and because of potential risks of the drugs to the fetus.

Ketoconazole should not be used in the treatment of fungal meningitis because it penetrates poorly into the cerebrospinal fluid (CSF).

Posaconazole is contraindicated with sirolimus, as it increases the sirolimus blood concentrations by approximately ninefold and can result in sirolimus toxicity. Posaconazole is also contraindicated with CYP3A4 substrates that prolong the QT interval. Concomitant administration of posaconazole with the CYP3A4 substrates pimozide and quinidine may result in increased plasma concentrations of these drugs, leading to QTc prolongation and rare occurrences of torsades de pointes.

Because voriconazole has been shown to cause fetal harm, it is not advised for women who are pregnant. Women are advised to use effective contraception during treatment with voriconazole.

Griseofulvin has been reported to worsen lupus symptoms in patients who have lupus erythematosus or lupuslike diseases. Griseofulvin should also be avoided in patients with severe liver disease.

Side Effects

Amphotericin B is associated with numerous side effects, with up to 90 percent of patients exhibiting some intolerance. Very often an acute reaction consisting of fever, shaking chills, low blood pressure, loss of appetite, nausea, vomiting, headache, shortness of breath, and rapid breathing can occur one to three hours after the infusion is completed. This reaction sometimes subsides with administration of additional doses of the drug and may in part be due to the release of histamine. An increase in prostaglandin synthesis may also play a role. In order to decrease the likelihood and severity of the symptoms, lower initial doses are recommended. The dose should then be increased slowly. Electrolyte disturbances can also occur. Lipid-based formulations have been developed to reduce the side effects of infusion-related reactions and kidney damage.

Natamycin may cause eye irritation, redness, or swelling.

Side effects are not common with nystatin but may include nausea, vomiting, gastrointestinal distress, diarrhea, facial swelling, or a rash (when applied to the skin).

Although side effects from butoconazole are not common, they can occur and may include burning, itching, soreness, and/or swelling in the vagina when cream is inserted; stomach or pelvic pain or cramping; fever; and foul-smelling discharge.

Clotrimazole side effects are uncommon but may occur. Lozenges may cause vomiting, upset stomach, unpleasant mouth sensations, or itching. Topical skin applications may cause stinging, blistering or burning, peeling, general skin irritation, swelling, or itching. Vaginal application may cause burning, irritation, or foul-smelling discharge.

Econazole may cause burning, itching, stinging, or redness. Skin rash with itching has occurred, but rarely.

Due to its side-effect profile, systemic ketoconazole has been superseded by newer antifungals, such as fluconazole and itraconazole. Its more common side effects include nausea, vomiting, blocked production of testosterone, and liver toxicity. Less common are headache, dizziness, sleepiness, abdominal pain, diarrhea, and severe itching. Topical ketoconazole has caused severe irritation, itching, and stinging. The shampoo has increased normal hair loss and has caused irritation, abnormal hair texture, loss of hair curl in "permed" hair, dry skin, itchiness, and oiliness or dryness of the hair and scalp.

Miconazole side effects are rare, but there have been isolated reports of irritation, burning or itching of the skin or vagina, foul-smelling vaginal discharge, stomach pain, or fever.

Oxiconazole side effects include itching, burning, stinging, eczema, reddening of the skin, dry or flaky skin, tingling, and folliculitis (inflammation of hair follicles).

Sulconazole side effects are not common but can include blistering, burning or stinging, itching, redness of the skin, peeling, dryness, or irritation of the skin.

Tioconazole side effects can include allergic reaction (shortness of breath, closing of the throat, or hives), vaginal swelling or redness, burning, itching, headache, abdominal pain or cramping, upper respiratory tract infection, increased need to urinate, and burning urination.

Fluconazole is generally well tolerated; more common side effects include headache, nausea, vomiting, abdominal discomfort, diarrhea, dizziness, changes in taste, and skin rash. Reversible hair loss has also been reported after long-term use of fluconazole.

Itraconazole is relatively well tolerated, although not as well tolerated as fluconazole or voriconazole, and the range of side effects it produces is similar to the other azole antifungals. The most common side effects include headache, dizziness, nausea, vomiting, diarrhea, abdominal pain, loss of appetite, fatigue, skin rash, and edema. Less common but more serious side effects are liver enzyme elevation, hepatitis, and high blood pressure.

Posaconazole side effects may include fever; headache; chills or shaking; dizziness; weakness; swelling of the hands, feet, ankles, or lower legs;

diarrhea; vomiting; stomach pain; constipation; heartburn; weight loss; rash; itching; back or muscle pain; sores on the lips, mouth, or throat; difficulty falling asleep or staying asleep; anxiety; increased sweating; nosebleeds; or coughing. More serious side effects, which should be reported to the patient's doctor immediately, include unusual bruising or bleeding; extreme tiredness; lack of energy; loss of appetite; nausea; pain in the upper right part of the stomach; yellowing of the skin or eyes; flulike symptoms; dark urine; pale stools; fast, pounding, or irregular heartbeat; sudden loss of consciousness; shortness of breath; or decreased urination.

Side effects most likely to occur with terconazole are headache and painful menstruation. Less frequently reported have been burning and itching. Less common side effects reported with terconazole include abdominal pain and fever.

Common side effects of voriconazole include blurred vision, increased eye sensitivity to light, or other visual disturbances; nausea, vomiting, abdominal pain or diarrhea; headache; swelling or water retention; fever; and respiratory disorder. Rare but life-threatening side effects include severe liver damage and allergic reactions to the medication.

More common side effects of naftifine cream include burning/stinging, dryness, and skin irritation. Side effects of the gel include burning/stinging, itching, rash, and tenderness.

Side effects from systemic terbinafine include rash, hives, itching, taste disturbances, diarrhea, indigestion, abdominal pain, nausea, and flatulence. Side effects from topical terbinafine include irritation, burning/tingling, itching, and dryness.

The echinocandins appear to be well tolerated and have relatively fewer side effects than polyene or azole antifungals. In clinical trials, the most common side effects from anidulafungin were lower than normal levels of potassium in the blood, diarrhea, liver function test abnormalities, and headache. Possible histamine-mediated symptoms have been reported infrequently with anidulafungin, including rash, hives, flushing, itching, breathing difficulties, and low blood pressure. Caspofungin can cause a serious allergic reaction. Signs of a serious allergic reaction are sudden problems breathing, swelling of lips or tongue, sudden cough, hives, and rash. Other side effects include fever, injection site reactions, nausea, flushing, and vomiting. Common side effects related to mycafungin include rash, mental confusion, itching, facial swelling, and relaxing of blood vessels. Mycafungin may also cause injection site reactions such as inflammation of the veins.

Central nervous system side effects are frequent with flucytosine and include confusion, hallucinations, psychosis, clumsiness, hearing loss, headache, burning/tingling, tremors, peripheral neuropathy, vertigo, and sedation. Skin reactions include rash, itching, and photosensitivity. Flucytosine may also cause gastrointestinal upset (nausea, vomiting, diarrhea).

Hypersensitivity reactions such as skin rashes and hives are the most common side effects of griseofulvin. Other occasional side effects include nausea, vomiting, diarrhea, headaches, fatigue, dizziness, insomnia, and mental confusion.

Interactions

Drinking alcohol, using medications that contain alcohol, or eating foods prepared with alcohol should be avoided while taking antifungals and for at least three days after finishing the medication, as alcohol may cause nausea, abdominal cramps, vomiting, headaches, and flushing.

Corticosteroids used along with amphotericin B increase the risk of potassium depletion and predispose patients to cardiac dysfunction.

Oral ketoconazole and itraconazole are best absorbed at highly acidic levels, so antacids, H_2 blockers, proton pump inhibitors, or sucralfate will lower these drugs' effectiveness. If itraconazole or ketoconazole must be used with antacids, it is recommended that at least two hours pass between the administration of each of these medications.

Ketoconazole and itraconazole may increase the effects of a number of drugs, including amiodarone; benzodiazepines; warfarin; buspirone; calcium channel blockers; clarithromycin; cyclosporine; digoxin; erythromycin; fluoxetine; protease inhibitors; oral drugs for diabetes such as glipizide, glimepiride, pioglitazone, and rosiglitazone; drugs for erectile dysfunction such as sildenafil, tadalafil, and vardenafil; methadone; methylprednisolone; mexiletine; paroxetine; phenytoin; pimozide; quinidine; quinine; sertraline; sirolimus; tacrolimus; tamoxifen; telithromycin; theophylline; trazodone; tricyclic antidepressants; and vincristine.

Ketoconazole, itraconazole, fluconazole, and voriconazole can interfere with the way some cholesterol-lowering medications (simvastatin, lovastatin, atorvastatin, rosuvastatin) are broken down by the body, which can increase the risk of serious side effects, such as muscle and liver toxicity. In fact, the use of simvastatin or lovastatin is not advised in patients taking either ketoconazole or itraconazole.

Posaconazole increases midazolam plasma concentrations by approximately fivefold. Increased plasma midazolam concentrations could increase and prolong hypnotic and sedative effects. The dose of other medicines may need to be adjusted when taken with posaconazole (e.g., cyclosporine, tacrolimus, ritonavir, or atazanavir). Because posaconazole and many medicines can interact with one another, it is important that the patient's doctor be apprised of all prescription and nonprescription medicines, vitamins, and herbal supplements the patient is taking or about to take. See also *When Not Advised (Contraindications.)* Posaconazole will work better if taken with a meal, within 20 minutes of eating a full meal, or with a liquid nutritional supplement.

Women who take warfarin and use a miconazole intravaginal cream or suppository may be at risk for developing an increased international normalized ratio (INR) and bleeding.

Caution is advised if taking certain other medications with fluconazole. Rifampin and phenytoin, for example, accelerate the metabolism of fluconazole in the liver and reduce

serum levels. In addition, fluconazole can cause a rise in serum levels of phenytoin and antidiabetic drugs such as chlorpropamide, glyburide, glipizide, and tolbutamide as well as the blood thinner warfarin. It also increases cyclosporine levels slightly.

Voriconazole interacts with many medications, including drugs given to suppress the immune system in transplant patients. Drugs that may decrease the effectiveness of voriconazole include rifampin, rifabutin, phenytoin, and carbamazepine. Voriconazole may increase the levels of antihistamines, methylprednisolone, sirolimus, cyclosporine, tacrolimus, ergotamine, warfarin, sulfonylureas, statins, midazolam and other benzodiazepines, vincristine, and some HIV drugs.

Rifampin may reduce the effectiveness of terbinafine. Cimetidine may increase terbinafine blood levels. Dosage adjustments or special monitoring during treatment may be needed if either of these medicines are being taken along with terbinafine.

Because the use of caspofungin with cyclosporin may temporarily increase liver enzymes, this combination should be used only when the potential benefit outweighs the potential risk. Caspofungin may increase levels of tacrolimus. Rifampin may reduce the effectiveness of caspofungin.

Flucytosine may increase the toxicity of amphotericin B and vice versa, although the combination may be life-saving and should be used whenever indicated. Cytarabine may inactivate the antifungal activity of flucytosine.

Other vaginal creams or douches should be avoided while using tioconazole.

The hydrogenated vegetable oil base used in terconazole may weaken certain latex products such as condoms or vaginal contraceptive diaphragms. Thus, such products should not be used within 72 hours of taking terconazole.

Combined use of ciclopirox with a systemic antifungal agent is not recommended. Also, nail polish and other cosmetic products should not be used on nails being treated with ciclopirox.

Griseofulvin may decrease the effectiveness of ANTICOAGULANTS such as warfarin, of oral contraceptives, of salicylates, and of cyclosporine. Barbiturates may decrease the blood levels of griseofulvin. The use of alcohol may increase the toxicity of griseofulvin.

Sales/Statistics

The world market for prescription antifungal drugs stood at more than $5.4 billion in 2004, according to Kalorama Information, a provider of market intelligence reports and services. Their study, "The World Market for Anti-Infectives, Volume I: Antifungals," found that systemic antifungal drugs continue to dominate over topical formulations in the market, accounting for more than 70 percent of total revenues. Another pharmaceutical industry market intelligence service, InPharm.com, had forecast revenue of $1.32 billion for triazole drugs used in systemic fungal infection treatment in the United States for 2011.

The RxList of Top 300 Prescriptions for 2004 (retail and mail order, excluding Wal-Mart) included several antifungal drugs: Diflucan, 7,107,234; nystatin (various brands), 5,111,085; fluconazole (various brands), 4,012,259; and Lamisil, 2,641,473. Also on the Top 300 list were two combination drugs that included an antifungal: clotrimazole/betamethasone, 3,886,738; and nystatin-triamcinolone, 2,348,605.

The 2010 *Drug Topics* Top 200 Generic Drugs by Retail Dollars listed fluconazole #116 ($127,763,760), ketoconazole topical #167 ($77,028,101), nystatin #170 ($74,709,149), and terbinafine #173 ($73,812,292). The 2010 *Drug Topics* Generic Drugs by Total Prescriptions listed fluconazole #47 (13,938,887 prescriptions), ketoconazole topical #155 (3,343,677 prescriptions), nystatin #173 (2,706,171 prescriptions), and terbinafine #189 (2,302,568 prescriptions).

Development History

Polyenes, the first antifungal agents, were developed in the 1950s. Nystatin was isolated from *Streptomyces noursei* in 1950 by Elizabeth Lee Hazen and Rachel Fuller Brown, who were doing research for the Division of Laboratories and Research of the New York State Department of Health. Hazen worked in New York City and Brown in Albany, sharing their tests and samples through the U.S. mail. The soil sample where they discovered nystatin was from the garden of Hazen's friends, called the Nourses; therefore, the strain was called *noursei*. Hazen and Brown named nystatin after the New York State Public Health Department. Amphotericin B was discovered in 1956. Natamycin was approved in 1978.

Azoles were developed to treat fungal infections that did not respond to polyenes. They have been used since the 1970s. Miconazole was originally approved by the FDA in 1974, and clotrimazole in 1975. Ketoconazole was discovered in 1976 and approved in 1985 as the first available oral treatment for fungal infections. Econazole was approved in 1982, tioconazole in 1983, terconazole in 1987, oxiconazole in 1988, sulconazole in 1989, fluconazole in 1990, itraconazole in 1992, butoconazole in 1995, voriconazole in 2002, and posaconazole in 2006.

Allylamines, developed in the 1980s, marked an advance in both the destruction and inhibition of fungi growth. Naftifine was approved by the FDA in 1988, topical terbinafine in 1992, butenafine in 1996, and systemic terbinafine in 1996.

Flucytosine was originally developed in the 1950s as a potential anticancer drug. Although ineffective against tumors, it was later found to have antifungal activity.

Caspofungin was the first approved drug (January 29, 2001) in the echinocandins class of antifungal agents. Micafungin received FDA approval on March 17, 2005.

Griseofulvin received FDA approval in 1959, and tolnaftate in 1965.

Ciclopirox was first approved in 1982. A stronger solution (8 percent) was approved in 1999, and a 1 percent shampoo in 2003.

Anidulafungin was approved by the FDA on February 21, 2006.

A number of antifungal agents are in development. Among them:

- Albaconazole, a unique broad-spectrum antifungal, showed promise in Phase II trials. According to news releases distributed by the developers, "It has shown potent activity against a broad range of organisms, including pathogens resistant to other antifungals (such as fluconazole or itraconazole). Albaconazole will be developed as an oral and topical formulation, and will be available to the medical community for a variety of dermatological indications and fungal infections, including vulvovaginal candidiasis. It is also well tolerated and has shown no significant adverse effects."

- Ravuconazole is a broad-spectrum triazole antifungal being developed for treatment of systemic fungal infections such as candidiasis, aspergillosis, and cryptococcal meningitis. Ravuconazole shows promise for the treatment of immunocompromised patients, such as those with HIV infection or cancer and organ transplant patients, who are at risk for developing serious fungal infections.

Adhikari, Raju. "Systemic Antifungal Market Still Enjoys the Sweet Smell of Success—a Commercial Insight." InPharm.com. Available online. URL: htttp://www.inpharm.com. Posted on December 8, 2004.

antigout agents Drugs used to treat gout, which is sometimes called gouty arthritis. Gout is a painful rheumatic disease resulting from deposits of needle-like crystals of uric acid in connective tissue, in the joint space between two bones, or in both. The deposits are a result of excess uric acid in the bloodstream (a condition called hyperuricemia), which may be due to increased production of uric acid or the kidney's inability to excrete uric acid efficiently. These deposits clog the joints, leading to inflammatory arthritis, which causes swelling, redness, heat, pain, and stiffness in the joints. In cases of chronic gout, the joint may become deformed and eventually be destroyed by the crystals. The term *arthritis* refers to more than 100 different rheumatic diseases that affect the joints, muscles, and bones as well as other tissues and structures. Gout usually attacks the big toe (approximately 75 percent of first attacks); however, it can also affect other joints such as the ankle, heel, instep, knee, wrist, elbow, fingers, and spine. Gout accounts for approximately 5 percent of all cases of arthritis and occurs in approximately 840 out of every 100,000 people. According to the National Institutes of Health (NIH), gout affects approximately 2.1 million people in the United States and is more common in men between the ages of 40 and 50. In women, incidence increases after menopause. The condition is rare in children and young adults.

Classes

Several classes of drugs are used to treat gout, some to treat symptoms of acute attacks and others to prevent future attacks.

- *Nonsteroidal anti-inflammatory drugs* (NSAIDs) The first line of therapy for acute gout attacks. *Examples:* indomethacin (Indocin), naproxen (Anaprox, Naprosyn), and sulindac (Clinoril). (See ANALGESICS.)

- *Miscellaneous* Colchicine is considered the second line of therapy for acute gout.

- *Corticosteroids* Considered the last line of therapy for acute gout, because they do not work as well as NSAIDs or colchicine. The most commonly prescribed corticosteroids for gout are prednisone (Meticorten, Orasone), prednisolone, and triamcinolone (Aristocort, Kenacort). (See CORTICOSTEROIDS.)

- *Uricosurics* Uric acid eliminators for chronic gout. *Examples:* probenecid and sulfinpyrazone (Anturane).

- *Xanthine oxidase inhibitors* Uric acid reducers for chronic gout. *Example:* allopurinol (Zyloprim) and febuxostat (Uloric).

How They Work

NSAIDs block the production of prostaglandins, hormones derived from fatty acids, which dilate blood vessels and cause the inflammation and pain of gout.

Colchicine works by attaching itself to a cell-scaffolding protein called tubulin, causing certain parts of a cell's architecture to crumble, and this action can interfere with a cell's ability to move around. Researchers suspect that in the case of gout, colchicine works by halting the migration of immune cells called granulocytes that are responsible for the inflammation characteristic of gout.

Corticosteroids also reduce the inflammation of gout by blocking the production of substances that cause inflammation, such as prostaglandins.

Uricosurics help the kidneys get rid of the excess uric acid produced in the body. By preventing the kidneys from reabsorbing uric acid, they increase the amount excreted in the urine.

Xanthine oxidase inhibitors decrease uric acid levels in the blood and urine by blocking xanthine oxidase, the enzyme responsible for production of uric acid.

Approved Uses

Indomethacin, naproxen, and sulindac are specifically labeled for the treatment of acute gouty arthritis. (See ANALGESICS for additional approved uses of NSAIDs.)

Colchicine is approved for treatment and relief of pain during attacks of acute gouty arthritis and as a preventive between attacks.

Corticosteroids are prescribed for people with gout who cannot take NSAIDs or colchicine. (See CORTICOSTEROIDS for their other approved uses.)

Probenecid is used to treat hyperuricemia associated with gout. Sulfinpyrazone is used to treat hyperuricemia and to lower blood uric acid in patients with chronic or intermittent gout.

In addition to treating the symptoms of and to prevent gout, allopurinol is used to prevent kidney stones as well as to treat elevated uric acid levels that occur in cancer patients receiving chemotherapy.

Febuxostat is approved for the chronic management of hyperuricemia in patients with gout.

Off-Label Uses

All other NSAIDs, in addition to those specifically labeled, are used to treat acute attacks of gout. (See ANALGESICS for additional off-label uses of NSAIDs.)

Colchicine is used to treat familial Mediterranean fever, cirrhosis of the liver, primary biliary cirrhosis (an autoimmune disease that affects primarily the bile ducts of the liver), Behget's disease (a rare autoimmune disorder that involves inflammation of blood vessels), amyloidosis (a tissue disorder), scleroderma (an autoimmune disease that involves the skin and connective tissue), acute inflammatory calcific tendonitis (calcium deposits in the tendons), and leukemia.

See CORTICOSTEROIDS for their off-label uses.

Sulfinpyrazone has been reported to be effective in reducing cardiac deaths during the first year after myocardial infarction.

Allopurinol has been found to be safe and effective in the treatment of Chagas' disease following heart transplantation. It is also used as a mouthwash to prevent inflammation of the mucous tissue of the mouth in cancer patients receiving fluorouracil treatment. In a 2003 study, allopurinol was reported to be effective for the treatment of aggressive behavior in patients with dementia.

Companion Drugs

Probenecid is used along with penicillins and cephalosporins to increase and prolong antibiotic blood levels.

Administration

NSAIDS are taken orally. Corticosteroids may be taken orally or injected into the affected joint. See ANALGESICS and CORTICOSTEROIDS.

Colchicine is available as tablets and as an intravenous injection.

Uricosurics and xanthine oxidase inhibitors are taken orally.

Cautions and Concerns

For cautions with NSAIDs, see ANALGESICS; for cautions with prednisone, see CORTICOSTEROIDS.

Colchicine should be administered with caution to elderly and debilitated patients, particularly to those with kidney, liver, gastrointestinal, or heart diseases. Periodic blood counts need to be done in patients receiving long-term colchicine therapy.

Uricosurics should be used with caution in patients with history of peptic ulcers. People taking uricosurics should consume liberal amounts of fluid to avoid kidney stones. Because probenecid may cause drowsiness, especially during the first few days, patients taking it need to use caution when driving or using machinery. Patients taking sulfinpyrazone should be kept under close medical supervision, with blood counts taken periodically.

An increase in acute attacks of gout has been reported during the early stages of allopurinol and febuxostat therapy; thus, maintenance doses of colchicine are generally recommended as a preventive when either of those drugs are begun. Liver and kidney function should be monitored periodically, especially during the first few months of allopurinol therapy. Liver function tests should be monitored periodically with febuxostat therapy. Because allopurinol may cause dizziness or drowsiness, patients taking it need to use caution when driving or using machinery.

Warnings

For warnings with NSAIDs, see ANALGESICS; for warnings with prednisone, see CORTICOSTEROIDS.

Colchicine arrests cell division in animals and plants and has adversely affected sperm production in humans and in some animal species. Increased colchicine toxicity may occur in patients with kidney or liver impairment. Colchicine should be discontinued if nausea, vomiting, or diarrhea occurs.

Severe allergic reactions have occurred with probenecid; in such cases, the drug should be discontinued. Exacerbation of gout during ther-apy with probenecid may occur; in such cases, a therapeutic dosage of colchicine or other appropriate therapy should be added. Sulfinpyrazone may precipitate acute attacks of gouty arthritis, especially in the initial stages of therapy.

Allopurinol should be discontinued at the first appearance of skin rash or other signs that may indicate an allergic reaction. The risk of skin rash may be higher in people with kidney disorders. Skin reactions can be severe, and on rare occasions fatal. Rarely, allopurinol can cause nerve, kidney, and bone marrow damage.

A higher rate of cardiovascular thromboembolic events was observed in patients treated with febuxostat than allopurinol in clinical trials. Therefore, patients taking febuxostat should be monitored for signs and symptoms of myocardial infarction (heart attack) and stroke.

When Not Advised (Contraindications)

For contraindications with NSAIDs, see ANALGESICS; for contraindications with prednisone, see CORTICOSTEROIDS.

Colchicine should not be given to patients with combined kidney and liver disease, nor to patients with serious kidney, liver, gastrointestinal, or heart disorders.

Probenecid should not be given to children under two years of age nor to patients with blood diseases or kidney stones. Probenecid should be avoided during acute gouty arthritis attacks because it can make the arthritis worse. Sulfinpyrazone should not be given to patients with active peptic ulcer or symptoms of gastrointestinal inflammation or ulceration nor to patients with blood diseases.

Febuxostat is contraindicated in patients being treated with azathioprine or mercaptopurine.

Side Effects

For side effects with NSAIDs, see ANALGESICS; for side effects with prednisone, see CORTICOSTEROIDS.

Side effects of colchicine include blood in the urine, difficulty breathing, fever, chills, sore throat, muscle weakness, nausea, vomiting, numbness and tingling in hands or feet, pain and difficulty passing urine, skin rash, itching, stomach pain, swelling of the face and mouth, bruising, bleeding, weakness, tiredness, diarrhea, loss of appetite, and hair loss.

Common side effects of probenecid include headache, loss of appetite, nausea, vomiting, frequent need to urinate, skin rash and itching (see *Warnings*), sore gums, flushing, dizziness, and anemia. The most frequent side effects of sulfinpyrazone are heartburn and stomach upset, which may be alleviated by taking with food, milk, or antacids. Other side effects include skin rash and itching, anemia, difficulty breathing, wheezing, and shortness of breath.

The most common side effect of allopurinol is skin rash, hives, and itching (see *Warnings*); loss of hair, fever, and feelings of unease may occur alone or in combination with a rash. Other side effects include headache, nausea, vomiting, taste loss, decreased kidney function, and drowsiness (see *Cautions and Concerns*).

The most common side effects with febuxostat are liver problems (see *Cautions and Concerns*), nausea, gout flares (see *Cautions and Concerns*), joint pain, and rash.

Interactions

For interactions with NSAIDs, see ANALGESICS; for interactions with prednisone, see CORTICOSTEROIDS.

Colchicine may increase sensitivity to the central nervous system depressants. Severe gastrointestinal side effects, liver toxicity, and kidney toxicity may occur when colchicine is administered along with cyclosporine or erythromycin.

Aspirin and other salicylates can prevent uricosurics from being fully effective. Probenecid may increase the actions of barbiturates, benzodiazepines, dapsone, NSAIDs, rifampin, and sulfonamides. Sulfinpyrazone taken along with acetaminophen can be damaging to the liver. Sulfinpyrazone may increase the effects of warfarin, which could lead to bleeding, and of tolbutamide, which could lead to low blood sugar levels. Sulfinpyrazone may decrease the

effects of theophylline and verapamil. Niacin may decrease the effects of sulfinpyrazone.

Patients receiving allopurinol along with either ampicillin or amoxicillin have been reported to have a higher rate of skin rash compared to patients who are receiving either allopurinol or ampicillin/amoxicillin alone. Similarly, there may be a higher risk of hypersensitivity among patients receiving both allopurinol and angiotensin-converting enzyme (ACE) inhibitors than among those receiving only allopurinol or only ACE inhibitors. Thiazide diuretics may increase the incidence of hypersensitivity reactions to allopurinol.

Based on a drug interaction study in healthy subjects, febuxostat altered the metabolism of theophylline (a substrate of XO). Therefore, caution should be used when coadministering febuxostat with theophylline.

Sales/Statistics

The RxList of Top 300 Prescriptions for 2005 (retail and mail order, excluding Wal-Mart) showed 9,828,000 allopurinol prescriptions. The 2010 *Drug Topics* Top 200 Generic Drugs by Total Prescriptions ranked allopurinol #54, with 12,550,481 prescriptions dispensed, and their Top 200 Generic Drugs by Retail Dollars listed allopurinol #137, with $105,860,532 in sales. Colchicine ranked #160 in prescriptions (3,258,225) and #182 in sales ($69,832,163).

Demographics and Cultural Groups

Gout is rare in children and young adults. Adult men, particularly those between the ages of 40 and 50, are more likely to develop gout than women, who rarely develop the disorder before menopause.

Development History

Colchicine was originally derived from the stem and seeds of the meadow saffron (autumn crocus). Colchicum extract was first described as a treatment for gout in *De Materia Medica* by the Greek physician Padanius Dioscorides in the first century A.D. The colchicine alkaloid was first isolated in 1820 by two French chemists. Lab experiments with colchicine led scientists to the drug's molecular target, a cell-scaffolding protein called tubulin.

Uricosurics were first used in the late 1800s; however, they were not widely used because of their side effects. In the 1950s, the first tolerable uricosurics were developed.

Allopurinol was first used in the United States in 1964. The chemists George Hitchings and Gertrude Elion were awarded the 1988 Nobel Prize in medicine for their work in developing a number of drugs, one of which was allopurinol. When it was approved in February 2009, Febuxostat because the first new FDA-approved prescription medicine for treating gout since allopurinol.

Future Drugs

Etoricoxib (Arcoxia) is a new COX-2 selective inhibitor from Merck & Co. being developed for the treatment of gout as well as rheumatoid arthritis, osteoarthritis, chronic low back pain, and ankylosing spondylitis. The FDA is requiring additional safety and efficacy data for etoricoxib before it will issue approval.

Savient Pharmaceuticals, Inc. has initiated Phase III trials for uricase (Puricase) for treatment-failure gout. Phase II trials demonstrated that uricase delivered substantial and sustained reduction of elevated plasma urate levels in treated patients.

antihistamines   Drugs used to reduce or eliminate effects caused by histamine, a chemical released within the body during allergic reactions to external agents such as pollen, mold, or animal dander. These allergic reactions can include itchy eyes, sneezing, and watery discharge from the eyes and nose. Allergic reactions can range from mild and annoying to sudden and life-threatening. Antihistamine drugs are also known as H_1 blockers because they block the action of histamine only on certain receptors, known as H_1 receptors. Many antihistamines are available over-the-counter (OTC); others only by prescription.

Classes

Antihistamines are classified on the basis of their chemical structure. Each class has slightly different actions, characteristics, and side effects.

First-generation antihistamines:

- *Alkylamines, nonselective Examples:* brompheniramine, chlorpheniramine (Chlor-Trimeton), dexchlorpheniramine, and triprolidine.

- *Ethanolamines Examples:* carbinoxamine, clemastine (Dayhist Allergy, Tavist Allergy), dimenhydrinate (Dramamine), diphenhydramine (Benadryl), and doxylamine.

- *Ethylenediamines Example:* pyrilamine.

- *Phenothiazines Example:* promethazine (Phenergan).

- *Piperazines, nonselective Examples:* cyclizine (Marezine), hydroxyzine (Atarax, Vistaril), and meclizine (Antivert).

- *Piperidines, nonselective Example:* cyproheptadine (Periactin).

Second-generation antihistamines:

- *Alkylamines, peripherally selective Example:* acrivastine.

- *Phthalazinones Example:* azelastine (Astelin, Optivar).

- *Piperazines, peripherally selective Example:* cetirizine (Zyrtec).

- *Piperidines, peripherally selective Examples:* desloratadine (Clarinex), fexofenadine (Allegra), and loratadine (Alavert, Claritin).

How They Work

Histamine is released in response to inflammation as part of the body's natural defense against infection (its immune system). However, sometimes this immune system overreacts—such as in people with allergies to such irritants as pollen, mold spores, and animal dander—and releases too much histamine. Excess amounts of histamine overstimulate the histamine receptors, causing allergic reactions. Antihistamines block (soak up) the histamine and thereby reduce or prevent most of those allergic reactions. By blocking the action of histamine on H_1 receptors, these drugs prevent dilation of the vessels, thus reducing the inflammation, watering, and swelling. Antihistamines do not prevent the release of histamine, nor do they bind with histamine after it has been released. All antihistamines work on the same allergy pathway, but different ones vary in potency and side effects.

Approved Uses

First-generation antihistamines are approved for hypersensitivity reactions, type 1, which includes perennial or seasonal allergic rhinitis (hay fever), vasomotor rhinitis (not related to allergic reactions, but having many of the same symptoms), allergic conjunctivitis (an eye inflammation), and hives. These agents can also be used as adjunctive anaphylactic therapy. Diphenhydramine is also used to treat angioedema (welts below the surface of the skin, especially around the eyes and lips) and to relieve allergic reactions after blood transfusions.

Dimenhydrinate and diphenhydramine are also used to treat motion sickness. Diphenhydramine is used as an antitussive (syrup only) to treat coughs caused by colds or allergy as well as to treat Parkinson's disease. Doxylamine is also used by itself as a short-term sleep aid, in combination with other drugs as a nighttime cold and allergy relief drug, and in combination with vitamin B6 (pyridoxine) to prevent morning sickness in pregnant women.

Promethazine is also used to treat and prevent motion sickness, for pre- and postoperative or obstetric sedation, for prevention and control of nausea and vomiting, and as adjunctive therapy for control of postoperative pain.

Cyclizine and meclizine are used to treat nausea, vomiting, and dizziness associated with motion sickness and vertigo. Hydroxyzine is also used to treat pruritus (severe itching), as a pre-operative sedative, as adjunctive analgesic before or after surgery or childbirth, and to control nausea and vomiting other than when associated with pregnancy.

Second-generation antihistamines are approved for certain allergic disorders. Studies have shown them to be as effective as first-generation antihistamines but without the sedative effect (although cetirizine does have a slight sedative effect).

The combination of acrivastine and pseudoephedrine (a DECONGESTANT) is used to prevent sneezing, itchy, watery eyes and nose, and other symptoms of allergies and hay fever as well as to treat nasal congestion and sinusitis (inflammation of the sinuses) associated with allergies, hay fever, and the common cold.

The intranasal formulation of azelastine is used to treat seasonal allergic rhinitis and vasomotor rhinitis, while the ophthalmic formulation is used to treat seasonal allergic conjunctivitis.

Cetirizine and desloratadine are used to treat perennial or seasonal allergic rhinitis as well as to reduce the occurrence, severity, and duration of chronic idiopathic urticaria (hives with no known cause). Fexofenadine is approved to treat seasonal allergic rhinitis and chronic idiopathic urticaria. Loratadine is approved to treat symptoms of seasonal allergic rhinitis.

Off-Label Uses

Cyproheptadine, dexchlorpheniramine, and diphenhydramine are used to induce sleep. Cyproheptadine may also be used to stimulate appetite. Loratadine is used off-label to treat chronic idiopathic urticaria in patients two years of age and older.

Administration

Most antihistamines are administered orally as tablets, capsules, chewables, suspension, and/or syrup. Diphenhydramine, hydroxyzine, and promethazine are also administered via injection. Promethazine is also available in suppository form. Azelastine is available as an intranasal spray and as an ophthalmic solution.

Cautions and Concerns

First-generation antihistamines have varying degrees of sedative effects, which may cause drowsiness and/or reduced mental alertness. Thus, patients taking them should not drive or operate machinery and should exercise caution when performing tasks requiring physical dexterity.

Antihistamines should be used with caution in patients predisposed to urinary retention and in patients with history of bronchial asthma, hyperthyroidism, or cardiovascular disease (especially hypertension).

Promethazine should be used with caution in patients with bone marrow depression and in patients with liver dysfunction.

Cetirizine, desloratidine, and loratadine should be used with caution in patients with liver or kidney dysfunction (lower starting doses are recommended in these patients). Fexofenadine should be used with caution in patients with kidney dysfunction (lower starting doses are recommended in these patients).

Warnings

The anticholinergic (drying) effects of antihistamines may thicken secretions and impair expectoration in patients with emphysema, chronic bronchitis, and asthma.

Antihistamines are more likely to cause dizziness, excess sedation, fainting, confusion, and low blood pressure in patients 65 years of age or older; lower doses may be necessary.

Promethazine may lower the seizure threshold in patients with seizure disorders.

When Not Advised (Contraindications)

First-generation antihistamines should not be used in newborn or premature infants, nursing mothers, or patients with narrow-angle glaucoma, peptic ulcer disease, bladder obstruction, or enlarged prostate.

Promethazine should not be used in children less than two years of age (because of the potential for causing respiratory depression).

Side Effects

The most common side effects of first-generation antihistamines include drowsiness; dry mouth, eyes, nose, or throat; gastrointestinal upset, stomach pain, or nausea; increased heart-rate; headache; blurred vision; increased appetite and weight gain; urinary retention; thickening of mucus; and worsened snoring. These drugs have also been shown to cause excitation in children.

Second-generation antihistamines may cause drowsiness, but to a lesser degree than the first-generation antihistamines (cetirizine tends to be the most sedating of these drugs). Azelastine may also cause headache, taste disturbances, dizziness, cough, nausea, dry mouth, or nasal burning, nose bleeds, or sneezing (for nasal spray). Cetirizine may cause headache, dizziness, stomach pain, dry mouth, diarrhea, nausea, vomiting, nose bleeds, or sore throat. Desloratadine may cause headache, dizziness, dry mouth, nausea, muscle pain, sore throat, or painful menstruation. Fexofenadine may cause headache, vomiting, dizziness, nausea, diarrhea, muscle pain, sore throat, cough, or painful menstruation. Loratadine may cause headache, dry mouth, stomach pain, or sore throat.

Interactions

Antihistamines can increase the sedative effects of alcohol, barbiturates, tranquilizers, and narcotic analgesics.

Monoamine oxidase inhibitor (MAOI) antidepressants may prolong and increase the effects of antihistamines and may cause tremors and muscle jerking with phenothiazines,

Cimetidine may increase the effects of azelastine.

Sales/Statistics

According to the U.S. General Accounting Office, in 2000, three oral antihistamines, Claritin, Allegra, and Zyrtec, accounted for 86 percent of all oral antihistamine sales, and all three of them were among the 15 most heavily advertised drugs.

Prescription antihistamine sales in the United States are approximately $5 billion annually and growing at a rate of approximately 20 percent per year, according to IMS Health, a pharmaceutical market research firm.

Development History

The first-generation antihistamines were developed during the 1940s, with ethylenediamines being the first group of clinically effective antihistamines and diphenhydramine being the first approved antihistamine in 1945. Hydroxyzine was approved by the FDA in 1957.

Terfenadine was the first second-generation antihistamine to be approved (1985). However, this drug was later removed from the market by the FDA due to the risk of cardiac arrhythmia caused by QT interval (length of the heart's electrical cycle) prolongation. Loratadine was approved in 1993, cetirizine and fexofenadine in 1995, azelastine in 1996, and desloratadine in 2001.

Future Drugs

Ebastine (Kestine) is a long-acting nonsedating antihistamine approved in more than 25 countries for treating seasonal and perennial allergic rhinitis and idiopathic chronic urticaria. Sanofi-Aventis is seeking FDA approval for marketing the drug in the United States.

A nasal spray form of epinastine is in clinical trials in the United States and Canada for the treatment or prevention of seasonal allergic rhinitis. Epinastine is a potent and fast-acting molecule that blocks multiple subtypes of histamine receptors, stabilizes mast cells, and affects proinflammatory mediators.

antihyperlipidemics Drugs used to treat hyperlipidemia, a group of diseases that involve an excess of lipids (fatty molecules) in the blood; also called cholesterol-lowering drugs, lipid-lowering drugs, antilipemics, or hypolipidemic agents. Hyperlipidemia can include high low-density lipoprotein (LDL) cholesterol (bad cholesterol), elevated triglycerides (TGs), and low high-density lipoprotein (HDL) cholesterol (good cholesterol). Hyperlipidemia is a key factor in atherosclerosis (hardening of the arteries); it increases the risk of heart attack, angina, stroke, and peripheral arterial disease. Hyperlipidemia may be acquired as a result of disease (e.g., diabetes mellitus, hypothyroidism, Cushing's syndrome, and certain types of renal failure), lifestyle (e.g., bad diet, lack of exercise, obesity, smoking), or taking certain medications (e.g., estrogens, CORTICOSTEROIDS, diuretics, and beta-blockers). Hyperlipidemia may also be an inherited (genetic) disorder. Some physicians prescribe cholesterol-lowering drugs to patients who already have or are at high risk for coronary artery disease, even when their cholesterol levels are in the normal range, as studies have shown that aggressively lowering cholesterol levels can dramatically increase their life expectancy. According to the American Heart Association, more than 105 million American adults have total blood cholesterol values of 200 mg/dl and higher, with 36.6 million American adults having levels of 240 mg/dl or above. A total cholesterol greater than 200 mg/dl is considered high.

Health, United States, 2006, the annual National Center for Health Statistics report on the health status of the nation, noted that "the percentage of the population with high serum cholesterol has been decreasing, in part due to the increased use of new cholesterol-lowering medications."

Classes

Antihyperlipidemics are classified according to their effects on lipids.

- *Bile acid sequestrants* Lower LDL cholesterol. *Examples:* colesevelam (WelChol), colestipol (Colestid), and cholestyramine (Prevalite, Questran).
- *Fibric acid derivatives* (also called fibrates) Increase HDL cholesterol levels and lower TG levels. *Examples:* fenofibrate (Antara, Lipofen, Lofibra, Tricor, Triglide) and gemfibrozil (Lopid).

- *HMG-CoA reductase inhibitors* (also called statins)   Primarily used to lower LDL cholesterol levels; may also modestly increase HDL cholesterol levels and lower TG levels. *Examples:* atorvastatin (Lipitor), fluvastatin (Lescol), lovastatin (Altoprev, Mevacor), pitavastatin (Livalo), pravastatin (Pravachol), rosuvastatin (Crestor), and simvastatin (Zocor).

- *Cholesterol absorption inhibitor*   Lowers LDL cholesterol levels. *Example:* ezetimibe (Zetia).

- *Niacin* (Niacor, Niaspan, Slo-Niacin) (also referred to as nicotinic acid or vitamin B_3)   Lowers LDL cholesterol and TG levels while increasing HDL cholesterol levels.

- *Omega-3-acid ethyl esters* (Lovaza)   Lowers TG levels. Omega-3-acid ethyl esters are obtained by esterification of the body oil of several fat fish species.

- *Combination products*   *Examples:* ezetimibe/simvastatin (Vytorin) and lovastatin/niacin (Advicor).

How They Work

Bile acid sequestrants bind with cholesterol-containing bile acids in the intestines, causing the acids to be eliminated in the stool rather than recycling repeatedly through the liver and the intestines. With fewer bile acids in circulation, the liver is forced to convert cholesterol into bile acids, thereby removing LDL cholesterol from the blood. The usual effect of bile acid sequestrants is to lower LDL cholesterol by about 10 to 20 percent. Bile acid sequestrants are sometimes prescribed with a statin or niacin to further lower LDL cholesterol.

Fibrates increase the breakdown of lipids and speed the removal of very-low-density lipoproteins from the bloodstream. They may also decrease very-low-density lipoprotein production by the liver. Fibrates are primarily effective in lowering TGs and, to a lesser extent, in increasing HDL cholesterol levels. The reductions in TGs generally are in the range of 20 to 50 percent with increases in HDL cholesterol generally being 10 to 15 percent. Gemfibrozil

can be very effective for patients with high TG levels. However, it is not very effective for lowering LDL cholesterol.

Statins inhibit an enzyme called HMG-CoA reductase, which controls the rate of cholesterol production in the body. These drugs lower cholesterol by slowing down the production of cholesterol and by increasing the liver's ability to remove the LDL cholesterol already in the blood. Statins work quickly, lowering cholesterol levels within one to two weeks. Studies using statins have reported 20 to 60 percent lower LDL cholesterol levels in patients on these drugs. Statins also reduce elevated TG levels and produce a modest increase in HDL cholesterol.

Ezetimibe acts by blocking the absorption of cholesterol, including dietary cholesterol, in the small intestine. In addition to this direct effect, decreased cholesterol absorption leads to an increase in LDL cholesterol uptake into cells, thus decreasing levels in the blood. Ezetimibe lowers LDL by approximately 20 percent.

Niacin is the water-soluble B-vitamin necessary for carbohydrate metabolism. When given in doses well above the vitamin requirement, it improves all lipoproteins. Niacin works by decreasing the production of very-low-density lipoproteins, which are used to synthesize LDL. Niacin reduces LDL cholesterol levels by 10 to 20 percent, reduces triglycerides by 20 to 50 percent, and raises HDL cholesterol by 15 to 35 percent.

The exact mechanism of action responsible for reducing TGs with omega-3-acid ethyl esters is not completely known. However, it may reduce the synthesis of TGs in the liver. The reduction in TGs seen with these drugs is approximately 50 percent.

Approved Uses

Bile acid sequestrants are used to treat elevated LDL cholesterol levels. Cholestyramine is also approved for the prevention of pruritus (itching) in patients with chronic liver disease due to the liver's inability to eliminate bile.

Fibrates are used to treat high very-low-density lipoprotein cholesterol, low HDL cholesterol, and dysbetalipoproteinemia, a rare lipid disorder characterized by high levels of blood cholesterol and TGs in adults. Fibrates are used primarily to treat people with exceptionally high levels of TGs.

Statins have been studied extensively in patients with no prior history of coronary heart disease (primary prevention trials) as well as in those with a history of coronary heart disease (secondary prevention trials). The results of these trials have shown that use of statins to lower an elevated LDL cholesterol level can substantially reduce coronary events and death from coronary heart disease in these patient populations. Certain studies have also demonstrated a benefit in people with normal cholesterol levels. Given their track record in these studies and their ability to lower LDL cholesterol, statins have become the drugs most often prescribed when a person with heart disease needs a cholesterol-lowering medicine.

Ezetimibe is used along with diet and exercise to lower levels of total cholesterol and LDL cholesterol. It is also used along with diet to treat homozygous sitosterolemia, an inherited disorder of sterol metabolism in which an excess of many plant sterols, including sitosterol, is absorbed and not enough is excreted (sterols are substances used to form hormones, vitamins, and membranes found in animal and plant lipids.) Ezetimibe in combination with fenofibrate is approved to treat mixed hyperlipidemia. Ezetimibe can be combined with a statin to further lower LDL cholesterol. The ezetimibe/simvastatin combination is used for treating high levels of cholesterol in the blood. It reduces total cholesterol and LDL cholesterol while it increases HDL cholesterol.

Niacin is used to treat high LDL and very-low-density lipoprotein cholesterol as well as dysbetalipoproteinemia. Niacin extended-release tablets are approved to reduce cholesterol and to reduce the risk of recurrent nonfatal heart attack in patients with a history of a previous heart attack and elevated cholesterol levels.

Omega-3-acid ethyl esters are approved as an adjunct to diet in patients with very high TG levels. Fish oils are available over the counter (OTC) and as a prescription product (Lovaza).

Off-Label Uses

Cholestyramine and colestipol have been used in the treatment of digitalis toxicity. These drugs prevent the further absorption of digoxin by interrupting circulation of bile from the liver and are especially effective in patients with significant kidney insufficiency.

There is a growing body of evidence supporting a role of omega-3 polyunsaturated fatty acids, such as omega-3-acid ethyl esters, for the prevention of coronary heart disease.

Administration

Bile acid sequestrants are available as powders (cholestyramine), granules (colestipol), or tablets (colestipol and colesevelam). The powders and granules must be mixed with water, noncarbonated beverage, or pulpy fruits (e.g., applesauce or crushed pineapple) and taken once or twice (rarely three times) daily with meals. Tablets must be taken with large amounts of fluids to avoid gastrointestinal symptoms.

Fibrates are available as tablets or capsules. Gemfibrozil is given twice daily, and fenofibrate is given once daily.

Statins are available in tablet form and are usually given in a single dose at the evening meal or at bedtime. Atorvastatin, pitavastatin, and rosuvastatin can be given at any time of the day. Lovastatin is most effective when given with a meal. The other statins are recommended to be taken at bedtime to take advantage of the fact that the body makes more cholesterol at night than during the day.

Ezetimibe comes in tablet form, is taken once a day, and can be taken with or without food.

There are three types of niacin: immediate release, timed release, and extended release. Niacin comes in tablets, capsules, and liquids. All forms should be taken with or following a meal to avoid stomach upset. The prescription product Niaspan is taken once daily. All niacin products except for Niaspan are available OTC.

Omega-3-acid ethyl esters are available as liquid-filled gel capsules, which are taken by mouth once or twice daily.

Cautions and Concerns

Bile acid sequestrants may interfere with normal fat absorption and digestion and may prevent absorption of fat-soluble vitamins (A, D, E, and K) and folic acid. The possible lack of proper vitamin absorption may have an effect on nursing infants; thus, caution should be exercised when administering bile-acid sequestrants to nursing women. Bile acid sequestrants can increase TGs (see *When Not Advised [Contraindications]*). Chronic use may increase bleeding tendencies associated with vitamin K deficiency. Bile acid sequestrants may produce or worsen preexisting constipation, may aggravate hemorrhoids, and may cause fecal impaction.

Fibrates can cause liver and muscle injury (see *Warnings*). Periodic blood counts are recommended during the first 12 months of therapy, as severe anemia, leukopenia, and bone marrow hypoplasia have occurred, although rarely.

Occasionally, statins will cause muscle degeneration, with the symptoms of pain and weakness (see *Warnings*). Statins should be used with caution in patients with alcohol disease, which independently predisposes to myopathy.

Very rarely, patients have experienced severe muscle problems while taking ezetimibe, usually when ezetimibe was added to statin therapy. On rare occasions, these muscle problems can be serious, with muscle breakdown resulting in kidney damage. (See *Warnings.*)

Diabetic patients taking niacin should notify their physicians if taking vitamins or other nutritional supplements containing niacin because of the risk of niacin causing loss of glucose control. Niacin can also cause liver and muscle injury.

In some patients, omega-3-acid ethyl esters have increased LDL cholesterol levels. Thus, LDL cholesterol levels should be monitored periodically during its use.

Warnings

Fibrates, statins, and niacin are associated with an increased risk of severe liver damage, requiring that the liver be checked regularly.

Rhabdomyolysis, a potentially fatal disease that destroys muscle, has been reported very rarely with ezetimibe monotherapy and very rarely with the addition of ezetimibe to agents known to be associated with increased risk of rhabdomyolysis, such as fibrates or statins. All patients starting therapy with ezetimibe should be advised of the risk of myopathy and told to report promptly any unexplained muscle pain, tenderness, or weakness. Risks of muscle injury can be minimized by prescribing at the lowest dose that achieves the goals of therapy. Patients having any unexplained muscle pain or weakness need to have a blood test performed to measure creatinine kinase. If these levels are elevated, the drug may need to be discontinued. Ezetimibe and any statin or fibrate that the patient is taking concomitantly should be immediately discontinued if myopathy is diagnosed or suspected.

Various forms of kidney failure have been reported in patients taking statins. Mild, transient proteinuria (or protein in the urine, usually from the tubules), with and without microscopic hematuria (minute amounts of blood in the urine), has occurred with statins.

Niacin is inexpensive and widely accessible to patients without a prescription but must not be used for cholesterol lowering without the monitoring of a physician because of the potential for causing liver damage and for making diabetes more difficult to control. Severe liver damage has occurred in patients who have substituted sustained-release niacin products for immediate-release niacin at equivalent doses. Rare cases of rhabdomyolysis have been associated with coadministration of lipid-altering doses (1 g/day or greater) of niacin and statins.

When Not Advised (Contraindications)

Bile acid sequestrants are contraindicated in individuals with bowel obstruction. Bile acid sequestrants should not be used in patients with hypertriglyceridemia, because these drugs can elevate TG levels.

Fibrates should be used with great caution in patients with preexisting gallbladder, liver, or kidney dysfunction, and especially in kidney transplant recipients.

Statins are contraindicated during pregnancy, as they may cause fetal harm, as well as in nursing mothers. Statins should not be used in patients with liver disease or unexplained persistent elevated liver function tests. Pitavastatin is contraindicated in anyone with liver disease; patients with severe kidney disease not on hemodialysis; women who are nursing, pregnant, or who may become pregnant; and in anyone currently taking cyclosporine.

Ezetimibe is not recommended for patients with moderate or severe liver disease.

Niacin should not be used in patients with active peptic ulcer disease or liver disease.

Omega-3-acid ethyl esters should not be given to patients with a known sensitivity or allergy to fish.

Side Effects

Bile acid sequestrants often cause constipation, bloating, nausea, abdominal pain, and gas. Colesevelam is believed to be associated with less gastrointestinal (GI) effects than cholestyramine or colestipol. These drugs may also increase triglyceride levels.

Statins, fibrates, and niacin may cause liver dysfunction and myopathy.

The most common side effects of fibrates are gastrointestinal, including diarrhea, nausea, bloating, and abdominal pain. They may also cause headache, fatigue, runny nose, rash, back pain, and muscle inflammation. They also appear to increase the likelihood of developing cholesterol gallstones.

Statins may produce upset stomach, gas, bloating, constipation, loose stools, and abdominal pain or cramps. These symptoms usually are mild to moderate in severity and generally go away as the body adjusts. Other side effects from

statins include headaches, rash, and fatigue. Clinical studies revealed the most common side effects of pitavastatin to be back pain, constipation, diarrhea, muscle pain, and pain in the legs or arms.

Ezetimibe side effects include stomach pain, fatigue, and joint pain. Less often, allergic reactions, including swelling of the face, lips, tongue, and/or throat that may cause difficulty in breathing or swallowing, rash, and hives may occur.

A common side effect of niacin is flushing or hot flashes, which are the result of blood vessels opening wide (dilating). Most patients develop a tolerance to flushing, and in some patients it can be decreased by taking the drug with meals, slowly increasing the niacin dose, and/or by taking aspirin or a nonsteroidal anti-inflammatory drug (NSAID) 30 to 60 minutes prior to taking the niacin. In addition, the risk of flushing can be minimized by avoiding ingestion of alcohol or hot beverages around the time of taking the niacin. The extended-release form may cause less flushing than the other forms. Also, a variety of gastrointestinal symptoms including nausea, indigestion, gas, vomiting, diarrhea, and the activation of peptic ulcers have been seen with the use of niacin. Risk of liver problems, gout, and high blood sugar increase as the dose of niacin is increased.

Nausea, belching, and fishy taste have been the most commonly reported adverse events with omega-3-acid ethyl esters.

Interactions

Although bile acid sequestrants are not absorbed, they may interfere with the absorption of other medicines if taken at the same time. Other medications therefore should be taken at least one hour before or four to six hours after the bile acid sequestrant. When compared with cholestyramine or colestipol, colesevelam is believed to be associated with fewer drug interactions.

Fibrates can increase the effect of ANTICOAGULANTS. Fenofibrate can increase the effect of cyclosporine, while gemfibrozil may decrease its effect. Both gemfibrozil and fenofibrate can interact with antidiabetic agents (particularly sulfo-nylureas) and increase the levels of these agents, which may predispose patients to hypoglycemia. Rhabdomyolysis has been associated with the administration of fibrates along with statins. This effect is greater with the use of gemfibrozil than with fenofibrate. Therefore, gemfibrozil is not to be used in combination with statins. If a fibrate is needed in a patient already receiving a statin, then fenofibrate should be used.

Consumption of grapefruit or grapefruit juice inhibits the metabolism of statins metabolized by the CYP3A4 enzyme (lovastatin, simvastatin, atorvastatin, and, to a small extent, rosuvas-tatin), which increases the levels of the statin and increases the risk of dose-related adverse effects (including myopathy/rhabdomyolysis and liver dysfunction). Consequently, consumption of grapefruit juice is not recommended in patients taking these statins. Rifampin and phenytoin may lower lovastatin, simvastatin, atorvastatin, and rosuvastatin levels enough to require dosage adjustment. Macrolides (erythromycin, clarithro-mycin), calcium channel blockers (verapamil, diltiazem), protease inhibitors, amiodarone, and azole ANTIFUNGALS may increase statin levels. The dose of lovastatin should not exceed 20 mg daily in patients also taking cyclosporine, a fibrate, or niacin or 40 mg daily in patients also taking amiodarone or verapamil; the dose of simvastatin should not exceed 10 mg daily in patients also taking cyclosporine, a fibrate, or niacin, or 20 mg daily in patients taking amiodarone or verapamil. Atorvastatin, fluvastatin, lovastatin, rosuvastatin, and simvastatin may enhance the effect of war-farin. Pravastatin is the only statin that does not interact with CYP450 system and is an appealing treatment option in patients when drug interac-tion may be a concern.

Cyclosporine increases the levels of ezetimibe and could lead to greater side effects of ezeti-mibe. Ezetimibe may also increase cyclosporine levels.

The blood pressure–lowering effect of antihy-pertensive medications may be increased while taking niacin.

Because some studies with omega-3-acids have demonstrated prolongation of bleeding time, patients receiving treatment with both omega-3-acid ethyl esters and ANTICOAGULANTS should be monitored periodically.

Sales/Statistics

Between 1995–96 and 2003–04, the rate of cho-lesterol-lowering drugs prescribed during medi-cal visits among those 55 to 64 years of age more than quadrupled, according to the U.S. Depart-ment of Health and Human Services *Chartbook on Trends in the Health of Americans* (2006). By 2003–04, the rate of cholesterol-lowering drugs prescribed among men age 55 to 64 years had increased from 25 to 111 drugs per 100 men. Over the same time period, the rate of cho-lesterol-lowering drugs prescribed for women increased from 25 to 92 drugs per 100 women.

In 2010, the overall percentage of generic prescriptions spending in the antihyperlipid-emics therapy class was 8 percent of overall drug spending, according to Express Scripts *2010 Generic Drug Usage Report.* Express Scripts is a drug benefit management company.

In 2005, HMG-CoA reductase inhibitors were the most commonly prescribed antihyperlip-idemic, accounting for just over 75 percent of all prescriptions in this class, according to the Express Scripts *2005 Generic Drug Usage Report.*

The "Top 200 Generic Drugs by Units in 2006" (*Drug Topics,* March 5, 2007) included four anti-hyperlipidemics: lovastatin at #35 (13,920,000 units, up 34.8 percent from 2005), simvastatin at #36 (13,162,000 units) and for the first time on the generics list, gemfibrozil at #75 (5,703,000 units) and pravastatin at #86 (4,480,000 units).

Four antihyperlipidemics appeared on the "Top 200 Generic Drugs by Retail Dol-lars in 2006" (*Drug Topics,* February 19, 2007): simvastatin at #2 ($1,390,479,000), lovas-tatin at #20 ($457,336,000), pravastatin at #22 ($429,217,000), and gemfibrozil at #78 ($121,684,000).

Lipitor was the number one brand-name drug in 2006 ("Top 200 Brand-Name Drugs by Units in 2006," *Drug Topics*, March 5, 2007) with 62,311,000 units sold. Other brand-name antihyperlipidemics in the top 200: Vytorin #17—15,765,000 units (93.3 percent increase since 2005), Zocor #18—14,678,000 units, Zetia #23—12,272,000 units, Crestor #27—11,410,000 units, Tricor #38—9,566,000 units, Niaspan #77—4,290,000 units, Pravachol #81—4,056,000 units, and Lescol XL #136—2,025,000 units.

Lipitor was also the number one brand-name drug in retail dollars in 2006 ("Top 200 Brand-Name Drugs by Retail Dollars in 2006," *Drug Topics*, February 19, 2007), with $6,577,810,000 in sales. Worldwide, Lipitor generated $12.9 billion in sales in 2006.

Other brand-name antihyperlipidemics in the U.S. top 200 in 2006: Zocor #8—$2,171,312,000, Vytorin #22—$1,469,209,000 (105.4 percent increase since 2005), Zetia #32—$1,139,638,000, Crestor #37—$1,058,160,000, Tricor #40—$965,680,000, Pravachol #65—$575,985,000, Niaspan #85—$473,755,000, and Lescol XL #151—$180,223,000.

According to a report from the IMS Institute for Healthcare Informatics, lipid regulators were the most often prescribed drug class in 2010, with 255.4 million prescriptions dispensed, and third-highest in sales ($18.8 billion). Among their top 20 drugs by prescriptions dispensed were simvastatin (#2, 94.1 million prescriptions) and Lipitor (#12, 45.3 prescriptions). In sales, Lipitor was their top-ranked drug ($7.2 billion), and Crestor ranked #8 ($3.8 billion). (Lipitor was scheduled to come off patent in November 2011.)

Demographics and Cultural Groups

Non-Hispanic blacks and Hispanics who qualify for cholesterol-lowering drug treatment are less likely than non-Hispanic whites to have their LDL cholesterol controlled to recommended levels, according to researchers who reported their findings at the American Heart Association's Scientific Sessions 2004. The National Heart, Lung, and Blood Institute–funded study involved 6,814 participants in six metropolitan areas. According to a report posted by the American Heart Asso-

ciation, the study measured prevalence and control of high cholesterol among the four ethnic groups and found the following differences in treatments.

- Among persons with high cholesterol, Hispanics were 36 percent less likely than non-Hispanic whites to have properly controlled cholesterol, and non-Hispanic blacks were 28 percent less likely. No difference was seen between Chinese Americans and non-Hispanic whites.

- Compared to non-Hispanic whites, Chinese Americans were 21 percent less likely to meet the criterion for drug therapy. Hispanics and non-Hispanic blacks were equally likely as non-Hispanic whites to qualify for drug therapy.

- Men were 28 percent more likely than women to qualify for drug therapy, but 22 percent less likely to receive treatment.

- Among those who met the recommendation for drug therapy, men were 30 percent less likely than women to have their cholesterol under control.

- Among all ethnic groups studied, only one in five Americans who qualify to take drugs to lower their high cholesterol levels have their LDL cholesterol under control.

Health, United States, 2006 (National Center for Health Statistics) reported that between 1988–1994 and 2001–04, the percentage of adults with elevated serum cholesterol levels greater than 240 mg/dL declined substantially for older adults. However, older women were more likely to have high serum cholesterol than men. In 2001–04, 26 percent of women age 65 to 74 years had high serum cholesterol, compared with 11 percent of men age 65 to 74 years.

Development History

The first lipid-lowering agent was a bile acid sequestrant, cholestyramine, which was approved by the FDA in 1964. Colestipol was approved in 1977; colesevelam in 2000.

Gemfibrozil was approved by the FDA in 1995; fenofibrate in 1998.

Lovastatin, the first HMG-CoA reductase inhibitor, was approved in 1987. It was followed by pravastatin and simvastatin in 1991, fluvastatin in 1993, atorvastatin in 1996, and rosuvastatin in 2003.

Nicotinic acid was first discovered from the oxidation of nicotine in 1867, but nothing was done with it until the late 1930s, when scientists showed that pellagra was prevented and cured by nicotinic acid. The term *niacin* came about in the decision to choose a name that would dissociate it from nicotine—thus avoiding any thinking either that smoking provided vitamins or that wholesome food contained a poison. The resulting name *niacin* was derived from nicotinic acid plus vitamin. In 1997, Kos Pharmaceuticals, Inc. received final FDA approval to market Niaspan as an antihyperlipidemic.

Ezetimibe, the first available 2-azetidinone compound, was approved by the FDA in 2002.

In 2004, omega-3-acid ethyl esters became the first marine-derived omega-3 polyunsaturated fatty acid product (fish oil) to be approved by the FDA as a prescription drug.

Pitavastatin was approved in August 2009.

Future Drugs

Isis Pharmaceuticals Inc., Carlsbad, California, is developing an injection drug (mipomersen) that blocks the production of an intermediate cholesterol molecule called ApoB-100. If proven safe and effective, it could be one of the first practical applications of a so far unproven drug technology called antisense, which aims to treat disease by blocking the function of individual genes.

Merck & Co. is developing anacetrapib, formerly known as MK-0859, which has more than doubled "good" HDL cholesterol in early clinical trials while not raising blood pressure, as the discontinued torcetrapib (Pfizer) did. Both drugs belong to a new class of drugs called CETP inhibitors, which act by blocking cholesterylcster

transfer protein (CETP), an enzyme that transforms good cholesterol into bad cholesterol.

antihypertensives Drugs that lower blood pressure; used to treat hypertension (HTN) (abnormally elevated blood pressure)—one of the risk factors for stroke, heart attack, heart failure, and arterial aneurysm and a leading cause of chronic kidney failure. Hypertension directly kills more than 40,000 Americans per year and is a contributing factor in more than 200,000 deaths. According to the Centers for Disease Control and Prevention (CDC), the percent of adults 55 to 64 years of age who have HTN increased from 42 to 50 percent between 1988–94 and 1999–2002. The prevalence of HTN increases with advancing age to the point that more than half of people 60 to 69 years of age and approximately three-fourths of those 70 years of age and older are affected. Data from the National Health and Nutrition Examination Survey (NHANES) have indicated that 50 million or more Americans have HTN warranting some form of treatment. As of December 1998, nearly 4,000 antihypertensive drug products (including all dosage forms and strengths) were reported to be on the market in the United States. According to a study of all medication groups, antihypertensives have a 65 percent noncompliance rate.

Classes

Antihypertensive drugs all lower blood pressure, but they vary by class in their mechanisms of action, potential side effects, suitability for patients who have other diseases and health problems along with HTN, and ability to protect against the long-term problems resulting from HTN. The classes of antihypertensive drugs include:

- *diuretics* Sometimes called water pills, diuretics are often used in combination with other antihypertensives. By December 1998, 950 diuretic drug products (including all dosage forms and strengths) were on the market in the United States. They are further subdivided into three classes:

- thiazide diuretics, such as chlorothiazide (Diuril), chlorthalidone (Thalitone), and hydrochlorothiazide (Esidrex, Microzide). Although it is not a true thiazide, metolazone (Zaroxolyn, Mykrox) is chemically related to the thiazide class of diuretics and works in a similar manner.

- potassium-sparing diuretics, such as amiloride and triamterene (Dyrenium).

- loop diuretics, such as bumetanide (Bumex), furosemide (Lasix), and torsemide (Demadex).

- *angiotensin-converting enzyme (ACE) inhibitors* By December 1998, 211 ACE inhibitors (including all dosage forms and strengths) were on the market in the United States. *Examples:* benazepril (Lotensin), captopril (Capoten), enalapril (Vasotec), fosinopril (Monopril), lisinopril (Prinivil, Zestril), moexipril (Univasc), perindopril (Aceon), quinapril (Accupril), ramipril (Altace), and trandolapril (Mavik).

- *angiotensin II receptor antagonists* Also called angiotensin receptor blockers (ARBs). *Examples:* candesartan (Atacand), eprosartan (Teveten), irbesartan (Avapro), losartan (Cozaar), olmesartan (Benicar), telmisartan (Micardis), and valsartan (Diovan).

- *beta-blockers* also called beta-adrenergic blocking agents. *Examples:* acebutolol (Sectral), atenolol (Tenormin), bisoprolol (Zebeta), carteolol (Catrol), carvedilol (Coreg), esmolol (Brevibloc), labetalol (Normodyne), metoprolol tartrate (Lopressor), metoprolol succinate (Toprol XL), nadolol (Corgard), penbutolol (Levatol), pindolol (Visken), propranolol (Inderal), and timolol (Blocadren). (See also ANTIANGINALS; ANTIARRHYTHMICS.)

- *aldosterone receptor antagonists Examples:* eplerenone (Inspra) and spironolactone (Aldactone).

- *calcium channel blockers (CCBs)* Also called calcium antagonists. *Examples:* amlodip-

ine (Norvasc), diltiazem (Cardizem, Cartia XT, Dilacor XR, Diltia XT, Taztia XT, Tiazac), felodipine (Plendil), isradipine (Dynacirc), nicardipine (Cardene), nifedipine (Adalat CC, Afeditab CR, Nifediac CC, Nifedical XL, Procardia), nisoldipine (Sular), and verapamil (Calan, Covera HS, Isoptin SR, Verelan). (See also ANTIANGINALS; ANTIARRHYTHMICS.)

- *centrally acting agents* Also called sympatholytics. *Examples:* clonidine (Catapres) and methyldopa (Aldomet).

- *alpha-1 adrenergic blockers* Also called alpha blockers. *Examples:* doxazosin (Cardura), prazosin (Minipress), and terazosin (Hytrin).

- *direct vasodilators Examples:* hydralazine (Apresoline) and minoxidil (Loniten).

- *direct remin inhibitors Examples:* aliskiren (Tekturna) and aliskiren HCT, a combination of aliskiren and hydrochlorotheazide (Tekturna HCT).

How They Work

Diuretics flush excess water, sodium, and chloride from the body by increasing urination. This reduces the amount of fluid in the blood and flushes sodium from the blood vessels so that they can open wider, increasing blood flow and thus reducing the blood's pressure against the vessels.

ACE inhibitors relax blood vessels by preventing formation of angiotensin II, a powerful hormone that causes the blood vessels to constrict. This narrowing of the blood vessels increases the pressure within the vessels and can cause HTN. ACE inhibitors prevent this narrowing so that blood pressure goes down.

Angiotensin II receptor antagonists produce the same effect as ACE inhibitors but by a different mechanism. Instead of preventing the production of angiotensin II, they block it from entering angiotensin II receptors in the body. As a result, the blood vessels relax and become wider, and blood pressure goes down.

Beta-blockers help the heart beat slower and with less force by blocking the effects of catecholamines on the beta receptors. Some block beta₁ receptors only (beta₁ selective), while the others are nonselective in that they block both beta₁ and beta₂ receptors. As the heart pumps less blood through the blood vessels, blood pressure goes down.

Aldosterone is a hormone that causes the body to retain salt and water. Aldosterone receptor antagonists block the receptors for this hormone in the kidneys, heart, blood vessels, and brain. This triggers the body to get rid of more salt and water in the form of urine. This, in turn, reduces the volume of blood in the body, lowering blood pressure.

Calcium channel blockers prevent calcium from entering the muscle cells of the heart and blood vessels, thus relaxing blood vessels and decreasing blood pressure.

Centrally acting agents selectively stimulate receptors in the brain that monitor catecholamine levels in the blood. By tricking the brain into believing that catecholamine levels are higher than they really are, these drugs cause the brain to reduce its signals to the adrenal medulla, which in turn lowers catecholamine production and blood levels. The result is a lowered heart rate and blood pressure.

Alpha-1 adrenergic blockers work by blocking alpha-1 receptors on the blood vessels, which causes their relaxation and lowering of blood pressure.

Direct vasodilators open (dilate) blood vessels by directly relaxing the muscle in the vessel walls, causing blood pressure to go down.

By inhibiting renin, aliskiren blocks the conversion of angiotensinogen to angiotensin I, which subsequently results in a reduction in angiotensin II concentrations. Unlike ACE inhibitors and ARBs, which reactively stimulate an increase in plasma renin activity, aliskiren suppresses the effects of renin and leads to a reduction in plasma renin activity. In clinical trials involving patients with mild to moderate hypertension, aliskiren provided antihypertensive efficacy that was comparable to that of an ARB. Combination therapy with aliskiren and an ARB may provide additional blood pressure–lowering effects compared with the respective monotherapies with each of the agents.

Approved Uses

In addition to HTN, diuretics are used to treat edema associated with congestive heart failure and to treat liver or kidney disease. Loop diuretics are the most powerful diuretics available and are particularly useful when less potent diuretics, such as the thiazides, have not worked. Because potassium-sparing diuretics do not cause the body to lose potassium, they are sometimes used to offset the potassium loss from thiazide and loop diuretics.

The Antihypertensive and Lipid-Lowering Treatment to Prevent Heart Attack Trial (ALLHAT), a large study that began in 1994 and lasted eight years, determined that patients who need to begin drug treatment should definitely try a thiazide diuretic initially. In 2003, the Seventh Report of the Joint National Committee on Prevention, Detection, Evaluation, and Treatment of High Blood Pressure (JNC 7) was approved by the National Heart, Lung, and Blood Institute (NHLBI) as a new guideline for the prevention and management of HTN. It stated that thiazide diuretics should be used as initial therapy for most patients with HTN, either alone or in combination with one of the other antihypertensive classes. The JNC 7 report also noted that "diuretics enhance the antihypertensive efficacy of multidrug regimens, can be useful in achieving blood pressure control, and are more affordable than other antihypertensive agents. Despite these findings, diuretics remain underutilized."

ACE inhibitors are effective alone or in combination with other antihypertensives, especially thiazide diuretics, in treating HTN. They are also used to treat chronic heart failure. The American Heart Association recommends ACE inhibitors as standard treatment following a myocardial infarction, and the American Diabetes Association recommends either an ACE inhibitor or angiotensin II receptor antagonist as standard treatment for diabetics with chronic kidney disease or HTN. For hypertensive people with chronic kidney disease, the guidelines from the National Kidney Foundation recommend that initial drug therapy include either an ACE inhibitor or angiotensin II receptor antagonist. Ramipril is also approved to reduce the risk of myocardial infarction, stroke, or death from cardiovascular causes in individuals at least 55 years of age who are at risk for these conditions. Perindopril is also approved to reduce the risk of myocardial infarction or death from cardiovascular causes in individuals with stable coronary artery disease.

Like ACE inhibitors, ARBs are also effective alone or in combination with other antihypertensives, especially thiazide diuretics, in treating high blood pressure. Irbesartan and losartan are also approved for the treatment of diabetic nephropathy (kidney damage due to diabetes) in patients with Type 2 diabetes and HTN. Both valsartan and candesartan can also be used for the treatment of chronic heart failure, especially in those patients who are intolerant of ACE inhibitors.

Beta-blockers can be used to treat HTN, angina, and certain types of arrhythmias (irregular heart rhythms). Both carvedilol and metoprolol CR/XL are approved for the treatment of stable, chronic heart failure. The FDA has approved propranolol and timolol for use in migraine prevention. Timolol is also used to improve survival after a heart attack.

Aldosterone receptor antagonists can be used alone or with other antihypertensives to treat HTN. Both spironolactone and eplerenone can also be used for the treatment of chronic heart failure. Eplerenone is specifically indicated for the management of congestive heart failure following an acute myocardial infarction. Spironolactone is also used in the management of hyperaldosteronism, a condition in which too much aldosterone is produced by the adrenal glands, which can lead to decreased levels of potassium.

Calcium channel blockers are used to treat HTN and angina. Verapamil and diltiazem are used to treat a type of arrhythmia called atrial fibrillation as well as paroxysmal supraventricular tachycardia (rapid heart rate that occurs from time to time).

Centrally acting agents are used to treat HTN. Injectable clonidine is used for severe pain in cancer patients.

Alpha-1 adrenergic blockers are used to treat HTN but may increase the risk of heart failure with long-term use. Their use for prostate problems is more common than their use for HTN.

Direct vasodilators are generally used as last-line agents to treat serious HTN that is not manageable with other hypertensives.

Aliskiren is a treatment option for patients with mild to moderate hypertension who are intolerant of first-line antihypertensive therapies. Aliskiren HCT can be used as the first medication to lower high blood pressure when more than one medicine is likely needed to reach the blood pressure goal.

Off-Label Uses

Because thiazide diuretics lower urinary calcium excretion, they have been used to prevent formation of calcium-containing kidney stones. Related to the lower calcium excretion, thiazides have been associated with an increase in bone mineral density and reduced risk of hip fracture in older patients. Thiazides are also used to treat nephrogenic diabetes insipidus, a condition in which the kidneys do not retain urine, resulting in excess urination and thirst and very watered-down urine.

ACE inhibitors have been shown in clinical trials to be useful in treating a number of conditions. Perindopril, both alone and along with a diuretic, has been shown to reduce the risk of stroke among patients with a history of stroke. Lisinopril has been shown to be effective in preventing migraines. Benazepril and ramipril have shown favorable effects on reducing the progression of nondiabetic nephropathy. ACE inhibitors have also shown effectiveness in managing Bartter syndrome, a genetic disease with low potassium levels, and in reversing kidney failure in scleroderma renal crisis.

Beta-blockers are used in a number of off-label treatments. Atenolol, metoprolol, and nadolol are used to prevent migraine headaches. Atenolol, esmolol, and metoprolol are used to treat unstable angina. Bisoprolol is used to treat stable, chronic heart failure. Nadolol and propranolol are used to treat Parkinsonian tremors. Propranolol is also used to treat generalized anxiety disorder.

Because they lower heart rate, beta-blockers have been used by some Olympic marksmen to provide more aiming time between heartbeats and to improve their scores. In 1986, the International Olympic Committee (IOC) added beta-blockers to its list of prohibited substances because of this usage. Some musicians and nervous public speakers have been reported to take beta-blockers to conquer stage fright and avoid tremor during auditions and performances. A number of calcium channel blockers have been prescribed for Raynaud's syndrome. Diltiazem and verapamil have been used to prevent migraine and cluster headaches. Nifedipine can be used to treat premature labor.

Because of its antiandrogen effect, the aldosterone receptor antagonist spironolactone has been used to treat hirsutism, an excessive growth of hair generally caused by increased androgens, particularly in women. Androgens are hormones that stimulate or control the development and maintenance of masculine characteristics. The combination of spironolactone and testolactone has been used for short-term treatment of familial male precocious puberty. Spironolactone has also been used to relieve premenstrual syndrome (PMS) symptoms as well as for short-term treatment of acne.

The centrally acting agent methyldopa is used off-label to treat HTN in pregnancy. Clonidine has had a number of off-label uses, including for alcohol withdrawal, attention-deficit/hyperactivity disorder (ADHD), growth delay in children, diabetic diarrhea, menopausal flushing, methadone/opiate detoxification, postherpetic neuralgia, psychosis in schizophrenic patients, allergic reactions in asthma patients, restless leg syndrome, smoking cessation, and ulcerative colitis.

Hydralazine is used off-label in the treatment of chronic heart failure (along with nitrates) and severe aortic insufficiency.

Administration

Antihypertensives are generally taken in tablet or capsule form. The medication typically begins to affect body systems within one to two hours after each dose. Extended-release tablets and capsules should be taken whole, not split, crushed, or chewed. Among the diuretics, chlorothiazide is also available as an oral suspension and intravenous injection; furosemide as a liquid or intravenous/intramuscular injection; torsemide and bumetanide as an intravenous injection. The ACE inhibitor enalapril is also available as an injection (as enalaprilat). The beta-blockers metoprolol tartrate, labetalol, and propranolol can also be administered intravenously. Esmolol is available only as an intravenous injection. The calcium channel blockers diltiazem, nicardipine, and verapamil can also be administered intravenously. The centrally acting agent clonidine is administered via injection or transdermal patch; methyldopa via tablets or intravenous injection. Hydralazine is also available as an injection.

Cautions and Concerns

Diuretics may cause fluid or electrolyte imbalances. Patients who take diuretics may lose potassium and magnesium because of increased urination and thus may need supplements. Diuretics should be used with caution in patients with severe kidney disease or liver impairment. Diuretics also can trigger gout attacks, increase the amount of sugar in the blood, and cause high cholesterol levels or high triglyceride levels. Diuretics may cause the skin to be more sensitive to sunlight than it is normally and cause sunburn.

Because diuretics have been associated with an increased risk of diabetes, which itself can lead to heart attacks and strokes, some physicians have expressed concern that diuretics' risks would cancel out their benefits. In the first long-term study to address this issue, Kostis et al. found that while diuretics may increase the risk of diabetes, the rate of death from heart attacks or strokes was nearly 15 percent lower in patients getting a diuretic (chlorthalidone) compared to those who were given placebo.

ACE inhibitors and ARBs may cause hyperkalemia (increased potassium) or worsening kidney function. Patients taking these drugs should not take potassium supplements or salt substitutes containing potassium unless they consult with their physician. Patients with impaired kidney function need to be closely monitored when these drugs are used.

Beta-blockers may mask signs and symptoms of low blood sugar. Studies have reported an increase of Type 2 diabetes in people who take these drugs. Beta-blockers may also mask clinical signs of hyperthyroidism, such as tachycardia. Abrupt withdrawal of beta-blockers should be avoided if possible, as this may cause a severe increase in blood pressure or even chest pain. If discontinuation is required, the dosage should be gradually tapered off. Asthmatics have been reported to have worsening symptoms when using beta-blockers. Beta-blockers can also severely impact the breathing of patients with chronic obstructive pulmonary disease (COPD). Dosages of certain beta-blockers need to be reduced in patients with severe kidney impairment and those on dialysis as well as adjusted in patients with liver disease.

Eplerenone and spironolactone should be used with caution in patients with mild to moderate renal impairment because of the increased risk for hyperkalemia. Eplerenone should also be used with caution in patients with congestive heart failure post–myocardial infarction who have diabetes and protein in their urine, as these patients are also at increased risk for hyperkalemia. Gynecomastia (breast enlargement in males) may develop with the use of spironolactone, although it usually reverses when therapy is discontinued.

Calcium channel blockers should be used with caution in patients who have impaired liver function. A dose reduction may be necessary in these patients. Mild to moderate peripheral edema may occur with these drugs.

Some centrally acting agent products contain sulfites that may cause allergic reactions in susceptible patients, particularly asthmatics. Blood and liver function tests should be performed before beginning therapy with methyldopa, followed by periodic testing during treatment.

The alpha-1 blocker doxazosin should be used with caution in patients with liver impairment or who are receiving other drugs known to influence liver metabolism. Alpha-1 blockers may cause dizziness, lightheadedness, or fainting when rising from a lying or sitting posture (known as orthostatic hypotension or postural hypotension). For this reason, they may need to be taken at bedtime.

The tachycardia that results with the use of hydralazine can cause anginal attacks and ECG changes of myocardial ischemia. Therefore, it must be used with caution in patients with suspected coronary artery disease. Hydralazine may also increase pulmonary artery pressure in patients with mitral valve rheumatic heart disease.

Hypertrichosis, a lengthening and thickening of fine body hair, develops within six weeks after starting minoxidil therapy in approximately 80 percent of patients. This new hair growth stops upon discontinuation of the drug, but it may take as long as six months for a return to pretreatment appearance.

Aliskiren can cause a serious reaction called angioedema, causing swelling of the face, lips, tongue, or throat. This may occur at any time during treatment and has occurred in patients with and without a history of angioedema with ACE inhibitors or angiotensin receptor antagonists. Patients who experience these effects, even without respiratory distress, require prolonged observation, because treatment with antihistamines and corticosteroids may not be sufficient to prevent respiratory involvement. Prompt administration of subcutaneous epinephrine solution and measures to ensure a patent airway may be necessary. Dizziness or lightheadedness may occur while using this medicine, especially if the patient has been taking a diuretic.

Warnings

Diuretics have been known to exacerbate or activate systemic lupus erythematosus (SLE). Intravenous chlorothiazide should be used only when the patient is unable to take oral medication or in an emergency. Diuretics should be used during pregnancy only when the potential benefits outweigh the potential hazards to the fetus. Patients with known sulfonamide sensitivity may show allergic reactions to loop and thiazide diuretics. Reversible and irreversible hearing loss have been reported in patients taking loop diuretics, usually associated with rapid injection, high doses, or severe kidney impairment. Potassium-sparing diuretics may cause hyperkalemia, which is potentially fatal if not corrected.

When pregnancy is detected, ACE inhibitor or ARB therapy must be discontinued as soon as possible. (See *When Not Advised [Contraindications]*.) Angioedema, a sudden and rapid allergic reaction that causes swelling of the eyes, skin, lips, throat, and/or tongue, has been reported with the use of ACE inhibitors. Involvement of the larynx or tongue may close off the throat, causing life-threatening airway obstruction. If this reaction occurs, ACE inhibitor therapy should never be restarted. ARBs should be used with extreme caution in patients who have a history of angioedema from ACE inhibitor therapy. Severe hypotension may occur with the use of ACE inhibitors, particularly in patients who are also taking diuretics or on dialysis. Neutropenia and bone marrow depression have occurred during therapy with ACE inhibitors, especially captopril.

Because beta-blockers reduce the volume of blood being pumped by the heart, they can precipitate or aggravate the symptoms of inadequate blood flow through the arteries in patients with peripheral vascular disease. Thus, these patients need to be observed closely for any signs of further arterial obstruction.

Exacerbation of angina and, in some cases, myocardial infarction have occurred after abrupt discontinuation of beta-blocker therapy. When discontinuing chronically administered timolol, particularly in patients with ischemic heart disease, the dosage should be gradually reduced over a period of one to two weeks, and the patient should be carefully monitored. If angina markedly worsens or acute coronary insufficiency develops, timolol administration should be reinstituted promptly, at least temporarily, and other measures appropriate for the management of unstable angina should be taken. Patients should be warned against interruption or discontinuation of therapy without the physician's advice. Because coronary artery disease is common and may be unrecognized, it may be prudent not to discontinue timolol therapy abruptly, even in patients treated only for hypertension.

Aldosterone receptor antagonists carry a risk for hyperkalemia, which may cause serious arrhythmias. Also, these drugs should be used during pregnancy only when the potential benefits outweigh the potential hazards to the fetus.

Abrupt withdrawal of CCBs may cause increased frequency and duration of chest pain. Because all CCBs, except for amlodipine and felodipine, reduce the ability of the heart to pump blood, symptoms may worsen in patients with heart failure who are receiving these drugs.

Vital signs should be monitored frequently, especially during the first few days of epidural clonidine therapy. Because severe low blood pressure may follow the administration of clonidine, it should be used with caution in all patients. Suddenly stopping clonidine treatment, regardless of the route of administration, has resulted in severely increased blood pressure, nervousness, agitation, headache, and tremor. If discontinuation of therapy is necessary, the dosage should be tapered off slowly.

Anemia and liver disorders may occur with methyldopa therapy, which could lead to potentially fatal complications unless properly recognized and managed. Occasionally, fever has occurred within the first three weeks of methyldopa therapy.

Alpha-1 blockers may cause low blood pressure and interrupt the baroreflex response, which regulates blood pressure. In doing so, they may cause dizziness, lightheadedness, or fainting when rising from a lying or sitting posture. Although it happens rarely, patients should be advised that alpha blockers have been associated with priapism (painful and sustained penile erection), which can lead to permanent impotence.

Patients given hydralazine over a period of six months or more may develop lupuslike symptoms that generally regress when the drug is discontinued, but residual effects have been detected years later. Long-term treatment with steroids may be necessary in patients who develop these lupuslike symptoms.

Minoxidil may produce serious adverse effects. It can cause pericardial effusion (an abnormal accumulation of fluid around the heart), occasionally progressing to tamponade (the fluid compressing the heart muscle and interfering with the normal pumping of blood), and can worsen angina. Minoxidil should be reserved for hypertensive patients who do not respond adequately to maximum therapeutic doses of other antihypertensive agents. Minoxidil must be administered under close supervision, usually along with a beta-blocker to prevent tachycardia and increased myocardial workload. Usually, it must also be given along with a diuretic to prevent serious fluid accumulation. Patients with malignant HTN (very high blood pressure with swelling of the optic nerve behind the eye) should be hospitalized when minoxidil is first administered so that they can be monitored to avoid too rapid decreases in blood pressure.

Drugs that act directly on the renin-angiotensin system can cause fetal and neonatal morbidity and death when administered to pregnant women. If aliskiren is used during pregnancy, or if the patient becomes pregnant while taking this drug, the patient should be apprised of the potential hazard to the fetus.

When Not Advised (Contraindications)

All diuretics are contraindicated in patients with anuria (inability to urinate). Aldosterone receptor antagonists are contraindicated in patients with severe renal impairment or hyperkalemia. When used for the treatment of hypertension, eplerenone is also contraindicated in patients with Type 2 diabetes with microalbuminuria (small amounts of albumin in the urine).

Use of any of the ACE inhibitors or ARBs during pregnancy, especially after the first three months, can cause low blood pressure, kidney failure, hyperkalemia, or even birth defects and death in newborns. They should be discontinued as soon as possible if pregnancy is detected. ACE inhibitors and ARBs are also contraindicated in patients with hyperkalemia. Patients with a history of angioedema from ACE inhibitors should never be rechallenged with this class of drugs.

Beta-blockers should not be used if any of the following conditions exist: cardiogenic shock or severe hypotension; severe bradycardia (heart rate less than 50 beats per minute); any type of second- or third-degree atrioventricular (AV) block or sick sinus syndrome (in the absence of a pacemaker); or severe reactive airway disease.

Calcium channel blockers are contraindicated if any of the following conditions exist: cardiogenic shock or severe hypotension; severe bradycardia (diltiazem and verapamil only); systolic heart failure (except for amlodipine and felodipine); any type of second- or third-degree AV block or sick sinus syndrome (in the absence of a pacemaker); or patients with atrial flutter or atrial fibrillation and an accessory bypass tract (e.g., Wolff-Parkinson-White, Lown-Ganong-Levine syndrome) except in the presence of a functioning ventricular pacemaker.

Epidural administration of clonidine is contraindicated in patients receiving anticoagulant therapy and is not recommended for most patients with severe cardiovascular disease. Methyldopa should not be used in patients with active liver disease.

Hydralazine is contraindicated in patients with mitral valve rheumatic heart disease. Minoxidil is contraindicated in pheochromocytoma (tumor of the adrenal glands) because it may stimulate secretion of catecholamines from the tumor through its antihypertensive action.

Side Effects

The most common side effects of thiazide and loop diuretics are hypokalemia (loss of potassium), hypomagnesemia (loss of magnesium), hypercalcemia (for thiazides), hypocalcemia (for loops), hyperuricemia, hyperglycemia, photosensitivity reactions, urinary incontinence, and dizziness. The main side effect of potassium-sparing diuretics is hyperkalemia, and excess potassium may result in irregular heart rate and heart palpitations.

The most common side effects of aldosterone receptor antagonists are hyperkalemia and renal dysfunction. Spironolactone may also cause inability to achieve or maintain an erection or breast enlargement in men and deep voice, menstrual irregularities, postmenopausal bleeding, or hirsutism in women.

A persistent dry cough is a relatively common side effect of ACE inhibitors. Patients who experience this cough and find it intolerable are often switched to an ARB. Other common side effects of ACE inhibitors include hyperkalemia, renal dysfunction, dizziness, and rash. Another potential serious side effect of ACE inhibitors is angioedema (see *Warnings*).

In general, ARBs are well-tolerated, with the most common side effects being hyperkalemia, renal dysfunction, and dizziness. Although the risk of angioedema with ARBs is less than with ACE inhibitors, there is still a risk.

Most beta-blocker side effects are temporary. The more common side effects include drowsiness, fatigue, lethargy, cold hands and feet, weakness, dizziness and lightheadedness upon standing, an abnormally slow heart rate (bradycardia), vivid dreams, and nightmares. Exercise capacity may be reduced. In addition to masking of hypoglycemia in patients with diabetes (see *Cautions and Concerns*), these drugs may also cause glucose intolerance in this patient population.

Calcium channel blockers may lead to a number of side effects, including constipation, headache, tenderness or bleeding of the gums, shortness of breath, skin rash, hair loss, swelling (edema) of feet, legs, or ankles, fainting, dizziness, or lightheadedness after getting up from a sitting or lying position, nausea, and numbness or tingling of hands and feet. Bradycardia can occur with diltiazem and verapamil. A rapid heart rate (tachycardia) can develop with the other CCBs.

Centrally acting agents can lower mood, which can trigger depression because of their role in depressing the central nervous system or by disrupting the balance of neurotransmitters. They may also cause drowsiness, sedation, confusion, and dry mouth.

Alpha-1 blockers can cause dizziness, fainting with the first dose, fluid retention, drowsiness, or headache.

Direct vasodilators can cause headache, tachycardia, fluid retention, nausea, vomiting, and rash. Long-term use of hydralazine may cause lupuslike symptoms (see *Warnings*). Hirsutism can occur with minoxidil (see *Cautions and Concerns*).

Because aliskiren does not significantly affect the cytochrome P450 system, it has been associated with few drug interactions. In clinical studies, aliskiren was well tolerated, and its adverse-effect profile was similar to that of placebo. Fatigue, headache, dizziness, diarrhea, nasopharyngitis, and back pain were the most commonly reported side effects.

Interactions

Neither prescription nor over-the-counter medicines for appetite control, colds, cough, sinus problems, or hay fever should be taken during treatment with antihypertensives without the physician's approval.

When taking potassium-sparing diuretics, ACE inhibitors, ARBs, or aldosterone receptor antagonists, patients should avoid eating large amounts of potassium-rich foods such as bananas, oranges, and green leafy vegetables.

Also, potassium supplements and salt substitutes that contain potassium should be avoided when taking any drugs in these classes.

The presence of low blood levels of potassium due to diuretics may increase the risk of arrhythmias in patients who are also taking digoxin.

The potential interaction with nonsteroidal anti-inflammatory drugs (NSAIDs) and COX-2 inhibitors exists particularly for all diuretics, ACE inhibitors, and ARBs. However, one could make an argument that NSAIDs and COX-2 inhibitors can attenuate the blood pressure–lowering effects of all antihypertensives because of their ability to cause sodium and water retention and to thus increase blood pressure.

Food appears to increase the absorption of spironolactone. The use of eplerenone with any of the following drugs is specifically contraindicated because of the increased risk of hyperkalemia: ketoconazole, itraconazole, nefazodone, troleandomycin, clarithromycin, ritonavir, and nelfinavir. For the treatment of HTN, its use is also contraindicated with potassium supplements or potassium-sparing diuretics. The dose of eplerenone needs to be reduced when patients are also receiving fluconazole, verapamil, saquinavir, or erythromycin.

Caution is recommended when ACE inhibitors are used with antacids, NSAIDs, aspirin, loop or thiazide diuretics, and lithium. Because food can decrease the absorption of captopril and moexipril, they should be taken one hour before or two hours after meals.

Caution is recommended when the angiotensin receptor blocker losartan is taken along with cimetidine, fluconazole, barbiturates, phenytoin, and rifampin.

Beta-blockers' effectiveness may be reduced by a number of drugs, including barbiturates, penicillins, rifampin, NSAIDs, and salicylates. Caution is recommended when using beta-blockers with other drugs that can slow the heart rate (diltiazem, verapamil, digoxin).

Verapamil and diltiazem can increase the effects of cyclosporine, tacrolimus, benzodiazepines, simvastatin, atorvastatin, lovastatin, theophylline, and digoxin. Among the types of medicines that can increase the effects of CCBs are fluconazole, clarithromycin, erythromycin, and protease inhibitors. Caution is recommended when using CCBs with other drugs that can slow the heart rate (beta-blockers, digoxin). The effects of CCBs may be decreased when used with carbamazepine, phenytoin, barbiturates, and rifampin.

Grapefruit juice interferes with the liver's ability to rid the body of some substances, which could result in a build-up of CCBs to toxic levels in the body. While the build-up is less likely if the juice is ingested four or more hours prior to the medicine, patients taking CCBs are advised to refrain from drinking grapefruit juice.

The use of clonidine with beta-blockers may cause bradycardia. In addition, the sudden discontinuation of clonidine while a patient is still receiving a beta-blocker can provoke a hypertensive crisis—a severe increase in blood pressure that can lead to a stroke or perhaps even death. Tricyclic antidepressants can block the blood pressure–lowering effects of clonidine, thereby causing blood pressure to rise. Clonidine can increase the sedating effects of narcotics, barbiturates, and sedatives.

Methyldopa may augment the antipsychotic effects of haloperidol as well as the central effects of levodopa in Parkinson's disease. Reduced doses of anesthetics may be required when a patient is taking methyldopa.

Patients taking alpha-1 blockers should avoid alcohol, as it may increase the risk of hypotension.

Concomitant use of aliskiren with potassium-sparing diuretics, potassium supplements, salt substitutes containing potassium, or other drugs that increase potassium levels may lead to increases in serum potassium. If concomitant use is considered necessary, caution should be exercised. When aliskiren was given with cyclosporine or itraconazole, the blood concentrations of aliskiren were significantly increased. Thus, aliskiren should not be used with cyclosporine or itraconazole.

Sales/Statistics

In October 2004, Piribo, a business intelligence firm that researches the pharmaceutical industry, reported that "the antihypertensive market accounted for almost $30 billion in the seven major markets in 2003 and this value is set to rise as prevalence increases. The increasing use of multiple drug therapy and the falling use of older drug classes in the absence of specific compelling indications are continuing to drive sales of the largest classes and will provide a growing market for new entrants."

A 2005 study by AARP's Public Policy Institute and the University of Minnesota found price increases for 110 brand-name drugs widely used by older Americans during the first three months of the year. The second biggest price increase, 5.9 percent, belonged to two types of blood pressure drugs, ARBs and CCBs.

Several studies have reported trends in the use of antihypertensives. Among those included by McCormack in his editorial:

- In 1982, thiazide diuretics accounted for 52 percent of all prescriptions for hypertension in the United States, but by 1993 thiazide diuretic use had declined to 27 percent.

- The use of beta-blockers decreased from 20 percent to 13 percent over this time period, while the use of CCBs and ACE inhibitors increased from 0.3 percent to 27 percent and 0.8 percent to 24 percent, respectively.

Then in "The Top 200 Prescription Drugs of 2004," *Pharmacy Times* reported that ARBs grew by 24 percent in 2004, and ACE inhibitors and CCBs saw declining and flat sales, respectively.

According to the Express Scripts *2004 Drug Trend Report,* generic drug use of antihypertensives "now approaches 50 percent of overall use, up from 14 percent in 2000."

According to a report from the IMS Institute for Healthcare Informatics, angiotensin II receptor antagonists were the 10th-highest drug class in U.S. sales in 2010 ($8.7 billion) and the 16th highest in prescriptions dispensed (83.7 million). Beta-blockers (plain and combo) ranked fourth (191.5 million prescriptions), ACE inhibitors fifth (168 million prescriptions), diuretics ninth (131 million prescriptions), and calcium antagonists (CCBs) 13th (97.9 million prescriptions). On the IMS individual top 20 drug rankings for 2010, lisinopril was third (87.4 million prescriptions dispensed), amlodipine fifth (57.2 million prescriptions), hydrochlorothiazide 10th (47.8 million prescriptions), furosemide 13th (43.4 million prescriptions), metropolol tartrate 14th (38.9 million prescriptions), atenolol 16th (36.3 million prescriptions), and metrolol succinate 18th (33 million prescriptions).

Demographics and Cultural Groups

Not all patients may respond in the same manner to the various classes of antihypertensives. Diuretics work very well to lower blood pressure in blacks, especially if their HTN has been caught early and is mild or moderate. Calcium channel blockers also work well in blacks who need more than a diuretic. The largest clinical trial ever conducted in blacks with kidney disease, the African-American Study of Kidney Disease and Hypertension (AASK), concluded in 2002 that ACE inhibitors are superior to CCBs and beta-blockers for slowing kidney disease due to hypertension. The ACE inhibitor (ramipril) reduced by 22 percent the risk of kidney failure, death, and a significant drop in kidney function compared to the beta-blocker (metoprolol) and by 38 percent compared to the CCB (amlodipine).

However, Berk noted that studies such as ALLHAT (see *Approved Uses* earlier in this chapter) have reported advantages for use of thiazide diuretics for initial therapy of HTN in both black and nonblack patients. "The discrepancy between these results and those from AASK, which found a significant benefit for ACE inhibition for prevention of renal failure, demonstrates the importance of organ-specific analysis in order to properly interpret therapeutic benefit."

Development History

The first antihypertensives, diuretics, were introduced for use in the United States in 1950s. Beta-blockers were first introduced in the 1960s to treat angina and to lower blood pressure. The alpha-1 blockers received approval for the treatment of HTN in the 1970s. Calcium channel blockers were first introduced in 1980. The ACE inhibitors were next, with captopril's FDA approval in 1981. The first ARB, losartan, was introduced to the United States in 1995. The first oral direct renin inhibitor, aliskiren, was approved in 2007. Aliskiren HCT followed in 2008.

Future Drugs

In March 2006, business intelligence firm Datamonitor reported that "innovation seen in other disease areas is scarce in antihypertensive R&D. Despite continued research into other hypertension targets—such as endothelin and vasopeptidase—a poor safety records, lack of efficacy compared to other classes, and a low patient potential, these agents promise to be no more than an academic interest rather than providing physicians with a real alternative in treating hypertension."

Berk, Bradford C. "AHA 2005: New Data and New Analyses of Old Data Concerning the RAS." Available online. URL: http://www.medscape.com/viewarticle/520163. Downloaded on April 27, 2006.

Express Scripts, *2004 Drug Trends Report*, June 2005. Available online. URL: http://www.express-scripts.com/ourcompany/news/industryreports/drugtrendreport/2004/.

Kostis, John, et al. "Long-term Effect of Diuretic-based Therapy on Fatal Outcomes in Subjects with Isolated Systolic Hypertension with and without Diabetes." *American Journal of Cardiology* 95, no. 1 (January 2005): 29–35.

McCormack, James. "ALLHAT—So What?" *Journal of Informed Pharmacotherapy* no. 12 (December 2003): 1. Available online. URL: http://www.informedpharmacotherapy.com/Issue12/Editorial/editorial12.htm.

Sanoski, Cynthia A. "Aliskiren: An Oral Direct Renin Inhibitor for the Treatment of Hypertension." *Pharmacotherapy* 29, no. 2 (February 2009): 193–212.

Wright, Jackson T., Jr., et al. "Effect of Blood Pressure Lowering and Antihypertensive Drug Class on Progression of Hypertensive Kidney Disease: Results from the AASK Trial." *Journal of the American Medical Association* 288, no. 19 (November 2002): 2,421–2,431. Available online. URL: http://jama.ama-assn.org/cgi/content/full/288/19/2421.

antimigraine agents Drugs used to prevent or reduce the severity of migraine headaches. Migraine is the most common recurring severe primary headache and affects at least 12 percent of the adult population in the United States, or more than 28 million people. Individual attacks are usually characterized by an intense pulsing or throbbing pain in one area of the head, often accompanied by extreme sensitivity to light and sound, nausea, and vomiting. Attacks vary in intensity, severity, and disability within and between patients. Patients suffering from migraine headaches report an average of one to five attacks per month of moderate to severe pain. Migraine is a leading cause of employee absenteeism; cost to American employers due to missed work and reduced productivity associated with migraine headaches is estimated at $13 billion per year. The World Health Organization now recognizes migraine as one of the world's most disabling medical conditions.

Classes

Antimigraine agents may be abortive, meaning they stop the migraine attack itself, relieving the pain and other symptoms, or prophylactic, meaning they are used to prevent migraines from developing. Abortive migraine treatments generally are classified as nonspecific (symptomatic) or migraine-specific. Nonspecific treatments include ANALGESICS and ANTIEMETICS, which relieve symptoms of migraine. Specific antimigraine drugs are in two classes:

- *selective serotonin receptor (5-HT₁) agonists*, also called *triptans Examples:* First-generation—sumatriptan (Imitrex); second-generation—almotriptan (Axert), eletriptan (Relpax), frovatriptan (Frova), naratriptan (Amerge), rizatriptan (Maxalt), and zolmitriptan (Zomig).

- *ergot alkaloids,* also called *ergots* Derived from ergot, a compound produced by a fungus (*Claviceps purpurea*) that grows on rye plants. *Examples:* dihydroergotamine (DHE-45, Migranal) and ergotamine tartrate (Ergomar).

Prophylactic migraine treatments attempt to reduce the frequency, severity, and duration of migraine attacks. Several classes of drugs are used for migraine prophylaxis: ANTICONVULSANTS, beta-blockers (see ANTIANGINALS; ANTIARRHYTHMICS; ANTIHYPERTENSIVES), calcium channel blockers (see ANTIANGINALS; ANTIARRHYTHMICS; ANTIHYPERTENSIVES), tricyclic ANTIDEPRESSANTS (TCAs), selective serotonin reuptake inhibitors (SSRIs) (see ANTIDEPRESSANTS), and nonsteroidal anti-inflammatory drugs (NSAIDs) (see ANALGESICS).

Combination drugs. *Example:* sumatriptan and naproxen sodium, an NSAID (Trefimet).

How They Work

Spierings noted that while the cause of migraines is not well understood, it seems to involve a complex process of widening and narrowing of the blood vessels in the brain, triggering changes in brain chemicals, inflammation, and pain.

Triptans work by stimulating particular subtypes of serotonin receptors, called 5-HT_{1B} and 5-HT_{1D}, located in the arteries of the brain. This narrows the dilated (enlarged) blood vessels, relieving the inflammation and increased blood flow that cause the pain of migraines. They are most effective if taken early during the migraine attack. Although the action of the various triptans is similar, they vary in speed of onset, rate of headache recurrence, and effectiveness among patients.

Ergots work by nonselectively stimulating $5HT_1$ receptors, which narrows blood vessels that are dilated during a migraine attack. Ergotamine works by narrowing blood vessels throughout the body, especially blood vessels in the head. Dihydroergotamine works in a similar way to ergotamine, but it does not narrow blood vessels throughout the body as much as ergotamine does. Because of this, dihydroergotamine is considered somewhat safer to use. Both ergotamine and dihydroergotamine are most effective when taken at the start of a migraine attack. However, the dihydroergotamine nasal spray can be used at any point during the course of a migraine attack.

NSAIDs, a class of analgesics, are suspected to act on the sterile inflammatory phase of migraine, although this has not been proven.

Anticonvulsants appear to reduce the frequency of migraines by several mechanisms, one of which probably includes intensifying the action of gamma-amino butyric acid (GABA), a neurotransmitter that carries messages between brain nerve cells. GABA slows down the transmission of nerve signals.

Beta-blockers are believed to reduce the frequency of migraines by preventing the blood vessels in the head from dilating and by increasing the release of oxygen to the surrounding tissues.

The mechanism by which calcium channel blockers prevent migraines is not completely understood, although it is believed that these drugs may prevent the narrowing (constriction) of blood vessels that may occur during the initial phase of migraine headaches.

TCAs prevent migraine headaches by altering norepinephrine and serotonin, the neurotransmitters that the nerves of the brain use to communicate with one another.

SSRIs work by preventing the reuptake (reabsorption) of serotonin by certain nerve cells in the brain.

The unique sumatriptan succinate and naproxen sodium formulation allows for the rapid disintegration of the sumatriptan but does not affect the disintegration of the naproxen sodium component. It works by targeting nerves and blood vessels believed to trigger a migraine and relieves the inflammation that can cause migraine pain.

Approved Uses

Triptans (including sumatriptan and naproxen sodium) are approved for the acute treatment of migraine with or without aura in adults. Sumatriptan injection is also approved for the acute treatment of cluster headache episodes.

Ergotamine is approved to abort or prevent migraine headaches. Dihydroergotamine is approved for the acute treatment of migraine headaches with or without aura; dihydroergotamine injection is also approved for the acute treatment of cluster headache episodes.

The FDA has approved two over-the-counter (OTC) products specifically to relieve the pain of migraine: Excedrin Migraine and Advil Migraine. Excedrin Migraine is a combination of aspirin, acetaminophen, and caffeine. Advil Migraine contains ibuprofen, which is an NSAID (see ANALGESICS).

Four prescription-only medications have been approved by the FDA to help prevent migraine: the beta-blockers propranolol and timolol (see ANTIHYPERTENSIVES) and the ANTICONVULSANTS topiramate and divalproex sodium (a derivative of valproic acid).

Off-Label Uses

Analgesics in general are medications given to relieve pain, and these drugs have long been used to treat patients who have infrequent migraine headaches or who cannot be treated with triptans. Analgesics most often used as acute treatment for migraines are aspirin, acetaminophen, and NSAIDS (e.g., naproxen and ibuprofen).

Antiemetics (e.g., prochlorperazine, metoclopramide) in general are medications given to stop vomiting, and these drugs are sometimes given to patients whose migraine headaches are accompanied by nausea and vomiting. When vomiting dominates the migraine symptoms, antiemetics may be given by suppository or injection. The earlier these drugs are taken in the attack, the better their effect. Metoclopramide, in particular, may also be prescribed to enhance the absorption of other medications taken by mouth, because migraines cause the digestive tract to slow down.

Beta-blockers that have been used off-label to treat migraines include nadolol, atenolol, and metoprolol.

The calcium channel blocker verapamil is sometimes used to treat patients who cannot take beta-blockers or who have also been diagnosed with hypertension.

TCAs are used off-label to prevent migraines. Amitriptyline has been shown in studies to be particularly effective, although imipramine, doxepin, nortriptyline, and protriptyline have also been used for preventive treatment. TCAs are often given to patients who are suffering from insomnia or depression as well as migraine.

SSRIs are not as effective for migraine prevention as TCAs, but a few small-scale studies have shown that fluoxetine, sertraline, and paroxetine benefit some patients.

NSAIDs are used for migraine prevention as well as acute treatment.

Administration

All triptans (including sumatriptan and naproxen sodium) are available in tablet form. Rizatriptan and zolmitriptan also are available as orally disintegrating tablets that rapidly dissolve when placed on the tongue. Sumatriptan and zolmitriptan are also available as nasal spray. Sumatriptan is also available as an injection, which can be administered subcutaneously (under the skin).

Ergotamine comes as a tablet that is placed under the tongue. Dihydroergotamine is available as a nasal spray and as an injection, which can be administered intravenously, intramuscularly, or subcutaneously.

All of the migraine preventive drugs must be taken daily to be fully effective; generally, it may take two to three months before positive results are seen with these drugs.

Cautions and Concerns

Chest, jaw, or neck tightness have occurred following treatment with triptans, as have pain, tightness, and pressure in the area of the heart. Although these have rarely been associated with arrhythmias or ischemic electrocardiographic (ECG) changes, patients experiencing these signs or symptoms should be further evaluated before receiving additional doses. All triptans may bind to melanin in the eye and accumulate over time, raising the possibility of toxicity in these tissues after extended use.

There have been rare reports of seizures following sumatriptan use; therefore, this drug should be used with caution in patients with a history of seizure disorders.

As many as 5 percent of patients using sumatriptan nasal spray have reported irritation in the nose and throat, including burning, numbness, paresthesia (tingling, tickling, itching), discharge, and pain or soreness. In 1 percent of patients treated, such symptoms were noted as severe. However, the symptoms were temporary, lasting less than two hours in 60 percent of the cases.

Individuals who have phenylketonuria (PKU), a genetic disorder, need to be made aware that rizatriptan and zolmitriptan orally disintegrating tablets contain phenylalanine (a component of aspartame).

Almotriptan and rizatriptan should be used with caution in patients with kidney or liver impairment. Eletriptan should be used with caution in patients with mild to moderate liver impairment. Frovatriptan, sumatriptan, and zolmitriptan should be used with caution in patients with liver impairment.

Because ergots may cause coronary arteries to constrict, patients who experience signs or symptoms suggestive of angina following its administration should be evaluated to determine if they are at risk for or have coronary artery disease before receiving additional doses. Similarly, patients who experience other symptoms or signs suggestive of decreased arterial flow, such as ischemic bowel syndrome or Raynaud's syndrome, following the use of ergots should be evaluated before receiving additional doses

Although signs and symptoms of ergotism (ergot poisoning) rarely develop even after long-term intermittent use of ergots, care should be exercised to remain within the limits of recommended dosage.

Taking symptom-relieving headache medicine more than a couple of days a week can set off a vicious cycle called rebound. As each dose of medicine wears off, the pain reappears, leading patients to take even more medicine. The overuse of medicine actually starts causing headaches. Rebound headaches can occur with any migraine drug, whether it is OTC or prescription.

For *Cautions and Concerns* regarding drugs used to prevent migraines, refer to their specific drug groups: ANTICONVULSANTS, ANTIANGINALS, ANTIARRHYTHMICS, ANTIHYPERTENSIVES, ANTIDEPRESSANTS, and ANALGESICS.

Warnings

Triptans may increase the risk of chest pain, stroke, abnormal heart rhythms, or heart attack in susceptible individuals. Patients who are intermittent long-term users of triptans who have or acquire risk factors predictive of coronary artery disease should undergo periodic cardiovascular evaluations during their continued use of these drugs. Significant increases in blood pressure, including hypertensive crisis, have been reported on rare occasions in patients both with and without a history of hypertension when taking triptans.

Hypersensitivity reactions to triptans have occurred on rare occasions, including severe anaphylaxis reactions.

Use of the triptans along with drugs that increase serotonin levels (e.g., serotonin norepinephrine reuptake inhibitors [e.g., venlafaxine, duloxetine]) may cause a potentially life-threatening condition called serotonin syndrome. If these drugs need to be used together, the patient should be observed closely.

Ergots should be used with caution in patients taking less potent CYP3A4 inhibitors (e.g., saquinavir, grapefruit juice, nefazodone, fluconazole, fluoxetine, fluvoxamine, zileuton, clotrimazole).

For *Warnings* regarding drugs used to prevent migraines, refer to their specific drug groups: ANTICONVULSANTS, ANTIANGINALS, ANTIARRHYTHMICS, ANTIHYPERTENSIVES, ANTIDEPRESSANTS, and ANALGESICS.

Sumatriptan succinate and naproxen sodium may increase the risk of heart attack, stroke, serious stomach and intestinal problems, such as bleeding and ulcers, and serious rash that may be fatal and occur without warning. Risk of stomach and intestinal problems increases in the elderly.

When Not Advised (Contraindications)

Triptans should not be used by patients who have a history of coronary artery disease, peripheral vascular disease (e.g., Raynaud's syndrome, ischemic bowel disease), stroke, transient ischemic attack (TIA), or uncontrolled hypertension. These drugs should also not be used to treat hemiplegic migraine (a type causing temporary paralysis on one side) or basilar migraine (a type associated with dizziness and tinnitus, a buzzing or ringing in the ear).

Rizatriptan, sumatriptan, and zolmitriptan should not be used within two weeks of a monoamine oxidase inhibitor (MAOI), which may increase the levels of these particular triptans.

Eletriptan should not be used within 72 hours of potent CYP3A4 inhibitors (e.g., clarithromycin, itraconazole, ketoconazole, nefazodone, nelfinavir, ritonavir, and troleandomycin), which may raise the eletriptan blood levels.

Eletriptan is contraindicated in patients with severe liver impairment. Naratriptan is contraindicated in patients with severe kidney or liver impairment.

Ergots should not be used by patients with a history of peripheral vascular disease (e.g., Raynaud' syndrome), stroke/TIA, coronary artery disease, uncontrolled hypertension, liver or kidney dysfunction, sepsis (blood poisoning), or basilar or hemiplegic migraine. Also, ergots may be harmful to unborn children or nursing infants and should not be taken by pregnant or nursing women.

Serious and/or life-threatening peripheral ischemia (restricted blood supply) has been associated with the coadministration of ergotamine derivatives with potent CYP3A4 inhibitors (e.g., nelfinavir, ritonavir, indinavir, erythromycin, clarithromcin, troleandomycin, ketoconazole, itraconazole). Because CYP3A4 inhibition elevates the serum levels of dihydroergotamine or ergotamine, the risk for vasospasm (sudden constriction of a blood vessel that reduces the blood flow) leading to cerebral ischemia and/or ischemia of the extremities is increased.

Triptans and ergotamine derivatives should not be used within 24 hours of each other because of the increased risk of prolonged vasospastic reactions.

For *Contraindications* regarding drugs used to prevent migraines, refer to their specific drug groups: ANTICONVULSANTS, ANTIANGINALS, ANTIARRHYTHMICS, ANTIHYPERTENSIVES, ANTIDEPRESSANTS, and ANALGESICS.

Side Effects

Common side effects of triptans include tightness in the throat or chest, redness or flushing of the face, feeling warm, numbness, tingling, dizziness, muscle weakness, fatigue, or nausea. Sumatriptan or zolmitriptan nasal spray may cause nose and throat irritation.

Common side effects of ergots include nausea and vomiting, tachycardia (increased heart rate), leg muscle pains, weakness in the legs, cold fingers or toes, and numbness and tingling of the fingers and toes. Dihydroergotamine nasal spray can cause sneezing and nasal stuffiness.

For *Side Effects* regarding drugs used to prevent migraines, refer to their specific drug groups: ANTICONVULSANTS, ANTIANGINALS, ANTIARRHYTHMICS, ANTIHYPERTENSIVES, ANTIDEPRESSANTS, and ANALGESICS.

Interactions

Triptans and ergots should not be taken within 24 hours of each other, as this may lead to excessive narrowing of the blood vessels (see *Contraindications*). Triptans and ergots should not be used along with other drugs that affect serotonin, such as fluoxetine, paroxetine, venlafaxine, or duloxetine (see *Warnings*). Certain triptans (rizatriptan, sumatriptan, and zolmitriptan) should not be taken within two weeks of an MAOI (see *Contraindications*).

Cimetidine may double the concentration of zolmitriptan in the blood by interfering with its elimination. Potent CYP3A4 inhibitors may increase concentrations of almotriptan. Oral contraceptives and propranolol may increase the effects of frovatriptan. Patients taking propranolol for migraine prevention should reduce the dosage of rizatriptan.

Eletriptan, ergotamine, and dihydroergotamine should not be used along with potent CYP3A4 inhibitors (see *Contraindications*).

For *Interactions* regarding drugs used to prevent migraines, refer to their specific drug groups: ANTICONVULSANTS, ANTIANGINALS, ANTIARRHYTHMICS, ANTIHYPERTENSIVES, ANTIDEPRESSANTS, and ANALGESICS.

Sales/Statistics

According to the "Top 200 Brand-Name Drugs by Retail Dollars in 2006" (*Drug Topics,* March 5, 2007), Imitrex Oral ranked #43 with sales of $858,252,000. Relpax ranked #140 with sales of $204,508,000 (up 26.2 percent). Maxalt ranked #190 with sales of $144,387,000 (up 17.7 percent from 2005), and Maxalt MLT ranked #195 with sales of $140,005,000 (up 12.4 percent). Zomig ranked #194 with sales of $140,265,000.

According to the "Top 200 Brand-Name Drugs by Units in 2006" (*Drug Topics,* March 5, 2007), Imitrex Oral ranked #73, with 4,535,000 prescriptions. Relpax ranked #166, with 1,499,000 prescriptions (up 18.9 percent).

Demographics and Cultural Groups

In 2003, severe headaches or migraines were more than twice as common among women as men (21 percent compared with 9 percent). The presence of severe headache or migraine diminished with age—from 25 percent among women age 18 to 44 years to 7 percent among women

age 75 years and over. (Source: *Health, United States, 2005,* National Center for Health Statistics).

Development History

Ergot has a long history of medicinal use; the basic chemical structure of the ergot alkaloids was determined in the early 1930s. Ergot derivatives were the primary oral drugs available to abort a migraine once it was under way until the introduction of the triptans.

On December 28, 1992, the FDA approved the injectable form of sumatriptan, the first of the triptans, which offered improved efficacy and tolerability over the ergots. The development of sumatriptan was quickly followed by a number of second-generation triptan compounds, which were developed to increase the drug's absorption through the digestive tract and thus relieve the migraine pain more quickly. These second-generation triptans were characterized by improved pharmacokinetic properties and/or tolerability profiles. Their order of approval: zolmitriptan (1997), rizatriptan (1998), naratriptan (1998), almotriptan (2001), frovatriptan (2001), and eletriptan (2002). The sumatriptan/naproxen combination drug was approved in 2008.

Future Drugs

According to data compiled by the National Headache Foundation (NHF), more than 20 drug companies had antimigraine products in the pipeline in 2006.

Unnamed antimigraine drugs that GlaxoSmithKline has in their pipeline include a transient receptor potential vanilloid-1 (TRPV1) antagonist (in Phase II trials in 2006), a selective iNOS inhibitor (in Phase II trials in 2006), and a gap junction blocker (in Phase I trials in 2006).

NHF noted that new delivery systems for antimigraine drugs are also being developed alongside the drugs themselves in an attempt to speed up pain relief. Alexza Molecular Delivery Corporation is developing a novel inhalation device called Stacatto, which uses heat to vaporize a drug into an odorless microparticulate mist that passes quickly through the lungs into the bloodstream. The hope is to provide relief within 60 seconds (compared to the typical 30 minutes for injections and two hours for tablets). With this delivery device, medication is vaporized and then inhaled and delivered immediately into the bloodstream. This device is being used with pro-chlorperazine, which is used often in the emergency room for the treatment of acute migraine and nausea and vomiting.

Brittania Pharmaceuticals is collaborating with Novartis Pharmaceuticals and developing a dihydroergotamine nasal powder. It is hoped that a nasal powder will be easier to administer than the current methods (subcutaneously or by nasal spray) and that the body will absorb it much faster.

Capnia is developing a device that delivers pressurized carbon dioxide into one nostril and out the other. The carbon dioxide would not be inhaled but rather is intended to permeate the mucous membranes of the nasal cavity, creating carbonic acid and preventing stimulation of neurons and the activation of the pain cycle. Completed Phase II studies found that about 30 percent of patients with migraine attacks were pain-free within two hours of treatment with the device. Phase III studies with this device are currently ongoing.

Reed, Lesley. "What's in the Future for the Treatment of Headache." *NHF Head Lines* 148 (January/February 2006): 1–4.

Spierings, E. L. "Mechanism of Migraine and Action of Antimigraine Medications." *Medical Clinics of North America* 85, no. 4 (July 2001): 943–958.

antineoplastics Sometimes referred to as chemotherapy agents, anticancer drugs, or oncology drugs, antineoplastic agents are widely used in cancer therapy. Antineoplastics are drugs that interfere with the development of malignant cells and neoplasms (tumors that may become cancerous) by disrupting cell division. They may also be called cytotoxic or cytostatic because they have the ability to kill actively growing cells. These therapies can be used alone or in combination. If these drugs are successful, the cancer is said to go into remission; however, a chance of a relapse, or recurrence of the cancer, remains. According to the Center for Drug Evaluation and Research (CDER), more than 300 oncology drugs have been approved since 1949, although not all are currently in use. See INTERFERONS for additional anticancer drugs.

Classes

Antineoplastic agents are classified according to their method of action and the types of cancer they treat.

- *Alkylating agents* The first anticancer drugs developed, and even though highly toxic, continue to be a major component of anticancer therapy. This group of drugs is comprised of the following subclasses: alkyl sulfonates, ethyleneimines, nitrogen mustards, nitrosoureas, triazenes, and miscellaneous. *Examples:* alkyl sulfonates: busulfan (Busulfex, Myleran); ethyleneimines: altretamine (Hexalen) and thiotepa; nitrogen mustards: chlorambucil (Leukeran), cyclophosphamide, ifosfamide (Ifex), mechlorethamine (Mustargen), and melphalan (Alkeran); nitrosoureas: carmustine (BiCNU, Gliadel), lomustine (CeeNU), and streptozocin (Zanosar); triazenes: dacarbazine (DTIC-Dome) and temozolomide (Temodar); miscellaneous: procarbazine (Matulane).

- *Antibiotics* Products of various strains of the soil fungus *Streptomyces;* also called antitumor antibiotics. *Examples:* bleomycin (Blenoxane), dactinomycin (Cosmegen), and mitomycin (Mutamycin).

- *Antimetabolites* Similar in structure to metabolites, which are required for normal biochemical reactions, yet different enough to interfere with the normal functions of cells. *Examples:* azacitidine (Vidaza), capecitabine (Xeloda), cladribine (Leustatin), cytarabine (Cytosar U, Depocyt [liposomal formulation]), decitabine (Dacogen), floxuridine (FUDR), fludarabine (Fludara, Oforta), fluorouracil (Adrucil, Carac, Efudex, Fluroplex), gemcitabine (Gemzar), hydroxyurea (Droxia, Hydrea), mercaptopurine (Purinethol), methotrexate (Trexall), pemetrexed (Alimta), pentostatin (Nipent), pralatrexate (Folotyn), and thioguanine (Tabloid).

- *Antimitotics* Also called antimicrotubule agents, mitotic inhibitors, and taxanes. *Examples:* docetaxel (Taxotere), estramustine (Emcyt), paclitaxel (Abraxane, Taxol), vinblastine, vincristine, and vinorelbine (Navelbine).

- *Epothilones* A novel class of cytotoxic compounds that function similarly to antimitotics. *Example:* ixabepilone (Ixempra).

- *Histone deacetylase (HDAC) inhibitors* Have been shown to alter the growth of several different forms of cancer. *Example:* vorinostat (Zolinza).

- *Hormones* Used to treat hormone-sensitive tumors. *Examples:* anastrozole (Arimidex), bicalutamide (Casodex), degarelix (trade name pending), exemestane (Aromasin), flutamide (Eulexin), fulvestrant (Faslodex), goserelin (Zoladex), histrelin (Vantas), letrozole (Femara), leuprolide (Lupron, Eligard), medroxyprogesterone (Depo-Provera, Provera), megestrol (Megace), nilutamide (Nilandron), tamoxifen (Nolvadex), toremifene (Fareston), and triptorelin (Trelstar).

- *Monoclonal antibodies* Antibodies made in the lab from a single clone that can recognize and target specific cancers. *Examples:* alemtuzumab (Campath), bevacizumab (Avastin), cetuximab (Erbitux), gemtuzumab (Mylotarg), ibritumomab tiuxetan (Zevalin), ofatumumab (Arzerra), panitumumab (Vectibix), rituximab (Rituxan), tositumomab and I-131 tositumomab (Bexxar), and trastuzumab (Herceptin).

- *mTOR inhibitors* Act against proteins (enzymes) called mammalian target of rapamycin (mTOR). *Examples:* everolimus (Afinitor) and temsirolimus (Torisel).

- *Platinum compounds* Also called heavy metal alkylating-like agents; derived from platinum. Examples: carboplatin (Paraplatin), cisplatin (Platinol-AQ), and oxaliplatin (Eloxatin).

- *Topoisomerase inhibitors* Also called DNA topoisomerase inhibitors; they act against rapidly dividing cells. They are comprised of three subclasses of drugs: anthracene derivatives, camptothecins, and epipodophyllotoxins. *Examples:* anthracene derivatives (anthracyclines), daunorubicin (Cerubidine), doxorubicin, doxorubicin liposomal (Doxil), epirubicin (Ellence), idarubicin (Idamycin PES), mitoxantrone (Novantrone), and valrubicin (Valstar); camptothecins: irinotecan (Camptosar) and topotecan (Hycamtin); podophyllotoxin derivatives: etoposide (VePesid, Toposar) and teniposide (Vumon).

- *Tyrosine kinase inhibitors* Act against chemical messengers (enzymes) called tyrosine kinases. *Examples:* dasatinib (Sprycel), erlotinib (Tarceva), gefitinib (Iressa), imatinib (Gleevec), lapatinib (Tykerb), nilotinib (Tasigna), pazopanib (Votrient), sorafenib (Nexavar), and sunitinib (Sutent).

- *Retinoids* Chemically related to or derived from vitamin A. *Examples:* bexarotene (Targretin), tretinoin (Vesanoid), and tretinoin topical (Atralin, Avita, Renova, Retin-A, Retin-A Micro, Tretin-X).

- *Proteasome inhibitors* Block the action of proteasomes, cellular complexes that break down proteins. *Example:* bortezomib (Velcade).

- *Miscellaneous examples:* aldesleukin (Proleukin), asparaginase (also called L-asparaginase) (Elspar), denileukin diftitox (Ontak), lenalidomide (Revlimid), and thalidomide (Thalomid).

How They Work

Alkylating agents interfere with cell division by attaching alkyl groups (small carbon compounds) to DNA (genetic material) bases in cells. This alteration results in the DNA being broken into pieces by enzymes as they attempt to repair and replace the alkylated bases, leading to their inability to replicate. Although the alkylated cell may not die, it also cannot further divide and produce more cancer cells. Because cancer cells generally grow and increase more than healthy cells do, cancer cells are more sensitive to the alkylated DNA damage.

Antibiotics work by interfering with normal cell functions, which damages the cancer cells and prevents them from multiplying. They either break up the DNA strands or inhibit DNA synthesis that cells need to grow. They may work in all phases of the cell cycle.

Antimetabolites work because they resemble metabolites, chemicals the cancer cells need for metabolism and growth. When the body tries to use the antimetabolites, however, it cannot make the DNA and RNA, which stops the growth of cancer cells and causes them to die. Antimetabolites work in the phase of the cell cycle when cells are dividing.

Antimitotic drugs block the final stage of the cell division process (mitosis) by interacting with tubulin, the major protein of mitotic spindles, and causing metaphase arrest. When this occurs, certain cellular signaling networks kill the cancer cell before it can divide to become two cells or repair the damage.

Epothilones function by disrupting the activity of microtubules, which are necessary for many cellular processes associated with cell growth and proliferation, including cell signaling and cell structure stability. Although they function in a similar fashion to paclitaxel, their mechanism of microtubule binding is different from that of paclitaxel, which makes epothilones an attractive drug class for patients with taxane-resistant malignancies.

Histone deacetylase inhibitors interfere with the regulation of gene expression (the process that takes the information contained in genes on DNA and turns that information into proteins) by inhibiting the activity of enzymes known as histone deacetylases. Although the precise mechanism through which these compounds work is not yet understood, it is believed that they inhibit cancer cell division and proliferation.

Hormone drugs work by keeping the body's own hormones from reaching the nucleus of the cancer cell, which prevents the cancer cell from using the hormone it needs to grow; by preventing the body from making the hormones, causing the cancer cells to stop growing and in some cases to shrivel up and die (self-destruction or apoptosis); or by substituting chemically similar agents for the active hormone, which cannot be used by the tumor cell to grow.

Monoclonal antibodies are proteins made in the laboratory that can locate and bind to substances in the body (e.g., epidermal growth factor receptor [EGFR] and vascular endothelial growth factor [VEGF]), targeting those substances that appear on cancer cells but rarely or never on normal cells. Many kinds of monoclonal antibodies exist, and each monoclonal antibody is made to find one substance. Monoclonal antibodies work by locating cancer cells and either killing them or delivering cancer-killing substances (e.g., drugs, toxins, or radioactive materials) to them without harming normal cells. For example, ibritumomab tiuxetan is combined with a radioactive substance and given with rituximab as a type of radioimmunotherapy. This therapeutic regimen targets tumor cells with a high dose of radiation, reducing the amount of full body radiation.

Mammalian target of rapamycin (mTOR) inhibitors work by blocking mTOR, an enzyme in cells that normally promotes their growth and division, thereby preventing an increase in the number of cancer cells.

Platinum compounds work by preventing the cell's production of DNA by forming links with the strands of DNA and in the process binding them together. This prevents the cancer cell from reproducing.

Topoisomerase inhibitors block topoisomerases (enzymes that break and rejoin DNA strands and are needed for cells to divide and grow). By stopping cancer cells from growing, these drugs cause the cells to die.

Tyrosine kinase inhibitors work by interfering with communication within cells, which stops the cancer cell from growing and dividing.

Retinoids help regulate, or control, the gene functions that help cells grow and divide. They activate certain retinoid receptors on the cancer cell, which work with other substances to control cancer cell growth and differentiation (change in a cell's size, shape, membrane potential, metabolic activity, and responsiveness to signals).

Proteasome inhibitors work by blocking proteasomes, which are found in all cells in the body and which help control the levels of certain proteins that are important for cell growth and survival. Bortezomib interferes with this process, which leads to a buildup of proteins in the cell, making the cell die. Cancer cells are more prone to this damage than are normal cells.

Asparaginase is an enzyme taken from the bacterium *Escherichia coli (E. coli)*. It breaks down the amino acid asparagine, which certain cancer cells need in order to grow. While normal cells can make more asparagine for themselves, these cancer cells cannot; therefore, they die.

Denileukin is a fusion protein (a combination of diphtheria toxin and interleukin-2) that selectively delivers the cell-killing activity of the diphtheria toxin to targeted cells.

Lenalidomide, a thalidomide analogue, and thalidomide are immunomodulatory agents (they affect the immune system) with antineoplastic properties that inhibit the growth of certain cancer cells. Also, their antiangiogenic properties are believed to help slow or stop the growth of new blood vessels (angiogenesis), which tumors need to grow and survive. The use of thalidomide in multiple myeloma patients is accompanied by an increase in the number of circulating natural killer cells and an increase in levels of certain cytokines associated with anticancer cell activity.

Approved Uses

Alkylating agents *Alkyl sulfonates:* Busulfan is used to treat chronic myelogenous leukemia (CML), a cancer of white blood cells. Busulfan injection is used in combination with cyclophoshamide as a conditioning regimen prior to progenitor cell transplantation for CML.

Ethyleneimines: Altretamine is used as a single agent in the palliative treatment (alleviating pain without curing) of patients with persistent or recurrent ovarian cancer following first-line therapy with a cisplatin- and/or alkylating agent–based combination. Thiotepa is used to treat lymphoma and cancers of the breast, ovary, and bladder and may also be used to control the fluid (effusions) that can build up in body spaces (such as the abdomen) where cancer has spread (mestastasized).

Nitrogen mustards: Chlorambucil is used in the treatment of chronic lymphocytic leukemia (CLL), Hodgkin's lymphoma, and non-Hodgkin's lymphoma (NHL). Cyclophosphamide is used for the treatment of lymphomas, leukemias, multiple myeloma, mycosis fungoides (a skin cancer), neuroblastoma, retinoblastoma, and breast, ovarian, testicular, and lung cancers. Ifosfamide is approved to treat testicular cancer. Mechlorethamine is used to treat Hodgkin's lymphoma, lymphosarcoma (cancer involving the lymphoid system), certain leukemias, mycosis fungoides, lung cancer, and metastatic carcinoma resulting in effusion. Melphalan is used for the palliative treatment of multiple myeloma (a type of cancer of the bone marrow) and ovarian cancer.

Nitrosoureas: Carmustine is used to treat brain tumors, multiple myeloma, Hodgkin's lymphoma, and NHL. The implantable wafer that contains carmustine is used to treat gliomas and glioblastoma multiforme, which are types of brain tumors. Lomustine is used to treat brain tumors and Hodgkin's lymphoma. Streptozocin is used to treat pancreatic cancer.

Triazenes: Dacarbazine is used to treat Hodgkin's lymphoma and metastatic malignant melanoma. Temozolomide is used to treat certain types of brain cancers in adult patients when the cancer has returned or has just been diagnosed.

Miscellaneous: Procarbazine is used to treat Hodgkin's lymphoma.

Antibiotics Bleomycin is used to treat testicular cancer, Hodgkin's lymphoma and NHL, and squamous cell carcinoma of the head, neck, and cervix. It is also used to treat cancer that has metastasized to the lungs to keep fluid (effusions) from building up between the lungs and chest wall. Dactinomycin is used to treat testicular cancer, sarcomas (cancers that grow from cartilage, fat, muscle, or bone), and Wilms' tumor (a cancer of the kidney found primarily in children). Mitomycin is used to treat stomach and pancreatic cancers.

Antimetabolites Azacitidine is used to treat myelodysplastic syndromes (MDS), which is a disease of the bone marrow, as well as chronic myelomonocytic leukemia. Capecitabine is used to treat metastatic breast, colon, or rectal cancer. Cladribine is used to treat hairy cell leukemia, a cancer of the blood and bone marrow. Cytarabine is used to prevent and treat meningeal leukemia (leukemia that has spread to the meninges, a membrane that envelops the brain and spinal cord), and to treat acute myeloid leukemia (AML), acute lymphoblastic leukemia (ALL), and CML. Liposomal cytarabine, a form of cytarabine contained inside liposomes (very tiny particles of fat) is approved to treat lymphomatous meningitis (lymphoma that has spread to the meninges). Floxuridine is used to treat gastrointestinal cancers that have metastasized to the liver. Fludarabine is used to treat B cell CLL. Fluorouracil is used to treat gastrointestinal cancers of the colon, rectum, breast, stomach and pancreas; it is used topically to treat a premalignant condition of scaly or crusty lesions on the face or bald scalp known as actinic or solar keratoses and some types of skin cancer. Gemcitabine is used to treat metastatic pancreatic, breast, ovarian, and non-small-cell lung cancers. Hydroxyurea is used to treat melanoma, CML, and recurrent, metastatic, or inoperable ovarian cancer. Hydroxyurea is also used along with radiation therapy for certain skin cancers of the head and neck. Hydroxyurea is also used to reduce the frequency of painful crises and the need for blood transfusions in adults with sickle-cell disease. Mercaptopurine is used for the treatment of ALL. Methotrexate is used to

treat choriocarcinoma (a cancer of the reproductive system, usually of the placenta), various leukemias, meningeal leukemia, osteosarcoma (bone cancer), NHL, and breast, lung, and head and neck cancers; to control symptoms of severe, disabling psoriasis (see *Warnings*); and to manage selective cases of rheumatoid arthritis (RA) and juvenile RA. Pemetrexed is used to treat metastatic non-small-cell lung cancer and malignant pleural mesothelioma (a cancer in the lining of the chest cavity around the lungs that is usually linked to asbestos exposure). Pentostatin is used to treat hairy cell leukemia. Pralatrexate is used to treat patients with relapsed or refractory peripheral T cell lymphoma (PTCL). Thioguanine is used to treat AML.

Antimitotics Docetaxel is used to treat breast cancer and metastatic non-small-cell lung, stomach, prostate, and head and neck cancers. Estramustine is used for the palliative treatment of advanced prostate cancer. Paclitaxel is used to treat breast, non-small-cell lung, and advanced ovarian cancers and acquired immunodeficiency syndrome (AIDS)–related Kaposi's sarcoma (a cancer of the skin and mucous membranes). Vinblastine is used to treat Hodgkin's lymphoma, Kaposi's sarcoma, breast cancer, choriocarcinoma, and testicular cancer. Vincristine is used to treat acute leukemia, Hodgkin's lymphoma, NHL, and several childhood cancers—rhabdomyosarcoma (cancer of connective tissues), neuroblastoma (cancer of the nervous system), and Wilms' tumor. Vinorelbine is used to treat non-small-cell lung cancer.

Epothilones Ixabepilone is used to treat advanced breast cancer.

Histone deacetylase inhibitors Vorinostat is used to treat cutaneous manifestations in patients with cutaneous T cell lymphoma that is progressive, persistent, or recurrent following two systemic therapies.

Hormones Anastrozole is used to treat breast cancer in postmenopausal women. Bicalutamide is used with a leuteinizing hormone-release hormone (LHRH) agonist to treat advanced prostate cancer. Degarelix is used to treat advanced prostate cancer. Exemestane is used to treat breast cancer in postmenopausal women. Flutamide is used with an LHRH agonist to treat advanced prostate cancer. Fulvestrant is used to treat advanced breast cancer in postmenopausal women. Goserelin is used to treat advanced prostate and breast cancers and also to treat endometriosis (endometrial tissúe found in areas of the body outside the uterus), a noncancerous condition. Letrozole is used to treat breast cancer in postmenopausal women. Leuprolide is used to treat advanced prostate cancer, uterine fibroids, endometriosis, central precocious puberty (CPP) (early onset of puberty before the age of eight in girls and nine in boys), and endometriosis.

Medroxyprogesterone is used to treat the symptoms of endometrial and kidney cancer, to treat secondary amenorrhea (absence or suppression of normal menstrual flow) or abnormal uterine bleeding due to hormonal imbalance, to prevent pregnancy, and to manage pain associated with endometriosis. Megestrol is used for the palliative treatment of advanced breast cancer and endometrial cancer as well as to improve appetite in people with anorexia, cachexia, or weight loss due to AIDS. Nilutamide is used in combination with surgical castration for the treatment of metastatic prostate cancer. Tamoxifen is used to prevent breast cancer in high-risk women; to decrease the risk of getting invasive breast cancer in women with ductal cancer in situ (DCIS) (a very early noninvasive form of breast cancer); to prevent cancer from coming back after surgery, radiation, and chemotherapy; and to treat metastatic breast cancer in women and men. Toremifene is used to treat advanced breast cancer in postmenopausal women. Triptorelin pamoate is used for the palliative treatment of advanced prostate cancer.

Monoclonal Antibodies Alemtuzumab is used to treat B cell CLL. Bevacizumab is used to treat metastatic colorectal, breast, and non-small-cell lung cancers as well as advanced glioblastoma. Bevacizumab has also been approved for the treatment of metastatic renal cell carcinoma in combination with interferon alfa. Cetuximab is used to treat head and neck cancer and metastatic colorectal cancer. Gemtuzumab ozogamicin is used to treat patients who are at least 60 years of age with relapsed CD33-positive AML who are not eligible for other chemotherapy regimens. Ibritumomab tiuxetan is used to treat certain types of B cell NHL in patients who have been treated with chemotherapy or with rituximab alone and have not gotten better or have had a relapse. Ibritumomab tiuxetan has also been approved for the treatment of previously untreated follicular NHL in patients who achieve a partial or complete response to first-line chemotherapy. Ofatumumab is used to treat CLL refractory to fludarabine and alemtuzumab. Panitumumab is used to treat metastatic colorectal cancer in patients who have failed standard chemotherapy treatment. Rituximab is used to treat certain types of CD20-positive NHL; it is also used with methotrexate to treat moderate-to-severe RA. Tositumomab is used to treat certain types of relapsed or refractory CD20-positive NHL. Trastuzumab is used to treat certain types of breast cancer.

mTOR inhibitors Everolimus is used to treat advanced kidney cancer that has progressed after treatment with sunitinib or sorafenib. Temsirolimus is used to treat advanced kidney cancer.

Platinum compounds Carboplatin is used to treat ovarian cancer. Cisplatin is used to treat advanced bladder cancer as well as metastatic testicular and ovarian cancers. Oxaliplatin is used with fluorouracil and leucovorin to treat advanced colon or colorectal cancer.

Topoisomerase inhibitors *Anthracene derivatives:* Daunorubicin is used to treat ALL and AML. Daunorubicin liposomal is used to treat advanced human immunodeficiency virus (HIV)–associated Kaposi's sarcoma. Doxorubicin is used to treat several cancers including ALL, AML, Wilms' tumor, Hodgkin's lymphoma, neuroblastoma, sarcomas, and breast, bladder, thyroid, stomach, lung, and ovarian cancer. Doxorubicin liposomal is used to treat ovarian cancer, AIDS-related Kaposi's sarcoma, and multiple myeloma. Epirubicin is used to treat breast cancer following surgery. Idarubicin is used to treat AML. Mitoxantrone is used to treat acute nonlymphocytic leukemias, advanced hormone-refractory prostate cancer, and certain forms of multiple sclerosis. Valrubicin is used to treat carcinoma in situ (CIS) of the urinary bladder that is refractory to treatment with Bacillus-Calmette-Guérin (BCG).

Camptothecins: Irinotecan is used either with or after failed therapy with fluorouracil and leucovorin for the treatment of metastatic colon or rectal cancer. Topotecan is used to treat ovarian, cervical, and small cell lung cancers.

Podophyllotoxin derivatives: Etoposide is used to treat testicular and small cell lung cancers. Teniposide is used to treat ALL in children.

Tyrosine kinase inhibitors Dasatinib is used to treat CML and Philadelphia chromosome-positive (Ph+) ALL. Erlotinib is used to treat metastatic pancreatic and non-small-cell lung cancers. Gefitinib is used to treat non-small-cell lung cancer after failure of both platinum compounds and docetaxel and is limited to patients who are benefiting or have benefited from gefitinib. (Gefitinib has not been shown to help people who have non–small cell lung cancer live longer. Because other medications are available that may help these patients live longer, only those who have already taken gefitinib and benefited from the medication are now approved to take it.) Imatinib is used to treat Ph+ CML and ALL, aggressive systemic mastocytosis (excessive accumulation of mast cells in different tissues, including bone marrow, the liver, spleen, and GI tract), dermatofibrosarcoma protuberans (a type of skin cancer), hypereosinophilic syndrome (persistently increased levels of eosinophils [white blood cells that play a role in the immune system] without any recognizable cause) and/or chronic eosinophilic leukemia (a disease in which too many eosinophils are found in the bone marrow, blood, and other tissues), gastrointestinal stromal tumors (a malignant cancer in the lining of the digestive tract), MDS, and myeloproliferative disease (a group of slow-growing blood cancers). Lapatinib is used to treat advanced or metastatic breast cancer in patients who have received prior therapy with an anthracycline, taxane, and trastuzumab. Nilotinib is used to treat chronic phase and accelerated phase Philadelphia chromosome-positive CML in patients who are refractory or intolerant to imatinib. Pazopanib is used to treat patients with advanced renal cell carcinoma. Sorafenib is used to treat advanced cancers of the kidney and liver. Sunitinib is used to treat advanced kidney cancer and gastrointestinal stromal tumor after disease progression on or intolerance to imatinib.

Retinoids Bexarotene is used to treat skin lesions caused by cutaneous T cell lymphoma in patients who have not responded to at least one previous treatment regimen. Tretinoin is used to induce remission of a specific form of acute promyelocytic leukemia. Topical formulations of tretinoin, which are not considered to be antineoplastics, are used to treat acne as well as wrinkles, hyperpigmentation, and roughness of the skin.

Proteasome inhibitors Bortezomib is used to treat cancers of the blood and bone marrow cancers, such as multiple myeloma and mantle cell lymphoma.

Miscellaneous Aldesleukin is used to treat metastatic skin and kidney cancers.

Asparaginase is used to treat ALL.

Denileukin is used to treat persistent or recurrent cutaneous T cell lymphoma, a type of NHL of the skin.

Lenalidomide is used to treat MDS and multiple myeloma.

Thalidomide is used to treat newly diagnosed multiple myeloma as well as for treatment of skin lesions associated with leprosy.

Off-Label Uses

Off-label use of antineoplastics is well documented and common. The National Cancer Institute (NCI) has noted that more than half of cancer patients receive at least one antineoplastic drug for an off-label indication. The NCI adds, "Cancer treatment is always evolving. Researchers continually conduct studies to determine new uses for already marketed drugs and to find effective combinations of drugs for new indications. The results of these studies are published in peer-reviewed medical journals. When a new treatment approach seems to produce better outcomes for patients, other doctors adopt it and it may become a new standard of care." Because of this constantly evolving and widespread off-label usage, the following such uses cannot be and are not intended to be all-inclusive but rather to provide current examples.

Alkylating Agents Thiotepa is used off-label to treat cancer in the membranes that cover and protect the brain and spinal cord (the meninges).

Chlorambucil is used off-label to treat ovarian and testicular cancers as well as autoimmune and inflammatory conditions such as RA and sarcoidosis.

Cyclophosphamide is used off-label for a variety of severe rheumatologic conditions, including Wegener's granulomatosis, progressive RA, and systemic lupus erythematosus. Cyclophosphamide has also been used to halt the progression of multiple sclerosis or decrease the frequency and duration of episodes and in the treatment of other autoimmune diseases, such as polyarteritis nodosa and polymyositis.

Ifosfamide is used off-label to treat lymphomas and leukemias as well as lung, breast, ovarian, pancreatic, gastric, and bladder cancers.

Melphalan is used off-label to treat breast cancer, testicular cancer, prostate cancer, and bone marrow transplantation.

Carmustine is used off-label to treat malignant melanoma.

Dacarbazine is used off-label in combination with other agents in the treatment of soft tissue sarcomas (a cancer of the connective tissue [muscles, tendons, joints, fat]) and cancer of the islet cells (a part of the pancreas).

Procarbazine is used off-label to treat NHL, brain tumors, small cell lung cancer, and melanoma.

Antibiotics Bleomycin is used off-label to treat bone cancer, mycosis fungoides, and AIDS-related Kaposi's sarcoma.

Dactinomycin is used off-label to treat Kaposi's sarcoma and osteosarcoma.

Mitomycin is used off-label to treat bladder cancer.

Antimetabolites Cladribine is used off-label to treat CLL, NHL, AML, mycosis fungoides, and autoimmune hemolytic anemia.

Decitabine is used off-label to treat acute leukemias.

Fludarabine is used off-label to treat NHL.

Hydroxyurea is used off-label to reduce platelet count and prevent thrombosis (blood clots) in high-risk patients with essential thrombocythemia (an excess amount of platelets in the blood due to a disorder of the bone marrow) and polycythemia vera (an abnormal increase in blood cells, primarily red blood cells, due to excess production of the cells by the bone marrow) and to manage psoriasis that does not respond to conventional treatment.

Methotrexate is used off-label as maintenance therapy for various autoimmune diseases such as ankylosing spondylitis, Crohn's disease, psoriatic arthritis, Wegener's granulomatosis, multiple sclerosis, ulcerative colitis, uveitis, systemic lupus erythematosus, and scleroderma.

Pentostatin is used off-label to treat certain lymphomas and leukemias.

Pralatrexate is used off-label to treat cutaneous T cell lymphoma.

Antimitotics Docetaxel is used off-label to treat ovarian cancer.

Paclitaxel is used off-label to treat head and neck cancer, small-cell lung cancer, NHL, and pancreatic cancer.

Vincristine is used off-label to treat breast cancer and bladder cancer.

Vinorelbine is used off-label to treat advanced esophageal cancer, advanced breast cancer, cervical cancer, and advanced Kaposi's sarcoma.

Histone deacetylase inhibitors Vorinostat is used off-label in combination with bortezomib for treatment of multiple myeloma.

Hormones Anastrozole is used off-label to treat male infertility.

Exemestane is used off-label to prevent prostate cancer.

Flutamide is used off-label to treat hirsutism (excessive hairiness) in women.

Medroxyprogesterone is used off-label to treat advanced breast cancer.

Tamoxifen is used off-label to treat malignant melanoma, brain tumors, uterine cancer, and male infertility and to stimulate ovulation in specially selected women desiring pregnancy.

Monoclonal antibodies Alemtuzumab has been used in phase 3 clinical trials to treat multiple sclerosis. This drug is also used off-label in bone marrow and kidney transplants.

Bevacizumab is used off-label to treat age-related macular degeneration.

Ofatumumab is used off-label to treat rheumatoid arthritis and multiple sclerosis.

Panitumumab is used off-label to treat advanced non-small-cell lung cancer, renal cell cancer, and prostate cancer.

Platinum compounds Carboplatin is used off-label to treat several cancers, including lung, head and neck, brain, testicular, prostate, endometrial, esophageal, bladder, and cervical.

Cisplatin is used off-label to treat several cancers, including head and neck, esophageal, stomach, lung, skin, prostate, lymphoma, and cervical.

Topoisomerase inhibitors Doxorubicin liposomal is used off-label to treat locally advanced or metastatic breast cancer.

Epirubicin is used in combination with other antineoplastics off-label to treat lung, gastric, and pancreatic cancers.

Mitoxantrone is used off-label to treat breast cancer and NHL.

Irinotecan is used off-label to treat various leukemias and lymphomas as well as lung, ovarian, stomach, breast, pancreatic, and cervical cancers.

Etoposide is used off-label to treat leukemias, Hodgkin's lymphoma, NHL, Kaposi's sarcoma, and neuroblastoma.

Retinoids Bexarotene is used off-label to treat breast and lung cancers.

Tyrosine kinase inhibitors Pazopanib is used off-label to treat patients with cancer of the ovary, fallopian tube, or peritoneum who have failed standard platinum-based therapy as well as to treat advanced thyroid cancer.

Miscellaneous Aldesleukin is used off-label to treat leukemias and lymphomas.

Asparaginase is used off-label to treat lymphomas.

Denileukin is used off-label to treat CLL.

Lenalidomide is used off-label to NHL and CLL.

Thalidomide is used off-label to treat graft-versus-host reactions after bone marrow transplantation, AIDS-related aphthous stomatitis, and several autoimmune diseases, such as Behget's disease, Crohn's disease, rheumatoid arthritis, and discoid lupus erythematosus.

Companion Drugs

Usually, a single antineoplastic agent will not cure cancer by itself, with combinations of drugs frequently superior to single-drug therapy. Antineoplastics may be used along with or following other treatments (e.g., surgery) as "adjuvant therapy," or two or more antineoplastics are often used effectively as "combination chemotherapy." As the American Cancer Society explains, "Different drugs attack cancer cells at varying stages of their growth cycles, making the combination a stronger weapon against cancerous cells. Furthermore, using a combination of drugs may reduce the chance of drug resistance." The specific drugs used in combination, when used (e.g., together or following each other according to a particular schedule), and for how long, is called a chemotherapy regimen. Regimens are established through ongoing scientific studies and clinical trials and may change as more information is learned and new drugs or new indications gain approval. Factors taken into consideration when selecting a regimen include the type of cancer, the cancer's stage or progression, the patient's age, and other health problems. Many dozens of drug regimens have been published for oncologists and pharmacists to use in their treatment choices. Some regimens are established and used universally. Others are less tested for some types of cancer, and the oncologist may make changes in a regimen's drug combination or schedule.

Administration

Alkylating agents Busulfan is administered orally as a tablet and also via intravenous infusion.

Altretamine is administered orally via capsules.

Thiotepa is administered via intravenous injection/infusion. It can also be given directly into the bladder using a urinary catheter or into a body cavity (e.g., the lining around the lungs, abdomen, or heart) for palliative treatment of metastatic carcinoma.

Chlorambucil is administered orally via tablets.

Cyclophosphamide can be administered orally via tablets or as an intravenous infusion.

Ifosfamide is administered via intravenous infusion.

Mechlorethamine is intended primarily for intravenous use and in most cases is given by this route. However, it can also be administered directly into a body cavity (e.g., the lining around the lungs, abdomen, or heart) for palliative treatment of metastatic carcinoma.

Melphalan is administered orally via tablets or via intravenous injection.

Carmustine is administered via intravenous injection/infusion or via wafer implants (into the brain).

Lomustine is administered orally via capsules.

Streptozocin is administered via intravenous injection/infusion.

Dacarbazine is administered via intravenous infusion.

Temozolomide is administered orally via capsules or via intravenous infusion.

Procarbazine is administered orally via capsules.

Antibiotics Bleomycin is administered via intramuscular or subcutaneous injection or by intravenous infusion. It can also be administered directly into the lining around the lungs to treat malignant pleural effusions.

Dactinomycin is administered via intravenous injection/infusion.

Mitomycin is administered via intravenous injection/infusion.

Antimetabolites Azacitidine is administered via intravenous infusion or subcutaneous injection.

Capecitabine is administered orally via tablets.

Cladribine is administered via intravenous infusion.

Cytarabine may be given by intravenous infusion or by subcutaneous, intramuscular, or intrathecal (into the fluid around the spinal cord) injection.

Decitabine is administered via intravenous infusion.

Floxuridine is infused into an artery that feeds directly into the liver.

Fludarabine is administered via intravenous infusion or orally via tablets.

Fluorouracil is administered via intravenous injection/infusion. It can also be applied to the skin as a topical cream or solution.

Gemcitabine is administered via intravenous infusion.

Hydroxyurea is administered orally via capsules or tablets.

Mercaptopurine is administered orally via tablets.

Methotrexate is administered orally via tablets, as intravenous injection/infusion, or as intramuscular, intrathecal, or subcutaneous injection.

Pemetrexed, pentostatin, and pralatrexate are administered via intravenous infusion.

Thioguanine is administered orally via tablets.

Antimitotics Docetaxel is administered via intravenous infusion.

Estramustine is administered orally via capsules.

Paclitaxel is administered via intravenous infusion.

Vinblastine and vincristine are administered via intravenous injection.

Vinorelbine is administered via intravenous injection/infusion.

Epothilones Ixabepilone is administered via intravenous infusion.

Histone deacetylase inhibitors Vorinostat is administered orally via capsules and with food.

Hormones Anastrozole is administered orally via tablets.

Bicalutamide is administered orally via tablets.

Degarelix is administered via subcutaneous injection.

Exemestane is administered orally via tablets.

Flutamide is administered orally via capsules.

Fulvestrant is administered via intramuscular injection.

Goserelin is administered via subcutaneous injection using an implant that slowly releases the drug over one to three months.

Histrelin is an implant that is placed under the skin and provides continuous release of the drug for 12 months.

Letrozole is administered orally via tablets.

Leuprolide is administered via intramuscular or subcutaneous injection.

Medroxyprogesterone is administered via intramuscular injection.

When megestrol is administered for cancer treatment, the tablet formulation is used; when administered to stimulate appetite, the oral suspension formulation is used.

Nilutamide, tamoxifen, and toremifene are administered orally via tablets.

Triptorelin pamoate is administered via intramuscular injection.

Monoclonal antibodies Monoclonal antibodies are administered via intravenous infusion.

mTOR inhibitors Everolimus is administered orally via tablets.

Temsirolimus is administered via intravenous infusion.

Platinum compounds Platinum compounds are administered via intravenous infusion.

Topoisomerase inhibitors Anthracene derivatives (except for valrubicin) are administered via intravenous infusion. Valrubicin is administered intravesically (placed directly into the bladder through a catheter).

Irinotecan is administered via intravenous infusion.

Topotecan is administered via intravenous infusion and orally via capsules.

Etoposide is administered via intravenous infusion and orally via capsules.

Teniposide is administered via intravenous infusion.

Tyrosine kinase inhibitors Tyrosine kinase inhibitors are administered orally; sunitinib and nilotinib are available as capsules and the others as tablets.

Retinoids Bexarotene is administered orally via capsules. It can also be applied to the skin as a topical gel.

Tretinoin is administered orally via capsules. It can also be applied to the skin as a topical gel or cream.

Proteasome inhibitors Bortezomib is administered via intravenous injection.

Miscellaneous Aldesleukin is administered via intravenous infusion.

Asparaginase is administered via intramuscular or intravenous injection.

Denileukin is administered via intravenous infusion.

Lenalidomide is taken orally via capsules.

Thalidomide is taken orally via capsules.

Cautions and Concerns

All chemotherapy drugs should be administered by experienced physicians, preferably oncologists. Administration of all chemotherapy drugs requires close supervision. If severe adverse reactions occur, most chemotherapy agents should be withheld and appropriate corrective measures taken.

Alkylating Agents The most consistent, dose-related toxicity with busulfan is bone marrow suppression (myelosuppression), which may manifest as anemia, leukopenia (abnormally low white blood count, which predisposes the patient to infection), thrombocytopenia (abnormally low platelet count in the blood, which predisposes the patient to bleeding), or any combination of these. It is imperative that patients be instructed to report promptly the development of fever, sore throat, signs of infection, bleeding from any site, or symptoms suggestive of anemia (e.g., general tiredness or weakness, dizziness, or shortness of breath). Any one of these findings may be a side effect of busulfan; however, they may also indicate transformation of the leukemia to an acute "blastic" form. Since busulfan may have a delayed effect, it is important to withdraw the medication temporarily at the first sign of an abnormally large or exceptionally rapid fall in any of the formed elements of the blood. Seizures have been reported in patients receiving busulfan.

With continuous high-dose daily altretamine, gradual onset of nausea and vomiting may occur. In most instances, this can be controlled with ANTIEMETICS; at times, however, the severity of nausea and vomiting requires altretamine dose reduction or, rarely, discontinuation.

If proper precautions, such as regular monitoring of blood counts, are not observed, thiotepa may cause myelosuppression. The patient should notify the physician in the case of any sign of bleeding (e.g., nosebleeds, easy bruising, change in color of urine, black stool) or infection (fever, chills) or for possible pregnancy to patient or partner.

Chlorambucil can cause leukopenia, especially in the weeks after the drug is given. Chlorambucil should not be given at full dosages before four weeks after a full course of radiation therapy or chemotherapy because of the vulnerability of the bone marrow to damage under these conditions.

Special attention to the possible development of toxicity should be exercised in patients being treated with cyclophosphamide if any of the following conditions are present: leukopenia, thrombocytopenia, tumor cell infiltration of bone marrow, previous X-ray therapy, previous therapy with other cytotoxic agents, impaired liver function, impaired kidney function.

Ifosfamide should be given cautiously to patients with impaired kidney function as well as to those with compromised bone marrow reserve, as indicated by leukopenia, extensive bone marrow metastases, prior radiation therapy, or prior therapy with other chemotherapy agents. Ifosfamide may interfere with normal wound healing.

Mechlorethamine can lower the white blood cell and red blood cell count as well as the number of platelets, especially in the weeks after the drug is given. Because of the toxicity of mechlorethamine and the unpleasant side effects following its use, the potential risk and discomfort from the use of this drug in patients with inoperable cancer or in the terminal stage of the disease must be balanced against the limited gain obtainable. Tumors of bone and nervous tissue have responded poorly to mechlorethamine therapy. Results are unpredictable in disseminated and malignant tumors of different types. Since drug toxicity, especially sensitivity to bone marrow failure, seems to be more common in CLL than in other conditions, mechlorethamine should be given in this condition with great caution, if at all.

Melphalan should be used with extreme caution in patients whose bone marrow reserve may have been compromised by prior radiation or chemotherapy or whose marrow function is recovering from previous cytotoxic therapy. Complete blood counts with differential should be performed during the course of treatment.

Nausea and vomiting frequently occur within two hours of carmustine intravenous administration and last four to six hours. Prior administration of ANTIEMETICS is effective in diminishing or preventing these side effects. Delayed wound healing may occur in wafer-treated patients.

Nausea and vomiting may occur three to six hours after taking lomustine and usually last less than 24 hours. ANTIEMETICS and/or fasting prior to dosing may diminish and sometimes prevent these effects.

If streptozocin accidentally seeps out of the vein into which it is injected (extravasation), it may cause severe tissue damage and scarring. Confusion, lethargy, and depression have been reported in a limited number of patients receiving a continuous intravenous infusion of streptozocin for five days. Patients should be informed that there may be a potential risk in driving or using complex machinery.

Extravasation with dacarbazine may result in tissue damage and severe pain. Local pain, burning sensation, and irritation at the site of injection may be relieved by locally applied hot packs.

Temozolomide capsules should not be opened. If capsules are accidentally opened or damaged, rigorous precautions should be taken with the capsule contents to avoid inhalation or contact with the skin or mucous membranes.

Undue toxicity may occur if procarbazine is used in patients with impaired kidney or liver function. When appropriate, hospitalization for the initial course of treatment should be considered. If radiation or a chemotherapeutic agent known to have bone marrow–depressant activity has been used, an interval of at least one month without such therapy is recommended before starting treatment with procarbazine. The length of this interval may also be determined by evidence of bone marrow recovery based on successive bone marrow studies. Procarbazine treatment should be stopped if any of the following occurs: abnormal skin sensations, confusion, leukopenia, thrombocytopenia, hypersensitivity reaction, mouth ulcer, diarrhea, or excess bleeding. Complete blood counts with differential should be performed during the course of treatment.

Antibiotics Lower doses of bleomycin may be required in patients with kidney dysfunction (see *Warnings*). Patients with creatinine clearance values of less than 50 mL/min should be treated with caution, and their kidney function should be carefully monitored during the administration of bleomycin, as an accumulation of the drug in the blood could occur in these patients.

Dactinomycin may cause hyperuricemia (increased levels of uric acid in the body), which can cause gout or kidney stones. Liver dysfunction may also occur. Dactinomycin may also cause decreased white blood cell, red blood cell, and platelet counts.

Acute shortness of breath and severe bronchospasm have been reported following the administration of vinca alkaloids (vinblastine, vincristine, vinorelbine) in patients who had previously or simultaneously received mitomycin. The onset of this acute respiratory distress occurred within minutes to hours after injection of these drugs. Bronchodilators, steroids, and/or oxygen have produced symptomatic relief. A few cases of adult respiratory distress syndrome have been reported in patients receiving mitomycin in combination with other chemotherapy.

Antimetabolites Treatment with azacitidine is associated with anemia, neutropenia (abnormally low number of a particular type of white blood cell called a neutrophil), and thrombocytopenia. Because azacitidine is potentially hepatotoxic in patients with severe preexisting hepatic impairment, caution is needed in patients with liver disease. Renal abnormalities ranging from elevated serum creatinine to kidney failure and death have been reported rarely in patients treated with intravenous azacitidine in combination with other chemotherapeutic agents for non-MDS conditions. Patients with renal impairment should be closely monitored for toxicity since azacitidine and its metabolites are primarily excreted by the kidneys.

Capecitabine can cause a condition known as hand-foot syndrome (palmar-plantar erythrodysesthesia or chemotherapy-induced acral erythema), in which the patient may experience pain, numbness, tingling, reddening, or swelling in the hands or feet. Peeling, blistering, or sores on the skin in these areas are also possible. Over time, hand-foot syndrome may cause a loss of fingerprints. Patients on long-term capecitabine maintenance therapy who travel internationally have been advised to carry a letter from their oncologist explaining their usage of this drug and this particular side effect. Damage to the heart observed with capecitabine includes myocardial infarction/ischemia, angina, arrhythmias, cardiac arrest, cardiac failure, heart failure, sudden death, and electrocardiographic changes. These adverse events may be more common in patients with a prior history of coronary artery disease. Patients with mild to moderate liver dysfunction due to cancer that has spread from the original (primary) tumor to the liver should be carefully monitored when capecitabine is administered.

For patients receiving cladribine, periodic assessment of blood counts, particularly during the first four to eight weeks posttreatment, is recommended to detect the development of anemia, neutropenia, and thrombocytopenia. Monitoring of kidney and liver function is also recommended, especially in patients with underlying kidney or liver dysfunction. Fever is a frequent side effect during the first month of treatment, especially in neutropenic patients. Antibiotics should be initiated when the fever is accompanied by infection. Given the known bone marrow suppressive effects of cladribine, practitioners should carefully evaluate the risks and benefits of administering this drug to patients with active infections (see *Warnings*). Rare cases of tumor lysis syndrome (a metabolic complication of chemotherapy) have been reported in patients with blood cancers who are treated with cladribine. Tumor lysis syndrome can occur after treatment of a fast-growing cancer, especially certain leukemias and lymphomas. As tumor cells die, they break apart and release their contents into the blood. This causes a change in certain chemicals in the blood, which may cause damage to organs, including the kidneys, heart, and liver.

Large doses of cytarabine frequently produce nausea and vomiting for several hours following the infusion. This problem tends to be less severe when the drug is infused over several hours or given by continuous infusion. Patients with kidney or liver function impairment may have a higher likelihood of central nervous system (CNS) toxicity after high-dose cytarabine treatment. Therefore, the drug should be used with caution and possibly at reduced dose in patients whose liver or kidney function is poor. Acute pancreatitis has been reported in a patient receiving cytarabine by continuous infusion and in patients being treated with cytarabine who have had prior treatment with L-asparaginase. Cytarabine may interfere with the normal menstrual cycle in women and may stop sperm production in men.

Because decitabine is associated with neutropenia and thrombocytopenia, complete blood and platelet counts should be performed as needed to monitor response and toxicity, but at a minimum, prior to each dosing cycle. Myelosuppression and worsening neutropenia may occur more frequently in the first or second treatment cycles and may not necessarily indicate progression of underlying MDS. Decitabine should be used with caution in patients with kidney or liver dysfunction, as no data exist on its use in these patients.

Floxuridine is a highly toxic drug with a narrow margin of safety. Severe hematological toxicity, gastrointestinal hemorrhage, and even death may result from the use of floxuridine despite meticulous selection of patients and careful adjustment of dosage. Therefore, patients should be carefully supervised since therapeutic response is unlikely to occur without some evidence of toxicity.

Fludarabine may lower the white blood cell and platelet counts. Tumor lysis syndrome has been reported with fludarabine treatment in patients with CLL who have large tumor burdens (i.e., the number of cancer cells, the size of a tumor, or the amount of cancer in the body). Fludarabine must be administered cautiously in patients with kidney insufficiency, as inadequate data on dosing of these patients exist.

Fluorouracil can cause hand-foot syndrome. Interruption of therapy is followed by gradual resolution of this side effect over five to seven days. Therapy should be discontinued promptly whenever one of the following signs of toxicity appears: inflammation of the mucous membrane of the mouth, rapidly falling white blood cell count, unmanageable vomiting, diarrhea, gastrointestinal ulceration and bleeding, low platelet count, or bleeding. Topical fluorouracil may have increased absorption through ulcerated or inflamed skin.

Hydroxyurea should be used with caution in patients with marked kidney dysfunction, as this drug is removed by the kidneys.

The safe and effective use of mercaptopurine demands close monitoring of the complete blood counts and patient clinical status. After selection of an initial dosage schedule, mercaptopurine therapy will frequently need to be modified depending upon the patient's response and manifestations of toxicity. Lower dosages are advisable in patients with impaired kidney function due to slower elimination of the drug and metabolites and a greater cumulative effect.

Because toxic effects from methotrexate can occur at any time during therapy, patients must be followed closely. Most adverse reactions are reversible if detected early. When such reactions do occur, the drug should be reduced in dosage or discontinued and appropriate corrective measures taken. Methotrexate has not been well studied in older individuals. Due to diminished liver and kidney function as well as decreased folate stores (a B vitamin) in the elderly population, relatively low doses should be considered, and these patients should be closely monitored for early signs of toxicity. Dizziness and fatigue sometimes caused by methotrexate may affect the ability to drive or operate machinery.

In pemetrexed clinical trials, skin rash was reported more frequently in patients who had not been pretreated with a corticosteroid. Pretreatment with dexamethasone (or equivalent) reduces the incidence and severity of skin reaction.

Pentostatin therapy requires regular patient observation and monitoring of blood counts and kidney function (see *Warnings*). Pentostatin treatment should be withheld or discontinued in patients showing evidence of nervous system toxicity.

Although pralatrexate has not been formally tested in patients with kidney impairment, caution is advised when administering it to patients with moderate to severe impairment. Liver function test abnormalities have been observed after pralatrexate administration. Persistent liver function test abnormalities may be indicators of liver toxicity and require dose modification. Kidney and liver function tests should be performed prior to the start of the first and fourth doses of a given cycle.

Complete blood counts should be obtained frequently while a patient is on thioguanine. Liver function tests should be routinely monitored during therapy with thioguanine. Patients with known preexisting liver disease or patients receiving other liver-toxic drugs should be monitored more frequently.

Antimitotics   Monitoring of blood cell counts, liver function, serum electrolytes, serum creatinine, heart function, and fluid retention is recommended for all patients receiving docetaxel. Side effects with docetaxel are experienced more frequently by elderly patients.

Worsening of preexisting peripheral edema (fluid in the ankles, feet, and legs) or congestive heart disease has been seen in some patients receiving estramustine. Other conditions that might be influenced by fluid retention, such as epilepsy, migraine, or kidney dysfunction, require careful observation. Estramustine may be poorly metabolized in patients with impaired liver function and should be administered with caution in such patients. Because estramustine may influence the metabolism of calcium and phosphorus, it should be used with caution in patients with metabolic bone diseases that are associated with hypercalcemia (high levels of calcium in the blood) or in patients with kidney impairment. Patients with prostate cancer and osteoblastic metastases are at risk for hypocalcemia (lower-than-normal blood calcium) and should have calcium levels closely monitored.

Excessive breast development and impotence may occur with estramustine due to its estrogen component. Allergic reactions and angioedema (manifested by swollen tongue, lips, and throat) at times involving the airway have been reported with this drug.

To avoid the occurrence of severe allergic reactions, all patients treated with paclitaxel should be premedicated (see *Warnings*). Hypotension, bradycardia, and hypertension have been observed during administration of paclitaxel but generally do not require treatment. Occasionally, paclitaxel infusions must be interrupted or discontinued because of initial or recurrent hypertension. Frequent monitoring of a patient's blood pressure and heart rate, particularly during the first hour of paclitaxel infusion, is recommended. Caution should be exercised when administering paclitaxel to patients with moderate to severe liver impairment, and dose adjustments should be considered. Injection site reactions may occur but are usually mild.

Leukopenia is the principal side effect with vinblastine. In patients with malignant-cell infiltration of the bone marrow, the leukocyte and platelet counts have sometimes fallen precipitously after moderate doses of vinblastine. Further use of the drug in such patients is inadvisable. Caution should be taken when administering vinblastine in patients with ischemic cardiac disease. Cardiac effects such as myocardial infarction, angina pectoris, and transient abnormalities of ECG related to coronary ischemia have been reported, but rarely.

Acute shortness of breath and severe bronchospasm may occur with vinblastine and vincristine, especially when used in combination with mitomycin C and may require aggressive treatment, particularly when there is preexisting lung disease. Progressive breathing difficulties requiring chronic therapy may occur. These drugs should not be readministered in these patients.

Kidney impairment has been reported with vincristine. Infections should be controlled before vincristine treatment starts. If CNS leukemia is diagnosed, additional agents may be required, because vincristine does not appear to cross the blood-brain barrier in adequate amounts. Particular attention should be given to dosage and neurologic side effects if vincristine is administered to patients with preexisting neuromuscular disease and when other drugs that might damage the nerves are also being used.

Vinorelbine should be used with extreme caution in patients whose bone marrow reserves have been reduced by previous radiation or chemotherapy treatment. Administration of vinorelbine to patients with prior radiation therapy may result in radiation recall reactions. Radiation recall occurs when certain chemotherapy agents cause skin in the area that had previously been treated with radiation therapy to turn red (ranging from very light to bright red). The skin may blister, peel, or be very painful. Patients with a prior history of neuropathy should be monitored for new or worsening signs and symptoms of neuropathy while receiving vinorelbine.

Epothilones Caution should be exercised when administering ixabepilone to patients with a history of cardiac disease, as the frequency of cardiac adverse reactions (myocardial ischemia and ventricular dysfunction) was higher in treatment groups receiving ixabepilone in combination with capecitabine than in the capecitabine alone treatment group. Discontinuation of ixabepilone should be considered in patients who develop cardiac ischemia or impaired cardiac function. Ixabepilone contains alcohol and may cause dizziness or drowsiness. Thus, activities that may be dangerous, such as driving or operating machinery, should be avoided until the patient knows how this drug affects him or her.

Histone deacetylase inhibitors Dose-related thrombocytopenia and anemia have occurred with vorinostat and may require dose modification or discontinuation. Gastrointestinal disturbances (e.g., nausea, vomiting, and diarrhea) have been reported with vorinostat. Patients may require ANTIEMETICS, ANTIDIARRHEALS, and fluid and electrolyte replacement to prevent dehydration. Hyperglycemia has been observed with vorinostat. Adjustment of diet and/or therapy for increased glucose may be necessary. An ECG should be monitored at baseline and periodically during treatment. Monitoring of blood cell counts and chemistry tests, including electrolytes, glucose, and serum creatinine, should be performed every two weeks during the first two months of therapy and monthly thereafter. Hypokalemia or hypomagnesemia should be corrected prior to administration of vorinostat, and consideration should be given to monitoring potassium and magnesium in patients with nausea, vomiting, diarrhea, fluid imbalance, or cardiac symptoms.

Hormones Anastrozole is not recommended for use in premenopausal women, as safety and efficacy have not been established.

Bicalutamide should be used with caution in patients with moderate to severe liver impairment, as this drug is extensively metabolized by the liver. Periodic liver function tests should be considered for patients with liver impairment who are on long-term therapy (see *Warnings*).

Exemestane should not be administered to premenopausal women and should not be coadministered with estrogen-containing agents, as these could interfere with its pharmacologic action. The safety of chronic dosing in patients with moderate or severe liver or kidney impairment has not been studied.

Swelling of the breasts may occur with flutamide treatment.

Safety and efficacy of fulvestrant have not been evaluated in patients with moderate to severe liver impairment.

Hypersensitivity, antibody formation, and acute anaphylactic reactions have been reported with LHRH agonists.

Patients receiving histrelin should refrain from wetting the arm for 24 hours and from heavy lifting or strenuous exertion of the inserted arm for seven days after implant insertion.

Because fatigue, dizziness, and sleepiness may occur with the use of letrozole, caution is advised when driving or using machinery.

Patients with spinal cord lesions and/or urinary tract obstruction should be closely observed during the first few weeks of leuprolide therapy, as their symptoms may worsen. Patients with known allergies to benzyl alcohol may experience symptoms of hypersensitivity in the form of redness and hardening of the skin at the injection site.

Because medroxyprogesterone may cause some degree of fluid retention, conditions that might be influenced by this condition, such as epilepsy, migraine, asthma, cardiac dysfunction, or kidney dysfunction, require careful observation. Patients who have a history of depression should be carefully observed and the drug discontinued if the depression recurs to a serious degree. Treatment with medroxyprogesterone may mask the onset of menopause.

Megestrol should be used with caution in patients with a history of blood clots, including deep vein thrombosis (DVT) and pulmonary embolus (PE) (clot in the lungs). Preexisting diabetes may be worsened by megestrol and may require increased insulin (see *Warnings*).

Patients receiving nilutamide have reported a delay in adaptation to dark, ranging from seconds to a few minutes, when passing from a lighted area to a dark area. This effect sometimes does not abate as drug treatment is continued. Patients who experience this effect should be cautioned about driving at night or through tunnels. This effect can be alleviated by the wearing of tinted glasses.

Thrombocytopenia has been occasionally reported in patients taking tamoxifen for breast cancer. Leukopenia has also been observed, sometimes in association with anemia and/or thrombocytopenia. There have been rare reports of neutropenia and pancytopenia (an abnormal deficiency in all blood cells) in patients receiving tamoxifen, which can sometimes be severe.

Patients with a history of blood clots, including DVT and PE, should generally not be treated with toremifene. In general, patients with preexisting endometrial hyperplasia (thickening or overgrowth of the lining of the uterus) should not be given long-term toremifene treatment. In women whose cancer has spread to the bones, calcium levels should be monitored closely for hypercalcemia (abnormally high levels of calcium in the blood) during the first weeks of treatment (see *Warnings*). Leukocyte and platelet counts should be monitored when using toremifene in patients with leukopenia and thrombocytopenia. Vaginal bleeding has been reported in patients using toremifene.

Patients with spinal cord lesions and/or urinary tract obstruction should be closely observed during the first few weeks of therapy with triptorelin (see *Warnings*). Hypersensitivity and anaphylactic reactions have been reported with this drug.

Monoclonal antibodies Complete blood counts and platelet counts should be done on a routine basis while patients are receiving alemtuzumab. Immunization during treatment with alemtuzumab is not recommended, as the T cell depletion during treatment increases the risk of infection from live vaccines.

Though rare, infusion reactions with the first dose of bevacizumab have included hypertension, hypertensive crises, wheezing, hypersensitivity, chest pain, headaches, shaking, and sweating. Bevacizumab therapy should not be initiated for at least 28 days following major surgery, and the surgical incision should be fully healed. Because of the potential for impaired wound healing, bevacizumab should be suspended prior to elective surgery (see *Warnings*).

Patients receiving cetuximab should limit sun exposure by using sunscreen and wearing hats during treatment and for two months following the last dose of the drug.

Electrolytes, liver function, complete blood counts, and platelet counts should be monitored during gemtuzumab ozogamicin therapy.

Complete blood counts and platelet counts should be monitored following ibritumomab tiuxetan therapy (see *Warnings*). During and after ibritumomab tiuxetan treatment, radiation exposure to patients and to medical personnel should be minimized.

Patients at high risk for hepatitis B should be screened prior to starting ofatumumab therapy. Patients with inactive hepatitis B infections should be monitored for reactivation. Obstruction of the small intestine can occur in patients receiving ofatumumab.

Exposure to sunlight can exacerbate skin reactions (see *Warnings*) in patients receiving panitumumab; thus, patients should wear sunscreen and hats and limit sun exposure while receiving this drug. Pulmonary fibrosis occurred rarely in patients enrolled in panitumumab clinical studies. Electrolytes (including magnesium and calcium) should be monitored periodically during and for eight weeks following completion of panitumumab therapy, as electrolyte depletion has occurred in patients during clinical trials.

Complete blood counts and platelet counts should be obtained at regular intervals during rituximab therapy and more frequently in patients who develop blood disorders.

As the iodine portion of tositumomab is radioactive, care should be taken to minimize exposure of medical personnel and other patients (see *Warnings*). Impaired kidney function may decrease the rate of excretion of the iodine portion of this drug regimen and increase patient exposure to the radioactive component. Complete blood counts and platelet counts should be obtained routinely during tositumomab therapy and more frequently in patients who develop blood disorders.

Patients receiving trastuzumab must be monitored frequently for deteriorating cardiac function (see *Warnings*), although monitoring may not identify all patients who will develop heart problems.

mTOR inhibitors At least half of all patients in everolimus clinical trials experienced anemia, leukopenia, high cholesterol, and high blood sugar.

Temsirolimus is likely to cause increases in triglyceride and cholesterol levels, which may require initiation or increase in the dose of lipid-lowering agents. Cholesterol and triglycerides should be tested before and during treatment. Temsirolimus has also been associated with abnormal wound healing.

Platinum compounds Needles or intravenous tubing containing aluminum parts that may come in contact with carboplatin should not be used for the preparation or administration of the drug. Aluminum can react with carboplatin, causing loss of potency.

Complete blood counts, platelet counts, and liver function should be monitored periodically during cisplatin therapy. A neurologic examination should also be performed regularly.

Complete blood counts and platelet counts should be obtained before each cycle of oxaliplatin. Premedication with ANTIEMETICS is recommended with oxaliplatin.

Topoisomerase inhibitors Daunorubicin requires close patient observation and frequent complete blood count and platelet monitoring. Heart, kidney, and liver function should be evaluated prior to each course of treatment. Daunorubicin may temporarily cause the urine to turn reddish in color.

Because doxorubicin and epirubicin are emetogenic (cause nausea and vomiting), patients should be premedicated with ANTIEMETICS. Doxorubicin may temporarily cause the urine to turn reddish in color.

Complete blood counts, including platelet counts, should be obtained frequently and at a minimum prior to each dose of doxorubicin liposomal. Doxorubicin liposomal may cause hand-foot syndrome, but in most patients this reaction is mild and resolves in one to two weeks, so that prolonged delay of therapy need not occur. Administration of doxorubicin liposomal to patients with prior radiation therapy may result in radiation recall reactions.

Facial flushing as well as redness streaking along the vein may be indicative of excessively rapid administration of epirubicin. It may precede phlebitis (inflammation of a vein) or thrombophlebitis (blood clots).

Appropriate measures must be taken to prevent hyperuricemia associated with the use of idarubicin.

Mitoxantrone requires frequent monitoring of blood counts. Mitoxantrone may cause the urine to become blue-green in color for about 24 hours. Also, the whites of the eyes may temporarily be blue-tinged.

Aseptic techniques must be used during administration of valrubicin to avoid introducing contaminants into the urinary tract or traumatizing unduly the urinary mucosa. Valrubicin should be used with caution in patients with severe irritable bladder symptoms. Bladder spasm and spontaneous discharge of the intravesical instillate may occur; clamping of the urinary catheter is not advised and, if performed, should be executed under medical supervision and with caution. Studies of the effects of valrubicin on male or female fertility have not been done.

Care should be taken to avoid extravasation of irinotecan during administration, and the infusion site should be monitored for signs of inflammation. Should extravasation occur, the administration site should be flushed with sterile water and ice applied. Because irinotecan is emetogenic, patients should be premedicated with ANTIEMETICS. Irinotecan commonly causes neutropenia and anemia, both of which may be severe, and therefore should not be used in patients with severe bone marrow failure. Patients must not be treated with irinotecan until resolution of any bowel obstruction. Patients with hereditary fructose intolerance should not be given irinotecan, as it contains sorbitol.

Extravasation of topotecan during administration has caused mild skin reactions such as redness and bruising. Frequent monitoring of complete blood counts and platelet counts during topotecan therapy is necessary (see *Warnings*).

Periodic complete blood counts and platelet counts should be done prior to each cycle of etoposide or teniposide therapy and at appropriate intervals during and after therapy. Patients with low serum albumin may be at an increased risk for etoposide-associated side effects.

Tyrosine kinase inhibitors With dasatinib, complete blood counts and platelet counts should be performed weekly for the first two months and then monthly thereafter or as clinically indicated. Myelosuppression (see *Warnings*) is generally reversible and usually managed by withholding dasatinib temporarily or reducing the dosage. Caution should be exercised if patients are required to take medications that inhibit platelet function or anticoagulants.

Cases of kidney failure or poor kidney function have occurred with erlotinib, sometimes following severe dehydration due to diarrhea, vomiting, and/or decreased appetite and at other times related to concurrent chemotherapy use. Patients at risk of dehydration should have their kidney function and electrolyte levels monitored periodically. Because erlotinib is broken down and deactivated in the liver, patients with liver disease should be closely monitored. Patients taking warfarin should be monitored regularly, as a few reports of gastrointestinal bleeding were reported in clinical studies, some associated with concomitant warfarin administration.

Elevation in liver function tests without any symptoms of liver damage has been observed in patients treated with gefitinib. Therefore, periodic liver function testing should be considered. In addition, liver impairment might cause more gefitinib than expected to remain in the body, which could lead to unwanted side effects.

Imatinib often causes edema and occasionally serious fluid retention. Patients should be weighed and monitored regularly for signs and symptoms of fluid retention, such as unexpected rapid weight gain. Various types of skin reactions, some serious, have occurred with imatinib. Because imatinib is associated with anemia, neutropenia, and thrombocytopenia, complete blood counts and platelet counts should be performed weekly for the first month, biweekly for the second month, and periodically thereafter. As liver damage, occasionally severe, may occur with imatinib, liver function should be monitored before beginning treatment and then monthly.

Caution should be taken when lapatinib is administered to patients who have a history of or are predisposed to left ventricular dysfunction, as this drug has been reported to decrease left ventricular ejection fraction. Because diarrhea, including severe diarrhea, has been reported during treatment with lapatinib, pretreatment with antidiarrheal agents is important.

Because nilotinib is associated with myelosuppression, complete blood counts should be done every two weeks for the first two months, then monthly. Nilotinib has not been studied in patients with liver impairment; thus, caution is recommended in these patients. Nilotinib can cause increases in serum lipase, and caution is recommended in patients with a history of pancreatitis. Serum lipase should be checked periodically.

Hypertension occurs early in the course of treatment with pazopanib. Blood pressure should be well controlled prior to initiating treatment, and patients should be monitored for hypertension and treated as needed with antihypertensive therapy. Because pazopanib may impair wound healing, its use should be stopped at least seven days prior to scheduled surgery. Since hypothyroidism was reported in 4 percent of patients during clinical trials, monitoring of thyroid function tests is recommended.

Mild to moderate hand-foot skin reaction and/or rash often occur with sorafenib, generally during the first six weeks of treatment. Patients taking warfarin should be monitored regularly, as infrequent bleeding or elevations in the international normalized ratio (INR) have been reported in these patients.

Treatment with sunitinib can induce hypothyroidism (a reduction in the level of thyroid hormone).

Retinoids Because of the relationship of bexarotene to vitamin A, patients should limit vitamin A supplements to avoid potential additive toxic effects. Caution should be used when administering bexarotene capsules in patients using insulin, agents enhancing insulin secretion (e.g., sulfonylureas), or insulin-sensitizers (e.g., thiazolidinediones). Based on the mechanism of action, bexarotene capsules could enhance the action of these agents, resulting in hypoglycemia. Retinoids as a class have been associated with photosensitivity, and bexarotene is a potential photosensitizing agent. Mild sunburn and skin sensitivity to sunlight have been observed in patients who were exposed to direct sunlight while taking bexarotene capsules. Patients should minimize exposure to sunlight and artificial ultraviolet light during the use of bexarotene. Sunlight, sun lamps, and tanning beds can cause severe sunburn. Patients need to wear SPF 15 or higher sunblock. Bexarotene capsules should be taken with food.

Because tretinoin has potentially significant toxic side effects in acute promyelocytic leukemia (APL) patients, those undergoing therapy should be closely observed for signs of respiratory compromise and/or leukocytosis (abnormal increase in the number of white blood cells in the blood). An increased risk of thrombosis exists during the first month of treatment with tretinoin. The ability to drive or operate machinery may be impaired in patients treated with tretinoin, particularly if they are experiencing dizziness or severe headache. Microdosed progesterone preparations ("minipill") may be an inadequate method of contraception during treatment with tretinoin (see *Warnings*). Tretinoin may make the skin more susceptible to sunburn and other adverse effects of the sun; patients should wear sunscreen.

Proteasome inhibitors Complete blood counts, including platelet counts, should be monitored frequently during treatment with bortezomib (see *Warnings*). Bortezomib treatment can cause nausea, diarrhea, constipation, and vomiting, sometimes requiring use of ANTIEMETICS and ANTIDIARRHEALS. Blockage of the intestine can occur. Fluid and electrolyte replacement should be administered to prevent dehydration.

Miscellaneous Aldesleukin has been associated with capillary leak syndrome (CLS), in which the body's small blood vessels become leaky. CLS begins immediately after aldesleukin treatment starts, and in most patients, this results in low blood pressure, fluid buildup, and poor blood flow to the internal organs. Careful monitoring of the patient's fluid status, blood pressure, and pulse along with proper management of these parameters is necessary. Kidney and liver function can be impaired during aldesleukin treatment. Alterations in mental status due to aldesleukin therapy may progress for several days before recovery begins. Rarely, patients have sustained permanent neurologic deficits. Exacerbation of preexisting autoimmune disease or initial presentation of autoimmune and inflammatory disorders has been reported following aldesleukin alone or in combination with interferon.

Asparaginase may cause glucose intolerance, which in some cases is irreversible. Blood sugar levels should be monitored. Asparaginase may rarely lower blood-clotting factors, which can increase the risk of bleeding.

Angioedema (a swelling similar to hives but located beneath the skin rather than on the surface) and serious, sometimes fatal, skin reactions have occurred with lenalidomide. Complications of tumor lysis syndrome may occur with lenalidomide, especially in patients with high tumor burden prior to treatment. These patients should be monitored closely and appropriate precautions taken.

Cases of bradycardia, some requiring medical treatment, have been reported with thalidomide. Serious skin reactions including Stevens-Johnson syndrome and toxic epidermal necrolysis, which may be fatal, have been reported. Thalidomide should be discontinued if a skin rash occurs and resumed only following appropriate clinical evaluation. Seizures, including grand mal convulsions, have been reported during use of thalidomide after the drug was approved during clinical use but not during actual monitored trials. Patients with a history of seizures or with other risk factors for the development of seizures should be monitored closely for clinical changes that could precipitate acute seizure activity.

Warnings

Antineoplastics in the IV form are highly toxic and must be handled and administered with care. Extreme caution must be used in their preparation in order to prevent contact with skin and mucous membranes.

Antineoplastics should not be administered during the first three months of pregnancy to avoid the risk of birth defects. Cancer drugs given after this time do not usually harm the fetus but may cause early labor and low birth weight. Effective contraception should be used during chemotherapy if either the patient or the partner is of childbearing potential.

If a patient develops a hypersensitivity reaction while receiving any infused antineoplastic drug, the infusion should be stopped and the appropriate supportive and symptomatic care should be administered.

Alkylating agents The most frequent, serious side effect of treatment with busulfan is the induction of bone marrow failure resulting in severe pancytopenia. The pancytopenia caused by busulfan may be more prolonged than that induced with other alkylating agents. The usual cause of busulfan-induced pancytopenia is generally believed to be the failure to stop administration of the drug soon enough; individual reaction to the drug does not seem to be an important factor. Busulfan should be used with extreme caution and exceptional vigilance in patients whose bone marrow reserve may have been compromised by prior irradiation or chemotherapy or whose bone marrow function is recovering from previous cytotoxic therapy. Although recovery from busulfan-induced pancytopenia may take from one month to two years, this complication is potentially reversible, and the patient should be vigorously supported through any period of severe pancytopenia. A rare, important complication of busulfan therapy is the development of bronchopulmonary dysplasia with pulmonary fibrosis (scarring of the lungs). Busulfan may cause abnormal cell growth in many organs in addition to the lung. The World Health Organization has concluded that there is a causal relationship between busulfan exposure and the development of secondary malignancies. Ovarian suppression and amenorrhea with menopausal symptoms commonly occur during busulfan therapy in premenopausal patients. Cardiac tamponade has been reported in a small number of patients with thalassemia (an inherited blood disorder in which the body makes an abnormal form of hemoglobin, the protein found in red blood cells) who received busulfan and cyclophosphamide as the preparatory regimen for bone marrow transplantation. In these patients, the cardiac tamponade was often fatal. Abdominal pain and vomiting preceded the tamponade in most patients.

Complete blood counts and platelet counts should be monitored routinely during the course of therapy with altretamine. Because of the possibility of altretamine-related neurotoxicity, neurologic examination should be performed regularly during therapy. Concurrent administration of altretamine and monoamine oxidase inhibitor (MAOI) antidepressants may cause severe orthostatic hypotension (low blood pressure when standing up).

Thiotepa is highly toxic to the bone marrow. A rapidly falling white blood cell or platelet count indicates the necessity for discontinuing or reducing the dosage of thiotepa. Weekly blood and platelet counts are recommended during therapy and for at least three weeks after therapy has been discontinued.

Chlorambucil can severely suppress bone marrow function. Both reversible and permanent sterility have been observed in both sexes receiving chlorambucil. Children with nephrotic syndrome and patients receiving high doses of chlorambucil may have an increased risk of seizures. Rare instances of skin rash progressing to erythema multiforme, toxic epidermal necrolysis, or Stevens-Johnson syndrome have been reported. Chlorambucil should be discontinued promptly in patients who develop skin reactions.

Secondary malignancies have developed in some patients treated with cyclophosphamide. Most frequently, they have been urinary bladder, myeloproliferative, or lymphoproliferative malignancies. In some cases, the second malignancy developed several years after cyclophosphamide treatment had been discontinued.

Cyclophosphamide may cause sterility in both sexes. Amenorrhea associated with decreased estrogen and increased gonadotropin secretion develops in a significant proportion of women treated with cyclophosphamide. Affected patients generally resume regular menses within a few months after cessation of therapy. Hemorrhagic cystitis may develop in patients treated with cyclophosphamide. Rarely, this condition can be severe and even fatal. A urinalysis should be obtained prior to each dose to examine the urine for red cells, which may precede hemorrhagic cystitis. Fibrosis of the urinary bladder, sometimes extensive, also may develop with or without accompanying cystitis. Forced fluid intake helps to assure an ample output of urine, necessitates frequent voiding, and reduces the time the drug remains in the bladder. In a few instances with high doses of cyclophosphamide, severe and sometimes fatal congestive heart failure has occurred after the first cyclophosphamide dose. Treatment with cyclophosphamide may cause significant suppression of immune responses. Serious, sometimes fatal, infections may develop in severely immunosuppressed patients. Cyclophosphamide treatment may not be indicated or should be interrupted or the dose reduced in patients who have or who develop viral, bacterial, fungal, protozoan, or helminthic infections. Cyclophosphamide may interfere with normal wound healing. Anaphylactic reactions have been reported; death has also been reported in association with this event. Possible cross-sensitivity with other alkylating agents has been reported.

Ifosfamide can cause hemorrhagic cystitis, so it should always be given with fluids and mesna, a drug that helps to protect the bladder wall. A urinalysis should be obtained prior to each dose to examine the urine for red cells, which may precede hemorrhagic cystitis. CNS toxicities such as confusion and coma have been associated with the use of ifosfamide. When urologic or CNS side effects occur, they may require cessation of ifosfamide therapy. Severe myelosuppression has been reported when ifosfamide is given in combination with other chemotherapy agents.

If extravasation occurs with mechlorethamine, tissue damage can occur, which can lead to painful inflammation, ulceration, and scarring.

Severe myelosuppression with resulting infection or bleeding may occur with melphalan. Hypersensitivity reactions, including anaphylaxis, have occurred after multiple courses of treatment. If a hypersensitivity reaction occurs, melphalan should not be readministered. Melphalan may increase the long-term risk of getting a secondary malignancy, such as leukemia, which, though rare, would likely occur years after the drug is used. The potential benefits from melphalan therapy must be weighed on an individual basis against the possible risk of the induction of a second malignancy. Melphalan causes suppression of ovarian function in premenopausal women, resulting in amenorrhea in a significant number of patients. Reversible and irreversible testicular suppression have also been reported.

Long-term use of nitrosoureas has been reported to be associated with the development of secondary malignancies.

Myelosuppression, notably thrombocytopenia and leukopenia, is the most common and severe of the toxic effects of carmustine. Because of delayed myelosuppression, blood counts should be monitored weekly for at least six weeks after a dose. Liver and kidney function tests should also be monitored periodically. Carmustine can cause pulmonary toxicity, such as pulmonary fibrosis. Delayed pulmonary toxicity can occur years after treatment and can result in death, particularly in patients treated in childhood.

Myelosuppression, notably thrombocytopenia and leukopenia, is the most common and severe of the toxic effects of lomustine. Blood counts should be monitored weekly for at least six weeks after a dose. At the recommended dosage, courses of lomustine should not be given more frequently than every six weeks. The bone marrow toxicity is cumulative; therefore, dosage adjustment must be considered on the basis of lowest blood counts from prior dose.

Streptozocin frequently causes dose-related kidney damage, which is cumulative and may be severe or fatal. Kidney function must be monitored before and after each course of therapy. Dose reduction or discontinuation of treatment is suggested if significant kidney damage occurs. Before using streptozocin in patients with preexisting kidney disease, physicians must weigh the potential benefit against the known risk of serious kidney damage. Other major toxicities are nausea and vomiting, which may be severe and at times treatment-limiting. In addition, liver dysfunction, diarrhea, and substantial reductions in white blood cell and platelet counts have been observed in some patients. Streptozocin can cause either hypo- or hyperglycemia, and although these mild to moderate abnormalities of glucose tolerance have generally been reversible, insulin shock with hypoglycemia has been observed.

Myelosuppression, notably leukopenia and thrombocytopenia (and occasionally anemia), is the most common toxicity with dacarbazine. These hematologic toxicities may be severe enough to cause death. The possible bone marrow depression requires careful monitoring of white blood cells, red blood cells, and platelet levels. Liver damage, accompanied by hepatic vein thrombosis and hepatocellular necrosis resulting in death, has been reported. Anaphylaxis can occur following the administration of this drug.

Patients treated with temozolomide, especially the elderly and women, may experience myelosuppression. Very rare cases of MDS and secondary malignancies, including leukemias, have also been observed. For treatment of newly diagnosed glioblastoma multiforme (a type of brain tumor), prophylaxis against *Pneumocystis jirovecii* pneumonia (PCP) is required for all patients receiving this drug along with radiotherapy for the 42-day regimen. There may be a higher occurrence of PCP when temozolomide is administered during a longer dosing regimen. However, all patients receiving temozolomide, particularly patients receiving steroids, should be observed closely for the development of PCP, regardless of the regimen.

To minimize CNS depression and possible potentiation, barbiturates, antihistamines, narcotics, hypotensive agents, or phenothiazines should be used with caution when using procarbazine. Alcohol should not be used during procarbazine therapy, since there may be a disulfiramlike reaction (e.g., flushing of the face or nausea). Because procarbazine exhibits some MAOI activity, epinephrine-related drugs, tricyclic antidepressant drugs (e.g., amitriptyline, imipramine), and foods with known high tyramine content, such as wine, yogurt, ripe cheese, and bananas, should be avoided.

Antibiotics Bleomycin should be used with extreme caution in patients with significant kidney impairment or compromised pulmonary function. Bleomycin causes serious lung problems in approximately 10 percent of treated patients. The most frequent presentation is pneumonitis (a form of pneumonia involving the connective tissue of the lung) occasionally progressing to pulmonary fibrosis. Approximately 1 percent of patients treated have died of pulmonary fibrosis. Pulmonary toxicity is both dose- and age-related, being more common in patients more than 70 years of age and in those receiving a total dose that exceeds 400 units; however, pulmonary toxicity has been observed in young patients and those treated with low doses. To monitor the onset of pulmonary toxicity, chest X-rays should be taken every one to two weeks during the course of therapy. A severe idiosyncratic reaction consisting of hypotension, mental confusion, fever, chills, and wheezing has been reported in approximately 1 percent of lymphoma patients treated with bleomycin. Kidney or liver toxicity, beginning as a deterioration in renal or liver function, have been reported infrequently. These toxicities may occur, however, at any time after initiation of therapy.

Dactinomycin is extremely corrosive to soft tissue. If extravasation occurs during intravenous use, severe damage to soft tissues will occur. In at least one instance, this has led to contracture (tightening of the tendons) of the arms. Reports indicate an increased incidence of secondary malignancies, including leukemia, following treatment with this drug.

Myelosuppression, notably thrombocytopenia and leukopenia, is the most common and severe side effect of mitomycin. Hemolytic uremic syndrome (HUS), a serious complication consisting primarily of anemia, thrombocytopenia, and irreversible kidney failure, has been reported in patients receiving mitomycin.

Antimetabolites Because azacitidine may cause birth defects when administered to a pregnant woman, women of childbearing potential should be advised to avoid becoming pregnant while receiving treatment. Also, men should be advised not to father a child while receiving treatment.

Patients receiving concomitant capecitabine and warfarin should have their anticoagulant response (INR) monitored frequently in order to adjust the anticoagulant dose accordingly. Patients with kidney impairment may require dose reduction of capecitabine and should be monitored for adverse events. Capecitabine can induce diarrhea, sometimes severe. Patients with severe diarrhea should be carefully monitored and given fluid and electrolyte replacement if they become dehydrated. Patients 80 years and older may experience a greater incidence of serious adverse events.

Myelosuppression, including neutropenia, anemia, and thrombocytopenia, should be anticipated with cladribine. This is usually reversible and appears to be dose-dependent. Serious neurological toxicity has been reported in patients who received cladribine injection by continuous infusion at high doses (four to nine times the recommended dose for hairy cell leukemia). Severe neurological toxicity has been reported rarely following treatment with standard cladribine dosing regimens. Acute kidney toxicity has been observed with high doses of cladribine, especially when given along with other agents damaging to the kidneys. Benzyl alcohol is a constituent of the recommended diluent for the seven-day infusion solution. Benzyl alcohol has been reported to be associated with a fatal "gasping syndrome" in premature infants.

Cytarabine is a potent bone marrow suppressant. Therapy should be started cautiously in patients with preexisting drug-induced myelosuppression. Patients receiving this drug for induction therapy (patients receiving initial cancer treatment) should have complete blood counts and platelet counts performed daily. Bone marrow biopsies should be performed frequently after blasts have disappeared from the peripheral blood. Experimental high dose therapy with cytarabine has resulted in incidences of cardiomyopathy (a disorder of the heart muscle) with subsequent death or sudden respiratory distress rapidly progressing to pulmonary edema as well as severe and at times fatal CNS, gastrointestinal, and pulmonary toxicity.

Decitabine may cause fetal harm when administered to a pregnant woman. Men should be advised not to father a child while receiving treatment with decitabine and for two months afterwards.

Because of the possibility of severe toxic reactions, all patients should be hospitalized for the first course of floxuridine therapy. Floxuridine should be used with extreme caution in patients with liver or kidney impairment, poor nutritional status, a history of high-dose pelvic radiation, or previous use of alkylating agents. The drug is not intended as an adjuvant to surgery. Any form of therapy that adds to the emotional or physical stress of the patient, interferes with nutrition, or depresses bone marrow function will increase the toxicity of floxuridine.

Fludarabine can severely suppress bone marrow function. When used at high doses in patients with acute leukemia, fludarabine was associated with severe neurological effects, including blindness, coma, and death. Instances of life-threatening and sometimes fatal autoimmune hemolytic anemia have been reported to occur after one or more cycles of treatment with fludarabine. Patients undergoing treatment with fludarabine should be evaluated and closely monitored for hemolysis (the breakdown of red blood cells).

Because of the possibility of severe toxic reactions, patients should be hospitalized at least during the initial course of therapy with fluorouracil injection. Fluorouracil injection should be used with extreme caution in patients with a history of high-dose pelvic radiation or previous use of alkylating agents, those who have a widespread involvement of bone marrow by metastatic tumors, or those with liver or kidney impairment. Rarely, unexpected, severe toxicity (e.g., stomatitis [inflammation of the mucous membrane of the mouth], diarrhea, neutropenia, and neurotoxicity) associated with fluorouracil has been attributed to deficiency of dihydropyrimidine dehydrogenase activity. Dihydropyrimidine dehydrogenase is an enzyme involved in the metabolism of uracil and thymine, components of fluorouracil.

Administering gemcitabine over longer than 60 minutes and more frequently than weekly doses have been shown to increase toxicity. Gemcitabine can cause myelosuppression. Pulmonary toxicity (including interstitial pneumonitis, pulmonary fibrosis, pulmonary edema, and adult respiratory distress syndrome) has been reported with the use of gemcitabine. In cases of severe lung toxicity, therapy should be discontinued immediately and appropriate supportive care measures instituted. HUS and/or kidney failure have been reported following one or more doses of gemcitabine. The majority of the cases of kidney failure leading to death have been due to HUS. Serious liver toxicity, including liver failure and death, has been reported very rarely in patients receiving gemcitabine alone or in combination with other potentially hepatotoxic drugs.

Myelosuppression may occur with hydroxyurea therapy, and leukopenia is generally its first and most common manifestation. Thrombocytopenia and anemia occur less often and are seldom seen without a preceding leukopenia. Recovery from myelosuppression is rapid when therapy is interrupted. Severe anemia

must be corrected before initiating therapy with hydroxyurea. Bone marrow depression is more likely in patients who have previously received radiation therapy or other antineoplastic agents; hydroxyurea should be used cautiously in such patients. Patients who have received radiation therapy in the past may have an exacerbation of postirradiation erythema (redness of the skin). In addition, kidney function, uric acid, and electrolytes as well as liver enzymes must be checked regularly. Elderly patients may be more sensitive to the effects of hydroxyurea and may require a lower dose regimen. In patients receiving long-term hydroxyurea for myeloproliferative disorders such as polycythemia vera and thrombocythemia, secondary leukemia has been reported. It is unknown whether this adverse effect is secondary to hydroxyurea or associated with the patient's underlying disease. Serious skin reactions, including leg ulcers and gangrene, have occurred in patients with myeloproliferative disorders during therapy with hydroxyurea. These toxicities were reported most often in patients with a history of or currently receiving interferon therapy. Hydroxyurea should be discontinued if leg ulcers develop.

The most consistent dose-related toxicity with mercaptopurine is myelosuppression, including anemia, leukopenia, and/or thrombocytopenia. Mercaptopurine can also cause hyperuricemia, which can worsen gout and cause serious kidney damage. Mercaptopurine can cause liver damage. A small number of deaths have been reported that may have been attributed to hepatic necrosis due to administration of mercaptopurine. Administration of mercaptopurine with other drugs damaging to the liver requires especially careful clinical and laboratory monitoring of liver function.

Deaths have been reported with the use of methotrexate in the treatment of malignancy, psoriasis, and RA. Patients should be closely monitored for bone marrow, liver, lung, and kidney toxicities. High-dose regimens for neoplastic diseases other than osteosarcoma are investigational, and a therapeutic advantage has not been established. Methotrexate elimination is reduced in patients with kidney impairment or with accumulation of fluid in the abdomen or lungs. Such patients require especially careful monitoring for toxicity and require dose reduction or, in some cases, discontinuation of methotrexate administration. Unexpectedly severe (sometimes fatal) myelosuppression, aplastic anemia (a blood disorder in which the body's bone marrow does not make enough new blood cells), and gastrointestinal toxicity have been reported with concomitant administration of methotrexate (usually in high dosage) along with some nonsteroidal anti-inflammatory drugs (NSAIDs). Methotrexate causes liver damage, fibrosis, and cirrhosis, but generally only after prolonged use. Periodic liver biopsies are usually recommended for patients with psoriasis or RA who are under long-term treatment. Methotrexate-induced lung disease is potentially dangerous and may occur at any time during therapy. It is not always fully reversible. Pulmonary symptoms, such as a dry, nonproductive cough, may require interruption of treatment and careful investigation. Diarrhea and stomach ulcers require interruption of therapy. Malignant lymphomas may occur in patients receiving low-dose methotrexate; these may regress following withdrawal of methotrexate and, thus, may not require cytotoxic treatment. Methotrexate may induce tumor lysis syndrome in patients with rapidly growing tumors. Severe, occasionally fatal, skin reactions have been reported following single or multiple doses of methotrexate. Reactions have occurred within days of oral methotrexate administration. Recovery has been reported with discontinuation of therapy. Potentially fatal opportunistic infections, especially PCP, may occur with methotrexate therapy. Methotrexate, given along with radiotherapy, may increase the risk of soft tissue and bone tissue death.

Patients treated with pemetrexed must be instructed to take folic acid and vitamin B_{12} as a preventive measure to reduce treatment-related blood and gastrointestinal toxicity. Pemetrexed can suppress bone marrow function, as manifested by neutropenia, thrombocytopenia, and anemia.

Higher than recommended doses of pentostatin have resulted in severe kidney, liver, lung, and CNS toxicities. Because initial courses of pentostatin treatment have been associated with worsening of neutropenia, frequent monitoring of complete blood counts during this time is necessary. If severe neutropenia continues beyond the initial cycles, patients should be evaluated for disease status, including a bone marrow examination. Kidney toxicity has occurred at higher doses of pentostatin. Rashes, occasionally severe, are common with pentostatin; they may worsen with continued treatment and may require withholding of treatment. Acute pulmonary edema and hypotension leading to death have been reported in patients treated with pentostatin in combination with carmustine, etoposide, and high-dose cyclophosphamide as part of the ablative regimen (kills any cancer cells that might remain in the bone marrow to make room for the new stem cells [from the bone marrow transplant] to grow) for bone marrow transplant.

Pralatrexate may cause myelosuppression manifested by thrombocytopenia, neutropenia, and anemia. Pralatrexate may cause mucositis (irritation or sores of the mucous membranes such as the lips, the mouth, and the digestive tract). Complete blood counts and severity of mucositis should be monitored weekly. Patients treated with pralatrexate should take folate and vitamin B_{12} supplements to potentially reduce treatment-related hematological toxicity and mucous membrane irritation.

Thioguanine is not recommended for long-term therapy because of the risk of liver toxicity. This liver toxicity is particularly prevalent in males. The most consistent dose-related toxicity is myelosuppression manifested by anemia, leukopenia, and/or thrombocytopenia. Since thioguanine may have a delayed effect, it is important to withdraw the medication temporarily at the first sign of an abnormally large fall in red blood cells, white blood cells, and/

or platelets. Individuals with an inherited deficiency of the enzyme thiopurine methyltransferase (TPMT) may be unusually sensitive to the myelosuppressive effects of thioguanine and prone to developing rapid myelosuppression following the initiation of treatment. Substantial dosage reductions may be required to avoid the development of life-threatening myelosuppression in these patients.

Antimitotics The incidence of treatment-related mortality associated with docetaxel therapy is increased in patients with liver impairment, in patients receiving higher doses, and in patients with non-small-cell lung carcinoma and a history of prior treatment with platinum-based chemotherapy who receive docetaxel as a single agent at a dose of 100 mg/m^2. Patients with liver impairment are at increased risk for the development of severe thrombocytopenia, severe stomatitis, severe skin toxicity, and death considered possibly or probably related to treatment. All patients receiving docetaxel should be premedicated with oral corticosteroids (such as dexamethasone) for three days to reduce the severity of fluid retention and hypersensitivity reactions. Severe hypersensitivity reactions characterized by generalized rash, hypotension and/or bronchospasm, or very rarely fatal anaphylaxis have been reported in patients who received the recommended three-day dexamethasone premedication. Severe fluid retention has also occurred in patients despite use of a three-day dexamethasone premedication regimen.

Patients taking estramustine have an increased risk of developing blood clots, congestive heart failure, and heart attacks. Because estramustine may decrease blood glucose tolerance, frequent blood glucose monitoring is recommended for diabetic patients. Blood pressure may also be increased with estramustine; therefore, blood pressure should be monitored periodically, especially in patients with a history of hypertension.

Anaphylaxis and severe allergic reactions characterized by breathing difficulty, hypotension, and hives have occurred in patients receiving paclitaxel. Fatal reactions have occurred in patients despite premedication. All patients should be premedicated with corticosteroids (such as dexamethasone), diphenhydramine, and H$_2$ antagonists (such as cimetidine or ranitidine). In order to monitor the occurrence of myelosuppression, primarily neutropenia, which may be severe, frequent complete blood cell counts should be performed on all patients receiving paclitaxel. Continuous cardiac monitoring is required in patients who develop conduction disturbances (e.g., bradycardia) during therapy.

Vinblastine, vincristine, and vinorelbine are for intravenous use only. Accidental administration of any of these drugs intrathecally may result in death. It is extremely important that the intravenous needle or catheter be properly positioned before any of these drugs is injected. Extravasation of any of these drugs may cause considerable tissue irritation. Vinorelbine has been reported to cause severe constipation, paralysis of the intestine, intestinal obstruction, necrosis, and/or perforation (tearing of the digestive lining). Some events have been fatal.

Epothilones Patients treated with ixabepilone should be monitored for symptoms of neuropathy, such as burning sensation, numbness, tingling, discomfort, or pain in the hands or feet. Ixabepilone, when used along with capecitabine or when used as monotherapy in patients who have liver impairment, may increase the risk of severe (sometimes fatal) myelosuppression and serious infection. All patients should be premedicated with an H$_1$ antagonist (e.g., diphenhydramine) and an H$_2$ antagonist (e.g., ranitidine) approximately one hour before ixabepilone infusion and should be observed for hypersensitivity reactions (e.g., flushing, rash, dyspnea, and bronchospasm).

Histone deacetylase inhibitors Pulmonary embolism and deep vein thrombosis have been reported with vorinostat; thus, patients should be monitored for pertinent signs and symptoms, particularly patients with a history of thromboembolic events. Vorinostat should be administered with particular caution in patients with congenital long QT (length of the heart's electrical cycle) syndrome and patients taking antiarrhythmic medicines or other medications that lead to QT interval prolongation.

Hormones Rare cases of death or hospitalization due to severe liver damage have been reported with the use of bicalutamide, generally within the first three to four months of treatment. Hepatitis or marked increases in liver enzymes led to drug discontinuation in a few cases during clinical trials.

Long-term use of degarelix may prolong the QT interval, which could increase the risk of developing a potentially fatal cardiac arrhythmia. Physicians should consider whether the benefits of therapy outweigh the potential risks in patients with congenital long QT syndrome, electrolyte abnormalities, or congestive heart failure and in patients taking certain ANTIARRHYTHMICS (e.g., quinidine, procainamide, amiodarone, sotalol) or other drugs known to prolong the QT interval.

Hospitalization and, rarely, death due to liver failure have occurred in patients taking flutamide. The liver injury was reversible after discontinuation of therapy in some patients. Approximately half of the reported cases occurred within the initial three months of treatment with flutamide. One metabolite of flutamide is 4-nitro-3-fluoro-methylaniline, which may cause aniline toxicity. Aniline is a manufactured chemical used by a number of industries to make a wide variety of products such as polyurethane foam, agricultural chemicals, synthetic dyes, antioxidants, stabilizers for the rubber industry, herbicides, varnishes, and explosives. The main effect of aniline by any route of exposure is a blood disorder in which oxygen delivery to the tissues is impaired. Several toxicities consistent with aniline exposure, including methemoglobinemia (decreased oxygen-carrying capability in the blood), anemia, and jaundice have been observed following flutamide administration. In patients susceptible to aniline toxicity (e.g., persons with glucose-6-phosphate dehydrogenase deficiency or hemoglobin M disease and smok-

ers), monitoring of methemoglobin levels should be considered.

Because fulvestrant is administered intramuscularly, it should not be used in patients with bleeding problems or thrombocytopenia or in patients on anticoagulants.

When used every 28 days, goserelin usually inhibits ovulation and stops menstruation; however, contraception is not ensured. During treatment, pregnancy must be avoided by the use of nonhormonal methods of contraception. Following the last goserelin injection, nonhormonal methods of contraception must be continued until the return of menstruation or for at least 12 weeks. When goserelin is first started, it may temporarily cause worsening of disease symptoms, including bone pain, blood in the urine for men, and vaginal bleeding for women. These disease "flares" usually stop within two weeks. Goserelin can cause hypercalcemia.

Women who have the potential to become pregnant while using letrozole, including women who are perimenopausal or who recently became postmenopausal, need to use adequate contraception until their postmenopausal status is fully established.

Disease signs and symptoms may worsen during the first weeks of leuprolide treatment. Worsening of symptoms may contribute to paralysis with or without fatal complications.

The use of medroxyprogesterone during the first four months of pregnancy is not recommended, as there is increased risk to the fetus. The drug should be discontinued immediately if the patient develops any signs or symptoms of blood clots. Medroxyprogesterone should also be discontinued if there is a sudden partial or complete loss of vision or if there is a sudden onset of visual impairment or migraine. This drug should also be discontinued at the first sign of liver impairment.

Clinical cases of new onset diabetes, worsening of preexisting diabetes, and overt Cushing's syndrome have been reported in association with the chronic use of megestrol. In addition, cases of adrenal insufficiency have been observed in patients receiving or being withdrawn from chronic megestrol therapy. The possibility of adrenal insufficiency should be considered in any patient receiving or being withdrawn from chronic megestrol therapy who experiences hypotension, nausea, vomiting, dizziness, or weakness.

Interstitial pneumonitis has been reported in 2 percent of patients exposed to nilutamide in controlled clinical trials. Reports of interstitial changes including pulmonary fibrosis that led to hospitalization and death have been rarely reported. Symptoms included difficulty breathing following exertion, cough, chest pain, and fever. Most cases occurred within the first three months of treatment with nilutamide, and most reversed with discontinuation of therapy. A routine chest X-ray should be performed prior to initiating treatment, and patients should be instructed to report any new or worsening shortness of breath that they experience while on this drug. If symptoms occur, nilutamide should be immediately discontinued until it can be determined if the symptoms are drug-related. Rare cases of death or hospitalization due to severe liver injury have been reported with the use of nilutamide.

Serious and life-threatening events associated with tamoxifen in women at high risk for cancer and women with DCIS include uterine cancer, stroke, and PE. Hypercalcemia has been reported in some breast cancer patients when the cancer has spread to the bone within a few weeks of starting treatment with tamoxifen. Tamoxifen has been associated with changes in liver enzyme levels and on rare occasions more severe liver abnormalities. A few of these serious cases included fatalities. An increased incidence of cataracts and the need for cataract surgery have been reported in patients receiving tamoxifen. Other vision problems may also occur.

Hypercalcemia and tumor flare (increased size of tumor lesions that later regress) have been reported in some breast cancer patients when the cancer has spread to the bone during the first weeks of treatment with toremifene. Tumor flare does not imply failure of treatment or represent tumor progression. If hypercalcemia occurs, appropriate measures should be instituted, and if hypercalcemia is severe, toremifene treatment should be discontinued. Endometrial hyperplasia has been reported in patients taking toremifene.

Initially, histrelin and triptorelin cause a temporary increase in testosterone levels. As a result, worsening of signs and symptoms of prostate cancer during the first weeks of treatment may occur. Patients may experience worsening of symptoms or onset of new symptoms, including bone pain, neuropathy, blood in the urine, or urethral or bladder outlet obstruction. Cases of spinal cord compression, which may contribute to paralysis with or without fatal complications, have been reported. If spinal cord compression or kidney impairment develops, standard treatment of these complications should be instituted and in extreme cases an immediate orchiectomy (surgical removal of one or both testicles) considered.

Monoclonal antibodies Serious hypersensitivity reactions, including some with fatal outcome, have been reported with monoclonal antibodies. Moreover, 10 to 30 percent of reactions to monoclonal antibodies are delayed and may occur with later infusions. Thus, it is important that patients receive proper premedication, close monitoring following administration, and prompt intervention when symptoms occur. Emergency supplies including drugs for the treatment of hypersensitivity reactions (e.g., epinephrine, antihistamines, and corticosteroids) should be available for immediate use in the event of an allergic reaction.

Serious, including fatal, pancytopenia/bone marrow hypoplasia, autoimmune idiopathic thrombocytopenia, and autoimmune hemolytic anemia can occur in patients receiving alemtuzumab. Large doses increase the incidence of pancytopenia. Alemtuzumab administration can result in serious, including fatal, infusion reactions (e.g., fainting, acute respiratory distress syndrome, respiratory arrest, cardiac arrhythmias, myocardial infarction, cardiac arrest, angioedema, and anaphylactoid shock). In clinical trials, the frequency of infusion reactions was highest in the first week of treatment. Premedication with diphenhydramine and acetaminophen 30 minutes prior to first infusion and each dose escalation may prevent or ameliorate infusion-related reactions. Serious, including fatal, infections can occur in patients receiving alemtuzumab.

Bevacizumab may cause perforation in the intestines, at times complicated by abscesses or fistula formation, and in some instances may be fatal. Bevacizumab interferes with wound healing because it inhibits the growth of blood vessels. Bevacizumab should be discontinued in patients with wound-healing complications. Bleeding complications have occurred with bevacizumab, including fatal hemorrhages. This drug may also cause severe hypertension or make existing high blood pressure worse and may cause congestive heart failure, especially in people who have received radiation to the chest or anthracene derivative chemotherapy drugs, such as doxorubicin or epirubicin.

Cetuximab has caused serious allergic reactions requiring medical intervention and immediate, permanent discontinuation of the drug. These reactions have included rapid onset of airway obstruction (bronchospasm, whistling sound while breathing, hoarseness), hypotension, shock, loss of consciousness, myocardial infarction, and/or cardiac arrest. Premedication is recommended with an H_1 antagonist such as diphenhydramine intravenously 30 to 60 minutes prior to the first dose of cetuximab; premedication should be administered for subsequent cetuximab doses based upon clinical judgment and presence/severity of prior infusion reactions. It is important to note that approximately 90 percent of severe allergic reactions occurred with the first treatment despite premedication with antihistamines. Rarely, patients with head and neck cancer who have received cetuximab along with radiation therapy have developed serious or fatal heart problems soon after treatment. Interstitial lung disease, including one

fatality, occurred rarely in patients receiving cetuximab in clinical trials. Acnelike skin rash is common during the first two weeks of treatment with cetuximab and in rare cases has developed into severe cases of skin rash, drying, fissuring, and infections requiring incision and drainage. Hypomagnesemia (abnormally low level of magnesium in the blood) occurred in more than half of patients receiving cetuximab in clinical trials and was severe in fewer than 20 percent of patients. Because hypomagnesemia and accompanying electrolyte abnormalities occurred days to months after initiation of treatment, patients should be periodically monitored for low levels of magnesium, calcium, and potassium.

Since there are no controlled trials demonstrating efficacy and safety using gemtuzumab ozogamicin in combination with other chemotherapeutic agents, this drug should be used only as single-agent chemotherapy and not in combination chemotherapy regimens outside clinical trials. Severe myelosuppression occurs when gemtuzumab ozogamicin is used at recommended doses. Gemtuzumab ozogamicin can cause allergic reactions, including anaphylaxis, especially during and right after the first treatment. Acetaminophen and diphenhydramine should be administered one hour before the infusion. Acetaminophen should then be repeated as needed every four hours for two additional doses. This drug can cause liver damage, which has resulted in a few deaths from liver failure. Extra caution should be exercised when administering gemtuzumab ozogamicin in patients with liver impairment.

The ibritumomab tiuxetan treatment regimen is more toxic than treatment with rituximab alone. Since ibritumomab is used only in combination with rituximab, the pretreatment regimen recommended is really intended to prevent the infusion-related reactions associated with rituximab. More than half of the patients in the ibritumomab tiuxetan clinical trials experienced serious leukopenia and thrombocytopenia that lasted for three to four weeks. Hemorrhages, some fatal, and life-threatening infections occurred in a small number of patients. Because of these concerns, the ibritumomab tiuxetan therapeutic regimen is approved only for patients who have failed other treatments. Ibritumomab tiuxetan may cause serious or fatal skin reactions, which may occur as soon as a few days after treatment or as long as four months after treatment. These reactions include blisters on the skin or on the inside of the mouth or nose, a rash, or peeling of the skin.

Serious infusion reactions, myelosuppression (severe neutropenia and thrombocytopenia), and infection, including progressive multifocal leukoencephalopathy (PML) and reactivation of hepatitis B virus infection (see *Cautions and Concerns*), were reported during clinical trials of ofatumumab. To decrease the risk of infusion reactions, patients should be premedicated with acetaminophen, an antihistamine, and a corticosteroid 30 minutes to two hours prior to each dose. Complete blood counts and platelet counts should be monitored at regular intervals during therapy. PML can be fatal with ofatumumab, and PML should be considered in any patient with new onset of or changes in preexisting neurological signs or symptoms (e.g., clumsiness, progressive weakness, and visual, speech, and personality changes). Ofatumumab should be discontinued if PML is suspected, and evaluation for PML including consultation with a neurologist, brain MRI, and lumbar puncture, should be initiated.

About 90 percent of patients in panitumumab clinical studies experienced skin reactions, including rash, acne, redness, dryness, and fissures. In about 16 percent of patients, these skin reactions were severe, resulting in sepsis, septic death, and abscesses requiring incisions and drainage. Though rare, infusion reactions have occurred with panitumumab, including anaphylactic reactions, bronchospasm, and hypotension.

Deaths within 24 hours of rituximab treatment have been reported. These fatal reactions followed a severe infusion reaction, typically during or within two hours of the first infusion. Pretreatment with acetaminophen and an antihistamine may lessen infusion reactions and is recommended before each infusion of rituximab. The rapid destruction of cancer cells leading to disturbances in metabolism has caused acute kidney failure requiring dialysis, which could be fatal. Rituximab may cause chest pain and an irregular heartbeat, particularly in patients having underlying cardiac conditions. Severe mucocutaneous (on the skin and/or mucous membrane) reactions, some with fatal outcome, have been reported in association with rituximab treatment. Serious viral infections, either new, reactivated, or exacerbated, have been identified in rituximab clinical studies or postmarketing reports. JC virus infection resulting in PML and death has been reported in patients treated with rituximab.

Premedication with acetaminophen and diphenhydramine should be given 30 minutes prior to administration of tositumomab. The majority of patients who receive the tositumomab therapeutic regimen experience severe thrombocytopenia and neutropenia. Because administration of the tositumomab therapeutic regimen may result in hypothyroidism, all patients must receive a thyroid-blocking agent (e.g., SSKI [saturated solution of potassium iodide], Lugol's solution, or potassium iodide); any patient who is unable to tolerate thyroid-blocking agents should not receive the tositumomab therapeutic regimen. Patients should be evaluated for signs and symptoms of hypothyroidism and have laboratory tests performed to screen for this disorder. The tositumomab therapeutic regimen contains a radioactive component and should be administered only by physicians and other health-care professionals qualified by training in the safe use and handling of therapeutic radionuclides and only by physicians who are in the process of being or have been certified by GlaxoSmithKline in dose calculation and administration of this regimen. Secondary malignancies have been reported with tositumomab therapy.

Trastuzumab may cause heart failure, especially if used with anthracene derivatives, and in people with heart disease or other risk factors such as advancing age. Infusion reactions, some serious and fatal, have occurred with trastuzumab, including fever and chills, nausea, vomiting, pain (in some cases at tumor sites), headache, dizziness, difficulty breathing, hypotension, rash, and loss of strength. Premedication with acetaminophen, diphenhydramine, and/or meperidine may be effective in managing the infusion reactions. Trastuzumab can result in serious and fatal lung damage (e.g., pneumonia, pulmonary fibrosis), especially in people with preexisting lung problems.

mTOR inhibitors Hypersensitivity reactions, including anaphylaxis, difficulty breathing, flushing, and chest pain may occur with temsirolimus. Pretreatment with an H_1-receptor antagonist (e.g., diphenhydramine) should be administered to reduce the risk of reactions. Temsirolimus is likely to raise blood glucose levels, which may result in the need for an increase in the dose of, or initiation of, insulin and/or oral hypoglycemic agent therapy. Patients should be advised to report excessive thirst or any increase in the volume or frequency of urination. Cases of interstitial lung disease, some resulting in death, occurred in patients who received temsirolimus. Because fatal bowel perforation has occurred in patients who received temsirolimus, patients should be advised to report promptly any new or worsening abdominal pain or blood in their stools. Cases of rapidly progressive and sometimes fatal acute kidney failure (not clearly related to disease progression) has occurred in patients who received temsirolimus. Some of these cases were not responsive to dialysis. In rare cases when patients have brain tumors or are taking blood-thinning drugs, temsirolimus may cause bleeding in the brain.

Platinum compounds Allergic reactions, which can be fatal, can occur within minutes of administration of platinum compounds and include rash, hives, redness of the skin, itching, bronchospasm, and hypotension. These reactions are usually managed with standard epinephrine, corticosteroid, or antihistamine therapy and may require discontinuation of therapy. Drug-related deaths associated with platinum compounds from anaphylaxis have been reported.

Platinum compounds may induce vomiting, which can be more severe in patients previously receiving drugs that also induce vomiting. The incidence and intensity of the vomiting have been reduced by using premedication ANTIEMETICS.

Myelosuppression (leukopenia, neutropenia, and thrombocytopenia) with carboplatin is dose-related and may be severe, resulting in infection and/or bleeding. Anemia may be cumulative and may require transfusion support. Carboplatin may cause damage to peripheral nerves, especially in patients older than 65 years and in patients previously treated with cisplatin. Loss of vision, which can be complete for light and colors, has been reported after the use of higher than recommended doses of carboplatin. Vision appears to recover totally or to a significant extent within weeks of stopping these high doses.

Cumulative kidney damage associated with cisplatin is severe. Other major dose-related toxicities are myelosuppression, nausea, and vomiting. Hearing damage, which may be more pronounced in children and appears as ringing in the ear and/or loss of high-frequency hearing and occasionally deafness, is significant. Because hearing damage is cumulative, audiometric testing should be performed prior to initiating therapy and prior to each subsequent dose of the drug. Cisplatin can cause severe damage to nerves and nervous system tissues, which may appear as tingling, numbness, and sometimes burning of the fingers and toes. Loss of motor function has also been reported with cisplatin.

Oxaliplatin can cause damage to nerves and nervous system tissues, which may appear as tingling, numbness, and sometimes burning of the fingers and toes. This nerve damage can be severe and gets worse in the cold. Oxaliplatin may also cause tightness or spasm in the throat, which is more likely to happen if the patient is exposed to cold food or drinks while receiving the drug. Oxaliplatin has been associated with pulmonary fibrosis, which may be fatal. In case of unexplained respiratory symptoms such as nonproductive cough or difficulty breathing, oxaliplatin should be discontinued until further pulmonary investigation excludes interstitial lung disease or pulmonary fibrosis.

Topoisomerase inhibitors Secondary leukemias have occurred in patients exposed to topoisomerase inhibitors when used in combination with other antineoplastic agents or radiation therapy.

If extravasation occurs with any of the anthracene derivatives, severe tissue damage could occur, which can cause pain, ulceration, and scarring. Potentially fatal congestive heart failure may occur either during anthracene therapy or months to years after termination of therapy. Severe myelosuppression occurs with these drugs. Dosage should be reduced in patients with liver or kidney impairment. Secondary leukemia has been reported in patients treated with anthracyclines.

Cardiac function should be monitored regularly in patients receiving daunorubicin liposome because of the potential risk for cardiac toxicity and congestive heart failure. Cardiac monitoring is advised, especially in those patients who have received prior anthracyclines, who have preexisting cardiac disease, or who have had prior radiotherapy encompassing the heart. Daunorubicin liposome dosage should be reduced in patients with impaired liver function. A triad of back pain, flushing, and chest tightness has been reported in some patients treated with daunorubicin liposomal, usually during the first five minutes of the infusion, subsiding with interruption of the infusion and generally not recurring if the infusion is then resumed at a slower rate.

Because doxorubicin may cause serious heart problems, the total amount of doxorubicin given to a patient over his or her entire lifetime is limited. The lifetime total dose should not exceed 550 mg/m^2 in patients with normal heart function. Patients receiving doxorubicin may develop serious cardiac arrhythmias.

Patients with preexisting myelosuppression as the result of prior drug therapy should not receive mitoxantrone unless it is felt that the possible benefit from such treatment warrants the risk of further myelosuppression. The safety of mitoxantrone injection in patients with liver impairment is not established. Mitoxantrone must not be given by intrathecal injection, as there have been reports of seizures leading to coma as well as paralysis with bowel and bladder dysfunction following intrathecal injection.

Patients should be informed that valrubicin has been shown to induce complete response in only about one in five patients with BCG-refractory CIS and that delaying cystectomy (bladder removal) could lead to development of metastatic bladder cancer, which is lethal. The exact risk of developing metastatic bladder cancer from such a delay may be difficult to assess but increases the longer cystectomy is delayed in the presence of persisting CIS. If there is not a complete response of CIS to valrubicin treatment after three months or if CIS recurs, cystectomy must be reconsidered. Valrubicin should not be administered to patients with a perforated bladder or to those in whom the integrity of the bladder mucosa has been compromised (see *Cautions and Concerns*). In order to avoid possible dangerous systemic exposure to valrubicin for patients undergoing transurethral resection of the bladder, the status of the bladder should be evaluated before the intravesical instillation of the drug. In case of bladder perforation, the administration of valrubicin should be delayed until bladder integrity has been restored.

Irinotecan can induce both early and late forms of diarrhea, either of which may be severe. Early diarrhea (occurring during or within 24 hours of administration) may be accompanied by cholinergic symptoms (i.e., runny nose, increased salivation, excess tears in the eyes, sweating, flushing, or abdominal cramps). These symptoms occur more frequently with higher doses. Early diarrhea and other cholinergic symptoms may be prevented or ameliorated by atropine. Late diarrhea (occurring more than 24 hours after drug administration) can be life-threatening as it may be prolonged and may lead to dehydration, electrolyte imbalance, or infection. Late diarrhea should be treated promptly with loperamide. Patients with diarrhea should be carefully monitored and given fluid and electrolyte replacement if they become dehydrated or antibiotic therapy if they develop intestinal blockage, fever, or severe neutropenia. Administration of irinotecan should be interrupted and subsequent doses reduced if severe diarrhea occurs. Severe myelosuppression may occur with irinotecan. Serious complications reported with irinotecan have included death due to infection following severe neutropenia; severe anaphylactic reactions; colitis complicated by ulceration, bleeding, blockage, and infection; rare cases of kidney impairment and kidney failure, usually following severe vomiting and/or diarrhea; and blood clots.

Myelosuppression (primarily neutropenia) is the most serious side effect commonly seen with topotecan and has been fatal. Neutropenia is not cumulative over time. Diarrhea, including severe diarrhea requiring hospitalization, has been reported during treatment with oral topotecan.

Severe myelosuppression with resulting infection or bleeding may occur with etoposide and teniposide. Patients being treated with these drugs must be frequently observed for myelosuppression both during and after therapy. Myelosuppression resulting in death has been reported. Anaphylactic reaction manifested by chills, fever, rapid heartbeat, bronchospasm, difficulty breathing, dyspnea, and hypotension may occur with etoposide or teniposide. Etoposide injection and teniposide should be given only by slow intravenous infusion (usually over a 30- to 60-minute period), as hypotension has been reported as a possible side effect of rapid intravenous injection.

Tyrosine kinase inhibitors Dasatinib may cause severe thrombocytopenia, neutropenia, and anemia. Severe gastrointestinal bleeding has occurred, requiring treatment interruptions and transfusions. Most bleeding events have been associated with severe thrombocytopenia. Dasatinib may cause fluid retention. In more severe cases, fluid may accumulate in the lining of the lungs, around the heart, or in the abdominal cavity. Dasatinib may cause cardiac arrhythmias.

Rarely during clinical trials, people taking erlotinib have had heart attacks or strokes; however, it is unknown whether these events occurred because of the drug. Erlotinib may cause inflammation or abscesses of the cornea of the eye.

Erlotinib and gefitinib may cause potentially fatal interstitial lung disease (pneumonia or inflammation of the lungs without infection). In the event of new or progressive unexplained pulmonary symptoms such as labored breathing, cough, and fever, erlotinib or gefitinib therapy should be interrupted pending diagnostic evaluation. If interstitial lung disease is diagnosed, these drugs should be discontinued.

Imatinib sometimes causes gastrointestinal irritation and should be taken with food and a large glass of water to minimize this problem. Gastrointestinal perforation, including fatalities, has occurred rarely. Imatinib has occasionally caused severe congestive heart failure. Most of the patients with reported cardiac reactions have had other risk factors, including advanced age and an underlying cardiac disease.

Lapatinib may cause liver dysfunction, which in rare cases may be serious or even life-threatening. Dose reduction should be considered in patients with severe preexisting liver impairment. Lapatinib has been associated with interstitial lung disease and pneumonitis. Lapatinib has also been shown to prolong the QT interval, which could increase the risk of potentially fatal cardiac arrhythmias. Any electrolyte abnormalities must be corrected prior to beginning therapy, and these electrolytes should be monitored periodically while taking lapatinib.

Nilotinib prolongs the QT interval. Sudden deaths have been reported in patients taking nilotinib. Nilotinib can cause a number of electrolyte abnormalities, including hypophosphatemia, hypokalemia, hyperkalemia, hypocalcemia, and hyponatremia. Any electrolyte abnormalities must be corrected prior to beginning therapy, and these electrolytes should be monitored periodically while taking nilotinib.

Severe and fatal liver damage has been observed in pazopanib clinical studies. Liver tests should be monitored every four weeks for at least the first four months, with periodic monitoring thereafter. Because QT interval prolongation has been seen with pazopanib, this drug should be used with caution in patients with a history of QT interval prolongation, in patients taking ANTIARRHYTHMICS or other medications that may prolong QT interval, and those with preexisting cardiac disease. Electrolyte abnormalities should also be corrected prior to use to minimize the risk for arrhythmias. Because heart attack and stroke have been observed with pazopanib, this drug should be used with caution in patients who are at increased risk for these events or who have had a history of these events. Gastrointestinal perforation or fistula has been reported rarely in patients taking pazopanib. Excessive protein (chicfly albumin but also globulin) in the urine has been reported with pazopanib; thus, baseline and periodic urinalysis during treatment is recommended.

Rarely, heart attack has been reported during sorafenib therapy. An increased risk of bleeding may occur following sorafenib administration. Blood pressure should be monitored weekly during the first six weeks of treatment, as hypertension was reported in nearly 17 percent of patients in one study. Hypertension was usually mild to moderate, occurred carly in the course of treatment, and was managed with standard antihypertensive therapy. Gastrointestinal perforation is an uncommon occurrence with sorafenib.

Sunitinib poses some risk of damage to the cardiovascular system. It has been shown to prolong the QT interval, which could increase the risk of potentially fatal cardiac arrhythmias. Sunitinib should not be used in people with congestive heart failure or uncontrolled extremely high blood pressure. Fatal tumor-related bleeding has occurred during treatment with sunitinib. Serious and sometimes fatal gastrointestinal complications have occurred in people with intra-abdominal tumors during treatment with sunitinib. One of the more common complications is gastrointestinal perforation.

Retinoids Bexarotene is associated with an extremely high risk of birth defects if either the male or female is taking it at the time of conception or during pregnancy. Men and women who are taking this drug need to use two kinds of birth control during treatment and for a month after treatment is done. Bexarotene capsules induce major lipid abnormalities (elevated triglycerides, elevated total and low-density lipoprotein cholesterol, and decreased high-density lipoprotein cholesterol) in most patients, which must be monitored and treated during long-term therapy. Acute pancreatitis has been reported rarely in patients taking bexarotene capsules. Bexarotene capsules have been associated with hypothyroidism in about half of all patients treated. Because bexarotene capsules may cause cataracts, patients who experience visual difficulties should have an appropriate ophthalmologic evaluation. Bexarotene may also cause neutropenia.

Patients with APL are at high risk for medical complications, in general, and can have severe adverse reactions to tretinoin. Approximately one-quarter of patients taking tretinoin develop retinoic-acid-APL (RA-APL) syndrome (also called APL differentiation syndrome), which is a reaction between the drug and the leukemia. Symptoms include fever, weight gain, difficulty breathing, lung and heart problems, and hypotension. The syndrome can occur from two days following treatment to a month later. Symptoms must be reported to the patient's physician immediately so that treatment can begin promptly. In rare cases, this syndrome is fatal. During tretinoin treatment, about 40 percent of patients will develop rapidly evolving leukocytosis. Patients with high white blood cell counts at diagnosis have an increased risk of a further rapid increase in these counts. Rapidly evolving leukocytosis is associated with a higher risk of life-threatening complications. If signs and symptoms of the RA-APL syndrome are present together with leukocytosis, treatment with high-dose corticosteroids should be initiated immediately. Due to the high risk of a severely deformed infant if tretinoin is administered during pregnancy, effective contraception must be used by all females during therapy and for one month following discontinuation of therapy. Contraception must be used even when there is a history of infertility or menopause, unless a hysterectomy has been performed. Whenever contraception is required, it is recommended that two reliable forms of contraception be used simultaneously unless abstinence is the chosen method. If pregnancy does occur during treatment, the physician and patient should discuss the desirability of continuing or terminating the pregnancy.

Proteasome inhibitors Bortezomib causes a peripheral neuropathy that has been serious in some cases. Patients should be monitored for symptoms of numbness, weakness, pain, burning sensation, tingling, sensitivity to cold in the hands or feet, or trouble walking or using the hands. Patients experiencing new or worsening peripheral neuropathy may require change in the dose and schedule of bortezomib. Hypotension and dizziness, especially when going from lying or sitting to standing, may occur with bortezomib. Caution should be used when treating patients with a history of fainting, patients taking drugs known to be associated with hypotension, and patients who are dehydrated. Development or worsening of congestive heart failure and other heart problems have been reported with bortezomib. Patients with risk factors for or existing heart disease should be closely monitored. Severe lung diseases have occurred rarely in patients receiving bortezomib. This drug is also associated with thrombocytopenia and neutropenia, especially in the weeks after the drug is given. Bortezomib may cause a rare, reversible brain disorder called reversible posterior leukoencephalopathy syndrome (RPLS). Symptoms of RPLS include seizures, hypertension, headache, trouble concentrating, confusion, and changes in vision. Cases of acute liver failure and hepatitis have been reported in patients receiving multiple drugs along with bortezomib and with serious underlying medical conditions.

Miscellaneous Adverse events are frequent, often serious, and sometimes fatal with aldesleukin. Thorough clinical evaluation should be performed to identify patients with significant cardiac, lung, kidney, liver, or CNS impairment in whom aldesleukin is contraindicated. Patients in whom these functions are normal may still experience serious, life-threatening, or fatal adverse events. Should adverse events, which require dose modification, occur, therapy should be withheld. Life-threatening events have included hypothermia, shock, bradycardia, myocardial ischemia (lack of blood flow to the heart), loss of consciousness, hemorrhage, atrial arrhythmia, phlebitis, gangrene, thrombosis, gastrointestinal hemorrhage, intestinal perforation, myelosuppression, paranoid reaction, convulsion, delirium, asthma, and kidney failure. Aldesleukin should be withheld in patients developing moderate to severe lethargy or sleepiness, as continued administration may result in coma.

Asparaginase frequently causes anaphylaxis and serious allergic reactions (e.g., difficulty breathing, itching, rash, swollen face, agitation, low blood pressure). This risk is higher in patients who have previously received asparaginase and with intravenous administration. Patients should be observed for one hour after administration of asparaginase with resuscitation equipment and other agents necessary to treat anaphylaxis (e.g., epinephrine, antihistamines, corticosteroids, oxygen) close at hand. Serious blood clots can occur in patients receiving asparaginase, and the drug should be discontinued in such cases. Pancreatitis, in some cases sudden or fatal, can occur with asparaginase. Patients with abdominal pain should be checked for evidence of pancreatitis, and, if found, asparaginase should be discontinued.

Serious and fatal infusion reactions have occurred with denileukin. Cardiopulmonary resuscitation equipment should be available during administration, and denileukin should be immediately stopped and permanently discontinued following a serious infusion reaction. Patients should be premedicated with an antihistamine and acetaminophen. CLS, resulting in death, has also occurred with denileukin. The onset of CLS symptoms may be delayed, occurring up to two weeks following infusion. Symptoms may persist or worsen after the cessation of the drug. Patients should be monitored for weight gain, new onset or worsening edema, and hypotension. Loss of sharpness of vision, usually with loss of color vision, has been reported following administration of denileukin. Recovery was reported in some of the affected patients; however, most patients reported permanent impairment.

If lenalidomide is taken during pregnancy, it may cause severe birth defects or death to an unborn baby; thus, females should be advised to avoid pregnancy. Women of childbearing age must use two forms of reliable birth control at the same time during treatment with lenalidomide as well as for four weeks before starting and four weeks after stopping the drug. Women who could become pregnant should take two pregnancy tests before starting the drug and again every two to four weeks throughout treatment. Lenalidomide is associated with significant myelosuppression. It has been associated with an increased risk of major blood clots in the veins of the legs or lungs.

Thalidomide can cause severe birth defects in humans (see *Contraindications*). Because thalidomide is present in the semen of males taking the drug, they must always use a latex condom during any sexual contact with women of childbearing potential. Thalidomide used to treat multiple myeloma results in an increased risk of major blood clots in the veins of the legs and lungs. This risk increases significantly when thalidomide is used in combination with standard chemotherapy agents including dexamethasone. Thalidomide frequently causes drowsiness and somnolence. Patients must be warned to use caution when performing tasks requiring

alertness. Peripheral neuropathy is a common, potentially severe, side effect of treatment with thalidomide that may be irreversible. Peripheral neuropathy generally occurs following chronic use over a period of months; however, reports following relatively short-term use also exist. Symptoms may occur some time after thalidomide treatment has been stopped. Patients should be examined at monthly intervals for the first three months of thalidomide therapy for any early signs of neuropathy, such as numbness, tingling, or pain in the hands and feet. Thalidomide may cause dizziness, especially when changing position, such as from sitting to standing. Thus, patients should sit upright for a few minutes prior to standing up from a recumbent position. Decreased white blood cell counts, including neutropenia, have been reported in association with thalidomide.

When Not Advised (Contraindications)

Alkylating agents Altretamine should not be used in patients with preexisting severe bone marrow depression or severe neurologic toxicity. Altretamine has been administered safely, however, to patients heavily pretreated with cisplatin and/or alkylating agents, including patients with preexisting cisplatin neuropathies. Careful monitoring of neurologic function in these patients is essential.

Thiotepa is usually contraindicated in cases of existing liver, kidney, or bone marrow damage. However, if the need outweighs the risk in such patients, thiotepa may be used in low dosage and accompanied by liver function, kidney function, and blood count tests.

There may be cross-hypersensitivity (skin rash) between chlorambucil and other alkylating agents.

Continued use of cyclophosphamide is contraindicated in patients with severely depressed bone marrow function.

Continued use of ifosfamide is contraindicated in patients with severely depressed bone marrow function (see *Warnings* and *Cautions and Concerns*).

The use of mechlorethamine is contraindicated in the presence of known infectious diseases.

Temozolomide is contraindicated in patients who have a history of hypersensitivity to dacarbazine, as both drugs are converted to the same active metabolite.

Procarbazine is contraindicated in patients with inadequate marrow reserve as demonstrated by bone marrow aspiration. Due consideration of this possible state should be given to each patient who has leukopenia, thrombocytopenia, or anemia.

Antibiotics Dactinomycin should not be given at or about the time of infection with chicken pox or herpes zoster because of the risk of severe generalized disease, which may result in death.

Mitomycin is contraindicated in patients with thrombocytopenia, coagulation disorder, or an increase in bleeding tendency due to other causes.

Antimetabolites Azacitidine is contraindicated in patients with a known hypersensitivity to azacitidine or mannitol and also in patients with advanced malignant liver tumors.

Capecitabine is contraindicated in patients who have a known hypersensitivity to fluorouracil, as cancer cells convert capecitabine into fluorouracil. Capecitabine is contraindicated in patients with known dihydropyrimidine dehydrogenase deficiency (a metabolic disorder) as well as in patients with severe kidney impairment.

Cytarabine liposome injection is contraindicated in patients with an active meningeal infection.

Floxuridine is contraindicated for patients in a poor nutritional state, those with depressed bone marrow function, or those with potentially serious infections.

Fludarabine is not recommended for patients with severe kidney impairment (see *Cautions and Concerns*).

Fluorouracil injection is contraindicated for patients in a poor nutritional state, those with depressed bone marrow function, or those with potentially serious infections.

Hydroxyurea is contraindicated in patients with marked bone marrow depression or severe anemia.

Patients with psoriasis or RA with alcoholism, alcoholic liver disease, or other chronic liver disease should not receive methotrexate. Patients with psoriasis or RA who have overt or laboratory evidence of immunodeficiency syndromes (e.g., acquired immunodeficiency syndrome [AIDS], hypogammaglobulinemia, or agammaglobulinemia) should not receive methotrexate. Patients with psoriasis or RA who have preexisting blood problems, such as bone marrow hypoplasia, leukopenia, thrombocytopenia, or significant anemia, should not receive methotrexate.

Antimitotics Docetaxel is contraindicated in patients with myelosuppression.

Estramustine should not be used in patients with allergic reactions to either estradiol or to nitrogen mustard or in patients who have a history of blood clots or a blood clotting disorder, except in those cases where the actual tumor mass is the cause of the blood clots and the benefits of therapy may outweigh the risks.

Paclitaxel is contraindicated in patients with solid tumors or AIDS-related Kaposi's sarcoma who have low neutrophil counts as well as in patients with low neutrophil or platelet counts and in patients who have a history of hypersensitivity reactions to drugs formulated in castor oil.

Vinblastine sulfate is contraindicated in patients who have significant granulocytopenia unless this is a result of the disease being treated. It should not be used in the presence of bacterial infections. Such infections must be brought under control prior to beginning therapy with vinblastine.

Patients with the demyelinating form of Charcot-Marie-Tooth syndrome (an inherited neurological disorder) should not be given vincristine.

Vinorelbine is contraindicated in patients with low pretreatment granulocyte counts.

Epothilones Ixabepilone is contraindicated in patients who have a history of hypersensitivity reactions to drugs formulated in castor oil. It is also contraindicated in patients who have a neutrophil count <1500 cells/mm³ or a platelet count <100,000 cells/mm³. Ixabepilone in combination with capecitabine is contraindicated in patients with severe liver impairment.

Hormones Bicalutamide has no indication for women and should not be used in this population.

Flutamide is contraindicated in patients with severe liver impairment.

Goserelin is contraindicated in those patients who have a known hypersensitivity to LHRH or LHRH agonist analogues (see *Cautions and Concerns*).

Histrelin is contraindicated in women and in pediatric patients.

Letrozole is contraindicated in premenopausal women (see *Warnings*).

Leuprolide is contraindicated in those patients who have a known hypersensitivity to LHRH or LHRH agonist analogues (see *Cautions and Concerns*). It is also contraindicated in women with abnormal vaginal bleeding.

Medroxyprogesterone is contraindicated in women with undiagnosed vaginal bleeding and in patients with active blood-clotting disorder, current or past history of blood clots or strokes, or significant liver impairment.

Nilutamide is contraindicated in patients with severe liver impairment or with severe respiratory insufficiency (when the respiratory system is unable to meet fully the demands of the body for the supply of extra oxygen).

Tamoxifen is contraindicated in women being treated to reduce the risk of breast cancer who are on warfarin therapy or those with a history of DVT or PE.

Triptorelin pamoate is contraindicated in individuals with a known hypersensitivity to other LHRH agonists or LHRH (see *Cautions and Concerns*).

Monoclonal antibodies No contraindications currently exist for this class of drugs.

mTOR inhibitors No contraindications currently exist for this class of drugs.

Platinum compounds Carboplatin is contraindicated in patients with a history of allergic reactions to any platinum-containing compound and in patients with severe bone marrow depression or significant bleeding.

Cisplatin is contraindicated in patients with preexisting kidney impairment, myelosuppression, or hearing impairment. Cisplatin is contraindicated in patients with a history of allergic reactions to any platinum-containing compound.

Oxaliplatin should not be administered to patients with a history of allergic reactions to any platinum-containing compound.

Topoisomerase inhibitors Doxorubicin and epirubicin are contraindicated in patients who have a history of congestive heart failure, arrhythmias (see *Warnings*), recent myocardial infarction, previous therapy with high cumulative doses of doxorubicin, daunorubicin, idarubicin, epirubicin, or mitoxantrone, severe liver impairment, or low neutrophil counts.

Doxorubicin liposomal is contraindicated in nursing mothers.

Idarubicin should not be used if the serum bilirubin exceeds 5 mg/dl.

Valrubicin is contraindicated in patients with known hypersensitivity to anthracyclines or to castor oil. Patients with concurrent urinary tract infections should not receive valrubicin. Valrubicin should not be administered to patients with a small bladder capacity, i.e., unable to tolerate a 75 mL instillation.

Irinotecan is contraindicated in patients concomitantly receiving ketoconazole or Saint-John's-wort.

Topotecan should not be used in patients with severe bone marrow depression.

Teniposide is contraindicated in patients with hypersensitivity to castor oil.

Tyrosine kinase inhibitors Nilotinib is contraindicated in patients with hypokalemia, hypomagnesemia, or long QT syndrome (see *Warnings*).

Retinoids Tretinoin should not be given to patients who are sensitive to parabens, which are used as preservatives in the gelatin capsule.

Proteasome inhibitors Bortezomib is contraindicated in patients with hypersensitivity to boron or mannitol.

Miscellaneous Aldesleukin is contraindicated in patients with an abnormal thallium stress test or abnormal pulmonary function tests and those with organ allografts. Retreatment with aldesleukin is contraindicated in patients who have experienced the following drug-related toxicities while receiving an earlier course of therapy: sustained ventricular tachycardia, cardiac arrhythmias not controlled or unresponsive to management, chest pain with ECG changes consistent with angina or myocardial infarction, cardiac tamponade, intubation for more than 72 hours, renal failure requiring dialysis for more than 72 hours, coma or toxic psychosis lasting more than 48 hours, repetitive or difficult to control seizures, bowel ischemia/perforation, or GI bleeding requiring surgery.

Asparaginase should not be used in patients with a history of pancreatitis, prior serious allergic reactions, blood clots, or serious bleeding events due to asparaginase (see *Warnings*).

Lenalidomide is contraindicated in pregnant women and women of childbearing potential (see *Warnings*).

Due to its known potential for severe birth defects or death to an unborn baby, even following a single dose, thalidomide is contraindicated in pregnant women and women of childbearing potential.

Side Effects

Nausea and vomiting caused by the administration of antineoplastics is one of the most common and distressing side effects of cancer treatment. Although most antineoplastics carry at least a mild emetic risk, the following drugs have a high risk (greater than 90 percent frequency without the use of antiemetics) of being emetogenic: altretamine, carmustine, cisplatin, cyclophosphamide, dacarbazine, mechloretha-

mine, procarbazine oral, and streptozocin. The following have a moderate risk (30 to 90 percent frequency without antiemetics) of being emetogenic: aldesleukin, azacitidine, busulfan, carboplatin, carmustine, cisplatin, cyclophosphamide, cyclophosphamide oral, cytarabine, dactinomycin, daunorubicin, doxorubicin, epirubicin, etoposide oral, idarubicin, ifosfamide, imatinib oral, irinotecan, lomustine, melphalan, methotrexate, oxaliplatin, temozolomide oral, and vinorelbine. *Note:* Drugs listed in both risk categories depend on the dosage being administered. Also, some drugs have a moderate or high risk only with certain dosing amounts.

Alkylating agents The most common side effect with busulfan is myelosuppression (see *Cautions and Concerns* and *Warnings*). Common side effects with busulfan injection include black, tarry stools, blood in urine or stools, cough or hoarseness, fever or chills, inflammation of the mouth, lower back or side pain, painful or difficult urination, pinpoint red spots on skin, unusual bleeding or bruising, abdominal pain, anxiety, general fatigue or muscle pain, headache, missed or irregular menstrual periods, nausea, vomiting, diarrhea, decreased appetite, rash, insomnia, and sudden weight loss. A common side effect with oral busulfan is hyperpigmentation (darkening of the skin), particularly in patients with a dark complexion.

Common side effects with altretamine include nausea and vomiting (see *Cautions and Concerns*), peripheral neuropathy, CNS symptoms (e.g., mood disorders, dizziness, vertigo), and myelosuppression (see *Warnings*).

Common side effects with thiotepa include myelosuppression (see *Cautions and Concerns*), nausea, vomiting, decreased appetite, and temporary or permanent sterility.

Common side effects with chlorambucil include black, tarry stools, blood in urine or stools, cough or hoarseness, fever or chills, lower back or side pain, painful or difficult urination, pinpoint red spots on skin, and unusual bleeding or bruising.

Common side effects with cyclophosphamide include leukopenia, hair loss, nausea, vomiting, diarrhea, decreased appetite, sores in mouth or on lips, stopping of menstrual periods in women, bladder irritation, blood in the urine, and decreased sperm production in men (see *Warnings*).

Common side effects with ifosfamide include nausea, vomiting, diarrhea, decreased appetite, hair loss, bladder irritation, blood in the urine (see *Warnings*), frequent or painful urination, kidney impairment, and myelosuppression.

Common side effects with mechlorethamine include nausea, vomiting, taste changes, decreased appetite, hair loss, and myelosuppression (see *Cautions and Concerns*).

Common side effects with melphalan include myelosuppression (see *Warnings*), nausea, vomiting, mouth ulcers, and injection site sores.

Common side effects with carmustine include nausea and vomiting (see *Cautions and Concerns*), decreased appetite, diarrhea, headache, pain along vein during administration, irritation of vein used for giving the drug, and myelosuppression (see *Warnings*).

Common side effects with lomustine include nausea and vomiting (see *Cautions and Concerns*) and myelosuppression (see *Warnings*).

Common side effects with streptozocin include kidney impairment, which usually improves when the drug is stopped (see *Warnings*), nausea, vomiting, liver impairment with yellowing of the skin or eyes (jaundice), and pain or burning in the vein where drug is given (see *Cautions and Concerns*).

Common side effects with dacarbazine include myelosuppression (see *Warnings*), nausea, vomiting, decreased appetite, irritation of vein used for giving the drug (see *Cautions and Concerns*), flulike illness for as long as a week after receiving the drug (fatigue, headache, muscle aches, fever), and hair loss.

Common side effects with temozolomide include myelosuppression (see *Warnings*), nausea, vomiting, diarrhea, constipation, decreased appetite, fatigue, and weakness.

Common side effects with procarbazine include myelosuppression and decreased platelet count with increased risk of bleeding (see *Cautions and Concerns*), nausea, vomiting, drowsiness, depression, difficulty sleeping, nightmares, nervousness, and flulike symptoms (fatigue, headache, muscle aches, fever, stuffy nose).

Antibiotics Common side effects with bleomycin include fever and chills, nausea, vomiting, decreased appetite, hair loss, sores in mouth or on lips, and skin changes, such as darkened, thickened areas, redness, rash, or dry skin peeling at the fingertips.

Common side effects with dactinomycin include nausea; vomiting; diarrhea; decreased appetite; sores in mouth or on lips, esophagus, or rectal area (worse if these areas have been recently treated with radiation—see *Interactions*); darkening of skin along the vein used for giving the drug; rash; and hair loss.

Common side effects with mitomycin include myelosuppression (see *Warnings* and *When Not Advised/Contraindications*), nausea, vomiting, decreased appetite, fever, fatigue, and hair loss.

Antimetabolites Common side effects with azacitidine include anemia; fatigue; nausea; vomiting; diarrhea; constipation; irritation, itching, or redness at the injection site; and fever.

Common side effects with capecitabine include diarrhea (see *Warnings*); nausea; vomiting; decreased appetite; stomach or abdominal pain; pain, swelling, or sores in mouth or on lips; numbness, tingling, or itching of hands and/or feet (see *Cautions and Concerns*); rash or dry skin; fatigue or weakness; and myelosuppression.

Common side effects with cladribine include anemia with increased fatigue, mild nausea, decreased appetite, rash, fever, and headache.

Common side effects with cytarabine include thinned or brittle hair, headache, weakness or achiness, decreased appetite or weight, mouth sores, tingling in the hands or feet, and myelosuppression (see *Warnings*).

Common side effects with decitabine include fatigue, fever, nausea, cough, red spots on the skin, constipation, diarrhea, and hyperglycemia.

Common side effects with floxuridine include decreased appetite, diarrhea, and numbness or tingling in hands and/or feet.

Common side effects with fludarabine include myelosuppression (neutropenia, thrombocytopenia and anemia) (see *Warnings*), fever and chills, infection, nausea, vomiting, and fatigue.

Common side effects with fluorouracil include myelosuppression, darkening of skin and nail beds, nausea, vomiting, decreased appetite, sores in mouth, lips, or throat, thinning hair, diarrhea, brittle nails, increased sensitivity to sun, and dry, flaky, cracking skin. Topical fluorouracil may cause irritation where applied.

Common side effects with gemcitabine include myelosuppression, nausea, vomiting, decreased appetite, and fatigue.

Myelosuppression (see *Warnings*) is a common side effect with hydroxyurea.

Myelosuppression (see *Warnings*) is a common side effect with mercaptopurine.

Common side effects with methotrexate include nausea, vomiting, sores in the mouth or on the lips, diarrhea, increased risk of sunburn, skin changes in areas previously treated with radiation, and decreased appetite.

Common side effects with pemetrexed include myelosuppression, fatigue, nausea, vomiting, diarrhea, constipation, sores in the mouth or on the lips, decreased appetite, rash, skin peeling or itching, and shortness of breath.

Common side effects with pentostatin include myelosuppression, nausea, vomiting, fever, chills, headache, and skin rash.

Common side effects with pralatrexate include mucositis, thrombocytopenia, neutropenia (see *Warnings*), fever, nausea, and fatigue.

Common side effects with thioguanine include nausea, vomiting, myelosuppression, headache, darkening of the skin, weakness, and aching.

Antimitotics   Common side effects with docetaxel include myelosuppression, swelling in hands or feet and shortness of breath (caused by fluid retention), nausea, diarrhea, hair loss, and weakness.

Common side effects with estramustine include breast enlargement (see *Cautions and Concerns*), nipple tenderness, decreased sex drive, itching, dry skin, and night sweats.

Common side effects with paclitaxel include myelosuppression; mild allergic reaction (fever, flushing, itching, rapid heart rate); numbness, tingling, or pain in the hands, feet, or elsewhere; nausea; vomiting; diarrhea; and hair loss.

Common side effects with vinblastine include myelosuppression, mouth sores, and fatigue.

Common side effects with vincristine include constipation, hair loss, and a tired feeling.

Common side effects with vinorelbine include constipation, nausea, vomiting, fatigue, weakness, and myelosuppression.

Epothilones   Common side effects with ixabepilone include fatigue, decreased appetite, hair loss, fever, anemia, joint and muscle pain, headache, nausea, vomiting, diarrhea, constipation, abdominal pain, sores on the lip, in the mouth, and in the esophagus, hand-foot syndrome, dry/peeling skin, and neuropathy (see *Warnings*).

Histone deacetylase inhibitors   The most common side effects with vorinostat are diarrhea, fatigue, nausea, thrombocytopenia, loss of appetite, and persistent abnormal taste.

Hormones   Common side effects with anastrozole include hot flashes, nausea, fatigue, weakness, bone pain, cough, and mood disturbances.

Common side effects with bicalutamide include swelling and tenderness of the breasts and hot flashes.

Common side effects with degarelix include injection site reactions (pain, redness, and swelling), hot flashes, increased weight, fatigue, and increases in some liver enzymes.

Common side effects with exemestane include fatigue and swelling of hands, feet, or ankles.

Common side effects with flutamide include hot flashes with sweating, swelling of the breasts, decreased sexual desire, nipple discharge, impotence, and diarrhea.

Common side effects with fulvestrant include nausea, fatigue, and weight gain.

Common side effects with goserelin include hot flashes, decrease in sexual desire, vaginal bleeding, discontinuation of menstrual periods, vaginal dryness, swelling of breasts in men, impotence, and prostate or breast cancer flare in the first two weeks of treatment (see *Warnings*).

Common side effects with histrelin include hot flashes and fatigue.

Common side effects with letrozole include pain in bones, joints, or muscles, nausea, cough, difficulty breathing, hot flashes, and fatigue (see *Cautions and Concerns*).

Common side effects with leuprolide include hot flashes, headache, dizziness, flare reaction at the start of treatment for prostate cancer, fatigue, bruising and burning reaction in the area of an implant, and discontinuation of menstrual periods in women (which may resume after treatment is stopped).

Common side effects with medroxyprogesterone include swelling from fluid retention, headache, irregular or absent periods, spotting, irritation at injection site, nausea, trouble sleeping, and weight gain or loss.

Common side effects with megestrol include swelling from fluid retention, increased appetite, and weight gain.

Common side effects with nilutamide include hot flashes, headache, insomnia, nausea, constipation, decreased appetite, difficulty breathing, impaired adaptation to the dark (see *Cautions and Concerns*), and back pain.

Common side effects with tamoxifen include fatigue, hot flashes, vaginal discharge, and loss of sex drive in men.

Common side effects with toremifene include hot flashes, sweating, nausea, and vaginal discharge.

Common side effects with triptorelin pamoate include hot flashes, decrease in sexual desire, and bone pain.

Monoclonal antibodies Common side effects with alemtuzumab include mild allergic reaction with first few infusions (e.g., fever, headache, chills, itching, hives, nausea, shortness of breath), myelosuppression (see *Warnings*), fever, nausea, and vomiting.

Common side effects with bevacizumab include high blood pressure (see *Warnings*), headache, mouth sores, diarrhea, constipation, decreased appetite, fatigue, weakness, abdominal pain, nosebleeds, and hair loss.

Common side effects with cetuximab include skin rash (see *Warnings*), headache, diarrhea, fatigue, weakness, low magnesium levels, and infection.

Common side effects with gemtuzumab ozogamicin include chills, fever, nausea, vomiting, and headache.

Common side effects with ibritumomab tiuxetan include nausea, vomiting, abdominal pain, fatigue, myelosuppression (see *Warnings*), dizziness, chills, and fever.

Common side effects with ofatumumab include neutropenia, pneumonia, fever, cough, diarrhea, anemia, fatigue, difficulty breathing, rash, nausea, bronchitis, and upper respiratory tract infections.

The most common side effects with panitumumab are skin rash (see *Warnings*), hypomagnesemia, fingernail and toenail infection, fatigue, abdominal pain, nausea, diarrhea, and constipation.

Common side effects with rituximab include mild to moderate infusion reactions consisting of fever and chills during the first treatment. Other frequent reaction symptoms include nausea, itching, hives, hypotension, headache, bronchospasm, throat irritation, runny nose, rash, vomiting, muscle pain, dizziness, and hypertension.

Common side effects with tositumomab include myelosuppression (see *Cautions and Concerns* and *Warnings*), fever, nausea, abdominal pain, and fatigue.

Common side effects with trastuzumab include fever, nausea, vomiting, diarrhea, infusion reactions (see *Warnings*), infection, cough, headache, fatigue, difficulty breathing, rash, neutropenia, anemia, and muscle pain.

mTOR inhibitors Common side effects with everolimus include mouth sores, weakness, diarrhea, decreased appetite, swelling, shortness of breath, cough, nausea, vomiting, rash, and fever.

Common side effects with temsirolimus include rash, loss of strength, mucositis, nausea, edema, and loss of appetite.

Platinum compounds Common side effects with carboplatin include myelosuppression (see *Warnings*), nausea and vomiting, taste changes, hair loss, weakness, dizziness, and fatigue.

Common side effects with cisplatin include kidney impairment (see *Warnings*); hypomagnesemia; hypokalemia; hypocalcemia; nausea; vomiting; taste changes, including metallic taste of foods; sensation of pins and needles or numbness in hands and/or feet; and swelling in hands, feet, or legs.

Common side effects with oxaliplatin include nausea and vomiting (see *Cautions and Concerns*), numbness and tingling in hands and/or feet due to nerve irritation (see *Warnings*), numbness of lips, skin disorder, diarrhea, abdominal pain, mouth sores, difficulty breathing, fever, and fatigue.

Topoisomerase inhibitors Common side effects with daunorubicin include myelosuppression (see *Warnings*), nausea, vomiting, hair loss, and darkened fingernails and toenails.

Common side effects with daunorubicin liposomal include myelosuppression, loss of appetite, nausea, diarrhea, headache, cough, difficulty breathing, and fatigue.

Common side effects with doxorubicin include myelosuppression (see *Warnings*), decreased appetite, mouth sores, darkening of nail beds and skin creases of hands, hair loss, nausea, and vomiting (see *Cautions and Concerns*).

Common side effects with doxorubicin liposomal include weakness, fatigue, fever, nausea, stomatitis, vomiting, diarrhea, constipation, loss of appetite, hand-foot syndrome (see *Cautions and Concerns*), rash, and myelosuppression.

Common side effects with epirubicin include low blood counts with myelosuppression (see *Warnings*), discontinuation of menstrual periods, nausea, vomiting (see *Cautions and Concerns*), mouth sores, diarrhea, and hair loss.

Common side effects with idarubicin include myelosuppression (see *Warnings*), nausea, vomiting, abdominal pain, decreased appetite, sores in mouth or on lips, hair loss, and skin rash.

Common side effects with mitoxantrone include myelosuppression (see *Warnings*), nausea, vomiting, headache, and sores in mouth or on lips.

The most common side effects with valrubicin are local to the bladder, usually occur during or shortly after instillation, and resolve within one to seven days after the instillate is removed from the bladder. These bladder problems include frequent urination, difficult or painful urination, urinary urgency, bladder spasm, blood in the urine, bladder pain, urinary incontinence, and cystitis.

Common side effects with irinotecan include diarrhea (see *Warnings*), nausea, vomiting, myelosuppression, hair loss, abdominal pain, decreased appetite, fatigue, and weakness.

Common side effects with topotecan include myelosuppression (see *Warnings*), nausea, vomiting, and hair loss.

Common side effects with etoposide include myelosuppression (see *Warnings*), nausea, vomiting, decreased appetite, and hair loss.

Common side effects with teniposide include myelosuppression (see *Warnings*), mouth sores, nausea, vomiting, and diarrhea.

Tyrosine kinase inhibitors Common side effects with dasatinib include swelling around the eyes or in the hands or feet, nausea, mild diarrhea, fatigue, headache, fever, muscle or bone pain, skin rash, shortness of breath, and myelosuppression (see *Warnings*).

Common side effects with erlotinib include skin rash, diarrhea, fatigue, and decreased appetite.

Common side effects with gefitinib include skin rash and diarrhea.

Common side effects with imatinib include nausea, vomiting, swelling around the eyes or feet (see *Cautions and Concerns*), weight gain, diarrhea, muscle aches and pains, skin rash, fatigue, headache, joint and bone pain, and abdominal pain.

Common side effects with lapatinib include diarrhea (see *Cautions and Concerns*), fatigue, nausea, and rash.

Common side effects with nilotinib include fatigue, rash, itching, nausea, vomiting, diarrhea, constipation, headache, and myelosuppression (see *Cautions and Concerns*).

Common side effects with pazopanib include diarrhea, hypertension (see *Cautions and Concerns*), hair color changes, nausea, loss of appetite, and vomiting.

Common side effects with sorafenib include diarrhea, fatigue, rash, itching, and redness, pain, swelling, or blisters on hands or feet (see *Cautions and Concerns*).

Common side effects with sunitinib include myelosuppression, nausea, vomiting, diarrhea, mouth sores, decreased appetite, fatigue, and yellowing of the skin.

Retinoids Common side effects with bexarotene include increased hyperlipidemia (see *Warnings*), headache, diarrhea, and with the gel, itching, rash, and pain where applied.

Common side effects with tretinoin include headache, fever, dry mouth, bone pain, nausea, vomiting, rash, and decreased appetite.

Proteasome inhibitors Common side effects with bortezomib include fatigue, weakness, nausea or vomiting and/or diarrhea (see *Cautions and Concerns*), constipation, and new or worsening peripheral neuropathy (see *Warnings*).

Miscellaneous Common side effects with aldesleukin include flulike symptoms (may include fever, chills, tiredness, headache, muscle and joint pain), low blood pressure (see *Cautions and Concerns*), nausea, vomiting, diarrhea, weakness, confusion, shortness of breath, flushing of the face, rash, itching, and low urine output.

Common side effects with asparaginase include allergic reactions, hyperglycemia (see *Cautions and Concerns*), pancreatitis (see *Warnings*), nausea, vomiting, loss of appetite, fatigue, drowsiness, depression, fever, and chills.

Common side effects with denileukin include infusion reactions (see *Warnings*), flulike symptoms (e.g., fever, chills, weakness, muscle aches), rash, loss of appetite, nausea, vomiting, edema, and low blood pressure.

Common side effects with lenalidomide include myelosuppression (see *Warnings*), diarrhea, itching, rash, and fatigue.

Common side effects with thalidomide include severe birth defects (see *Warnings*), sleepiness, dizziness, headache, fever, and rash.

Interactions

Additive myelosuppression may result when myelosuppressive antineoplastics are used with other drugs that cause myelosuppression (e.g., basiliximab, clozapine, zidovudine).

Alkylating agents Itraconazole decreases busulfan clearance (the rate at which the active drug is removed from the body) by up to 25 percent; phenytoin increases the clearance of busulfan by 15 percent or more.

Concurrent administration of altretamine and MAOIs may cause severe orthostatic hypotension (see *Warnings*).

It is not advisable to combine, simultaneously or sequentially, cancer chemotherapeutic agents or a cancer chemotherapeutic agent and a therapeutic modality having the same mechanism of action. Therefore, thiotepa combined with other alkylating agents such as nitrogen mustard or cyclophosphamide or thiotepa combined with irradiation would serve to intensify toxicity rather than to enhance therapeutic response. If these agents must follow each other, it is important that recovery from the first agent, as indicated by white blood cell count, be complete before therapy with the second agent is instituted. Other drugs known to produce myelosuppression should be avoided along with thiotepa.

Cyclophosphamide can increase the effects of succinylcholine, a drug used for anesthesia during surgery. Daunorubicin taken along with cyclophosphamide can increase the risk of heart damage. Doxorubicin given along with cyclophosphamide may increase the risk of bleeding in the bladder. Cyclophosphamide can also be harmful if taken with colchicine or probenecid.

Severe kidney failure has been reported in patients treated with a single dose of intravenous melphalan followed by standard oral doses of cyclosporine. Cisplatin may affect melphalan by inducing kidney impairment and subsequently reducing melphalan clearance. Intravenous melphalan may also reduce the threshold for carmustine lung toxicity. There are no known drug/drug interactions with oral melphalan.

Greater myelotoxicity (e.g., leukopenia and neutropenia) have been reported when carmustine was combined with cimetidine.

Phenytoin may reduce the effects of streptozocin. Drugs that are eliminated by the kidney may increase the risk of kidney impairment if they are taken during the same time as streptozocin (e.g., medicines for pain, inflammation, and fever [such as aspirin and NSAIDs]). A reduction of the doxorubicin dosage should be considered in patients receiving streptozocin concurrently, as streptozocin may prolong the elimination half-life of doxorubicin and may lead to severe myelosuppression.

Administration of valproic acid decreases clearance of temozolomide by about 5 percent. The clinical implication of this effect is not known. Because food reduces the rate and extent of oral temozolomide absorption, consistency of administration with respect to food is recommended.

For interactions with procarbazine, see *Warnings.*

Antibiotics Because bleomycin is eliminated predominantly through the urine, the administration of drugs toxic to the kidneys with bleomycin may affect its kidney clearance.

An increased incidence of gastrointestinal toxicity and myelosuppression has been reported with combined therapy incorporating dactinomycin and radiation. Moreover, the normal skin as well as the mouth and throat mucus may show early erythema (redness). Erythema from previous radiation therapy may be reactivated by dactinomycin alone, even when radiotherapy was administered many months earlier and especially when the interval between the two forms of therapy is brief. This potentiation of radiation effect represents a special problem when the radiotherapy involves the mucous membrane.

For interactions with mitomycin, see *Cautions and Concerns.*

Antimetabolites Capecitabine must be taken with food to slow down its absorption into the body. If taken without food, it reaches higher levels in the body, which may increase dangerous side effects. Aluminum- and magnesium-containing antacids may increase concentrations of capecitabine. Capecitabine may interact with warfarin and increase bleeding risk (see *Warnings*). Concomitant use of leucovorin may increase the risk of capecitabine toxicity. Capecitabine may increase phenytoin levels, and the phenytoin dose may need to be reduced.

Cytarabine may decrease digoxin absorption and blood levels even several days after stopping chemotherapy.

The use of fludarabine in combination with pentostatin is not recommended due to the risk of severe pulmonary toxicity.

Leucovorin calcium may enhance the toxicity of fluorouracil.

When allopurinol and mercaptopurine are administered concomitantly, the dose of mercaptopurine must be reduced to one-third to one-quarter of the usual dose to avoid severe side effects. Because methotrexate increases blood levels of mercaptopurine, the dose of mercaptopurine may need to be reduced. Mercaptopurine may decrease the anticoagulant effect of warfarin.

NSAIDs and salicylates may elevate the effects of methotrexate to potentially harmful levels (see *Warnings*). Probenecid is known to inhibit the excretion of methotrexate through the kidneys. Toxicity may be increased when methotrexate is used along with either phenytoin or sulfonamides. In the treatment of patients with osteosarcoma, caution must be exercised if high-dose methotrexate is administered in combination with cisplatin or other antineoplastics toxic to the kidneys. Because methotrexate increases blood levels of mercaptopurine, this combination may require mercaptopurine dose reduction. Penicillin given along with methotrexate increases the risk of a severe adverse reaction. Methotrexate may decrease the clearance of theophylline. Vitamin preparations containing folic acid or its derivatives may decrease responses to methotrexate.

Ibuprofen can decrease the clearance of pemetrexed. Caution should be used when administering ibuprofen concurrently with pemetrexed to patients with mild to moderate kidney impairment. Patients with mild to moderate kidney impairment should avoid taking other NSAIDs with short elimination half-lives (e.g., aspirin, diclofenac, flurbiprofen, ketoprofen) for a period of two days before, the day of, and two days following administration of pemetrexed.

The combined use of pentostatin and fludarabine phosphate is not recommended because it may be associated with an increased risk of fatal pulmonary toxicity. Acute pulmonary edema and hypotension leading to death have been re^mbination with carmustine, etoposide, and high-dose cyclophosphamide (see *Warnings*).

Probenecid, NSAIDs, and trimethoprim/sulfamethaxazole may result in delayed renal clearance of pralatrexate.

Aminosalicylate derivatives (e.g., olsalazine, mesalazine, or sulfasalazine) inhibit the TPMT enzyme and should be administered with caution to patients receiving thioguanine therapy.

Antimitotics The metabolism of docetaxel may be modified by the concomitant administration of compounds that induce, inhibit, or are metabolized by cytochrome P450 3A4, such as cyclosporine, ketoconazole, and erythromycin. Caution should be exercised with these drugs when treating patients receiving docetaxel, as there is a potential for a significant interaction. Milk, milk products, and calcium-rich foods or drugs may impair the absorption of estramustine.

In some cases, bone suppression has been more profound when paclitaxel has been given after cisplatin than when given before cisplatin. Clinical reports suggest that blood levels of doxorubicin (and its active metabolite) may be increased when paclitaxel and doxorubicin are used in combination.

The simultaneous administration of phenytoin and vinblastine or vincristine has been reported to lead to reduced blood levels of phenytoin and to have increased seizure activity. Hearing impairment may be enhanced when vinblastine or vincristine are used with other drugs that affect the ear (e.g., platinum-containing antineoplastic agents, such as cisplatin, and aminoglycosides).

Acute pulmonary reactions have been reported with vinorelbine used in conjunction with mitomycin. The use of vinorelbine and paclitaxel, either concomitantly or sequentially, may increase the risk of neuropathy.

Epothilones Ketoconazole, itraconazole, voriconazole, atazanavir, saquinavir, ritonovir, fosamprenavir, indinavir, nelfinavir, delaviridine, clarithromycin, erythromycin, telithromycin, and nefazodone may interfere with the breakdown (metabolism) and increase the toxicity of ixabepilone. Grapefruit juice may increase blood levels of ixabepilone and should be avoided. Dexamethasone, phenytoin, carbemazepine, phenobarbital, rifampin, rifapentin, rifabutin, and Saint-John's-wort can lower blood levels of ixabepilone and decrease its effectiveness.

Histone deacetylase inhibitors Prolongation of the INR has been observed in patients receiving vorinostat concomitantly with warfarin. Severe thrombocytopenia and gastrointestinal bleeding have been reported with concomitant use of vorinostat and other HDAC inhibitors (e.g., valproic acid). Platelet counts should be monitored every two weeks for the first two months when two HDAC inhibitors are used concomitantly. Vorinostat should not be used concomitantly with drugs that cause QT interval prolongation.

Hormones Drugs that contain estrogen and tamoxifen should not be used with anastrozole, as they may reduce the action of anastrozole.

Bicalutamide can increase the risk of bleeding when taken with warfarin.

Drugs that are CYP 3A4 inducers, such as rifampin, phenytoin, carbamazepine, phenobarbital, and Saint-John's-wort, may lead to increased clearance and decreased effects of exemestane.

Increases in prothrombin time have been noted in patients receiving warfarin therapy and flutamide.

Tamoxifen may reduce blood levels of letrozole.

Nilutamide can increase the risk of bleeding when taken with warfarin. Because of the possibility of an intolerance to alcohol (facial flushes, malaise, hypotension) following ingestion of nilutamide, it is recommended that intake of alcoholic beverages be avoided by patients who experience this reaction. This effect has been reported in about 5 percent of patients treated with nilutamide.

Tamoxifen can interfere with the effects of warfarin (see *When Not Advised/Contraindications*). When other cytotoxic agents are used in combination with tamoxifen, there is an increased risk of thromboembolic events (blood clots).

Toremifene may increase the effects of warfarin.

Monoclonal antibodies Rituximab may interact with cisplatin to cause kidney impairment.

Due to the frequent occurrence of severe and prolonged thrombocytopenia with tositumomab, the potential benefits of medications that interfere with platelet function and/or anticoagulation should be weighed against the potential increased risk of bleeding and hemorrhage.

In clinical trials, trastuzumab remains in the body longer when combined with paclitaxel.

mTOR inhibitors Ketoconazole, itraconazole, clarithromycin, atazanavir, indinavir, nefazodone, nelfinavir, ritonavir, saquinavir, telithromycin, and voriconazole may increase blood levels of temsirolimus and should be avoided. Grapefruit juice may also increase levels of temsirolimus and should be avoided. Dexamethasone, phenytoin, carbamazepine, rifampin, rifabutin, rifapentin, phenobarbital, and Saint-John's-wort may decrease blood levels of temsirolimus and should be avoided.

Platinum compounds Drugs that cause damage to the kidneys or hearing may have increased effect when used with platinum compounds.

Cisplatin may lessen the effectiveness of anticonvulsants (e.g., phenytoin, fosphenytoin, and carbamazepine).

Topoisomerase inhibitors Use of daunorubicin in a patient who has previously received doxorubicin increases the risk of heart damage. Cyclophosphamide used concurrently with daunorubicin may also result in increased heart damage. Dosage reduction of daunorubicin may be required when used concurrently with other myelosuppressive agents.

Drugs that may increase the levels/effects of doxorubicin include certain antibiotics (clarithromycin, erythromycin), chloroquine, dolasetron, droperidol, foscarnet, drugs used to control heart rhythm (e.g., amiodarone), drugs used for mental problems, psychosis, or depression (e.g., amitriptyline, chlorpromazine, fluphenazine, haloperidol, pimozide, prochlorperazine, risperidone, thioridazine, ziprasidone), methadone, paclitaxel, progesterone, verapamil, cyclosporine, cytarabine, streptozocin, or saquinavir. An increased risk of bleeding in the bladder may occur if doxorubicin is given with cyclophosphamide. Phenobarbital lowers the effectiveness of doxorubicin.

Cimetidine and verapamil can raise the levels and risk of toxicity of epirubicin.

Phenytoin, phenobarbital, carbamazepine, and Saint-John's-wort may decrease the effects of irinotecan. Saint-John's-wort should be discontinued at least two weeks prior to the first cycle of irinotecan and is contraindicated during irinotecan therapy. Ketoconazole may increase the effects of irinotecan. Patients should discontinue ketoconazole at least one week prior to starting irinotecan, and ketoconazole is contraindicated during irinotecan therapy. The adverse side effects caused by irinotecan, such as myelosuppression and diarrhea, may be increased by other antineoplastics having similar adverse effects. Patients who have previously received pelvic/abdominal radiation are at increased risk of severe myelosuppression following the administration of irinotecan. Laxative use during irinotecan treatment can be expected to worsen the incidence or severity of diarrhea. Diuretics should be withheld during treatment with irinotecan and, certainly, during periods of active vomiting or diarrhea.

Cyclosporine, ketoconazole, ritonavir, and saquinavir may increase the amount of topotecan in the blood.

Etoposide may increase the effects of warfarin. Cyclosporine may increase blood levels of etoposide.

Tolbutamide may increase blood levels of teniposide.

Tyrosine kinase inhibitors Because the stomach needs acid to absorb dasatinib, antacids should be taken at least two hours before or after taking dasatinib. Other drugs commonly used to treat heartburn, reflux, or ulcers, including H_2 antagonists and proton pump inhibitors, also reduce acid levels in the stomach and may decrease dasatinib levels. Saint-John's-wort may decrease blood levels of dasatinib and should not be taken along with this drug. Aspirin, warfarin, clopidogrel, ticlopidine, and vitamin E could affect the body's ability to stop bleeding when taken along with dasatinib. Dasatinib may increase blood levels of alfentanil, cyclosporine, fentanyl, pimozide, quinidine, simvastatin, sirolimus, tacrolimus, and ergotamine.

Atazanavir, clarithromycin, indinavir, itraconazole, nefazodone, nelfinavir, ritonavir, saquinavir, telithromycin, ketoconazole, voriconazole, and grapefruit juice may increase blood levels of erlotinib. Cigarette smoking has been shown to reduce the effectiveness of erlotinib. Patients should be advised to stop smoking; however, if they continue to smoke, a cautious increase in the dose of erlotinib may be considered while monitoring the patient's safety.

Gefitinib increases the effect of metoprolol and may increase the risk of bleeding in patients taking warfarin. Cimetidine, phenytoin, rifampin, ranitidine, and sodium bicarbonate may decrease the effectiveness of gefitinib.

Imatinib may increase blood levels of cyclosporine, dihydropyridine calcium channel blockers, eletriptan, pimozide, simvastatin, triazolam, alprazolam, and warfarin. Acetaminophen and alcohol should not be used with imatinib to avoid stressing the liver. Saint-John's-wort, carbamazepine, dexamethasone, phenobarbital,

phenytoin, rifabutin, and rifampin may reduce the effectiveness of imatinib. Grapefruit juice, clarithromycin, erythromycin, itraconazole, ketoconazole, voriconazole, and aprepitant may increase blood levels of imatinib.

Ketoconazole, itraconazole, clarithromycin, atazanavir, indinavir, nefazodone, nelfinavir, ritonavir, saquinavir, telithromycin, voriconazole, and grapefruit juice may increase blood levels of lapatinib and pazopanib and should be avoided. Dexamethasone, phenytoin, carbamazepine, rifampin, rifabutin, rifapentin, phenobarbital, and Saint-John's-wort may decrease blood levels of lapatinib and should be avoided.

Sorafenib may increase blood levels of docetaxel and doxorubicin. Both increases and decreases in the exposure of fluorouracil were observed when used along with sorafenib; thus, caution is recommended when sorafenib is coadministered with fluorouracil/leucovorin. Saint-John's-wort, carbamazepine, dexamethasone, phenobarbital, phenytoin, rifabutin, and rifampin may reduce the effectiveness of sorafenib.

Ketoconazole, itraconazole, voriconazole, nelfinavir, ritonavir, saquinavir, clarithromycin, telithromycin, nefazodone, and grapefruit juice may increase blood levels of sunitinib. Dexamethasone, phenytoin, carbamazepine, phenobarbital, rifampin, rifabutin, and Saint-John's-wort may reduce blood levels of sunitinib.

Retinoids Retinoids must not be administered in combination with vitamin A because symptoms of hypervitaminosis A (an abnormal condition resulting from taking vitamin A excessively), such as nausea and vomiting, headache, dizziness, blurred vision, and muscular incoordination, could be aggravated. Retinoids should always be taken with food; failure to do so will significantly decrease absorption.

Ketoconazole, itraconazole, erythromycin, gemfibrozil, and grapefruit juice may increase the effects of bexarotene. Rifampin, phenytoin, and phenobarbital may decrease the effects of bexarotene. Because concomitant administration of bexarotene capsules and gemfibrozil have caused substantial increases in blood levels of bexarotene, these drugs should not be used together.

Proteasome inhibitors Ketoconazole and ritonavir may increase the effects of bortezomib.

Miscellaneous Reduced kidney and liver function secondary to aldesleukin treatment may delay elimination of concomitant medications and increase the risk of adverse events from those drugs. Hypersensitivity reactions have been reported in patients receiving combination regimens containing sequential high dose aldesleukin and dacarbazine, cisplatin, tamoxifen, and interferon-alfa. Myocardial infarction, myocarditis, ventricular dysfunction, and severe rhabdomyolysis appear to be increased in patients receiving aldesleukin and interferon-alfa concurrently.

Thalidomide may enhance the sedative activity of alcohol, ethanol, phenobarbital, reserpine, and chlorpromazine. Medications known to be associated with peripheral neuropathy (e.g., ribavirin, metronidazole, altretamine, bortezomib, didanosine, etravirine, stavudine) should be used with caution in patients receiving thalidomide.

Sales/Statistics

According to a MarketResearch.com report in December 2008, the total antineoplastics market was forecast to be valued at $43 billion in 2013. The IMS Institute for Healthcare Informatics (the public reporting arm of IMS, a pharmaceutical market intelligence firm) later reported oncologics to be the number-one drug class by spending in 2010, with $307.4 billion in sales. IMS listed two antineoplastics on their top 20 drug products by spending—#14, Avastin ($3.1 billion), and #20, Rituxan ($2.8 billion).

Demographics and Cultural Groups

According to the American Cancer Society's *Cancer Facts & Figures for African Americans 2011–2012,* "African Americans have the highest death rate and shortest survival of any racial and ethnic group in the United States for most cancers. The causes of these inequalities are complex and are thought to reflect social and economic disparities more than biologic differences associated with race. These include inequalities in work, wealth, income, education, housing, and overall standard of living, as well as barriers to high-quality cancer prevention, early detection, and treatment services."

Development History

The beginnings of antineoplastics can be traced back to the battlefields of Italy in 1943 and the chemical warfare agent nitrogen mustard. After an accident had exposed civilians and soldiers to the mustard gas, subsequent autopsies revealed profound lymphoid and myeloid suppression in those exposed. Pharmacologists hired by the U.S. Department of Defense to investigate potential medical applications of chemical warfare agents

CANCER INCIDENCE RATES BY RACE		
Race/Ethnicity	Male	Female
All Races	541.8 per 100,000 men	408.5 per 100,000 women
White	544.3 per 100,000 men	420.5 per 100,000 women
Black	633.7 per 100,000 men	398.9 per 100,000 women
Asian/Pacific Islander	349.1 per 100,000 men	287.5 per 100,000 women
American Indian/Alaska Native	331.0 per 100,000 men	302.2 per 100,000 women
Hispanic	409.7 per 100,000 men	312.5 per 100,000 women

Source: SEER Cancer Statistics Review, 1975–2006, National Cancer Institute. Bethesda, Md., http://seer.cancer.gov/csr/1975_2006/, based on November 2008 SEER data submission, posted to the SEER Web site, 2009. Available online. URL: http://seer.cancer.gov/statfacts/html/all.html. Downloaded on April 17, 2009.

reasoned that mustard gas might have possible use as a treatment for Hodgkin's lymphoma. Further research resulted in the drug mechlorethamine, which was approved by the Food and Drug Administration (FDA) on March 15, 1949.

The next major advance in antineoplastics occurred following World War II, when Dr. Sidney Farber, a pediatric pathologist at Harvard Medical School, studied the effects of folic acid on children with leukemia. Spurred on by the results, Farber worked with the Research Division of Lederle Laboratories, which had been seeking drugs that resembled folic acid. Their collaboration resulted in the development of methotrexate, which was approved by the FDA in 1953.

In the meantime, Dr. Joseph Burchenal, an oncologist at Memorial Sloan-Kettering Cancer Center in New York, worked with chemists at the Burroughs Wellcome Company to develop an antimetabolite. Their work culminated in the discovery of mercaptopurine, which gained FDA approval on September 11, 1953.

In response to these early successes, the U.S. Congress created a National Cancer Chemotherapy Service Center (NCCSC) at the National Cancer Institute to promote drug discovery for cancer. Up to that point, pharmaceutical companies had not shown great interest in developing antineoplastics. The NCCSC developed methodologies, cell lines, and other tools crucial for drug development in this field.

With more incentive and interest in discovering new cancer treatments, drug companies began developing antineoplastics in earnest.

Approval Time Line for Other Antineoplastics Described in this Section

Busulfan—June 26, 1954
Chlorambucil—March 18, 1957
Thiotepa—March 9, 1959
Cyclophosphamide—November 16, 1959
Medroxyprogesterone—September 23, 1960
Fluorouracil injection—April 25, 1962 (topical fluorouracil—July 29, 1970)

Vincristine—July 10, 1963
Melphalan tablet—January 17, 1964 (melphalan injection—1992)
Dactinomycin—December 10, 1964
Vinblastine—November 5, 1965
Thioguanine—January 18, 1966
Hydroxyurea—December 7, 1967
Cytarabine—June 17, 1969
Procarbazine—July 22, 1969
Floxuridine—December 18, 1970
Megestrol—August 18, 1971
Bleomycin—July 31, 1973
Dacarbazine—May 27, 1975
Lomustine—August 4, 1976
Carmustine injectable—March 7, 1977 (wafer implant—September 23, 1996)
Cisplatin—December 19, 1978
Daunorubicin—December 19, 1979
Mitomycin—August 24, 1981
Estramustine—December 24, 1981
Streptozocin—May 7, 1982
Etoposide—November 10, 1983
Leuprolide—April 9, 1985
Doxorubicin—May 20, 1985
Tamoxifen—December 10, 1985
Mitoxantrone—December 23, 1987
Ifosfamide—December 30, 1988
Carboplatin—March 3, 1989
Goserelin—December 29, 1989
Idarubicin—September 27, 1990
Altretamine—December 26, 1990
Fludarabine—April 22, 1991
Pentostatin—October 11, 1991
Aldesleukin—May 5, 1992
Teniposide—July 14, 1992
Paclitaxel—December 29, 1992
Cladribine—February 26, 1993
Asparaginase—February 1, 1994
Vinorelbine—December 23, 1994
Bicalutamide—October 4, 1995
Doxorubicin liposomal—November 17, 1995
Tretinoin—November 22, 1995
Anastrozole—December 27, 1995
Daunorubicin liposomal—April 30, 1996
Gemcitabine—May 2, 1996
Docetaxel—May 14, 1996

Topotecan—May 28, 1996 (capsule form—
    October 15, 2007)
Irinotecan—June 14, 1996
Flutamide—September 19, 1996
Nilutamide—September 19, 1996
Toremifene—May 30, 1997
Letrozole—July 30, 1997
Rituximab—November 26, 1997
Capecitabine—April 30, 1998
Thalidomide—July 16, 1998
Trastuzumab—September 25, 1998
Valrubicin—Ocotber 1998 (Valrubicin was
    originally approved by the FDA for CIS
    in October 1998 and marketed by Anthra
    Pharmaceuticals, Inc. In 2002, Anthra vol-
    untarily withdrew the medication from the
    U.S. market because of a formulation issue
    with an inactive component. On February
    27, 2009, Indevus Pharmaceuticals, Inc.,
    the previous owner of Valstar, received FDA
    approval to reintroduce the drug after mod-
    ifying the formulation. On March 23, 2009,
    Endo acquired Indevus and began prepar-
    ing to relaunch the drug.)
Denileukin—February 5, 1999
Temozolomide—August 11, 1999
Epirubicin—September 16, 1999
Exemestane—October 21, 1999
Bexarotene capsules—December 29, 1999
    (gel—June 28, 2000)
Gemtuzumab ozogamicin—May 18, 2000
Triptorelin pamoate—June 15, 2000
Alemtuzumab—May 7, 2001
Imatinib—May 10, 2001
Ibritumomab tiuxetan—February 19, 2002
Fulvestrant—April 25, 2002
Oxaliplatin—August 12, 2002
Gefitinib—May 5, 2003
Bortezomib—May 13, 2003
Tositumomab—June 27, 2003
Pemetrexed—February 5, 2004
Cetuximab—February 12, 2004
Bevacizumab—February 26, 2004
Azacitidine—May 19, 2004
Histrelin—October 13, 2004
Erlotinib—November 18, 2004

Sorafenib—December 20, 2005
Lenalidomide—December 27, 2005
Sunitinib—January 26, 2006
Decitabine—May 2, 2006
Dasatinib—June 28, 2006
Panitumumab—September 27, 2006
Vorinostat—October 6, 2006
Lapatinib—March 13, 2007
Temsirolimus—May 30, 2007
Ixabepilone—October 16, 2007
Nilotinib—October 29, 2007
Degarelix—December 24, 2008
Everolimus—March 30, 2009
Pralatrexate—September 25, 2009
Pazopanib—October 19, 2009
Ofatumumab—October 26, 2009

Future Drugs

The Office of Oncology Drug Products (OODP), established in 2005, is responsible for making safe and effective drug and therapeutic biologic treatments for cancer available to the U.S. public. According to Richard Pazdur, M.D., OODP director, Investigational New Drug (IND) applications for cancer drugs have increased dramatically in recent years, rising from 925 in 2003 to more than 1,400 in 2008.

In April 2009, the National Cancer Institute listed more than 8,000 clinical trials actively soliciting participants to test new drugs or new indications for current drugs.

The following is but a representative sample of some of the new drugs in development.

Archexin, also known as RX-0201 (Rexahn Pharmaceuticals, Inc.), is a first-in-class signal inhibitor that directly blocks the production of Akt, a protein kinase that plays a key role in cancer progression. Archexin is in clinical trials for advanced pancreatic and kidney cancers.

Deforolimus, also known as AP23573 and MK-8669 (ARIAD Pharmaceuticals), is an mTOR inhibitor. At least five cancer indications will be pursued for deforolimus, including sarcomas and endometrial, prostate, breast, and non-small-cell lung cancers.

MDV3100 (Medivation Inc.) is an investigational novel small-molecule androgen receptor antagonist that is one of a series of small molecule compounds, known as the MDV300 series, being developed to treat castration-resistant and hormone-sensitive prostate cancer.

NPI-2358 (Nereus Pharmaceuticals, Inc.) is a vascular disrupting agent. The formation of new blood vessels (angiogenesis) is an important component of tumor growth, and vascular disrupting agents are intended to target the differences between these tumor blood vessels and the blood vessels in normal tissues. In addition, NPI-2358 causes cell apoptosis. It is in clinical trials for the treatment of non-small-cell lung cancer.

Picoplatin (Poniard Pharmaceuticals, Inc.) is a new generation platinum agent that has an improved safety profile compared to existing platinum-based compounds and was designed to overcome platinum resistance. It causes apoptosis (cell death) by binding to DNA and interfering with DNA replication and transcription. Picoplatin is in trials for the treatment of patients with recurrent small-cell lung cancer.

antiobesity agents Drugs used to reduce weight and control obesity, or the accumulation of body fat. Obesity is a chronic disease that often requires long-term treatment to promote and sustain weight loss. The World Health Organization has estimated that worldwide, more than 1 billion adults are overweight, with at least 300 million of them being obese. Nearly 134 million American adults (66 percent of the population) are considered overweight (body mass index [BMI] of 25–29.9 kg/m^2) or obese (BMI of $\geq$ 30 kg/m^2), with nearly one-third (63.6 million or 31.4 percent) in the obese range. Body mass index is a measure of weight in relation to height. A BMI of 18.5 to 24.9 kg/m^2 is considered normal. Results from the 2001–2004 National Health and Nutrition Examination Survey (NHANES) indicated that an estimated 17.5 percent of children (age six

to 11) and 17 percent of adolescents (age 12 to 19) are overweight. This represents a 54 percent increase from the overweight estimates obtained from NHANES III (1988–94). (NHANES I, II, and III were survey cycles conducted in the 1970s, 1980s, and early 1990s. Since 1999, NHANES has become a continuous survey.) The data for adolescents are of notable concern because overweight adolescents are at increased risk to become overweight adults. The 2001–04 findings for children and adolescents suggest the likelihood of another generation of overweight adults who may be at risk for subsequent overweight- and obesity-related health conditions.

Classes

Antiobesity agents are divided into two classes, according to their mechanism of action:

- *Anorexiants* (also called anorectants, anorexigenics, appetite suppressants) These reduce the desire to eat. *Examples:* benzphetamine (Didrex), diethylpropion, phendimetrazine (Bontril, Plegine), phentermine (Adipex-P, Ionamin), and sibutramine (Meridia).

- *Lipase inhibitors* These reduce the body's ability to absorb dietary fat. *Example:* orlistat (Xenical).

Amphetamines are also a type of appetite suppressant. However, these drugs are currently not recommended for the treatment of obesity because of their strong potential for abuse and dependence.

How They Work

Anorexiants promote weight loss by decreasing appetite or increasing the feeling of being full. They make the person feel less hungry by changing levels of one or more brain chemicals (called neurotransmitters) that control mood and appetite. It is not known exactly how all anorexiants work, but they are believed to work in part by acting on the appetite center in the brain to cause a temporary reduction in hunger or craving for food. Sibutramine works to suppress the appetite primarily by inhibiting the reuptake of the neurotransmitters norepinephrine and serotonin.

Orlistat works by reducing the body's ability to absorb dietary fat by about 30 percent. It does this by blocking the enzyme lipase, which breaks down dietary fat for use by the body. When fat is not broken down, the body cannot absorb it, so fewer calories are taken in.

Approved Uses

Because these drugs are intended to alter one of the fundamental processes of the human body, prescription antiobesity drugs are approved only for those with a BMI of ≥ 30 kg/m^2, or for those with a BMI of ≥ 27 kg/m^2 if they have obesity-related conditions, such as hypertension (high blood pressure), dyslipidemia (abnormal amounts of cholesterol in the blood), or Type 2 diabetes.

Anorexiants are to be used as a short-term (a few weeks) supplement to calorie restriction and exercise in the management of obesity. Sibutramine is approved for longer-term use, although its safety and effectiveness have not been tested beyond two years.

Orlistat is approved for obesity management including weight loss and weight maintenance when used along with a reduced-calorie diet. Orlistat is also approved to reduce the risk for weight regain after prior weight loss. The safety and effectiveness of orlistat have not been tested beyond four years.

Off-Label Uses

The use of more than one weight-loss medication at a time (combined drug treatment) is considered an off-label use. Little information is available about the safety or effectiveness of drug combinations for weight loss, including fluoxetine/phentermine, phendimetrazine/phentermine, orlistat/sibutramine, herbal combinations, or others. Using weight-loss medications other than sibutramine or orlistat for more than a few weeks is also considered off-label use.

Administration

Antiobesity drugs are administered orally as tablets, capsules, or sustained-release tablets/capsules.

Cautions and Concerns

With any antiobesity agent, the potential exists for misuse in inappropriate patient populations (e.g., patients with anorexia nervosa or bulimia).

Insulin requirements in diabetes mellitus may change in association with use of antiobesity drugs and the accompanying dietary restrictions.

Psychological disturbances have been reported in patients who receive an anorexiant together with a calorie-restricted diet.

Caution should be taken in prescribing anorexiants for patients with even mild hypertension. The least amount feasible should be prescribed or dispensed at one time in order to minimize the possibility of overdosage or abuse.

Currently, all anorexiants are controlled substances, meaning doctors need to follow certain restrictions when prescribing them. Anorexiants are chemically and pharmacologically related to amphetamines and have abuse potential. Although abuse and dependence are not common with nonamphetamine appetite-suppressant medications, doctors should be cautious when they prescribe these drugs for patients with a history of alcohol or other drug abuse. If psychological dependence or severe social dysfunction occurs while using anorexiants, the dosage should be gradually reduced to avoid withdrawal symptoms.

Anorexiants may produce dizziness, extreme fatigue, and depression after abrupt discontinuation of prolonged high-dose therapy. Therefore, patients should observe caution while driving or performing other tasks requiring alertness.

Patients with a history of seizure disorders who are receiving diethylpropion may experience a recurrence of seizures. During clinical testing, seizures were reported in < 0.1 percent of patients receiving sibutramine. Thus, sibutramine should be used cautiously in patients with a history of seizure disorders and should be discontinued in any patient who develops seizures.

Bruising and prolonged bleeding have been reported in patients taking sibutramine. Although the cause has not been determined, caution is advised in patients predisposed to bleeding events and those taking medications known to affect platelet function.

Sibutramine can cause dilation of the pupils and hence should be used with caution in patients with narrow-angle glaucoma.

Gastrointestinal events (see *Side Effects*) may increase when orlistat is taken with a diet high in fat. The daily intake of fat should be distributed over three main meals. If orlistat is taken with any one meal very high in fat, the possibility of gastrointestinal effects increases.

The use of orlistat may lead to impaired absorption of fat-soluble vitamins (A, D, E, and K). Therefore, patients should be instructed to take a daily multivitamin supplement at least two hours before or after the orlistat.

Weight-loss induction by antiobesity drugs may be accompanied by improved metabolic control in patients with diabetes, which might require a dosage reduction of oral hypoglycemic medications (e.g., sulfonylureas, metformin, etc.) or insulin.

Warnings

Tolerance to anorexiants may develop within a few weeks. If tolerance does develop, the recommended dose should not be exceeded in an attempt to increase the effect; rather, the drug should be discontinued.

Sibutramine may cause increased blood pressure and heart rate. The FDA recommends that all patients taking sibutramine have their blood pressure monitored on a regular basis.

Organic causes of obesity (e.g., hypothyroidism) should be excluded before prescribing antiobesity drugs.

When Not Advised (Contraindications)

People with a history of cardiovascular disease (coronary artery disease, congestive heart failure, stroke, cardiac arrhythmias), hyperthyroidism, or glaucoma should not use anorexiants.

Phendimetrazine, phentermine, sibutramine, and orlistat have not been well studied in pregnant patients and should be used only if the potential benefits greatly outweigh the potential hazards. Benzphetamine is contraindicated during pregnancy. Abuse with diethylpropion during pregnancy may result in withdrawal symptoms in the newborn infant.

Patients with chronic malabsorption syndrome or cholestasis (a condition in which little or no bile is secreted or the flow of bile into the digestive tract is obstructed) should not take orlistat.

Side Effects

Benzphetamine, diethylpropion, phendimetrazine, and phentermine may cause hypertension, tachycardia, nausea, diarrhea, insomnia, nervousness, and euphoria (feeling of well-being).

The most common side effects associated with sibutramine are dry mouth, headache, dizziness, nervousness, constipation, loss of appetite, insomnia, tachycardia, and hypertension.

The most common side effects of orlistat include cramping, intestinal discomfort, passing gas, diarrhea, and leakage of oily stool.

Interactions

Interactions of anorexiants include increased risk of serotonin syndrome (see How Drugs Work in the Body, p. xxi) when used with selective serotonin reuptake inhibitors (SSRIs) and monoamine oxidase (MAO) inhibitors. Anorexiants should not be used within 14 days of these drugs. Anorexiants may enhance the effects of tricyclic antidepressants. Anorexiants should not be taken with medications that may increase blood pressure, such as over-the-counter (OTC) weight-loss, allergy, asthma, sinus, cough, or cold products that contain the sympathomimetic drugs pseudoephedrine or phenylephrine. Erythromycin, clarithromycin, itraconazole, ketoconazole, protease inhibitors, quinidine, or verapamil may increase the effects of sibutramine. The risk of serious side effects will be increased if sibutramine is taken with other appetite suppressants, antidepressants, or antimigraine agents. Extreme drowsiness may occur when sibutramine is taken with central nervous system depressants, such as alcohol, antihistamines, barbiturates, benzodiazepines, muscle relaxants, narcotics, and phenothiazines.

Orlistat may decrease the blood levels of cyclosporine. Therefore, to minimize the potential for this interaction, cyclosporine should be taken at least two hours before or after orlistat. In addition, more frequent monitoring of cyclosporine levels should be performed throughout the course of therapy with orlistat.

Sales/Statistics

In their January 2007 report on "Commercial and Pipeline Perspectives: Obesity," Datamonitor noted that although the obesity "epidemic" is taking place to a certain extent in all the major markets, with no signs of slowing down in the near future, the antiobesity drug market growth "does not follow the growth of obesity prevalence. The major cause for the lack of growth in most of the major markets is lack of reimbursement for pharmacological management of obesity." Also, the report stated, "The drugs currently available in the major markets for treatment of obesity have significant unmet needs and do not meet the expectations of obese patients."

In the United States, one antiobesity agent was listed among the "Top 200 Generic Drugs by Retail Dollars in 2006" (*Drug Topics*, February 19, 2007)—phentermine, ranked #87 with $108,202,000 in sales. It was ranked #107 among the "Top 200 Generic Drugs by Unit Sales in 2006," with 3,523,000 units. In 2010, the phentermine numbers had increased to $167,256,528 in sales (ranking 91st) and 6,403,366 prescriptions dispensed (ranking 92nd). No antiobesity agent was listed among the top 200 brand name drugs in either year.

Demographics and Cultural Groups

Currently, 133.6 million American adults (20+ years old) are overweight or obese (66 percent

of the adult population). According to gender, these numbers break down as women: 65 million (61.6 percent), and men: 68.3 million (70.5 percent). Nearly one-third of U.S. adults are obese—63.6 million (31.4 percent), which breaks down as women: 35 million (33.2 percent), and men: 28.6 million (29.5 percent).

The age-adjusted prevalence of combined overweight and obesity (BMI $\geq$ 25 kg/m^2) in racial/ethnic minorities—especially minority women—is generally higher than in whites in the United States: non-Hispanic black women: 79.6 percent; Mexican-American women: 73 percent; non-Hispanic white women: 57.6 percent; non-Hispanic black men: 67 percent; Mexican-American men: 74.6 percent; non-Hispanic white men: 71 percent.

Development History

Diethylpropion and phentermine were approved by the FDA in 1959, benzphetamine in 1960, phendimetrazine in 1982, and sibutramine in 1997.

In April 1999, the FDA approved orlistat for long-term use.

On February 7, 2007, the FDA approved orlistat (60 mg capsules) for OTC use as a weight-loss aid for overweight adults. Orlistat also remains available as a prescription drug for obesity at a higher dose than the OTC formulation.

Future Drugs

Encinosa et al. wrote that "there are about twenty-two new anti-obesity drug compounds in the pharmaceutical pipeline, with two currently in Phase III development." Of the two drugs furthest along in development, rimonabant works by blocking the cannabinoid receptors in the brain, and ciliary neurotrophic factor (CNTF) acts directly within muscles to increase the body's metabolism to burn fat. Both drugs simultaneously suppress appetite.

Rimonabant, being developed by Sanofi-Aventis, not only causes weight loss but reverses the metabolic effects of obesity such as insulin resistance and dyslipidemia. Although it was approved in Europe in June 2006 for use as an adjunct to diet and exercise for obese or overweight patients with associated risk factors, such as Type 2 diabetes or dyslipidemia, rimonabant has had some difficulty in getting through the U.S. regulatory system. In June 2007, an FDA advisory panel recommended that the FDA not approve rimonabant for sale because of the psychiatric side effects associated with it, including suicidal thinking. The panel said additional safety data were needed before the FDA should consider approving the drug. The company withdrew its application but said it plans to resubmit it at a future date.

Merck is developing taranabant and began a Phase III study in 2006. Early studies showed that taranabant can help people lose weight but did link it to an increase in psychiatric side effects. Taranabant is in the same drug class as rimonabant.

Ciliary neurotrophic (or nerve-nourishing) factor is a nerve growth factor that protects against some of the effects of obesity by activating an enzyme, skeletal muscle activated protein kinase (MAPK), which increases the ability of the body to metabolize fat and sugar. In a human study examining the usefulness of CNTF for treatment of motor neuron disease, reported on in 2001, CNTF produced an unexpected and substantial weight loss in the study subjects. Further investigation revealed that CNTF could reduce food intake without causing hunger or stress. Research led by Dr. Greg Steinberg, a Canadian scientist at the University of Melbourne, Australia, showed how CNTF activates similar pathways to those stimulated by exercise. "While hormones such as leptin were initially thought to be the cure-all for weight loss, they were later found to be ineffective in obesity due to the presence of proteins which inhibit their ability to stimulate fat metabolism," Dr. Steinberg said. "Fortunately, CNTF's effects on fat burning are maintained." Obesity treatments from neurotrophic factors such as CNTF are several years away, but this research opens the door to further studies.

Encinosa, William E., Didem M. Bernard, Claudia A. Steiner, and Chi-Chang Chen. "Use and Costs of Bariatric Surgery and Prescription Weight-loss Medications." *Health Affairs* 24, no. 4 (July–August 2005): 1,039–1,046.

antiparkinson agents Drugs used to provide relief from the symptoms of parkinsonism, a group of motor system disorders with similar features and symptoms that result from the loss of dopamine-producing brain cells. The most common form of parkinsonism is Parkinson's disease (PD). While no cause has yet been found for most forms of parkinsonism, there are some cases for which the cause is known or suspected or in which the symptoms result from another disorder. For example, parkinsonism may result from changes in the brain's blood vessels. The four main symptoms are tremor, or trembling in hands, arms, legs, jaw, or head; rigidity, or stiffness of the limbs and trunk; bradykinesia, or slowness of movement; and postural instability, or impaired balance. These symptoms usually begin gradually and worsen with time. As they become more pronounced, patients may have difficulty walking, talking, or completing other simple tasks. Parkinson's disease was first described in 1817 by James Parkinson, a British physician, who published a paper on what he called "the shaking palsy." In this paper, he set forth the major symptoms of the disease that would later bear his name. The associated biochemical changes in the brains of patients were identified in the 1960s. Researchers believe that at least 500,000 people in the United States currently have PD, although some estimates are as high as 1.5 million. One study states that PD affects one out of every 100 Americans older than the age of 60; another notes that 60,000 new cases are diagnosed each year. The total cost to the nation is estimated to exceed $6 billion annually. The risk of PD increases with age, so analysts expect the financial and public health impact of this disease to increase as the population gets older. At present, no drug will cure PD, replace lost nerve cells, or stop progression of the disease, but a variety of medications provide dramatic relief from the symptoms, making movement easier and allowing patients to function effectively for many years.

Classes

Antiparkinson agents are divided into classes according to how they treat the motor symptoms of parkinsonism. Some directly or indirectly increase the level of dopamine in the brain. Some affect other neurotransmitters (chemicals) in the body.

- *Dopamine precursors*—increase the level of dopamine in the brain. *Example:* levodopa/carbidopa (Parcopa, Sinemet).

- *Dopamine agonists*—mimic the role of dopamine in the brain. *Examples:* apomorphine (Apokyn), bromocriptine (Parlodel), pramipexole (Mirapex), and ropinirole (Requip).

- *Monoamine oxidase type B (MAO-B) inhibitors*—inhibit dopamine breakdown. *Examples:* rasagiline (Azilect) and selegiline (Eldepryl, Zelapar).

- *Catechol-O-methyltransferase (COMT) inhibitors*—inhibit dopamine breakdown. *Examples:* entacapone (Comtan) and tolcapone (Tasmar).

- *Anticholinergics*—decrease the action of acetylcholine. *Examples:* benztropine (Cogentin), biperiden (Akineton), diphenhydramine (Benadryl), procyclidine (Kemadrin), and trihexyphenidyl (Artane).

- *Miscellaneous*—Amantadine (Symmetrel) is an antiviral drug that reduces symptoms in PD. Stalevo (levodopa/carbidopa/entacapone) is a combination drug that enhances the benefits of levopoda.

How They Work

Dopamine precursors are converted by the brain to dopamine, a chemical involved in controlling movement. Levodopa/carbidopa is the most widely used medicine for PD. Levodopa (also called L-dopa) is the cornerstone of therapy for PD. Nerve cells can use levodopa to make dopamine and replenish the brain's dwindling supply. People cannot simply take dopamine pills because dopamine does not easily pass through the blood-brain barrier, a lining of cells inside blood vessels that regulates the transport of oxygen, glucose, and other substances into the brain. When added to levodopa, carbidopa delays the conversion of levodopa into dopamine until it reaches the brain, thereby preventing or diminishing some of the side effects that often accompany levodopa therapy. Carbidopa also reduces the amount of levodopa needed.

Dopamine agonists directly stimulate nerves in the brain that are not naturally being stimulated by dopamine. By mimicking the role of dopamine in the brain, they cause the neurons to react as they would to dopamine.

MAO-B inhibitors inhibit the enzyme MAO-B, which breaks down dopamine in the brain. MAO-B inhibitors cause dopamine to accumulate in surviving nerve cells and reduce the symptoms of PD.

COMT inhibitors prevent the breakdown of levodopa and therefore increase the amount of levodopa that is available to cross the blood-brain barrier and be converted into dopamine.

Anticholinergics decrease the activity of the neurotransmitter acetylcholine and help to reduce tremors and muscle rigidity.

Researchers are not certain how amantadine reduces parkinsonism symptoms, but it is thought to work by causing dopamine to be released from nerve endings of the brain cells along with stimulation of norepinephrine response.

Approved Uses

Levodopa/carbidopa is used to reduce tremors and muscle rigidity and to improve movement. It allows the majority of people with PD to extend the period of time in which they can lead relatively normal, productive lives. Although levodopa helps most people with PD, not all symptoms respond equally to the drug. Levodopa usually helps most with bradykinesia and rigidity. Problems with balance and other nonmotor symptoms may not be alleviated at all with levodopa. Levodopa is often so effective that some people may temporarily forget they have PD during the early stages of the disease. Levodopa/carbidopa is also approved to treat postencephalitic parkinsonism, a disease that is believed to have been caused by a viral illness, and symptomatic parkinsonism, which may follow injury to the nervous system by carbon monoxide and manganese intoxication.

Dopamine agonists are used alone or in conjunction with levodopa. They may be used in the early stages of the disease or later on in order to lengthen the duration of response to levodopa in patients who experience wearing-off or on-off effects. Wearing off means the period of effectiveness after each dose begins to shorten. The on-off effect refers to sudden, unpredictable changes in movement, from normal to parkinsonian movement and back again. Dopamine agonists arc generally less effective than levodopa in controlling rigidity and bradykinesia. Apomorphine is considered a "rescue" drug, intended for the acute, intermittent treatment of hypomobility and "off" episodes associated with advanced PD while waiting for the effect of other medications to begin. Its onset of effect is approximately 10 minutes and lasts approximately 90 minutes. Bromocriptine is also used to treat amenorrhea (absence of normal menstrual flow), infertility, galactorrhea (spontaneous flow of milk from the breast not associated with childbirth or nursing), hypogonadism (inadequate functioning of the ovaries or testes), acromegaly, and pituitary tumors. Ropinirole and pramipexole are the only medications in the United States with an FDA-approved indication for the treatment of restless legs syndrome.

MAO-B inhibitors are used as a supplement to levodopa and can also be used as monotherapy in patients with early PD. Studies supported by the National Institute of Neurological Disorders and Stroke (NINDS) have shown that selegiline can delay the need for levodopa therapy by up to a year or more. When selegiline is given with levodopa, it appears to enhance and prolong the response to levodopa and thus may reduce wearing-off fluctuations. Rasagiline can be used in early PD to reduce the severity or delay worsening of symptoms. When used with levodopa, rasagiline may help reduce the motor fluctuations that occur in advanced stages of PD, especially reducing the off time. Selegiline has also been approved by the FDA as a transdermal patch for the treatment of major depression (see ANTIDEPRESSANTS).

COMT inhibitors can decrease the duration of hypomobility (off periods), and they usually make it possible to reduce the patient's dose of levodopa. Their main use is to prolong the relief gained from levodopa/carbidopa. These drugs must be used with levodopa/carbidopa.

Anticholinergics were the principal treatment for PD prior to the development of levodopa and are now used to help control tremor and rigidity in all forms of parkinsonism.

Amantadine can help reduce symptoms of PD and levodopa-induced dyskinesia, or involuntary movements, such as twitching, twisting, and writhing. It is often used alone in the early stages of the disease. It also may be used with an anticholinergic drug or levodopa. After several months, amantadine's effectiveness wears off in up to half of the patients taking it. Amantadine is also used to treat symptomatic parkinsonism following injury to the nervous system by carbon monoxide intoxication. Symmetrel was originally approved as an antiviral drug for the treatment of influenza A virus.

Off-Label Uses

Levodopa/carbidopa has been used to relieve herpes zoster (shingles) pain and restless legs syndrome.

Bromocriptine is used to treat addiction to cocaine, a drug that exhibits its own effects by blocking dopamine reuptake. Pramipexole is used off-label to treat cluster headaches.

Selegiline is sometimes used off-label to treat narcolepsy. It has also been reported to positively affect libido, particularly in older males.

Administration

Levodopa/carbidopa is available in tablet form; sustained release and orally disintegrating tablets are also available.

Dopamine agonists are administered orally via tablets except for apomorphine, which is an injection. Apomorphine should be administered by subcutaneous injection only, with the site of injection rotated. Parlodel is also available as capsules.

MAO-B inhibitors are administered orally via tablets or capsules. Selegiline is also available as orally disintegrating tablets.

COMT inhibitors are available in tablet form.

Anticholinergics are available in tablet form; benztropine is also available as an injection for psychotic patients with dystonic reactions (involuntary, sustained muscle contractions) or other reactions that make it difficult to administer oral medication.

Amantadine is administered orally via capsules, tablets, or syrup.

Cautions and Concerns

Common side effects of antiparkinsonian drugs may impair driving performance; these include excessive daytime sleepiness, lightheadedness, dizziness, blurred vision, and confusion.

Dyskinesias commonly develop in people who take large doses of levodopa/carbidopa over an extended period. These movements may be either mild or severe and either very rapid or very slow. The dose of levodopa is often reduced in order to lessen these drug-induced movements. However, the PD symptoms often reappear even with lower doses of medication. Doctors and patients must work together closely to find a tolerable balance between the drug's benefits and side effects. Because dyskinesias tend to occur with long-term use of levodopa/carbidopa, doctors often start younger PD patients on other dopamine-increasing drugs and switch to levodopa/carbidopa only when those drugs become ineffective.

Other troubling and distressing problems may occur with long-term use of levodopa/carbidopa.

Patients may begin to notice more pronounced symptoms before their first dose of medication in the morning, and they may develop muscle spasms or other problems when each dose begins to wear off. Wearing-off and on-off effects probably indicate that the patient's response to the drug is changing or that the disease is progressing. One approach to alleviating these side effects is to take levodopa/carbidopa more often and in smaller amounts. Patients with PD should never stop taking levodopa/carbidopa without their physician's knowledge or consent because rapidly withdrawing the drug can have potentially serious side effects, such as immobility or difficulty breathing.

Levodopa/carbidopa should be used with caution in diabetic patients, as the levodopa may affect blood glucose control.

A sudden fall in blood pressure when standing up, causing dizziness and lightheadedness (called postural or orthostatic hypotension), has been reported with the use of dopamine agonists and levodopa/carbidopa. These drugs may also cause sudden and unpredictable episodes of extreme drowsiness.

Severe nausea and vomiting is to be expected at recommended doses of apomorphine; thus, use of an antiemetic such as trimethobenzamide three days prior to the initial dose of apomorphine and continued for at least the first two months of therapy is advised. Because of its ability to reduce blood pressure, apomorphine should be used with caution in patients with known cardiovascular and cerebrovascular disease. Apomorphine should also be used with caution in patients with kidney or liver impairment.

A single case of rhabdomyolysis occurred in a 49-year-old male with advanced PD treated with pramipexole. The symptoms resolved with discontinuation of the medication. Because pramipexole is eliminated through the kidneys, caution should be exercised when prescribing this drug to patients with renal insufficiency.

Because patients with liver impairment may have higher plasma levels and lower clearance, ropinirole should be titrated with caution in these patients.

When used as an adjunct to levodopa therapy, MAO-B inhibitors may exacerbate levodopa-associated side effects. These effects may be mitigated by reducing the dose of levodopa/carbidopa by 10 to 30 percent.

Patients taking rasagiline should be monitored for melanomas frequently and on a regular basis. In trials, postural hypotension was reported in some patients treated with rasagiline, occurring most frequently in the first two months of rasagiline treatment and tending to decrease over time.

In clinical trials, an increased frequency of mild oropharyngeal abnormality (e.g., swallowing pain, mouth pain, ulceration) occurred in patients taking selegiline orally disintegrating tablets.

Because COMT inhibitors enhance the effects of levodopa, their use requires a reduction of levodopa/carbidopa to prevent the occurrence of levodopa-related side effects, such as orthostatic hypotension, loss of appetite, nausea, vomiting, drowsiness, and hallucinations. It may be necessary to adjust the levodopa/carbidopa dosage within the first days to first weeks following the initiation of COMT inhibitor treatment.

Anticholinergics should be used with caution in patients with tachycardia, cardiac arrhythmias, hypertension, hypotension, any tendency toward urinary retention, liver or kidney disorders, or obstructive disease of the gastrointestinal (GI) or genitourinary (GU) tract. From 19 to 30 percent of patients given anticholinergics develop depression, confusion, delusions, or hallucinations. Large doses of benztropine may cause weakness and inability to move particular muscle groups, necessitating dosage adjustment. Anhidrosis (lack of sweating) may occur during hot weather with anticholinergic therapy, necessitating decreased dosage until the ability to maintain body heat equilibrium by perspiration is not impaired. Fatal hyperthermia has occurred. If dry mouth is so severe that it makes swallowing or speaking difficult, anticholinergic

dosage should be reduced or the drug discontinued temporarily.

Withdrawing or reducing amantadine may cause life-threatening high fever with disturbances in blood pressure, breathing, and heart rates. Because amantadine increases the amount of dopamine in the brain, patients with a history of epilepsy or other seizure disorders should be carefully monitored—particularly the elderly and patients with kidney disease. Amantadine may cause visual disturbances and affect mental alertness and coordination.

Warnings

Dyskinesias will occur at lower dosages and sooner during therapy with the sustained release form of levodopa/carbidopa. Because mental disturbances have been reported with levodopa therapy, patients should be observed for depression with suicidal tendencies. Levodopa/carbidopa should be used with caution in patients with current or past psychoses.

Patients taking dopamine agonists may not experience any warning signs of sudden sleep onset and should be warned about this possibility at the commencement of therapy, when increasing doses, or when switching agents. Elderly patients taking dopamine agonists have experienced hallucinations five to seven times more often than younger patients on these drugs, and the incidence of hallucinations appears to increase with age. Apomorphine has been associated with QT interval (length of the heart's electrical cycle) prolongation and should be used with caution in patients at risk for torsade de pointes. Patients with moderate to severe kidney disease should take reduced doses of pramipexole.

Rasagiline or selegiline treatment at any dose may be associated with a hypertensive crisis if the patient ingests tyramine-rich foods, beverages, or dietary supplements or amines (from over-the-counter medications). Hypertensive crisis, which in some cases may be fatal, consists of marked systemic blood pressure elevation and requires immediate treatment/hospitalization. Tyramine-rich foods and beverages to avoid include air dried, aged, and fermented meats, sausages, and salamis; pickled herring; fava bean pods; aged cheeses; beers that have not been pasteurized so as to allow for ongoing fermentation; red wines; sauerkraut; and most soybean products (including soy sauce and tofu). These drugs/substances should be avoided for at least two weeks after discontinuation of rasagiline or selegiline.

In a few rare cases, tolcapone has caused severe liver disease. Because of this, tolcapone should be used only after other medications have failed. In addition, liver function tests are recommended at baseline and at regular intervals.

Narrow-angle glaucoma may be precipitated by anticholinergics; thus, eye pressure needs to be monitored regularly. Patients over 60 years of age require strict dosage regulation, as they frequently develop increased sensitivity to anticholinergics, resulting in confusion, disorientation, agitation, or hallucinations.

Patients with kidney disease must have their doses of amantadine lowered or take them less frequently.

When Not Advised (Contraindications)

Levodopa/carbidopa should not be used in patients who have narrow-angle glaucoma or those with suspicious, undiagnosed skin lesions or history of melanoma.

Apomorphine should not be used in patients receiving 5HT3 antagonists (e.g., ondansetron, granisetron, dolasetron, palonosetron, alosetron), as this drug combination may lead to a significant reduction in blood pressure and a possible loss of consciousness.

Bromocriptine should not be used in patients with uncontrolled hypertension or sensitivity to any ergot alkaloids. When bromocriptine is being used in patients who subsequently become pregnant, a decision should be made as to whether the therapy continues to be medically necessary or can be withdrawn. If it is continued, the drug should be withdrawn in those who may experience hypertensive disorders of pregnancy (including eclampsia, preeclampsia, or pregnancy-induced hypertension) unless withdrawal of bromocriptine is considered to be medically contraindicated. Bromocriptine should not be used during the postpartum period in women with a history of coronary artery disease and other severe cardiovascular conditions unless withdrawal is considered medically contraindicated.

Rasagiline should not be used in patients with moderate or severe liver impairment. Rasagiline and selegiline should not be used in patients receiving meperidine, tramadol, methadone, or propoxyphene, as a severe reaction (i.e., coma, severe hypertension or hypotension, seizures, respiratory depression) may result if these drugs are used together. As with other MAO inhibitors, patients taking rasagiline or selegiline should not undergo elective surgery requiring general anesthesia. Also, they should not be given cocaine or local anesthesia containing sympathomimetic vasoconstrictors. Rasagiline and selegiline should be discontinued for at least 14 days before a patient undergoes surgery requiring general anesthesia. Rasagiline and selegiline should not be used with the antitussive agent dextromethorphan, as the combination of MAO inhibitors and dextromethorphan has been reported to cause brief episodes of psychosis or bizarre behavior.

Tolcapone is contraindicated in patients with liver disease, in patients with a history of nontraumatic rhabdomyolysis (breakdown of skeletal muscle) or abnormally high fever and confusion possibly related to medication, and in patients already suffering from low blood pressure.

Anticholinergics are not advised for patients with glaucoma, bowel or duodenal obstruction, peptic ulcer disease, bladder obstruction, or myasthenia gravis.

Side Effects

Side effects caused by levodopa/carbidopa include gastroesophageal reflux disease, nausea, vomiting, low blood pressure, involuntary facial movements, nightmares, and restlessness. The drug also can cause drowsiness or sudden sleep onset, which can make driving and other activities dangerous. Long-term use of levodopa sometimes causes hallucinations and psychosis. The nausea, vomiting, constipation, drowsiness, palpitations, and flushing caused by levodopa are greatly reduced by combining levodopa and carbidopa, which enhances the effectiveness of a lower dose.

Many of the potential side effects of dopamine agonists are similar to those associated with the use of levodopa, including drowsiness, sudden sleep onset, low blood pressure, hallucinations, confusion, dyskinesias (tics and other involuntary movements), edema (swelling due to excess fluid in body tissues), nightmares, and vomiting. In rare cases, they can cause compulsive behavior, such as an uncontrollable desire to gamble, hypersexuality, or compulsive shopping. Bromocriptine may also cause fibrosis, or a buildup of fibrous tissue, in the heart valves or the chest cavity. Fibrosis usually goes away once bromocriptine is discontinued.

MAO-B inhibitors are usually well tolerated, although side effects may include nausea, dizziness, confusion, dry mouth, low blood pressure, abdominal pain, or insomnia. Studies have reported balance difficulties, anorexia, vomiting, and weight loss with rasagiline.

The most common side effect of COMT inhibitors is diarrhea. The drugs may also cause nausea, sleep disturbances, dizziness, urine discoloration, abdominal pain, back pain, low blood pressure, abnormal involuntary movements, or hallucinations.

Anticholinergic side effects include dry mouth, constipation, urinary retention, hallucinations, memory loss, blurred vision, drowsiness, dizziness, heat stroke (see *Cautions and Concerns*), muscular weakness and cramping, and confusion.

Amantadine's side effects include insomnia, mottled skin, edema, agitation, hallucinations, nausea, dizziness, anxiety, impaired concentration, and confusion.

Interactions

A high-protein diet can interfere with the absorption of levodopa, so some physicians recommend that patients taking levodopa/carbidopa restrict their protein consumption during the early parts of the day or avoid taking their medications with protein-rich meals.

Levodopa/carbidopa therapy may require dosage adjustment of antihypertensives in patients taking these drugs. Concomitant therapy with dopamine agonists, COMT inhibitors, or selegiline and levodopa/carbidopa can cause a sudden fall in blood pressure upon standing not attributable to levodopa/carbidopa alone. Adverse reactions, including hypertension and dyskinesia, have been reported with the concomitant use of tricyclic antidepressants and levodopa/carbidopa.

Dopamine D_2 receptor antagonists (e.g., phenothiazines, butyrophenones, risperidone) and isoniazid may reduce the therapeutic effects of levodopa. In addition, the beneficial effects of levodopa in PD have been reported to be reversed by phenytoin and papaverine.

Apomorphine should not be given with antiemetics of the selective 5-HT$_3$ receptor antagonists class, such as dolasetron, granisetron, ondansetron, and palonosetron, because of reports of profound low blood pressure and loss of consciousness. Caution should be used when taking with drugs that also prolong the QT/QTc interval. Apomorphine used along with alcohol, ANTIHYPERTENSIVES, and vasodilators (particularly nitrates) may increase effects on blood pressure.

Erythromycin, risperidone, and ritonavir may greatly increase the effects of bromocriptine.

Dopamine antagonists, such as neuroleptics (phenothiazines, butyrophenones, thioxanthines) or metoclopramide, ordinarily should not be administered concurrently with dopamine agonists, as they may lessen the effectiveness of the agonists. Because pergolide is approximately 90 percent bound to plasma proteins, caution should be exercised if pergolide is administered along with other drugs known to affect protein binding.

Cimetidine may increase the effects of pramipexole.

Smoking can make ropinirole less effective; alcohol can increase some of its side effects. Ciprofloxacin may increase the amount of ropinirole in the blood.

Rasagiline should not be combined with other MAO inhibitors nor with the analgesic meperidine, the antidepressant mirtazapine, the muscle relaxant cyclobenzaprine, or Saint-John's-wort. It should be avoided with tricyclic antidepressants, selective serotonin reuptake inhibitors, and serotonin-norepinephrine reuptake inhibitors. Rasagiline and selegiline should not be taken with the antidepressant fluoxetine, the analgesic mepiridine, or dextromethorphan (see *When Not Advised [Contraindications]*).

Entacapone taken along with isoproterenol, epinephrine, norepinephrine, dopamine, dobutamine, alpha-methyldopa, apomorphine, isoetherine, and bitolterol may cause increased heart rates, possibly arrhythmias, and abrupt changes in blood pressure.

Phenothiazines may increase the incidence of anticholinergic side effects. Anticholinergics taken along with haloperidol may worsen schizophrenic symptoms, decrease haloperidol serum concentrations, and cause development of tardive dyskinesia. Digoxin serum levels may be increased by anticholinergics when digoxin is administered as a slow dissolution oral tablet. Cannabinoids, barbiturates, opiates, and alcohol may have additive effects when taken with anticholinergics.

Amantadine taken along with anticholinergics may increase incidence of anticholinergic side effects. When taken along with amphetamines or decongestants, amantadine may cause increased central nervous stimulation or increase the likelihood of seizures. Amantadine adds to the sedating effects of alcohol, benzodiazepines, tricyclic antidepressants, and some ANTIHISTAMINES.

Kava, derived from a South Pacific plant and sold as a tea and herbal supplement, acts as a dopamine antagonist and therefore may increase tremor and make antiparkinson agents less effective in persons with PD.

Sales/Statistics

The "Top 200 Generic Drugs by Units in 2006" (*Drug Topics*, March 5, 2007) included two antiparkinson agents: levodopa/carbidopa at #143 (2,479,000 units) and benztropine at #156 (2,266,000 units).

One antiparkinson agent appeared on the "Top 200 Generic Drugs by Retail Dollars in 2006" (*Drug Topics*, February 19, 2007): levodopa/carbidopa at #95 ($98,128,000).

Requip ranked #113 in brand-name drugs for 2006 ("Top 200 Brand-Name Drugs by Units in 2006," *Drug Topics*, March 5, 2007), with 2,661,000 units sold; Mirapex ranked #165, with 1,524,000 units sold.

Requip ranked #122 among the "Top 200 Brand-Name Drugs by Retail Dollars in 2006," (*Drug Topics*, February 19, 2007), with $260,813,000 in sales. Mirapex ranked #145, with $197,457,000 in sales.

By 2010, only levodopa/carbidopa remained on these lists, ranking #150 in sales ($91,535,681) and #182 in units (2,504,723 prescriptions).

Demographics and Cultural Groups

Van Den Eeden et al. noted that whether or not PD frequency varies by race/ethnicity or gender has been a source of controversy for many decades. In their study to address this issue, they looked at the incidence of PD in a large prepaid health maintenance organization with a multiethnic population of sufficient size to increase precision and without economic barriers limiting access to care. According to their findings, the PD incidence rates were highest among Hispanics, followed by non-Hispanic whites, Asians, and blacks. In all groups other than Asians, the incidence of PD among men was approximately twofold higher than the incidence among women. Among Asians, however, PD incidence was slightly lower among men than women.

Development History

Levodopa was introduced in the 1960s. The Swedish scientist Arvid Carlsson had first shown in the 1950s that administering levodopa to animals with Parkinsonian symptoms would cause a reduction of the symptoms. In 1961, a Vienna group reported that small doses of levodopa provided some improvement in 20 PD cases. Then in 1967, George Constantin Cotzias, M.D., of the Brookhaven National Laboratories, Upton, New York, and his coworkers reported more impressive benefits using large oral doses of levodopa. These studies led to the widespread introduction of levodopa as a treatment for PD and revolutionized management of the disease. The controlled-release form of levodopa/carbidopa—formulated to help keep blood levels of levodopa more constant throughout the day, possibly preventing on-off fluctuations—was approved for use by the FDA in 1991.

Bromocriptine was originally approved by the FDA in 1978 for the treatment of amenorrhea/galactorrhea, then subsequently approved for infertility and PD. Pramipexole was approved for PD in July 1997 and for restless leg syndrome in November 2006. FDA approval of ropinirole for PD was first granted in September 1997, with its approval to treat restless leg syndrome following in May 2005. Apomorphine received approval for PD in April 2004.

Selegiline was the first selective MAO-B inhibitor approved for use in PD in the United States, which occurred in January 1989. In May 2006, the FDA approved rasagiline to be used along with levodopa.

Tolcapone was the first COMT inhibitor approved by the FDA for PD, in January 1998; entacapone followed in October 1999.

Botanical preparations with anticholinergic properties had been used to treat Parkinson's disease for more than a century. Diphenhydramine was originally approved by the FDA in 1946. Biperiden was synthesized by the German chemist W. Klavehn from Knoll AG, Germany; in March 1953, a patent was applied for in Germany and subsequently in many other countries.

Amantadine was approved by the FDA in 1966 for the treatment of influenza virus A in adults. It was serendipitously discovered to benefit patients with PD when it was prescribed for a woman to prevent flu but also relieved some of her Parkinson symptoms and made her generally feel better.

Among the anticholinergics, trihexyphenidyl received FDA approval in 1949, benztropine in 1954, and procyclidine in 1955.

Future Drugs

In December 2006, the Pharmaceutical Research and Manufacturers of America (PhRMA) showed 31 antiparkinson drugs in various stages of development, with about two-thirds of those in late clinical trials. Among these:

- Acadia Pharmaceuticals is developing pimavanserin (ACP-103) for treatment of the psychiatric and motor dysfunction that frequently results from current PD therapies. ACP-103 is given orally and blocks the activity of the 5-HT2A receptor.

- Vasogen, Inc. is developing VP025, the first candidate in a new class of phospholipid-based drugs designed to aid in regulating cytokine levels and controlling inflammation within the central nervous system, which is associated with a number of neurological diseases, including Alzheimer's disease, PD, and amyotrophic lateral sclerosis (Lou Gehrig's disease).

- Juvantia Pharma, Ltd. is developing fipamezole, the first in a potential new class of drugs, alpha-2 adrenoceptor antagonists. Fipamezole is designed to counteract the loss of noradrenergic neurons in the locus ceruleus and generalized depletion of noradrenaline in the brain. These losses may contribute significantly to the nonmotor syndromes in PD and may also make dopaminergic terminals more susceptible to drug-induced damage.

Van Den Eeden, Stephen K. et al. "Incidence of Parkinson's Disease: Variation by Age, Gender, and Race/Ethnicity." *American Journal of Epidemiology* 157, no. 11 (November 2003): 1,015–1,022.

antiplatelets Drugs that stop blood particles called platelets from clumping together to form a harmful clot (thrombus). Platelets are blood cells that circulate through the blood vessels and help stop bleeding by sticking together to seal small cuts or breaks in tiny blood vessels. In many instances, platelets play this positive role; however, too much platelet activity, called platelet aggregation, can lead to formation of blood clots inside blood vessels that increase the risk of heart attack and stroke. Antiplatelets can prevent this process from occurring and thus reduce the risk of a heart attack, stroke, transient ischemic attack (TIA) (a temporary interruption of the blood flow to an area of the brain ["mini-stroke"]), and peripheral arterial disease (PAD) (narrowed arteries that decrease blood flow to the extremities, primarily the legs). In general, antiplatelet drugs may be given to people who have had or are at risk for a heart attack or stroke/TIA, who have had a stent placed in a coronary artery, or who have angina.

The term *antithrombotics* includes ANTICOAGU-LANTS, antiplatelets, and THROMBOLYTICS.

Classes

Antiplatelets are divided into several classes according to their method of action.

- *Aspirin*—usually thought of for its effects on fever, pain, and inflammation, aspirin also has an inhibitory effect on platelets in the blood.
- *Thienopyridines*—adenosine diphosphate (ADP) receptor antagonists. *Examples:* clopido-grel (Plavix), prasugrel (Effient), and ticlopi-dine (Ticlid).
- *Cyclo-pentyl-triazolo-pyrimidines (CPTPs)*—reversibly binding P2Y12 receptor antagonists—*Example:* ticagrelor (Brilinta).
- *Glycoprotein IIb/IIIa inhibitors*—*Examples:* abcix-imab (ReoPro), eptifibatide (Integrilin), and tirofiban (Aggrastat).
- *Phosphodiesterase inhibitors*—*Examples:* cilo-stazol (Pletal) and dipyridamole (Persantine).

- *Combination product*—Dipyridamole/aspirin (Aggrenox).

How They Work

The American Heart Association explains that blood platelets are actually fragments of cells—meaning they do not contain all the necessary cellular equipment. When a person gets a cut or scratch, platelets release thromboxane A2, a chemical that signals other platelets to "help out." Without the release of thromboxane A2, the platelets will not come together, no clot will form, and the cut will continue to bleed. In the case of a wound, thromboxane A2 is an indis-pensable self-sealing material, but for a stroke or heart attack victim, thromboxane's A2 ability to round up or "help" to form a blood clot becomes potentially life-threatening.

Low-dose, long-term aspirin irreversibly blocks the formation of thromboxane A2 in platelets, producing an inhibitory effect on platelet aggre-gation. Higher doses of aspirin tend to have more anti-inflammatory and analgesic effects.

Thienopyridines work by irreversibly blocking the ADP receptor on platelet cell membranes. This receptor, named P2Y12, is important in platelet aggregation, the cross-linking of plate-lets by fibrinogen. The blockade of this receptor ultimately inhibits platelet aggregation by block-ing activation of the glycoprotein IIb/IIIa (GPIIb/IIIa) pathway.

Unlike thienopyridines, which irreversibly bind to the P2Y12 receptor for the lifetime of the platelet, ticagrelor binds reversibly to the ADP receptor and exhibits rapid onset and offset of effect, which closely follow drug exposure levels.

Glycoprotein IIb/IIIa inhibitors prevent plate-let aggregation and thrombus formation by pre-venting the binding of fibrinogen to the GPIIb/IIIa receptor on the surface of the platelets.

Cilostazol inhibits phosphodiesterase III (PDE III), which leads to increased concentrations of cyclic adenosine monophosphate (cAMP), a platelet inhibitor and vasodilator. The precise mechanism of action for dipyridamole has not been determined. In addition to decreasing the action of the enzyme phosphodiesterase, it may also work by inhibiting the red blood cell uptake of adenosine. Both of these effects lead to inhibition of platelet aggregation and vasodilation.

Approved Uses

The blood-thinning property in low-dosage aspirin makes it useful for reducing the incidence of heart attacks as well as for preventing strokes/TIA after percutaneous coronary intervention (includes angioplasty, stent implantation) or coronary artery bypass graft (CABG) surgery.

The thienopyridines appear modestly more effective than aspirin in preventing serious vascular events in high-risk patients. Clopidogrel was initially FDA-approved in 1997 to reduce the risk of heart attack, stroke, or PAD in patients with a history of these conditions. Since that time, clopidogrel has also been approved for the treatment of non-ST-segment elevation acute coronary syndrome (NSTE ACS) or ST-segment-elevation myocardial infarction (STEMI). Prasugrel is used along with aspirin to prevent serious or life-threatening problems with the heart and blood vessels in people who have had a heart attack or severe chest pain and have been treated with angioplasty (a procedure to open the blood vessels that supply blood to the heart). Ticlopidine is used to help prevent thrombotic strokes in patients who have already had a stroke or a TIA. It is also approved for patients who have received an intracoronary stent (placed in a coronary artery) to prevent blood clot formation around the stent. Because of the risk of side effects with ticlopidine (primarily blood abnormalities), clopidogrel is the thienopyridine that is used most often in practice.

Ticagrelor is approved to reduce cardiovascular death and heart attack in patients with acute coronary syndromes (ACS). ACS includes a group of symptoms for any condition, such as unstable angina or heart attack, that could result from reduced blood flow to the heart.

The GPIIb/IIIa inhibitors, eptifibatide and tirofiban, are both approved for the treatment of NSTE ACS. Both epitifibatide and abciximab are approved for use during percutaneous coronary intervention (PCI), a procedure performed to open up blocked arteries in the heart. Such procedures may include angioplasty or implanting an intracoronary stent.

Cilostazol is FDA-approved for the reduction of symptoms of intermittent claudication (pain in the legs that develops during exercise caused by decreased oxygen supply to the calf muscles). This drug allows people with this condition to exercise longer before developing their characteristic leg pain and to walk longer before they must stop because of the pain.

Oral dipyridamole is used with anticoagulants to reduce the risk of blood clots following heart valve replacement. Intravenous dipyridamole can be used during a cardiac stress test (in place of exercise) so that blood flow to the heart can be evaluated.

Dipyridamole/aspirin is used to reduce the risk of stroke in patients who have had a TIA or an ischemic stroke due to thrombosis.

Off-Label Uses

Clopidogrel is widely used (off-label) along with aspirin in patients who have had coronary stents (bare metal or drug-coated) implanted to prevent blood clots from forming around the stents. Ticlopidine has been used off-label to improve distance and pain-free walking in cases of intermittent claudication.

Companion Drugs

Glycoprotein IIb/IIIa inhibitors should be used with heparin. Clopidogrel is usually used with aspirin for the prevention of cardiovascular events or to prevent blood clot formation around an intracoronary stent.

Prasugrel should be used along with aspirin. After an initial higher "loading" dose of aspirin (usually 325 mg), ticagrelor is taken with a daily aspirin maintenance dose of 75 to 100 milligrams unless aspirin is contraindicated.

Administration

Aspirin is most widely used in tablet form but is also available as caplets, gum, and suppositories.

Thienopyridines are taken orally in tablet form. Administration of ticlopidine with food is recommended to maximize gastrointestinal tolerance.

Ticagrelor is taken orally in tablet form with or without food.

Glycoprotein IIb/IIIa inhibitors are administered via intravenous injection.

Both cilostazol and dipyridamole are available as tablets. Dipyridamole is also available as an intravenous injection. Dipyridamole/aspirin is available as extended release capsules.

Cautions and Concerns

Side effects from antiplatelets may be increased in patients who have high blood pressure, asthma, allergies, or nasal polyps. Patients undergoing any surgical procedure while taking an antiplatelet agent should consult with their physician to determine if they will need to discontinue the drug prior to the procedure.

For cautions and concerns regarding aspirin, see ANALGESICS.

Heart patients who have received drug-coated stents to hold open an artery and who stop taking clopidogrel to reduce blood clotting may face more than double the risk of death or heart attack than patients who continue on the drug, according to an analysis by Duke Clinical Research Institute investigators.

Thienopyridines prolong bleeding time and therefore should be used with caution in patients who may be at risk of increased bleeding from trauma, surgery, ulcers, or coadministration with nonsteroidal anti-inflammatory drugs (NSAIDs) or warfarin. Thienopyridines should also be used with caution in patients with liver or kidney disease.

Shortness of breath (dyspnea) was reported more frequently with ticagrelor than with clopidogrel. Dyspnea was usually mild to moderate in intensity and often resolved during continued treatment. If a patient develops new, prolonged, or worsened dyspnea during treatment with ticagrelor, other causes that may require treatment should be ruled out. If dyspnea is determined to be related to ticagrelor, no specific treatment is required, and ticagrelor can be continued without interruption. Since ticagrelor has not been studied in patients with moderate hepatic impairment, physicians should consider the risks and benefits of treatment, noting the probable increase in exposure to ticagrelor.

Because of the potential for bleeding, it is important to monitor platelet counts, hemoglobin, hematocrit, serum creatinine (for tirofiban and eptifibatide), and prothrombin time (PT)/activated partial thromboplastin time (aPTT) prior to treatment with GPIIb/IIIa inhibitors within six hours following infusion and at least daily thereafter during treatment.

Rare cases of thrombocytopenia (low platelet count) or leukopenia (low white blood cell count) have been reported with the use of cilostazol; if either of these conditions develops, the cilostazol should be immediately discontinued to prevent progression to agranulocytosis (severely low levels of white blood cells). Cilostazol should be used with caution in patients taking itraconazole, ketoconazole, erythromycin, diltiazem, or omeprazole.

Dipyridamole should be used with caution in patients with abnormally low blood pressure. Because dipyridamole may cause dizziness, patients should exercise caution when driving, operating machinery, or performing other hazardous activities.

Warnings

For warnings regarding aspirin, see ANALGESICS.

Thrombotic thrombocytopenic purpura (TTP), defined as low platelet counts with spontaneous bleeding and clotting, has been reported rarely following use of thienopyridines (less frequently with clopidogrel), sometimes after a short exposure. TTP is a serious condition that can be fatal and requires urgent treatment including plasma exchange. Prasugrel may cause serious or life-threatening bleeding and should be discontinued at least seven days prior to any surgery, including dental surgery. Additional risk factors for bleeding include body weight under 132 pounds, propensity to bleed, and concomitant use of medications that increase the risk of bleeding (e.g., warfarin, heparin, nonsteroidal inflammatory [NSAID] medications). Ticlopidine may cause neutropenia, a severe decrease in the number of certain white blood cells (neutrophils).

Like other blood-thinning agents, ticagrelor increases the rate of bleeding and can cause significant, sometimes fatal, bleeding. Watch for bleeding in any patient who is hypotensive and has recently undergone coronary angiography, percutaneous coronary intervention (PCI), heart bypass surgery, or other surgical procedures while taking ticagrelor. If possible, bleeding should be managed without discontinuing ticagrelor, as stopping ticagrelor increases the risk of subsequent cardiovascular events. Maintenance doses of aspirin above 100 mg reduce the effectiveness of ticagrelor and should be avoided.

Thrombocytopenia is a rare but known serious risk with GPIIb/IIIa inhibitors. Major and minor bleeding events are the most common complications occurring during treatment with these drugs; therefore, patients must be monitored for potential bleeding.

Several drugs with the same pharmacologic effect as cilostazol have caused decreased survival compared with placebo in patients with moderate to severe heart failure.

When Not Advised (Contraindications)

Antiplatelet medicines may not be appropriate for some people because they increase the risk of bleeding.

For contraindications regarding aspirin, see ANALGESICS.

Thienopyridines are contraindicated in patients with active pathologic bleeding, such as peptic ulcer or intracranial hemorrhage, or with a history of TTP. Prasugrel is generally not rec-

ommended in patients 75 years of age or older and is contraindicated in patients with active pathological bleeding or a history of transient ischemic attack or stroke. Ticlopidine should not be used in patients with severe liver disease.

Ticagrelor is contraindicated in patients with a history of intracranial hemorrhage, in patients with active bleeding such as peptic ulcer or intracranial hemorrhage, and in patients with severe hepatic impairment.

GPIIb/IIIa inhibitors should not be used in patients who have active internal bleeding or a history of bleeding or stroke within the previous 30 days, who have a history of thrombocytopenia, who have had a major surgical procedure or severe physical trauma within the previous month, or who have severe hypertension.

Cilostazol is contraindicated in patients with heart failure of any severity.

Side Effects

Antiplatelet agents may cause internal bleeding that can lead to anemia.

Common side effects of aspirin include skin bruising, particularly in older patients, irritation of the stomach lining, gastrointestinal tract bleeding, and allergic reaction.

Common side effects of thienopyridines include nausea and vomiting, diarrhea, skin rash, itching, and ringing in the ears (tinnitus). Bleeding is the most common side effect of prasugrel, followed by hypertension, hypercholesterolemia/hyperlipidemia, headache, and back pain.

Various types of bleeding (e.g., hematoma, nosebleed, gastrointestinal, subcutaneous, or dermal) are the most common side effect of ticagrelor, followed by shortness of breath, headache, cough, dizziness, nausea, and atrial fibrillation.

The most common side effects of GPIIb/IIIa inhibitors are bleeding (especially gastrointestinal) and thrombocytopenia. Nonbleeding side effects with abciximab include low blood pressure, nausea, vomiting, back pain, chest pain, and headache. Hypotension may also occur with eptifibatide. Nonbleeding side effects with tirofiban include bradycardia (abnormally slow heart rate) and dizziness.

The most commonly reported side effects of cilostazol are headache, abnormal stool, diarrhea, rhinitis, dizziness, tachycardia (abnormally fast heart rate), and palpitations.

Common side effects of dipyridamole and dipyridamole/aspirin are dizziness, upset stomach, nausea, vomiting, headache, or rash.

Interactions

The use of antiplatelet agents with NSAIDs or anticoagulants may increase a patient's risk of bleeding. Antiplatelets should not be taken with these drugs unless advised by a physician.

For interactions regarding aspirin, see ANALGESICS.

Coadminstration of prasugrel and warfarin increases the risk of bleeding; concurrent use with NSAIDs (used chronically) may increase the risk of bleeding.

Strong inhibitors of the liver enzyme CYP3A4 (e.g., ketoconazole, itraconazole, voriconazole, clarithromycin, nefazodone, ritonavir, saquinavir, nelfinavir, indinavir, atazanavir, and telithromycin) increase blood plasma levels of ticagrelor and consequently can lead to bleeding and other adverse effects. Conversely, drugs that are metabolized by CYP3A4 (e.g., simvastatin and lovastatin) show increased blood levels and more side effects if combined with ticagrelor. CYP3A4 inductors (e.g., rifampicin dexamethasone, phenytoin, carbamazepine, and phenobarbital) can reduce the effectiveness of ticagrelor.

Administration of ticlopidine after antacids may result in a decrease in plasma levels of ticlopidine. Cimetidine may increase plasma levels of ticlopidine. Ticlopidine may decrease the digoxin levels by about 15 percent. Ticlopidine may increase the effects of phenytoin and theophylline.

Concurrent use of GPIIb/IIIa inhibitors with heparin and aspirin has been associated with an increase in bleeding.

Administration of ketoconazole, itraconazole, erythromycin, diltiazem, or omeprazole may increase plasma levels of cilostazol.

Theophylline may reduce the effects of dipyridamole.

Sales/Statistics

Americans are reported to consume 16,000 tons of aspirin tablets a year, equaling 80 million pills.

Worldwide sales of Plavix reached $5.9 billion in 2005, according to IMS Health, Inc., up 59 percent from two years earlier, making it the second highest drug brand in sales (Lipitor, a cholesterol-lowering drug, being the highest). In the United States, Plavix ranked seventh ("Top 200 Brand-Name Drugs by Retail Dollars in 2006," *Drug Topics,* February 19, 2007), with $2,231,825,000 in sales. It ranked #15 on the "Top 200 Brand-Name Drugs by Units in 2006" list (*Drug Topics,* March 5, 2007), with 16,248,000 prescriptions. Aggrenox ranked #185 in retail dollars ($151,976,000) and #200 in units (1,175,000 prescriptions).

Cilostazol appeared on the "Top 200 Generic Drugs by Retail Dollars in 2006" (*Drug Topics,* February 19, 2007) at #118 ($74,961,000) and on the "Top 200 Generic Drugs by Units in 2006" list (*Drug Topics,* March 5, 2007) at #192 (1,466,000 prescriptions).

In 2010, the IMS Institute for Healthcare Informatics ranked antiplatelets #13 in their top 20 drug classes by spending, with $7.1 billion in sales in the United States. Among individual drug spending, Plavix ranked #3, with $6.1 billion in sales.

Development History

A powder extracted from willow bark has been used since ancient times in many cultures to ease pain and reduce fever; that powder became the basis for aspirin in the early 19th century. But it was not until 1971 that John Robert Vane, who was then employed by the Royal College of Surgeons in London, first showed that aspirin suppresses the production of prostaglandins and thromboxanes.

Ticlopidine was approved by the FDA in October 1991, while clopidogrel was approved in November 1997 and prasugrel din July 2009.

Ticagrelor was approved in July 2011.

The development of GPIIb/IIIa inhibitors arose from the understanding of Glanzmann's thrombasthenia, a condition in which the GPIIb/IIIa receptor on platelets is lacking. Abciximab was approved by the FDA in December 1994; eptifibatide and tirofiban in May 1998.

Dipyridamole was first approved in the early 1960s and cilostazol in January 1999. The combination drug dipyridamole/aspirin was approved in November 1999.

Future Drugs

Regado Biosciences, a drug development company headquartered in Basking Ridge, N.J., but whose technology was invented at Duke University, is focused on validated platelet receptor targets involved in platelet adhesion and activation. Regado's REG3 program consists of a specific GPVI inhibitor and its active control agent (RB571 and RB515, respectively). REG3 was slated to enter Phase I human clinical testing in 2011 and will be indicated for antiplatelet therapy.

Tezampanel, a molecule invented by Dr. Charles Lowenstein and Dr. Craig Morrell of the University of Rochester in New York and developed by Eli Lilly, has been licensed to Raptor Pharmaceutical Corp. in Novato, Calif. Tezampanel has been shown to inhibit human platelet activation, subsequent human platelet aggregation, and thrombosis in mice. The company Web site states, "Tezampanel has been extensively tested in Phase I clinical trials. The drug candidate has been demonstrated to be safe over a wide range of doses, without any serious adverse events and without any major abnormal laboratory tests. Human pharmacokinetics of tezampanel are well characterized. In collaboration with Dr. Lowenstein and Dr. Morrell, Raptor is conducting a Phase I clinical trial in healthy volunteers to determine the efficacy of tezampanel in blocking platelet activation and aggregation."

Seligsohn, Uri. "Glanzmann Thrombasthenia: A Model Disease Which Paved the Way to Powerful Therapeutic Agents." *Pathophysiology of Haemostasis and Thrombosis* 32, no. 5–6 (September–December 2002): 216–217.

antipsychotics Medications used to treat symptoms of severe psychiatric disorder (or psychosis), a broad category of mental disorders often rendering an individual incapable of staying in contact with reality, such as schizophrenia or paranoia. People with psychosis may hear voices or have strange and illogical ideas (for example, thinking that others can hear their thoughts or are trying to harm them or that they are the president of the United States or some other famous person). They may get excited or angry for no apparent reason or spend a lot of time by themselves or in bed sleeping during the day and staying awake at night. The person may neglect appearance, not bathing or changing clothes, and may be hard to talk to—barely talking or saying things that make no sense. They often are initially unaware that their condition is an illness. These kinds of behaviors are symptoms of a psychotic illness such as schizophrenia.

Antipsychotic medications act against these symptoms. These medications cannot "cure" the illness, but they can take away many of the symptoms or make them milder, thus making it possible for the persons with the disorders to function more effectively. In some cases, they can shorten the course of an episode of the illness as well. According to the National Institute of Mental Health (NIMH), approximately 3.2 million Americans have schizophrenia, which affects men and women with equal frequency. Schizophrenia often first appears earlier in men, usually in their late teens or early twenties, than in women, who are generally affected in their twenties or early thirties. Antipsychotic drugs are sometimes called major tranquilizers or neuroleptics, although *major tranquilizers* is becoming less used, as the newer antipsychotics tend to not have strong sedating properties. In the past these drugs have also been called psychotropics. Because everyone responds differently to antipsychotics, several different drugs may need to be tried before the right one is found.

Classes

Two main types of antipsychotics currently exist—typical antipsychotics, sometimes referred to as conventional antipsychotics, and atypical antipsychotics.

Typical antipsychotics are the older antipsychotics, which were introduced in the 1950s.

- The major class (or family) of typical antipsychotics is the *phenothiazines. Examples:* chlorpromazine (Thorazine), fluphenazine (Prolixin), perphenazine (Trilafon), prochlorperazine (Compazine), thioridazine (Mellaril), and trifluoperazine (Stelazine).

- Structurally related are the *thioxanthenes. Example:* thiothixene (Navane, Taractan).

- Other classes in the typical group include:

  - *butyrophenones—Example:* haloperidol (Haldol).

  - *diphenylbutylpiperidones—Example:* pimozide (Orap).

  - *dibenzoxazepines—Example:* loxapine (Loxitane), structurally related to clozapine (an atypical antipsychotic), but a member of the typical group.

  - *dihydroindolones—Example:* molindone (Moban).

Atypical antipsychotics were introduced in the 1990s. Each atypical antipsychotic has a unique side effect profile, but, in general, these medications are better tolerated than the conventional drugs. Because they have fewer side effects than the older drugs, they are often used as a first-line treatment even though the typical group drugs are off-patent and thus available in less costly generic versions. Atypical antipsychotics fall into three classes based on their chemical structure:

- *dibenzepines—Examples:* clozapine (Clozaril), olanzapine (Zyprexa), and quetiapine (Seroquel).

- *benzisoxazoles—Examples:* iloperidone (Fanapt), risperidone (Risperdal), lurasidone (Latuda), and ziprasidone (Geodon).

- *quinolinone—Example:* aripiprazole (Abilify).

How They Work

Antipsychotics affect neurotransmitters that allow communication between nerve cells. It is believed that in psychotic disorders, the brain cells release too much of one such neurotransmitter, dopamine, causing overstimulation of brain activity. Dopamine is thought to be relevant to schizophrenia symptoms. Antipsychotics block the stimulatory actions of dopamine. These drugs can also block other receptors, such as serotonin. The main differences among antipsychotics are in the potency—that is, the dosage (amount) prescribed to produce therapeutic effects—and the side effects. The higher the dose of medication prescribed does not necessarily mean the more serious the illness.

Aripiprazole possesses a novel mechanism of action when compared to other atypical antipsychotics, appearing to mediate its antipsychotic effects primarily by partial agonism at the receptors, meaning that it activates the dopamine and serotonin receptors but does not cause as much of a physiological change as does a full agonist.

Antipsychotic medications have helped many patients with psychosis lead a more normal and fulfilling life by alleviating such symptoms as hallucinations, both visual and auditory, and paranoid thoughts.

Just as people vary in their responses to antipsychotic medications, they also vary in how quickly they improve. Some symptoms may diminish in days; others take weeks or months. Many people see substantial improvement by the sixth week of treatment.

Approved Uses

All antipsychotics except pimozide have been approved to treat schizophrenia, although clozapine and thioridazine are approved only for patients who have failed to respond adequately to other antipsychotic drugs.

In 2002, clozapine was also approved for reducing the risk of suicide in schizophrenic patients judged to be at chronic risk for suicidal behavior.

Haloperidol and pimozide are approved to treat Tourette's syndrome, haloperidol for controlling tics and vocal utterances in both children and adults, and pimozide for those patients who have not responded adequately to other treatment.

Chlorpromazine and haloperidol are used to treat severe behavioral problems in children, including certain symptoms of hyperactivity, such as aggression and extreme agitation.

Olanzapine has been approved for the treatment of schizophrenia, acute mania in bipolar disorder, and agitation associated with schizophrenia and bipolar disorder and as short-term maintenance treatment in bipolar disorder.

Prochlorperazine and trifluoperazine are approved for short-term treatment of nonpsychotic anxiety, but only after the preferred ANTI-ANXIETY AGENTS have proven ineffective.

Chlorpromazine is approved for treating restlessness and apprehension prior to surgery and as part of tetanus treatment and for intractable hiccups.

Chlorpromazine, perphenazine, and prochlorperazine are approved as treatment to control severe nausea and vomiting.

Off-Label Uses

A three-part investigative series by Knight Ridder Newspapers in 2003 found that nearly two-thirds of antipsychotics prescribed during 2002–03 were for off-label use. Among the specific antipsychotic off-label statistics cited in their research:

- **Olanzapine**
  Off-label uses: dementia, depression, anxiety, cancer pain, Huntington's disease
  Percent of this drug's prescriptions that are for off-label uses: 42 percent
  Annual off-label sales: $913 million

- **Quetiapine**
  Off-label uses: depression, anxiety, sleep disorders, Parkinson's symptoms
  Percent of this drug's prescriptions that are for off-label uses: 78 percent
  Annual off-label sales: $778 million

- **Risperidone**
  Off-label uses: autism spectrum disorders, Tourette's syndrome, stuttering
  Percent of this drug's prescriptions that are for off-label uses: 65 percent
  Annual off-label sales: $929 million

Yang and Koo's research also found widespread international off-label use of antipsychotics: "A recent survey of the VA Connecticut Health Care System showed that over a four month period, 42.8 percent of prescribed atypical antipsychotics were given for off-label indications. Patients prescribed off-label antipsychotics were mostly being treated for non-psychotic conditions such as major affective disorder, post-traumatic stress syndrome, Alzheimer's dementia, and dysthymia. Another survey, conducted at an Austrian pharmacy, examined the indications for antipsychotics prescribed to patients at a particular pharmacy. In this survey, 66.5 percent of the patients reported that they were taking antipsychotics for off-label indications. Furthermore, another study conducted by IMS (Intercontinental Marketing Services) Health in 2001 for the National Disease and Therapeutic Index (NTI), illustrated the international prevalence of off-label antipsychotic prescriptions."

Pimozide is used outside the United States to treat schizophrenia, although it has not been approved by the Food and Drug Administration (FDA) for such use.

Chlorpromazine and prochlorperazine are occasionally used off-label for treatment of severe migraine headache.

On April 11, 2005, the FDA issued a public health advisory to alert health care providers, patients, and patient caregivers to new safety information concerning off-label use of atypical antipsychotic drugs to treat behavioral disorders in elderly patients with dementia—with clinical studies showing a higher death rate associated with their use compared to patients receiving a placebo (sugar pill). The FDA requested that the manufacturers of all of these kinds of drugs add a boxed warning to their drug labeling describing this risk and noting that these drugs are not approved for the treatment of behavioral symptoms in elderly patients with dementia. Because the increase in mortality was seen with atypical antipsychotic medications in all three chemical classes, the FDA concluded that the effect is probably related to the common pharmacologic effects of all atypical antipsychotic medications, including those that have not been studied in the dementia population.

Companion Drugs

If people with schizophrenia become depressed, it may be necessary to add an antidepressant to their drug regimen.

Administration

Unlike many prescription drugs, which must be taken several times during the day, some antipsychotic medications can be taken just once a day. In order to reduce daytime side effects such as sleepiness, some can be taken at bedtime. Some antipsychotic medications, such as haloperidol, fluphenazine, and risperidone, are available in a long-acting form called a depot that can be injected once or twice a month. A depot in the body is a storage place, such as a fat depot or drug depot. Depot doses, then, remain in long-term storage in the body. Those medications administered in this manner have been formulated to allow for a slow release of the active drug when given as a deep, intramuscular injection. This has the advantage of providing reliable dosing for a person who has trouble with compliance—either forgetting or skipping daily doses. Also, some patients who do not respond well to oral (tablet) antipsychotics do have better results with depot form. Depot injections can also be used for involuntary treatment of patients to ensure compliance with a legal treatment order when the patient would refuse to take daily oral medication. For practical reasons, depot preparations are limited to high-potency antipsychotics, so the treating physician has a limited choice. It is therefore preferable to use oral medications if the cooperation and compliance of the patient can be obtained.

If a person is feeling better or even completely well, the medication should not be stopped without talking to the doctor. It may be necessary to stay on the medication to continue feeling well. If, after consultation with the doctor, the decision is made to discontinue the medication, it is important to continue to see the doctor while tapering off medication. Many people with bipolar disorder, for instance, require antipsychotic medication only for a limited time during a manic episode until mood-stabilizing medication takes effect. On the other hand, some people may need to take an antipsychotic medication for an extended period of time. These people usually have chronic (long-term, continuous) schizophrenic disorders or have a history of repeated schizophrenic episodes and are likely to become ill again. Also, in some cases, a person who has experienced one or two severe episodes may need medication indefinitely. In these cases, medication may be continued in as low a dosage as possible to maintain control of symptoms. This approach, called maintenance treatment, prevents relapse in many people and removes or reduces symptoms for others.

Cautions and Concerns

A major concern with antipsychotics is patient noncompliance. In September 2005, the National Institute of Mental Health (NIMH)-funded CATIE (Clinical Antipsychotic Trials of Intervention Effectiveness) study compared four atypical antipsychotics and one typical antipsychotic in 1,493 patients from the United States with schizophrenia over 18 months. Overall, this study demonstrated that 74 percent of patients discontinued their medication before 18 months. Several factors, such as adequacy of symptom relief, tolerability of side effects, and treatment cost influenced the patients' willingness and ability to stay on their medication.

Antipsychotic drugs are used with caution in patients with liver damage, kidney disease, and cardiovascular disease.

Use of antipsychotics in the elderly, many of whom are in nursing homes, is widespread and controversial, as they are often used to quiet and control residents instead of as antipsychotics. Also, the phenothiazines class may cause cognitive deficits leading to dementia.

During initial treatment, drowsiness and impaired judgment may affect motor skills and thinking. Thus, extra caution needs to be taken when driving, operating machinery, or executing other tasks requiring mental alertness.

Iloperidone and lurasidone should be used with caution in patients with a history of seizures or having conditions that lower seizure threshold. Dizziness, tachycardia, and fainting can occur on standing, especially early in treatment.

Warnings

Because of the potential side effect of a serious blood disorder—agranulocytosis (loss of the white blood cells that fight infection)—patients who are on clozapine must have blood tests every week for the first six months, with tests every other week after that if the blood counts are initially stable. The inconvenience and cost of blood tests and the medication itself have made maintenance on clozapine difficult for many people. Clozapine, however, continues to be the drug of choice for treatment-resistant schizophrenia patients.

An increased incidence of cerebrovascular adverse events (e.g., stroke, transient ischemic attack) has been seen in elderly patients with dementia-related psychoses treated with atypical antipsychotic drugs. Also, studies have shown that older adults with dementia who take antipsychotics have an increased risk of death during treatment.

When Not Advised (Contraindications)

Most antipsychotics should be avoided during pregnancy, unless essential. Because the safety of typical antipsychotics during breast-feeding has not been established, breast-feeding should be discontinued during treatment, particularly when taking aripiprazole, clozapine, haloperidol, loxapine, olanzapine, quetiapine, risperidone, or ziprasidone.

Coadministration of lurasidone with a strong CYP3A4 inhibitor (e.g., ketoconazole) or inducer (e.g.,rifampin) is contraindicated.

Side Effects

The older typical antipsychotics can cause extrapyramidal side effects, such as rigidity, persistent muscle spasms, tremors, and restlessness.

Long-term treatment with one of the typical antipsychotics may cause a person to develop tardive dyskinesia (TD), a condition characterized by involuntary movements, most often around the mouth. It may range from mild to severe. In some people, it cannot be reversed, while others recover partially or completely. Tardive dyskinesia is sometimes seen in people with schizophrenia who have never been treated with an antipsychotic medication; this is called spontaneous dyskinesia. However, it is most often seen after long-term treatment with older antipsychotic medications. The risk has been reduced with the newer atypical medications. There is a higher incidence in women, and the risk rises with age. The possible risks of long-term treatment with an antipsychotic medication must be weighed against the benefits in each case. The risk for TD is 5 percent per year with older medications; it is less with the newer atypical medications.

Most side effects of atypical antipsychotic medications are mild. Many of the most common side effects, such as drowsiness, rapid heartbeat, and dizziness when changing position, lessen or disappear after the first few weeks of treatment.

Some people gain weight while taking these drugs and need to pay extra attention to diet and exercise to control their weight.

Other side effects may include a decrease in sexual ability or interest, problems with menstrual periods, sunburn, or skin rashes.

Neuroleptic malignant syndrome, or NMS, is a rare but potential side effect with all antipsychotics. NMS is characterized by fever, muscle rigidity, autonomic dysfunction, and altered mental status; it can be fatal. Treatment includes discontinuation of the offending agent and supportive care.

Interactions

Antipsychotic medications can produce unwanted effects when taken with other medications. Therefore, the doctor should be told about all medicines being taken, including over-the-counter medications and vitamin, mineral, and herbal supplements, and the extent of alcohol use. Some antipsychotic medications interfere with ANTIHYPERTENSIVES, ANTICONVULSANTS, and medications used for Parkinson's disease. Other antipsychotics add to the effect of alcohol and other central nervous system depressants such as ANTIHISTAMINES, ANTIDEPRESSANTS, barbiturates (see ANTIANXIETY AGENTS), some sleeping and pain medications, and narcotics.

Sales/Statistics

A University of Pennsylvania study of Medicaid patients over a five-year period found that atypical antipsychotics were used by 39 percent of these patients and constituted 41 percent of all antipsychotic agents prescribed compared to 59 percent for typical agents. Duration on a typical agent was eight months versus 7.4 months for atypicals, with duration 11 months for those on clozapine.

Cooper et al. found that the number of children prescribed antipsychotics jumped fivefold between 1995 and 2002, to an estimated 2.5 million. That is an increase from 8.6 out of every 1,000 children in the mid-1990s to nearly 40 out of 1,000.

According to a 2004 Pharmacor marketing study, U.S. sales of antipsychotics will fall from $2.3 billion in 2008 to $1.5 billion in 2013 as drugs lose the patent protection and go generic.

Antipsychotics were the fifth-highest selling drug class in the United States in 2010, according to the IMS Institute for Healthcare Informatics, with sales of $16.1 billion. In the IMS top 20 individual drug listings, Abilify ranked fifth ($4.6 billion), Seroquel sixth ($4.4 billion), and Zyprexa 17th ($3 billion).

Demographics and Cultural Groups

Following a review of recent literature in psychiatric clinical trials, pharmacology, drug safety, toxicology, obstetrics and gynecology, and pediatrics, Seeman concluded that optimal maintenance regimens of antipsychotics for women and men are not the same. "The pharmacokinetics and pharmacodynamics of antipsychotic drugs differ in women and men and are influenced by gender-specific factors such as body build, diet, smoking, concurrent medication, exercise, substance use, and hormonal transitions. In general, and for some drugs in particular, women require lower doses in order to stay well. Because preliminary drug testing is not done in pregnant women, the issue of effective dosing during pregnancy is unstudied, and safety for fetuses and nursing infants may not become evident until a drug is widely used. Specific adverse effects on issues crucial to women (e.g., parenting) have not been well studied, but some side effects, such as weight gain, passivity, hypotension, and hyperprolactinemia, are reported to be particularly problematic for women."

Kuno and Rothbard found ethnic disparities in antipsychotic prescription patterns among 2,515 adult Medicaid recipients treated for schizophrenia. Black patients were less likely than white patients to receive clozapine (8 percent versus 15 percent, respectively) and risperidone (25 percent versus 31 percent, respectively) and more likely to receive depot antipsychotics (26 percent versus 14 percent, respectively). In general, black patients were more likely to receive typical antipsychotic medications. In terms of the number of months that patients received any type of antipsychotic medication, black patients had significantly shorter treatment durations than did white patients.

Rothbard et al. found that atypical antipsychotic drug users were more likely to be younger white men with higher use of inpatient and ambulatory mental health services compared to those on typical medications.

Development History

Shen wrote, "The history of antipsychotic drug development has had a long and torturous course, often based on chance findings that bear little relationship to the intellectual background driving observations. In 1891, Paul Ehrlich observed the antimalarial effects of methylene blue, a phenothiazine derivative. Later, the phenothiazines were developed for their antihistaminergic properties. In 1951, Laborit and Huguenard administered the aliphatic phenothiazine, chlorpromazine, to patients for its potential anesthetic effects during surgery. Shortly thereafter, Hamon et al. and Delay et al. extended the use of this treatment in psychiatric patients and serendipitously uncovered its antipsychotic activity. Between 1954 and 1975, about 15 antipsychotic drugs were introduced in the United States and about 40 throughout the world."

However, these early antipsychotic medications often have unpleasant side effects, such as muscle stiffness, tremor, and abnormal movements, leading researchers to continue their search for better drugs.

Clozapine was developed by Sandoz in 1961 and introduced in Europe 10 years later. In 1975, after reports of agranulocytosis that led to death in some patients, clozapine was voluntarily withdrawn by the manufacturer. However, in 1989, when studies demonstrated that clozapine was more effective against treatment-resistant schizophrenia than other antipsychotics, the FDA approved its use only for treatment-resistant schizophrenia and required blood monitoring.

During the 1990s, risperidone (1993), olanzapine (1996), and quetiapine (1997) were introduced, with ziprasidone (2001) and aripiprazole (2002) soon following.

Future Drugs

According to industry watchers, a new wave of antipsychotics that focus on drug delivery and pharmacokinetics are progressing though the pipeline. Among them:

Ocaperidone is a new benzisoxazol antipsychotic with particularly beneficial effects in schizophrenia being developed by Neuro3d, a French drug discovery and development company that hopes for the drug's approval in Europe and the United States. No change in mean weight gain compared to baseline was seen in patients receiving ocaperidone in one placebo-controlled Phase II trial. In a second study comparing ocaperidone against a standard atypical antipsychotic compound, weight gain was statistically significantly higher in patients treated with the reference compound. Also, no serious adverse effects or cardiovascular events were observed with ocaperidone.

Cariprazine (RGH-188) is an antipsychotic drug being developed by Forest/Gedeon Richter. An atypical antipsychotic, it works as a dopamine receptor antagonist, with high selectivity toward D3 receptors. Phase III studies for schizophrenia and mania in bipolar disorder I were expected by the end of 2011. Phase II studies for bipolar depression are also in progress. It may also be useful as an add-on therapy in major depressive disorder. The developers describe the drug as a "dopamine stabilizer."

Blonanserin (AD 5423) is a combined D and 5-HT receptor antagonist currently undergoing development in Japan (Dainippon Sumitomo Pharmaceutical). According to *Primary Psychiatry,* "Blonanserin is unrelated structurally to typical antipsychotics or to newer agents such as risperidone. It is hoped that the combination of receptor blockade possessed by blonanserin will be effective against both the positive and negative symptoms of schizophrenia, with a low tendency to cause EPS (extrapyramidal symptoms). Blonanserin is expected to have minimal sedative and hypotensive effects, as its adrenaline receptor-blocking function is weak. Dainippon is conducting phase III clinical trials with oral formulations (tablet and powder) of the compound in psychotic disorders in the United States."

Cooper, William, et al. "Trends in Prescribing of Antipsychotic Medications for U.S. Children." *Ambulatory Pediatrics* 6, no. 2 (March–April 2006): 79–83.

Glick, Ira D., and Eric D. Peselow. "New Antipsychotic Agents." *Primary Psychiatry* 15, no. 12 (2008): 57–64. Available online. URL: http://www.primarypsychiatry.com/aspx/articledetail.aspx?articleid=1908. Accessed August 3, 2011.

Kuno, Eri, and Aileen B. Rothbard. "Racial Disparities in Antipsychotic Prescription Patterns for Patients with Schizophrenia." *American Journal of Psychiatry* 159, no. 4 (April 2002): 567–572.

Rothbard, Aileen B., Eri Kuno, and K. Foley. "Trends in the Rate and Type of Antipsychotic Medications Prescribed to Persons with Schizophrenia." *Schizophrenia Bulletin* 29, no. 3 (2003): 531–540.

Seeman, M. V. "Gender Differences in the Prescribing of Antipsychotic Drugs." *American Journal of Psychiatry* 161, no. 8 (August 2004): 1,324–1,333.

Shen, W. W. "A History of Antipsychotic Drug Development." *Comprehensive Psychiatry* 40, no. 6 (November–December 1999): 407–414.

Yang, Aparche, and John Y. Koo. "Non-psychotic Uses for Antipsychotics." *Journal of Drugs in Dermatology* 3, no. 2 (March–April 2004): 162–168.

antiresorptives Drugs that slow the progressive thinning of bone in osteoporosis. Osteoporosis is a disease that reduces bone density, weakening the bones to the point that they become fragile and break easily. Particularly susceptible to fracture are bones in the hip, spine, pelvis, upper arm, and wrist. Fractures related to osteoporosis are frequently associated with chronic pain and decreased quality of life as well as significant morbidity and mortality. About 80 percent of those affected by osteoporosis are women; approximately 8 million women in the United States have osteoporosis, and 22 million have low bone mineral density (BMD—also referred to as bone quantity or bone mass) of the hip. More than 2 million men in the United States also have osteoporosis, and 14 million more have low bone mass. The lifetime risk of experiencing an osteoporotic fracture in men over the age of 50 is estimated to be 30 percent, similar to the lifetime risk of developing prostate cancer. Although postmenopausal women are at particular risk, osteoporosis can strike at any age and is responsible for more than 1.5 million fractures annually in the United States. As many as half of all women older than 50 will break a bone due to osteoporosis. A combination of genetic, dietary, hormonal, age-related, and lifestyle factors all contribute to osteoporosis. Women are at higher risk for osteoporosis because they have smaller bones, and they lose bone more rapidly than men because of hormone changes that occur after menopause. Some children and adolescents develop osteoporosis that has no known cause, known as idiopathic juvenile osteoporosis (IJO). Young people who have this rare form of osteoporosis usually recover completely within two to four years. Antiresorptive therapies reduce bone loss, stabilize the microarchitecture (interior structure) of the bone, and decrease bone turnover (also called remodeling, or the continual process of bone breakdown and formation)—all leading to a reduction in fractures. These drugs increase BMD because the resorption (breakdown) spaces in bone get refilled with new bone and the amount of mineral in the bone increases. Antiresorptives do not build bone beyond what is produced to help fill the remodeling spaces. Antiresorptives are also used to reduce fractures, spinal cord compression, and other skeletal events in patients with bone metastases (the spread of cancerous cells from the original site to bone).

Classes

Antiresorptive drugs are classified according to their mechanisms of action.

- *Bisphosphonates*—phosphate-based, nonhormonal compounds that have been shown to increase BMD and decrease fractures. *Examples:* alendronate (Fosamax), etidronate (Didronel), ibandronate (Boniva), pamidronate (Aredia), risedronate (Actonel), tiludronate (Skelid), and zoledronic acid (Reclast, Zometa).

- *Selective estrogen receptor modulators (SERMs)*—interact with estrogen receptors located throughout the body. *Example:* raloxifene (Evista).

- *Estrogen therapy*—Estrogen is a hormone that is important throughout life for bone development and maintenance in both men and women. Estrogen therapy is the oldest prescribed treatment for osteoporosis, but it is the most controversial because of its health risks. *Examples:* conjugated estrogen (Premarin), estradiol (Alora, Climara, Estrace, Estraderm, Menostar, Vivelle, Vivelle Dot), and estropipate (Ogen, Ortho-Est).

- *RANK ligand inhibitors*—RANK ligand (RANKL) is a protein that acts as the primary signal to promote bone removal. In many bone loss conditions, RANK ligand overwhelms the body's natural defense against bone destruction. *Example:* denosumab (Prolia, Xgeva).

- *Other*—calcitonin (Fortical, Miacalcin), a hormone produced by the thyroid gland when serum calcium is elevated that acts primarily on bone. The drug calcitonin is derived from salmon.

In addition to prescription drugs, the National Institute of Arthritis and Musculoskeletal and Skin Diseases (NIAMS) stresses that adequate calcium and vitamin D are essential for minimizing bone loss and maintaining bone health. Calcium is the most important nutrient for preventing osteoporosis and for reaching peak bone mass. The body depends on dietary calcium to build healthy new bone and avoid excessive loss of calcium from bone to meet other needs. Adults need 1,000 milligrams of calcium per day, and the recommendation increases to 1,200 milligrams after age 50.

Many people in the United States consume much less than the recommended amount of calcium in their diets. Good sources of calcium include low-fat dairy products; dark green leafy vegetables, including broccoli, bok choy, collards, and turnip greens; sardines and salmon with bones; soy beans, tofu, and other soy products; and calcium-fortified foods such as orange juice, cereals, and breads. Those who have trouble getting enough calcium in their diet may need to take a calcium supplement such as calcium carbonate or calcium citrate.

How They Work

Bisphosphonates attach to the surfaces of bones and reduce the ability of osteoclasts (bone cells that break down [erode] bone tissue) to bind to and break down the bone. This process allows the osteoblasts (cells that build bone tissue) to work more effectively.

Raloxifene mimics the action of estrogen on the bones, protecting against bone loss, and blocks estrogen from binding to breast and uterine tissues.

Estrogen therapy slows bone loss and prevents osteoporosis when taken after menopause.

RANK ligand inhibitors work by decreasing bone breakdown and increasing bone strength and density.

Calcitonin is a hormone that inhibits the activity of osteoclasts, thus reducing bone breakdown. By causing less bone tissue to be reabsorbed, it slows the rate of bone destruction and decreases the amount of calcium released into the blood. Salmon calcitonin is 30 times more potent than that secreted by the human thyroid gland.

Approved Uses

Bisphosphonates are used to slow bone loss, reduce fracture risk, and in some cases increase bone density. Specifically, alendronate, ibandronate, and risedronate are indicated for the treatment and prevention of osteoporosis in postmenopausal women. Alendronate and risedronate are approved for the treatment of osteoporosis in men. Alendronate and risedronate are also approved for the treatment (both drugs) and prevention (risedronate only) of osteoporosis due to corticosteroids in men and women who have low BMD and are receiving a daily dosage equivalent to at least 7.5 mg of prednisone for the management of chronic diseases.

Bisphosphonates are also used in treating Paget's disease, cancer metastatic to bone, and other bone diseases with high bone resorption. Specifically, etidronate, pamidronate, risedronate, tiludronate, and zoledronic acid are approved to treat Paget's disease. Etidronate is also used to treat heterotopic ossification (abnormal formation of bone in soft tissues) after total hip replacement or due to spinal cord injury. Pamidronate and zoledronic acid are used to treat hypercalcemia of malignancy. Pamidronate is also approved to treat osteolytic bone metastases of breast cancer and osteolytic lesions of multiple myeloma in conjunction with standard ANTINEOPLASTIC therapy. Zoledronic acid is also approved for treatment of patients with multiple myeloma and patients with documented bone metastases from solid tumors in conjunction with standard antineoplastic therapy.

Raloxifene is approved for the treatment and prevention of osteoporosis in postmenopausal women.

Estrogen is approved for the treatment of menopausal symptoms and prevention of osteoporosis.

Under the brand name Prolia, denosumab is approved to treat postmenopausal women with osteoporosis at high risk for fracture and patients who have failed or are intolerant to other available osteoporosis therapy. In postmenopausal women with osteoporosis, Prolia reduces the incidence of vertebral, nonvertebral, and hip fractures. Under the brand name Xgeva, denosumab is approved to prevent skeletal-related events in patients with bone metastases from solid tumors.

Calcitonin nasal spray and injection are approved for the treatment of osteoporosis in women who are at least five years past menopause. Only the injection is approved for the treatment of Paget's disease and hypercalcemia (increased levels of calcium in the blood).

Off-Label Uses

Although etidronate is not approved by the Food and Drug Administration (FDA) for osteoporosis, it is used in Canada and Europe for this purpose. It is also used in the United States off-label for the treatment and prevention of osteoporosis in postmenopausal women and for prevention of corticosteroid-induced osteoporosis.

Pamidronate is used off-label to treat hyperparathyroidism and to reduce pain in patients with prostate cancer.

Following a large trial comparing raloxifene versus tamoxifen, the National Comprehensive Cancer Network in 2007 added raloxifene to its treatment guidelines as a breast cancer risk reduction agent for healthy postmenopausal women at increased risk of breast cancer. It is being considered by the FDA for breast cancer prevention in this particular group of women.

Calcitonin is used off-label to alleviate bone pain in cancer patients.

Administration

Alendronate, etidronate, ibandronate, risedronate, and tiludronate are available in tablet form—alendronate in daily and weekly doses; risedronate in daily, weekly, and monthly doses; ibandronate in a daily or monthly dose. Alendronate is also available as an oral solution. Also, ibandronate, pamidronate, and zoledronic acid are administered via intravenous injection.

Alendronate is also available in combination with cholecalciferol, a form of vitamin D (Fosamax Plus D). Risedronate is also available as a product called Actonel and Calcium, which contains risedronate tablets as well as calcium carbonate tablets.

Raloxifene is available as oral tablets.

Estrogen therapy is available in oral tablets or capsules or as a transdermal (skin) patch.

Denosumab is given as a subcutaneous injection every six months when treating osteoporosis and every four weeks when treating patients whose cancer has spread to the bones.

Calcitonin is not effective when given orally; it is available for injection or in a nasal spray.

Cautions and Concerns

Physicians should proceed cautiously when prescribing oral bisphosphonates to patients with a known history of narrowing or ulcers of the esophagus or long-term problems with stomach ulcers and heartburn that require medication.

According to guidelines published in the *Journal of the American Dental Association* (ADA), a small but growing number of reports have linked bisphosphonates to the development of osteonecrosis of the jaw (dead bone tissue). Therefore, the ADA recommends that dental patients who are receiving oral bisphosphonates discuss with their dentists the risks they face when undergoing procedures that involve the jaw bone, such as tooth extraction or placing implants. Patients with risk factors for osteonecrosis should undergo dental examination and preventive dentistry prior to starting bisphosphonate therapy. The ADA further states that patients currently receiving intravenous bisphosphonates should avoid invasive dental procedures if possible. The risk of osteonecrosis of the jaw in patients using oral bisphosphonates following dental surgery appears to be low. The ADA notes that dentists, generally, will not need to modify dental treatments based solely on bisphosphonate therapy. Further, patients should understand that the risk for developing osteonecrosis of the jaw is considered very small and that the vast majority of patients receiving a bisphosphonate do not develop any oral complication.

Patients taking oral bisphosphonates should take calcium and vitamin D supplements; however, because calcium supplements may interfere with the body's ability to absorb bisphosphonates, they should not be taken at the same time of day.

Wysowski and Chang describe more than 100 reports received by the FDA of severe bone, joint, and muscle pain in patients being treated with alendronate for osteoporosis. Many patients were unable to walk, climb stairs, or perform usual activities, and some of them became bedridden. Many of them had numerous diagnostic tests with mostly normal findings. A majority of the patients experienced relief from pain after the drug was discontinued. This improvement was gradual in most of the patients, although some did show immediate improvement. The article also notes that the FDA has received similar reports for risedronate, suggesting a possible class effect. The article states that pain in patients treated with bisphosphonates is likely to be underreported because of its subjective nature and because physicians may attribute the pain to the osteoporosis itself. Patients should be instructed to report severe bone, joint, or muscle pain that starts shortly after beginning bisphosphonate therapy, and physicians should consider discontinuing the drug if that happens.

To be effective, bisphosphonate therapy for osteoporosis must continue for at least a year, yet studies have shown that nearly half of all patients on oral bisphosphonates stop therapy, according to Sayler. "Short-term use not only thwarts the treatment but has the opposite effect intended," putting patients at increased risk of fracture.

With that being said, there are concerns about long-term use of older bisphosphonates such as etidronate, with animal studies suggesting increased risk of fracture. This has not been seen in animal studies with risedronate and alendronate. It appears that alendronate may be safely taken for 10 years; however, it is not clear whether there is any benefit from taking bisphosphonates continuously for longer than five years, according to Terri L. Levien, Pharm. D, writing in *Arthritis Self-Management* magazine (March/April 2006).

Raloxifene has not been adequately studied with concurrent use of estrogen or hormone replacement therapy or lipid-lowering agents in women with a prior history of breast cancer or in men.

Estrogen therapy may cause breast tenderness, weight gain, fluid retention, gall bladder disease, vaginal bleeding, and an increased risk of breast or endometrial cancers. This therapy may also increase the risk of heart attack, stroke, or blood clots.

In clinical trials, infections associated with denosumab occurred at a higher rate than with placebo. Green writes: "The suggested mechanism of the increased risk of infection may be attributable to RANKL inhibition, because RANKL can be found on T and B lymphocytes and in lymph nodes. Therefore, patients taking immunosuppressant agents or patients with impaired immune systems may be at a higher risk for infections, including serious infections" when taking denosumab therapy.

A nasal examination should be performed prior to starting patients on calcitonin nasal spray because of the potential for the drug to cause nasal abnormalities (e.g., nose bleeds, runny nose, ulcers).

Daily calcium intake should not exceed 2,500 milligrams, because too much calcium can cause problems such as kidney stones. Calcium coming from food sources provides better protection from kidney stones. Anyone who has had a kidney stone should increase their dietary calcium and decrease the amount from supplements as well as increase fluid intake.

Warnings

Oral bisphosphonates can cause serious digestive problems if they are not taken properly. All bisphosphonates are poorly absorbed and therefore should be taken alone first thing in the morning on an empty stomach with a full glass of water. These drugs should be taken at least 30 minutes (60 minutes for ibandronate, two hours for tiludronate and etidronate) before consuming any food, drink (other than water), or medications. Patients should not lie down for at least 30 minutes (60 minutes for ibandronate) after taking the medication to prevent irritation of the esophagus.

The bisphophosphonate drugs zoledronic acid and pamidronate can cause deterioration in kidney function, which may progress to kidney failure. The true incidence of this severe complication is unknown. Because of the widespread use of bisphosphonates, experts advise monitoring of renal function, especially prior to each dose. As progressive myeloma can also cause kidney deterioration and the standard duration of bisphosphonate usage is indefinite, a constant risk/benefit assessment is warranted.

In clinical trials, raloxifene-treated women showed an increased risk of deep vein thrombosis (DVT) and pulmonary embolism. The greatest risk for thromboembolic events occurs during the first four months of treatment. Patients should be advised to move around frequently during prolonged travel experiences. Because of the increased potential for clot formation, raloxifene should be discontinued if the patient experiences a prolonged period of immobility. The risk-to-benefit balance should be considered in women at risk of these clotting conditions, such as those with congestive heart failure and/or active malignancy.

The Women's Health Initiative (WHI) study reported increased risks of heart attack, stroke, invasive breast cancer, and blood clots in the lungs and in the legs in postmenopausal women during five years of treatment with conjugated estrogens combined with medroxyprogesterone acetate. Because of the availability of safer medications for osteoporosis, estrogen therapy should be considered only for women at significant risk for osteoporosis who are not able to take these non-estrogen-containing medications.

Hypocalcemia must be corrected before initiating denosumab (see *Contraindications*), as it may worsen, especially in patients with renal impairment. Patients must supplement denosumab with calcium and vitamin D. Serious infections, including skin infections, may occur, including those leading to hospitalization (see *Cautions and Concerns*). Patients should seek prompt medical attention if they develop signs or symptoms of infection, including cellulitis.

When Not Advised (Contraindications)

Bisphosphonates should not be given to patients with severe kidney disease or hypocalcemia (low calcium levels in the blood). Patients with abnormalities of the esophagus should not take alendronate. Patients who cannot stand or sit upright for at least 30 minutes should not take alendronate or risendronate. Patients who cannot stand or sit upright for at least 60 minutes should not take ibandronate.

Raloxifene should not be used in women who are pregnant or breast-feeding. This drug also should not be used in women who have a history of blood clots. The safety of raloxifene in premenopausal women has not been established, and its use is not recommended in this patient group.

Women with a personal or family history of breast cancer or those who are pregnant should not take estrogens. Estrogen therapy is also contraindicated in patients with a history of blood clots, heart attack, stroke, or liver disease. Estrogens should also not be used in women experiencing unusual vaginal bleeding that has not been checked by a doctor.

Denosumab is contraindicated in patients who have hypocalcemia.

Because the drug calcitonin is derived from salmon, it should not be used in patients with a salmon allergy.

Side Effects

The most common side effects of oral bisphosphonates include nausea, heartburn, and stomach pain, which can be minimized or prevented by remaining seated upright for 30 to 60 minutes after taking the medication. Intravenous bisphosphonates can also cause fever and flulike symptoms after the first infusion. Pamidronate, particularly at dosages above 60 mg, may cause chills, confusion, muscle spasms, sore throat, constipation, and decreased appetite.

The most common side effects with raloxifene include hot flashes, leg cramps, nausea, weight gain, and fluid retention.

Estrogen therapy may cause breast tenderness, weight gain, fluid retention, gall bladder disease, and vaginal bleeding.

The most common side effects reported with denosumab are back pain, pain in arms or legs, muscle pain, hypercholesterolemia, and cystitis.

Calcitonin injection may cause nausea, vomiting, and flushing of the hands or face; the nasal spray is most frequently associated with back pain or a runny or stuffy nose.

Interactions

Calcium supplements, iron supplements, and antacids interfere with the absorption of all oral bisphosphonates. The oral bisphosphonates should be taken at least 30 minutes (60 minutes for ibandronate, two hours for tiludronate and etidronate) before these particular medications. Aspirin and nonsteroidal anti-inflammatory drugs may increase the risk for developing esophageal or gastrointestinal irritation with the oral bisphosphonates. Aspirin can significantly decrease the absorption of tiludronate, while indomethacin can significantly increase the absorption of tiludronate. Therefore, tiludronate should not be taken within two hours of either of these medications.

Cholestyramine may decrease the absorption of raloxifene; if used together, the raloxifene should be taken either one hour before or four to six hours after the cholestyramine.

No drug-drug interaction studies have been conducted with denosumab.

Potent CYP3A4 inhibitors (e.g., clarithromycin, erythromycin, itraconazole, ketoconazole, ritonavir, and grapefruit juice) may increase the blood levels of estrogens and increase the patient's potential for developing side effects. Drugs that induce CYP3A4 (e.g., carbamazepine, Saint-John's-wort, rifampin, phenobarbital, and phenytoin) may decrease the blood levels of estrogens.

Sales/Statistics

GlobalData's report, *Osteoporosis—Pipeline Assessment and Market Forecasts to 2017*, noted that "the global osteoporosis therapeutics market was valued at $9.6 billion in 2009. It is expected to grow to $18.2 billion by 2017."

In the United States, Fosamax ranked #23 among the "Top 200 Brand-Name Drugs by Retail Dollars in 2006" (*Drug Topics*, February

19, 2007), with $2,480,042,000 in sales. Actonel ranked #48 ($780,529,000); Evista #77 ($507,954,000); Boniva #119 ($270,321,000). Fosamax ranked #14 among the "Top 200 Brand-Name Drugs by Units in 2006" (*Drug Topics,* March 5, 2007), with 16,720,000 total prescriptions; Actonel #41; Evista #66; Boniva #100; and Miacalcin #199.

Boniva ranked #72 among the "2010 Top 200 Branded Drugs by Retail Dollars" (*Drug Topics,* June 2011), with $480,470,301 in sales. Evista ranked #77 ($469,013,238), and Actonel 150 #122 ($264,858,113). In the "2010 Top 200 Branded Drugs by Prescriptions," Boniva ranked #62, with 3,524,839 prescriptions dispensed, Evista ranked #69 (3,296,079), and Actonel ranked #83 (2,558,636). Alendronate was the only generic antiresoptive on the 2010 lists, ranking #50 in sales ($288,712,684) and #41 in prescriptions (16,177,014).

Demographics and Cultural Groups

According to Miller, "Twenty percent of non-Hispanic white and Asian women age 50 and older are estimated to have osteoporosis and 52 percent are estimated to have low bone mass. The corresponding figures for non-Hispanic black women are 5 percent and 35 percent (for osteoporosis and low bone mass, respectively); these figures are slightly higher in Hispanic women (10 percent and 49 percent). One out of every two white women will experience an osteoporosis-related fracture (i.e., a fracture in which the associated trauma would not have resulted in a fracture of normal bone; also called a fragility fracture)."

Development History

According to *Bone Health and Osteoporosis: A Report of the Surgeon General* (U.S. Department of Health & Human Services, October 2004), Fuller Albright, a clinical researcher in the 1930s, observed that most of his patients with osteoporosis were postmenopausal women. Given this, Albright proposed that estrogen triggers a buildup of calcium reserves in bone during adolescence to provide for later reproductive needs (pregnancy and lactation) and that bone is lost after menopause when estrogen levels decrease. Many subsequent observations have confirmed the theory that "replacing" estrogen in postmenopausal women prevents bone loss, and thus this approach naturally seemed to be an effective way to stave off the effects of menopause on bone.

The FDA approved estrogen in 1942 in the form of conjugated equine estrogens (CEE), derived from the urine of pregnant horses, for the relief of menopausal symptoms. The use of hormone therapy by postmenopausal women increased dramatically during the 1960s, and, in 1972, the FDA approval was extended to postmenopausal osteoporosis. This latter approval was based on evidence from trials that evaluated the impact of estrogen therapy on bone mass, not on fracture reduction. However, by the early 1970s, it also became clear that estrogen alone (without progestin) was associated with an increased risk of endometrial (uterine) cancer. Since this time, only women who have had their uterus removed by hysterectomy are prescribed estrogen alone; women with an intact uterus should receive estrogen combined with some form of progesterone, another hormone, to protect the uterus.

Bisphosphonates were first synthesized in Germany in 1865, but their original use was industrial, mainly in the textile, fertilizer, and oil industries, according to Fleisch. Their nonmedical use over the years included water softening in irrigation systems used in orange groves and in washing powders. The first medical potential for bisphosphonates was reported in 1968, when they were investigated for use in disorders of bone metabolism. The initial rationale for their use in humans was their potential in preventing the dissolution of hydroxyapatite, the principal bone mineral, and hence arresting bone loss. Etidronate was approved for treatment of Paget's disease in 1977, pamidronate in October 1991, tiludronate in 1997, risedronate in 1998, and zoledronic acid in 2007. Alendronate was approved for the management of osteoporosis in September 1995, risedronate in March 1998, and ibandronate in May 2003. Zoledronic acid received FDA approval in 2001 for hypercalcemia of malignancy and in 2002 for bone metastases. Pamidronate received FDA approval in 1998 to treat osteolytic bone metastases of breast cancer in conjunction with standard antineoplastic therapy and in 2002 to treat hypercalcemia associated with malignancy, with or without bone metastases.

Denosumab was the first RANK ligand inhibitor to be approved by the FDA. It was approved for osteoporosis treatment in June 2010 and for bone cancer therapy in November 2010.

Calcitonin was purified in 1962 by Copp and Cheney. While it was initially considered a secretion of the parathyroid glands, it was later identified as the secretion of the C-cells of the thyroid gland. The FDA approved the first drug based on salmon calcitonin in an injectable form in 1975. Though the calcitonin in drugs is based chemically on salmon calcitonin, it is now made synthetically in the lab in a form that copies the molecular structure of the fish gland extract. Synthetic calcitonin offers a simpler, more economical way to create large quantities of the product.

The interest in developing a SERM for the prevention and treatment of osteoporosis occurred when it was observed that the antineoplastic tamoxifen has estrogenlike effects on bone. Raloxifene was approved by the FDA for the prevention of postmenopausal osteoporosis in 1997 and for the treatment of postmenopausal osteoporosis in 1999.

Future Drugs

According to reports at medical meetings in 2006, investigational antiresorptives are not likely to increase bone mineral density any more so than the current bisphosphonates; however, they may be easier for patients to take. The hope is that new methods of action and new dosing regimens may improve patient compliance.

A newer class of antiresorptive drugs (known as integrin inhibitors) prevent osteoclasts from anchoring to bone surfaces and thereby absorbing the underlying bone. Early studies with this therapy are encouraging with respect to both safety and effectiveness, according to the Surgeon General's 2004 report. One such drug, L-000845704, is being investigated by Merck Research Laboratories.

An oral version of salmon calcitonin is in clinical trials. Thus far, poor absorption and rapid proteolytic degradation have impeded the clinical development of an orally administered salmon calcitonin drug product, according to Lee and Sinko. Early in 2007, Novartis Pharma AG and its development partner Nordic Bioscience initiated a Phase III clinical trial for the treatment of osteoporosis with salmon calcitonin formulated in a tablet form using a novel delivery technology developed by Emisphere Technologies, Inc., a biopharmaceutical company. Emisphere's eligen® technology makes it possible to orally deliver a therapeutic molecule across biological membranes such as the small intestine without altering its chemical form or biological integrity.

Copp, D. H., and B. Cheney. "Calcitonin—A Hormone from the Parathyroid Which Lowers the Calcium-level of the Blood." *Nature* 193 (January 27, 1962): 381–382.

Fleisch, Herbert. "Development of Bisphosphonates." *Breast Cancer Research* 4, no. 1 (2002): 30–34.

Green, Wendy. "Denosumab (Prolia) Injection: A New Approach to the Treatment of Women with Postmenopausal Osteoporosis." *Pharmacy and Therapeutics* 10, no. 35 (October 2010): 553–559. Available online. URL: http://www.ncbi.nlm.nih.gov/pmc/articles/PMC2957751/. Accessed August 3, 2011.

Lee, Y. H., and P. J. Sinko. "Oral Delivery of Salmon Calcitonin." *Advanced Drug Delivery Reviews* 42, no. 3 (August 31, 2000): 225–238.

Mehrotra, Bhoomi, and Salvatore Ruggiero. "Bisphosphonate Complications Including Osteonecrosis of the Jaw." *Hematology* (2006): 356–360. Available online. URL: http://www.asheducationbook.org/cgi/content/full/2006/1/356. Downloaded on February 27, 2007.

Miller, Redonda G. "Osteoporosis in Postmenopausal Women." *Geriatrics* 61, no. 1 (January 2006): 24–30.

Sayler, Mary Harwell. *The Encyclopedia of the Back and Spine Systems and Disorders.* New York: Facts On File, 2007.

Wysowski, Diane K., and Jennie T. Chang. "Alendronate and Risedronate: Reports of Severe Bone, Joint and Muscle Pain." *Archives of Internal Medicine* 165 (February 14, 2005): 346–347. Available online. URL: http://www.fda.gov/cdrh/psn/show-54-alendronate.html. Downloaded on February 27, 2007.

antiretrovirals Drugs used in the treatment of infection by retroviruses, primarily human immunodeficiency virus (HIV); also called anti-HIV drugs. Antiretrovirals are used to control the reproduction of the HIV virus and to slow the progression of HIV-related disease. By killing or damaging cells of the body's immune system, HIV progressively destroys the body's ability to fight infections and certain cancers. The combination of several (typically three or four) antiretroviral drugs is known as Highly Active Anti-Retroviral Therapy (HAART) and is the recommended treatment for HIV infection. Antiretrovials do not cure HIV infection, and individuals taking these medications can still transmit HIV to others. Human immunodeficiency virus causes AIDS (acquired immunodeficiency syndrome), which was first reported in the United States in 1981 and has since become a major worldwide epidemic. The term AIDS applies to the most advanced stages of HIV infection. People diagnosed with AIDS may get life-threatening diseases called opportunistic infections, which are caused by microbes such as viruses or bacteria that usually do not make healthy people sick. In 2006, more than 1 million persons were living with HIV/AIDS in the United States.

Classes

Antiretrovirals are classified according to the way they attack HIV and help the body fight infection:

- *Nucleoside/nucleotide reverse transcriptase inhibitors (NRTIs)—Examples:* abacavir (Ziagen), abacavir/lamivudine (Epzicom), abacavir/lamivudine/zidovudine (Trizivir), didanosine (Videx), emtricitabine (Emtriva), emtricitabine/tenofovir (Truvada), etravirine (Intelence), lamivudine (Epivir), lamivudine/zidovudine (Combivir), stavudine (Zerit), tenofovir DF (Viread), and zidovudine (Retrovir).

- *Nonnucleoside reverse transcriptase inhibitors (NNRTIs)—Examples:* delavirdine (Rescriptor), efavirenz (Sustiva), nevirapine (Viramune), and rilpivirine (Edurant).

- *Protease inhibitors (PIs)—Examples:* atazanavir (Reyataz), darunavir (Prezista), fosamprenavir (Lexiva), indinavir (Crixivan), lopinavir/ritonavir (Kaletra), nelfinavir (Viracept), ritonavir (Norvir), saquinavir (Invirase), and tipranavir (Aptivus).

- *Entry and fusion inhibitors—Examples:* enfuvirtide (Fuzeon) and maraviroc (Selzentry).

- *Integrase inhibitors—Example:* raltegravir (Isentress).

- *Miscellaneous*—Fixed dose combinations containing two or more anti-HIV medications from more than one drug class. *Example:* efavirenz/emtricitabine/tenofovir (Atripla).

How They Work

Antiretrovirals attack the HIV virus directly and cripple the ability of the virus to make copies of itself. Different classes of antiretroviral drugs act at different stages of the HIV life cycle. When the HIV virus enters a healthy cell, it attempts to make copies of itself by using an enzyme called reverse transcriptase. Without reverse transcriptase, HIV cannot make new virus copies of itself.

The NRTIs, which are faulty versions of the building blocks (nucleosides) used by reverse transcriptase, work by blocking that enzyme. When HIV uses an NRTI instead of a normal building block, reproduction of the virus is stalled.

NNRTIs also prevent HIV from using reverse transcriptase to make copies of itself, but in a different way. NNRTIs bind to and disable reverse transcriptase.

Once HIV has infected a cell and makes copies of itself, it uses an enzyme called protease to process itself correctly so it can be released from the cell to infect other cells. PIs work by blocking or disabling protease.

The fusion and entry inhibitors work by stopping the HIV virus from getting into the body's healthy cells in the first place. Enfuvirtide disrupts the HIV-1 molecular machinery at the final stage of fusion with the target cell, preventing uninfected cells from becoming infected. Maraviroc blocks the cell surface protein CCR5 to prevent the virus from entering cells.

Integrase inhibitors work by blocking integrase, a protein that HIV needs to insert its viral genetic material into the genetic material of an infected cell.

Approved Uses

Antiretrovirals are used in combination with one another in order to get the best results. The goal is to get the viral load as low as possible for as long as possible.

Except in very special circumstances, anti-HIV drugs should never be used one or two at a time. Using only one or two drugs at a time can fail to control the viral load and let the virus adapt (or become resistant) to the drugs. Once the virus adapts to a drug, the drug will not work as well against the virus and may not work at all.

HIV treatment guidelines in the United States are set by the Department of Health and Human Services (DHHS). For example, guidelines for adults and adolescents stated on January 29, 2008, included:

- Antiretroviral therapy is recommended for the following groups of patients:
  - all patients with a history of an AIDS-defining illness regardless of CD4 cell count. (CD4 is a primary receptor used by HIV to gain entry into host T cells. The Centers for Disease Control and Prevention [CDC]'s definition of AIDS includes all HIV-infected people with a CD4 count less than 200

cells/mm^3. Healthy adults usually have CD4 counts of 1,000 cells/mm^3 or more.)
  - patients with a CD4 count less than 350 cells/mm^3
  - pregnant women infected with HIV (regardless of CD4 cell count)
  - patients with HIV-associated nephropathy (regardless of CD4 cell count)
  - patients with HIV who are also infected with hepatitis B virus and require therapy for the hepatitis (regardless of CD4 cell count)
- Antiretroviral therapy may be considered in certain patients with CD4 counts greater than 350 cells/mm^3.

A combination antiretroviral regimen in treatment-naïve patients generally contains one NNRTI + two NRTIs or a single PI (with or without ritonavir boosting) + two NRTIs. The Office of AIDS Research Advisory Council (OARAC) cautions that specific drug regimens for managing HIV evolve rapidly, and for this reason guidelines are updated regularly and posted on the AIDS*info* Web site at http://AIDSinfo.nih.gov.

Ritonavir boosting is an approach using ritonavir in combination with other PIs. Studies have shown that small amounts of ritonavir can "boost" or increase the strength and effectiveness of these drugs and may overcome drug and food interactions. In some cases, ritonavir boosting reduces the number of pills necessary or how often they are taken.

Lamivudine is also used to treat chronic hepatitis B associated with evidence of hepatitis B viral replication and active liver inflammation.

Administration

Most antiretrovirals come as pills, capsules, or coated tablets. Abacavir, emtricitabine, fosamprenavir, lamivudine, lopinavir/ritonavir, nevirapine, ritonavir, stavudine, and zidovudine are also available as oral solutions or suspensions. Nelfinavir is also available as an oral powder. Zidovudine is also available as an intravenous injection. Enfuvirtide is available only as a subcutaneous injection.

Malabsorption can occur if certain antiretroviral agents are taken improperly with regard to meals. Didanosine should be taken on an empty stomach, at least 30 minutes before or two hours after eating. Efavirenz should also be taken on an empty stomach, as high-fat or high-calorie meals may increase blood levels. Etravirine should be taken after meals. Rilpivirine is taken with a meal. The protease inhibitors atazanavir, darunavir, nelfinavir, and ritonavir should be taken with food. If not administered with ritonavir, indinavir should be taken either one hour before or two hours after a meal. If indinavir is taken with ritonavir, it can be given with or without food. In addition, it is important to drink plenty of fluids (at least 1.5 liters per day) during treatment with indinavir. The lopinavir/ritonavir oral solution should be taken with food; however, the tablet formulation can be taken without regard to food. When taken with ritonavir, saquinavir should be taken within two hours after a meal.

Darunavir, saquinavir, and tipranavir must be administered (boosted) with ritonavir, as the bioavailability of these PIs is poor when given as monotherapy. Other PIs may be administered with or without ritonavir.

Cautions and Concerns

Redistribution and accumulation of body fat (called lipodystrophy) has been observed in patients receiving antiretroviral therapy. Fat may accumulate on the back of the neck and upper shoulders (often described as "buffalo hump"), the abdomen, the breasts (in both men and women), or as lipomas (fatty growths in different parts of the body). The mechanism and long-term consequences of these occurrences are unknown, although recent evidence suggests that lipodystrophy is linked to taking NRTIs (primarily stavudine) and PIs at the same time.

Skin rash may occur with NNRTIs, NRTIs, and PIs. NNRTIs cause the majority of skin rashes, with nevirapine causing the most severe rashes. Women appear to be at higher risk for developing nevirapine-associated skin rashes than men. Abacavir may cause a rash that is a symptom of a severe drug hypersensitivity (allergic) reaction (see *Warnings*). Rare cases of serious skin reactions such as Stevens-Johnson syndrome and erythema multiforme have been reported with etravirine. Darunavir, fosamprenavir, and tipranavir are the PIs associated with the highest risk of a rash. Women taking birth control pills that contain estrogen may be more likely to develop a rash when taking tipranavir.

Peripheral neuropathy, a form of nerve damage manifested by numbness, tingling, or pain in the hands or feet, has been reported in patients receiving didanosine or stavudine therapy. Peripheral neuropathy has occurred more frequently in patients with advanced HIV disease and in patients with a history of neuropathy.

Serious psychiatric adverse experiences (severe depression, suicidal ideation, nonfatal suicide attempts, aggressive behavior, paranoid reactions, and manic reactions) have been reported in patients treated with efavirenz. People who take efavirenz may falsely test positive for marijuana use.

Caution should be given to prescribing rilpivirine with drugs that may reduce the exposure of rilpivirine. In healthy subjects, supratherapeutic doses of rilpivirine (75 mg once daily and 300 mg once daily) have been shown to prolong the QTc interval of the electrocardiogram. Rilpivirine should be used with caution when coadministered with a drug having known risk of torsade de pointes.

All patients taking PIs are at risk of developing hyperglycemia and diabetes.

Some PIs can raise blood lipid (fat) levels (hyperlipidemia). These increases can lead to heart disease and pancreatitis. Ritonavir is particularly likely to cause hyperlipidemia.

In clinical trials, atazanavir caused very high levels of bilirubin in nearly a third of patients who took it. Bilirubin is produced by the liver when old red blood cells are broken down. High levels of bilirubin can cause yellow skin or eyes, called jaundice. About 10 percent of patients using atazanavir got jaundice. Atazanavir may also cause changes in heart rhythm.

Darunavir and tipranavir are both sulfa drugs and should be used with caution in patients with a known sulfonamide allergy.

Two maraviroc Phase III studies reported possible liver problems (cirrhosis or failure, cholestatic jaundice [yellowing of the skin]) and cardiac events (including myocardial ischemia and/or infarction), an increased risk for upper respiratory tract and herpes virus infections, and a slight increase in cholesterol levels.

Warnings

All NRTIs, NNRTIs, and PIs are associated with hepatotoxicity, a general term for liver damage. Several specific conditions fall within the general category of hepatotoxicity. These conditions include hepatitis (inflammation of the liver), hepatic necrosis (death of liver cells), and hepatic steatosis (too much fat in the liver).

All NRTIs are associated with the development of lactic acidosis (accumulation of lactate in the blood, which causes the blood to become acidic and potentially harmful to the body's cells) and hepatic steatosis; however, didanosine, stavudine, and zidovudine are associated with the highest incidence of these potentially life-threatening side effects.

A higher incidence of hepatotoxicity occurs with nevirapine than with other NNRTIs, including serious and even fatal cases of hepatic necrosis.

Serious and sometimes fatal hypersensitivity reactions have been associated with abacavir, including fever, rash, nausea, vomiting, diarrhea, abdominal pain, malaise or fatigue, achiness, loss of appetite, and respiratory symptoms such as sore throat, cough, and shortness of breath. Abacavir should be discontinued as soon as hypersensitivity reaction is suspected. Any product containing abacavir should be permanently discontinued if hypersensitivity cannot be ruled out, even when other diagnoses are possible, because more severe symptoms can occur within hours after restarting abacavir and may include life-threatening low blood pressure and death.

Fatal and nonfatal pancreatitis have occurred with didanosine alone or in combination with other antiretroviral agents.

Severe acute exacerbations of hepatitis B have been reported in patients coinfected with hepatitis B and HIV who discontinued emtricitabine, tenofovir, and lamivudine-containing products.

Renal impairment, including cases of acute kidney failure, have been reported in association with the use of tenofovir. The majority of these cases occurred in patients with underlying systemic or kidney disease or in patients taking agents that are harmful to the kidneys; however, some cases occurred in patients without identified risk factors.

Nevirapine can cause severe, life-threatening liver damage, skin reactions (including Stevens-Johnson syndrome), and allergic reactions. These reactions occur most often during the first 18 weeks of treatment but can occur later. A patient who stops taking nevirapine because of a serious skin, allergic, or liver reaction should never take nevirapine again.

Severe depressive disorders (depressed mood, depression, dysphoria, major depression, mood altered, negative thoughts, suicide attempt, suicidal ideation) have been reported in patients taking rilpivirine. Patients with severe depressive symptoms should seek immediate medical evaluation to assess the possibility that the symptoms are related to rilpivirine and, if so, to determine whether the risks of continued therapy outweigh the benefits.

In clinical trials and post-marketing experience, drug-induced hepatitis has been reported in patients receiving combination therapy with darunavir/ritonavir. Appropriate laboratory testing should be conducted prior to initiating therapy with this combination, and patients should be monitored during treatment, especially during the first several months of treatment.

Indinavir can cause kidney stones. A doctor should be notified if an individual (especially a child) taking this medication experiences symptoms of kidney stones, which include severe side or back pain or blood in the urine. Drinking at least 1.5 liters of water per day while taking indinavir will lessen the chance of developing kidney stones.

Coadministration of ritonavir with certain nonsedating antihistamines, sedative hypnotics, antiarrhythmics, or ergot alkaloids may result in potentially serious or life-threatening adverse events. (See *Interactions.*)

Tipranavir can make liver problems worse. Patients with hepatitis B or hepatitis C should have careful monitoring of liver blood tests. Some patients taking tipranavir developed hepatitis and, in rare cases, liver failure.

Tipranavir coadministered with 200 mg twice daily ritonavir has been associated with reports of clinical hepatitis and hepatic decompensation (failure of the liver to repair itself from injury, resulting in a decrease in liver functions), including some fatalities.

In 2006, several cases of intracranial bleeding were reported in patients taking tipranavir. Some of these were fatal.

Hepatotoxicity has been reported with maraviroc use. Evidence of a systemic allergic reaction prior to the development of hepatotoxicity may occur. Patients with signs or symptoms of hepatitis or allergic reaction following use of maraviroc should be evaluated immediately, with discontinuation of the drug considered.

Spontaneous bleeding has occurred in patients with hemophilia A or B treated with PIs.

When Not Advised (Contraindications)

As studies in monkeys have shown that efavirenz and nelfinavir are likely to cause birth defects, pregnant women should not take these drugs, especially during the first three months of pregnancy.

Side Effects

Anyone beginning any antiretroviral therapy may have temporary side effects such as headaches, high blood pressure, or a general sense of feeling ill. These side effects usually get better or disappear over time.

The most common side effects of abacavir are headache, nausea, and vomiting.

The most common side effects of didanosine are diarrhea, nausea, vomiting, and rash. The most serious side effects of didanosine are peripheral neuropathy (see *Cautions and Concerns*), pancreatitis, hepatic steatosis, and lactic acidosis. (See *Warnings.*)

The most common side effects of emtricitabine include nausea, vomiting, diarrhea, headache, rash, and skin discoloration.

In addition to skin rash (see *Cautions and Concerns*), etravirine may cause nausea, diarrhea, abdominal pain, vomiting, fatigue, peripheral neuropathy, headache, and high blood pressure.

The most common side effects of lamivudine are nausea, vomiting, diarrhea, abdominal pain, insomnia (difficulty sleeping), and headache.

The most serious side effects of stavudine are peripheral neuropathy, lipodystrophy, pancreatitis, lactic acidosis, and hepatic steatosis. (See *Cautions and Concerns* and *Warnings*).

The most common side effects of tenofovir are nausea, vomiting, diarrhea, loss of appetite, and headache. Tenofovir can reduce bone mineral density—especially in people with osteopenia or osteoporosis—which may be helped by calcium or vitamin D supplements.

The most common side effects of zidovudine are headache, malaise, nausea, loss of appetite, vomiting, insomnia, lactic acidosis, and hepatic steatosis (*see Warnings*).

The most common side effect of delavirdine is a skin rash, which develops in about a third of people taking the drug. Headache is also a common side effect of delavirdine. Both delavirdine and efavirenz can elevate liver function tests.

Central nervous system symptoms are common in patients taking efavirenz and may include dizziness, somnolence, insomnia, abnormal dreams, confusion, abnormal thinking, impaired concentration, amnesia, agitation, depersonalization, hallucinations, and euphoria. Dizziness can be avoided by taking efavirenz at bedtime.

The most common side effect of nevirapine is a skin rash, which develops in up to one-quarter of people taking the drug and is much more common for women than for men.

The most common side effects with rilpivirine of at least moderate to severe intensity were depression (see *Warnings*), insomnia, headache, and rash.

The most common side effects associated with protease inhibitors include nausea, diarrhea, and other gastrointestinal symptoms. These drugs are also associated with endocrine disturbances (e.g., onset or worsening of diabetes and abnormal amounts of cholesterol in the blood) and can cause changes in body fat. In addition, protease inhibitors can interact with other drugs, resulting in serious side effects (see *Interactions*).

In addition to gastrointestinal side effects, the most common side effects of atazanavir include headache and rash.

In addition to gastrointestinal side effects, the most common side effects of darunavir include headache and a common cold. Some people may get a skin rash, which in rare cases could be serious. Darunavir may also be associated with Stevens-Johnson syndrome.

In addition to gastrointestinal side effects, fosamprenavir may cause numbness around the mouth and headache. About 1 percent of people get serious skin reactions, including Stevens-Johnson syndrome. The diarrhea in most cases can be controlled with over-the-counter medications. Fosamprenavir may also cause headache as well as elevated liver function tests.

In addition to gastrointestinal side effects, indinavir may cause dizziness or drowsiness, general feeling of weakness, headache, stomach pain, and trouble sleeping.

In addition to gastrointestinal side effects, lopinavir/ritonavir may cause headache, rash, trouble sleeping, and weakness. Diarrhea may occur more frequently in patients taking lopinavir/ritonavir once daily.

In addition to the common gastrointestinal side effects, some people taking ritonavir also experience tingling or numbness around the mouth or find that foods taste strange. Ritonavir can also cause hepatitis.

In addition to gastrointestinal side effects, saquinavir may cause anxiety, change in sense of taste, depression, dizziness, eczema, generalized muscle pain or weakness, headache, mouth sores, trouble sleeping, numbness, pain or tingling in the hands or feet, rash, and unusual tiredness.

In addition to the gastrointestinal side effects, the most common side effects of tipranavir include fatigue and headache. Women taking birth control pills that contain estrogen may be more likely to develop a skin rash. About 10 percent of patients develop a rash or sensitivity to the sun, sometimes with joint pain or stiffness, itching, or tightness in the throat. Tipranavir may also be associated with Stevens-Johnson syndrome.

Enfuvirtide may cause severe allergic reactions such as trouble breathing, chills and fever, rash, blood in urine, nausea, vomiting, and low blood pressure. Enfuvirtide has also been associated with the development of bacterial pneumonia. Local skin reactions at the injection site are also possible. The most common other side effects of enfuvirtide are headache, pain and numbness in feet or legs, dizziness, and loss of sleep.

The most common side effects seen in maraviroc studies have included cough, fever, dizziness, headache, lowered blood pressure, nausea, and bladder irritation (See also *Cautions and Concerns* and *Warnings*).

The most common side effects seen in raltegravir clinical trials have been diarrhea, nausea, headache, and fever.

Interactions

Any three-drug combination of NRTIs should be avoided except for abacavir/lamivudine/zidovudine or possibly zidovudine/lamivudine + tenofovir.

Peripheral neuropathy, lactic acidosis, and pancreatitis have occurred when stavudine was taken with didanosine. Use of these two drugs together should be avoided. Stavudine should also not be taken with zidovudine, as zidovudine may reduce the effects of stavudine.

Blood levels of lamivudine may be increased by trimethoprim/sulfamethoxazole.

Tenofovir results in higher blood levels of didanosine. Tenofovir blood levels increase if it is taken with atazanavir, lopinavir/ritonavir, or darunavir, which can increase the risk of tenofovir side effects. However, atazanavir levels also decrease when used with tenofovir; therefore, it is recommended that if these two drugs are used together, ritonavir be used as part of the regimen. Ganciclovir or cidofovir may also increase levels of tenofovir.

Methadone may increase blood levels of zidovudine, increasing zidovudine's side effects. Ribavirin should be avoided in patients taking zidovudine.

NNRTIs and PIs should not be taken with Saint-John's-wort.

Delavirdine should not be taken within one hour of taking didanosine or antacids. Delavirdine should not be taken along with simvastatin, lovastatin, rifabutin, rifampin, H_2 blockers, proton pump inhibitors, alprazolam, midazolam, triazolam, dihydroergotamine, ergotamine, ergonovine, methylergonovine, fosamprenavir, carbamazepine, phenobarbital, or phenytoin. Delavirdine may increase the blood levels of methadone and erectile dysfunction (ED) drugs, such as sildenafil, vardenafil, and tadalafil.

Efavirenz may decrease blood levels of rifabutin, atorvastatin, lovastatin, simvastatin, methadone, and warfarin. Blood levels of efavirenz may be reduced by rifampin, rifabutin, carbamazepine, phenytoin, and phenobarbital. Efavirenz should not be taken with midazolam, triazolam, dihydroergotamine, ergotamine, ergonovine, methylergonovine, or voriconazole.

Etravirine should not be used with rifampin, Saint-John's-wort, unboosted PIs, ritonavir-boosted atazanavir, fosamprenavir, tipranavir, other NNRTIs, carbamazepine, phenobarbital, or phenytoin. Etravirine may increase blood levels of voriconazole, fluvastatin, warfarin, and diazepam. Concentrations of itraconazole, ketoconazole, atorvastatin, lovastatin, simvastatin, cyclosporine, tacrolimus, sirolimus, and sildenafil may be reduced with etravirine.

Nevirapine lowers blood levels of estrogen-containing birth control medications, which could make them ineffective. Nevirapine may also decrease blood levels of methadone. Blood levels of nevirapine may be increased by fluconazole and voriconazole. Nevirapine blood levels may be reduced by rifabutin. Nevirapine should not be used with rifampin or ketoconazole. PIs should not be taken along with simvastatin, lovastatin, rifampin, midazolam, triazolam, dihydroergotamine, ergotamine, ergonovine, methylergonovine, or fluticasone. Most PIs may increase the blood levels of ED drugs.

Rilpivirine is contraindicated with the following drugs, as significant decreases in rilpivirine plasma concentrations may occur due to CYP3A enzyme induction or gastric pH increase, which may result in loss of virologic response and possible resistance to rilpivirine or to the class of NNRTIs: the anticonvulsants carbamazepine, oxcarbazepine, phenobarbital, phenytoin; the antimycobacterials rifabutin, rifampin, rifapentine; proton pump inhibitors, such as esomeprazole, lansoprazole, omeprazole, pantoprazole, rabeprazole; the glucocorticoid systemic dexamethasone (more than a single dose); and Saint-John's-wort.

Atazanavir should not be taken with indinavir (due to increased risk of jaundice), irinotecan, proton pump inhibitors, or H_2 blockers. Atazanavir may increase blood levels of fluconazole, ketoconazole, voriconazole, clarithromycin, rifabutin, or calcium channel blockers. Fluconazole, ketoconazole, and voriconazole may also increase the blood levels of atazanavir. Carbamazepine, phenobarbital, and phenytoin may decrease blood levels of atazanavir.

Darunavir should not be taken with carbamazepine, phenytoin, or phenobarbital. Darunavir may increase blood levels of fluconazole, ketoconazole, and clarithromycin. Darunavir/ritonavir may decrease blood levels of paroxetine, sertraline, and estrogen-containing birth control pills. Fluconazole, ketoconazole, and voriconazole may also increase the blood levels of darunavir.

Fosamprenavir should not be used with delavirdine or estrogen-containing birth control pills. Fosamprenavir may increase blood levels of itraconazole, ketoconazole, voriconazole, rifabutin, or atorvastatin. Fosamprenavir may decrease blood levels of methadone. Carbamazepine, phenobarbital, and phenytoin may decrease blood levels of fosamprenavir.

Indinavir should not be taken with amiodarone or atazanavir. Itraconazole or ketoconazole may increase blood levels of indinavir. Rifabutin, carbamazepine, and grapefruit juice may decrease blood levels of indinavir. Indinavir may increase blood levels of clarithromycin, rifabutin, atorvastatin, or calcium channel blockers.

Lopinavir/ritonavir should not be used with flecainide or propafenone. Lopinavir/ritonavir may increase blood levels of itraconazole, ketoconazole, clarithromycin, rifabutin, or atorvastatin. Lopinavir/ritonavir may decrease blood levels of estrogen-containing birth control pills and methadone. Phenytoin may decrease blood levels of lopinavir.

Nelfinavir may increase blood levels of itraconazole, ketoconazole, and voriconazole; these antifungal drugs may also increase nelfinavir levels. Nelfinavir may also increase blood levels of rifabutin and atorvastatin. Blood levels of estrogen-containing birth control pills and methadone may be reduced by nelfinavir. Nelfinavir levels may be decreased by carbamazepine, phenytoin, and phenobarbital.

Ritonavir should not be used with amiodarone, flecainide, propafenone, quinidine, and alfuzosin. Voriconazole should also not be used with higher doses of ritonavir (> 800 mg/day). Ritonavir may increase blood levels of itraconazole, ketoconazole, clarithromycin, rifabutin, atorvastatin, carbamazepine, desipramine, and trazodone. Ritonavir may decrease levels of estrogen-containing birth control pills, methadone, and theophylline.

Saquinavir should not be taken along with garlic supplements. Saquinavir may increase blood levels of itraconazole, ketoconazole, and voriconazole; these antifungal drugs may also increase saquinavir levels. Saquinavir may also increase blood levels of clarithromycin, rifabutin, and atorvastatin. Saquinavir/ritonavir may decrease levels of methadone. Clarithromycin and grapefruit juice may increase blood levels of saquinavir. Rifabutin, carbamazepine, phenobarbital, phenytoin, and dexamethasone may decrease levels of saquinavir.

Tipranavir should not be used with amiodarone, flecainide, propafenone, quinidine, and higher doses of fluconazole (> 200 mg/day). Tipranavir capsules contain alcohol; therefore, to avoid a disulfiram-like reaction (e.g., flushing, headache, nausea, vomiting), use of metronidazole should be avoided. Tipranavir may increase blood levels of itraconazole, ketoconazole, rifabutin, and atorvastatin. Clarithromycin may increase levels of tipranavir. Tipranavir/ritonavir may decrease levels of estrogen-containing birth control pills, methadone, abacavir, zidovudine, and loperamide. Carbamazepine, phenobarbital, phenytoin, and antacids may decrease levels of tipranavir.

No clinically significant drug-drug interactions have been identified with enfuvirtide to date.

Maraviroc should not be taken with rifampin or Saint-John's-wort. Itraconazole, ketoconazole, and clarithromycin may increase levels of maraviroc. Rifabutin, carbamazepine, phenobarbital, and phenytoin may decrease levels of maraviroc.

Rifampin, efavirenz, tipranavir/ritonavir, and rifabutin may decrease blood levels of raltegravir.

Sales/Statistics

A 2006 report by the World Health Organization (WHO) and the Joint United Nations Program on HIV/AIDS (UNAIDS) showed that the number of people on HIV antiretroviral treatment in low- and middle-income countries more than tripled to 1.3 million in December 2005 from 400,000 in December 2003.

In the United States, 10 antiretrovirals were listed among the "Top 200 Brand-Name Drugs by Retail Dollars in 2006" (*Drug Topics*, February 19,

2007). Truvada ranked #66, with $569,618,000 in sales, Reyataz #94 ($372,790,000), Combivir #99 ($355,848,000), Kaletra #100 ($352,013,000), Sustiva #110 ($300,944,000), Fuzeon #123 ($256,183,000), Norvir #125 ($249,522,000), Viread #135 ($223,659,000), Trizivir #136 ($222,562,000), and Epzicom #150 ($181,391,000). Didanosine was the only antiretroviral in the "Top 200 Generic Drugs by Retail Dollars in 2006," ranking #184, with $38,291,000 in sales.

In 2010, according to the IMS Institute for Healthcare Informatics (the public reporting arm of IMS), antiretrovirals were the ninth-largest therapeutic drug group in the United States, with $9.2 billion in sales. On the 2010 *Drug Topics* lists of top brand-name drugs, Truvada had climbed to #44 in sales ($813,944,833), Reyataz to #86 ($412,293,572), Norvir to #111 (287,102,342), and Epzicom to #140 ($221,406,518). Prezista ranked #135, with $230,406,897 in sales. Viread had dropped to #143 ($216,264,393), Kaletra to #144 ($212,723,964), and Combivir to #184 ($163,406,344).

Demographics and Cultural Groups

The HIV/AIDS epidemic is growing most rapidly among minority populations and is a leading killer of African-American males ages 25 to 44. According to the Centers for Disease Control and Prevention (CDC), AIDS affects nearly seven times more African Americans and three times more Hispanics than whites. In recent years, an increasing number of African-American women and children are being affected by HIV/AIDS. In 2003, two-thirds of U.S. AIDS cases in both women and children were among African Americans.

Development History

NRTIs were the first type of drug available to treat HIV. Zidovudine was the first drug approved for the treatment of HIV, on March 19, 1987. NRTIs to follow were: didanosine, October 9, 1991; stavudine, June 24, 1994; lamivudine, November 17, 1995; lamivudine/zidovudine,

September 27, 1997; abacavir, December 17, 1998; abacavir/lamivudine/zidovudine, November 14, 2000; tenofovir DF, October 26, 2001; emtricitabine, July 2, 2003; abacavir/lamivudine, August 2, 2004; emtricitabine/tenofovir, August 2, 2004; and etravirine, January 18, 2008.

Nevirapine was the first NNRTI to be approved by the FDA, on June 21, 1996, followed by delavirdine on April 4, 1997, efavirenz on September 17, 1998, and ripilvirine on May 20, 2011.

Saquinavir was the first PI to be approved by the FDA, on December 6, 1995, followed by ritonavir, March 1, 1996; indinavir, March 13, 1996; nelfinavir, March 14, 1997; lopinavir/ritonavir, September 15, 2000; atazanavir, June 20, 2003; fosamprenavir, October 20, 2003; tipranavir, June 22, 2005; and darunavir, June 23, 2006.

Enfuvirtide was the first fusion inhibitor drug approved for HIV treatment on March 13, 2003; maraviroc followed on August 6, 2007.

Raltegravir, the first integrase inhibitor, was approved on October 12, 2007.

Efavirenz/emtricitabine/tenofovir was approved by the FDA on July 12, 2006.

Future Drugs

Among NRTIs in development: Apricitabine (Avexa Limited, Australia), also known as AVX754 or SPD754, is being studied for the treatment of HIV infection in treatment-experienced patients and has been granted fast-track status by the FDA. Elvucitabine (Achillion Pharmaceuticals) is similar to lamivudine and may be effective in treating patients infected with HIV strains resistant to lamivudine. Elvucitabine is also being studied for the treatment of hepatitis B virus (HBV) infection. KP-1461 (Koronis Pharmaceuticals), also known as SN1461 and SN1212, works by introducing changes to HIV's genetic makeup that eventually kill the viral particles. Fozivudine tidoxil is being developed by a German company, with once-daily doses under study. Racivir (Pharmasset, Inc.), also known as RCV, is being studied for the treatment of HIV infection as part of a combination regimen.

Among the fusion and entry inhibitors in development: AMD070, also known as AMD11070, is a CXCR4 inhibitor being developed by Genzyme Corporation. PRO 140, which binds to the CCR5 receptor and interferes with HIV's ability to enter the cell, is being developed as an intravenous formulation by Progenics Pharmaceuticals, Inc. Another intravenous formulation, ibalizumab (TMB-335, previously known as TNX-335), which binds to CD4 and prevents entry of HIV into target cells, is being studied by Tanox, Inc. Vicriviroc, also known as SCH-D, blocks HIV from attaching to the CCR5 receptor, preventing the virus from entering and infecting the cell. SCH-D, being developed by Schering-Plough Corp., was granted fast-track status by the FDA in 2005, but was pulled from ongoing studies in July 2010 due to poor results.

GS 9137 (elvitegravir) is an integrase inhibitor being developed by Gilead Sciences Inc.

antitussives Drugs that relieve coughing by suppressing the cough reflex; also called cough suppressants. Antitussives are used to suppress dry coughs, not the productive coughs that expel mucous, which are encouraged (see EXPECTORANTS). Dry coughing may be caused by underlying conditions such as cough-variant asthma, gastroesophageal reflux disease (GERD), allergies, common cold, and some lung diseases. Also, smoking, pollutants, dry air from heating and air-conditioning systems, and some medications (such as angiotensin-converting enzyme inhibitors) can lead to dry coughing. If persistent enough, dry coughing can interfere with normal activities or sleep, leading to exhaustion. Continual severe coughing can cause fatigue fractures of lower ribs and costochondritis, an inflammation of the connective tissue between the breastbone and the ribs. It can also lead to fainting spells when coughs are prolonged and forceful. In certain cases, it can even lead to abdominal or pelvic hernias. Some antitussives must be prescribed by a physician or other qualifying medical person; however, many are available over-the-counter (OTC).

Classes

Antitussives can be divided into two classes:

- *Opioids*—All opioids (see ANALGESICS) have antitussive properties, but codeine and hydrocodone are the ones most often used as cough suppressants.
- *Nonnarcotic antitussives*—Nonaddictive. *Examples:* benzonatate (Tessalon) and dextromethorphan (Robitussin, Vicks 44).

How They Work

Opioids work by suppressing the cough reflex in the brain. They do this by acting directly on receptors in the cough center of the medulla (the lower part of the brain). By depressing these receptors, they raise the threshold for incoming cough impulses. The cough suppression effect of opioids can be achieved at lower doses than those required to provide pain relief (analgesia).

Benzonatate anesthetizes the stretch receptors in respiratory passages, lungs, and pleura (a thin membrane around the lungs and inner walls of the chest) that link to the cough reflex, dampening their activity and reducing the cough reflex at its source.

Dextromethorphan, a semisynthetic morphine derivative, works similarly to the opioids in suppressing cough by acting on the cough center in the medulla, However, unlike the opioids, dextromethorphan does not have analgesic or addictive properties.

Approved Uses

As antitussives, codeine and hydrocodone are used to reduce coughing induced by chemical or mechanical irritation of the respiratory system and to relieve the dry cough caused by the common cold.

For other uses of codeine and hydrocodone, see ANALGESICS.

Benzonatate is used to treat cough due to the common cold, bronchitis, pneumonia, or other lung infections. Dextromethorphan temporarily relieves cough caused by minor throat and bronchial irritation as may occur with the common cold or inhaled irritants.

Benzonatate as well as products containing codeine or hydrocodone require a prescription, while dextromethorphan-containing products are available over-the-counter.

Companion Drugs

Used as an antitussive, hydrocodone may be combined with phenylephrine, pseudoephedrine, guaifenesin, pyrilamine, pheniramine, or chlorpheniramine. Nearly 50 antitussive preparations contain hydrocodone. Codeine is also combined with a variety of drugs in antitussive preparations.

Dextromethorphan is found in more than 120 OTC cold medications, either alone or in combination with other drugs such as ANALGESICS, ANTIHISTAMINES, DECONGESTANTS, and/or EXPECTORANTS.

Administration

Antitussives are administered orally. Codeine as a cough suppressant is taken via tablets and oral solution. Hydrocodone is commonly available in tablet, capsule, and syrup form.

Benzonatate is administered orally via softgel capsules.

Dextromethorphan is available in gelcap, lozenge, liquid, and syrup form.

Cautions and Concerns

Antitussives containing codeine or hydrocodone can cause drowsiness and impairment. Caution should be taken when performing activities requiring mental alertness and physical coordination.

Benzonatate is chemically related to anesthetic agents of the para-aminobenzoic acid class (e.g., procaine, tetracaine) and has been associated with adverse CNS effects.

Dextromethorphan can cause drowsiness and taken in large doses can produce hallucinations and bizarre behavior. These effects are increased when combined with antihistamines. According to the Office of Diversion Control, Drug Enforcement Administration, dextromethorphan is often abused in high doses by adolescents to generate euphoria and visual and auditory hallucinations.

Some hydrocodone and dextromethorphan products contain tartrazine, which may cause allergic-type reactions (including bronchial asthma) in certain susceptible people. This reaction is sometimes seen in patients who also have aspirin sensitivity.

Some formulations of opioid antitussives contain sulfites, which may cause allergic-type reactions, including anaphylaxis and life-threatening or less severe asthmatic episodes, in certain susceptible individuals.

Warnings

Possible tolerance, psychologic dependence, and physical dependence may occur following prolonged administration of opioid antitussives.

Severe hypersensitivity reactions (including bronchospasm, laryngospasm, and cardiovascular collapse) have been reported with benzonatate. Such reactions may have resulted from ingesting local anesthesia after sucking or chewing the liquid-filled capsules instead of swallowing them whole. Severe reactions have required intervention with vasopressor therapy and supportive measures. Isolated instances of bizarre behavior, including mental confusion and visual hallucinations, have also been reported in patients taking benzonatate in combination with other prescribed drugs.

Side Effects

Codeine in antitussive dosages can cause nausea, vomiting, drowsiness, dizziness, palpitation, intense itching, and constipation (with repeated doses). Side effects occurring with usual hydrocodone antitussive dosages may include lightheadedness, dizziness, drowsiness, nausea, vomiting, and constipation.

Side effects of benzonatate may include drowsiness, headache, dizziness, mental confusion, visual hallucinations, constipation, nausea, gastrointestinal upset, itchiness, skin eruptions, nasal congestion, sensation of burning in the eyes, vague "chilly" sensation, and numbness of the chest.

Dextromethorphan in usual doses can cause confusion, excitability, nervousness, and irritability. Other common side effects associated with this drug include upset stomach and vomiting.

Interactions

Taking opioid antitussives along with sedatives and tranquilizers may cause greater drowsiness than is caused by the products used alone. Opioid antitussives may increase the antidepressant effect of monoamine oxidase inhibitors (MAOIs) and tricyclics.

Dextromethorphan taken in combination with MAOIs can cause a severe reaction, with fever, hypotension, abnormal muscle movement, and coma; thus, coadministration should be avoided. Also, dextromethorphan should not be used for two weeks after stopping MAOIs. Similarly, sibutramine should not be taken along with dextromethorphan, as the combination may cause motor weakness, central nervous system irritability, hypertensive crises, and altered consciousness.

Sales/Statistics

In the United States, dextromethorphan has been reported to account for 75 percent of OTC sales of antitussives.

Benzonatate ranked #175 in the 2010 "Top 200 Generic Drugs by Retail Dollars" (*Drug Topics*, June 2011), with $73,396,360 in sales, and #119 in the 2010 "Top 200 Generic Drugs by Total Prescriptions" (*Drug Topics*, June 2011), with 4,613,236 prescriptions. The generic combination of promethazine/codeine ranked #161 in retail dollars and #91 in prescriptions in the 2006 list.

Development History

Codeine is a naturally occurring alkaloid of opium, which is obtained from the unripe seedpods of the poppy. First isolated by the French chemist Pierre-Jean Robiquet in 1832, codeine may be extracted directly from opium, but most codeine is produced from morphine, another opium derivative. Codeine was officially approved by the FDA in 1939.

Hydrocodone is semisynthetic, derived from two of the naturally occurring opiates, codeine and thebaine.

Benzonatate was approved by the FDA in 1958.

Dextromethorphan was first patented in the United States on April 20, 1954, and received FDA approval for OTC sale as a cough suppressant in 1958. In the 1960s, a tablet form of dextromethorphan, Romilar, was marketed in the United States as an alternative to codeine. However, it was soon discovered that large doses of dextromethorphan had psychedelic effects on those who used codeine. In 1973, Romilar was taken off the shelves after a burst in sales due to common recreational use. It was then replaced by cough syrup in an attempt to cut down on recreational usage. Around 2000, gel capsule forms began reappearing as well as several generic forms of dextromethorphan. Due to abuse and theft concerns, many retailers have moved dextromethorphan-containing products behind the counter so that one must ask a pharmacist to receive them or be of adult age to purchase them.

antivirals Drugs used specifically for dealing with infections caused by viruses. Van Regenmortel and Mahy note that "viruses occupy a unique position in biology. Although they possess some of the properties of living systems such as having a genome, they are actually nonliving infectious entities and should not be considered microorganisms." Viruses are difficult to treat because they reproduce so quickly. Antivirals are one type of antibiotics (also called antimicrobials), a larger group of drugs that also includes ANTIBACTERIALS, ANTIFUNGALS, and ANTIRETROVIRALS (antiviral agents used to treat human immunodeficiency virus [HIV] infections). Antivirals are fairly new drugs, having been developed only since the 1980s. Unlike other types of antibiotics, antiviral agents tend to be narrow in spectrum, targeting specific viruses. In addition to being specific, antiviral drugs can both prevent infection and treat illness.

Classes

Antivirals are classified according to the viruses they target.

- *Anticytomegalovirus agents*—Cytomegalovirus (CMV) is a common virus that infects between 50 and 80 percent of adults in the United States by 40 years of age. Cytomegalovirus infection is usually harmless and rarely causes illness, as a healthy immune system can hold the virus in check. However, if a person's immune system is seriously weakened in any way (immunosuppressed), the virus can become active and cause CMV disease. Cytomegalovirus is the most common virus transmitted to a pregnant woman's unborn child. *Examples of anticytomegalovirus agents:* cidofovir (Vistide), foscarnet (Foscavir), ganciclovir (Cytovene, Vitrasert), and valganciclovir (Valcyte),

- *Antihepatitis agents*—Agents effective against hepatitis B virus (HBV) and hepatitis C virus (HCV). According to the Centers for Disease Control and Prevention (CDC), approximately 1.25 million Americans are chronically infected with the HBV virus. Hepatitis B has been estimated by the World Health Organization to be the ninth most common cause of death worldwide. Approximately 350 million people, 5 percent of the world's population, have chronic infection with the hepatitis B virus, and about one third of these individuals are at risk for serious progressive liver disease. Hepatitis B virus can cause lifelong infection, cirrhosis (scarring) of the liver, liver cancer, liver failure, and death. Both HBV and HCV are transmitted primarily through activities that involve contact with blood or blood-derived fluids. Such activities can include unprotected sex with an HBV- or

HBC-infected partner; shared needles used for injection of illegal drugs; work in health-care fields (medical, dental, laboratory, or other) that entails direct exposure to human blood; receiving blood transfusions that have not been screened for HBV or HCV; or having dental, medical, or cosmetic (e.g., tattooing or body piercing) procedures with needles or other equipment that are contaminated with HBV or HCV.

Hepatitis C is a liver disease caused by a virus found in the blood of persons who have the disease. Hepatitis C virus infection results in chronic hepatitis in 50 to 80 percent of cases, with possible further progression to cirrhosis and liver cancer in 20 to 50 percent of infected individuals. Hepatitis C virus is currently the leading cause of liver transplantation in the United States and causes 8,000 to 10,000 deaths per year. *Examples of antihepatitis agents:* adefovir dipivoxil (Hepsera), entecavir (Baraclude), lamivudine (Epivir-HBV), and ribavirin (Copegus, Rebetol, Ribasphere, RibaPak).

- *Antiherpes agents*—Herpes simplex virus (HSV) is a common viral infection. Herpes simplex virus type 1 most commonly infects the mouth and lips, causing sores known as fever blisters or cold sores. It is also an important cause of sores to the genitals. Herpes simplex virus type 2 is the usual cause of genital herpes, but it also can infect the mouth through oral sex. According to the CDC, one out of five American teenagers and adults is infected with HSV-2. Women are more commonly infected than men. In the United States, one out of four women is infected with HSV-2. Since the late 1970s, the number of people with genital herpes infection has increased 30 percent nationwide. The largest increase has been among teens and young adults.

Varicella-zoster virus is a herpes family virus that causes chicken pox and shingles. Chicken pox, also called varicella, is a highly contagious disease in which a rash usually develops on the scalp and body, then spreads to the face, arms, and legs. Chicken pox spreads from person to person through the air by coughing or sneezing. It can also be spread through direct contact with the fluid from a blister of a person infected with chicken pox or from direct contact with a sore from a person with shingles. Until a vaccine became available, there were an estimated 4 million cases of chicken pox per year. Since the vaccine has been available, the number of cases of chicken pox has fallen by about 90 percent. Shingles, also called herpes zoster, is a painful skin rash often accompanied by blisters. Shingles is most common in people age 50 and older. It is also more common in people whose immune systems are weakened because of a disease, such as cancer, or drugs, such as steroids or chemotherapy. At least 1 million people a year in the United States get shingles. Only someone who has had a case of chicken pox—or received the chicken pox vaccine—can get shingles. *Examples of antiherpes agents:* acyclovir (Zovirax), famciclovir (Famvir), foscarnet (Foscavir), penciclovir (Denavir), valacyclovir (Valtrex).

- *Antiinfluenza agents*—Influenza (also called flu) is a contagious respiratory illness caused by influenza viruses. It can cause mild to severe illness and at times can lead to death. Every year in the United States, on average, 5 to 20 percent of the population get the flu; more than 200,000 people are hospitalized due to flu complications, and about 36,000 people die from flu. *Examples of antiinfluenza agents:* amantadine (Symmetrel), oseltamivir (Tamiflu), rimantadine (Flumadine), and zanamivir (Relenza).

How They Work

All anticytomegalovirus agents suppress active viral replication, meaning they prevent the virus from reproducing but do not eliminate the virus. Cidofovir suppresses CMV replication by selective inhibition of viral DNA synthesis. Foscarnet works by inhibiting the binding of pyrophosphate at viral-specific DNA polymerases. Ganciclovir works by blocking the action of a viral component called DNA polymerase. This compound is required by the virus for it to copy genetic material (from RNA to DNA), a process that is needed for the virus to multiply and survive. Ganciclovir is also incorporated into the viral DNA. By blocking the action of DNA polymerase and disrupting viral DNA, ganciclovir prevents CMV from multiplying. Valganciclovir is changed into ganciclovir in the body.

Adefovir dipivoxil helps stop HBV from multiplying by blocking HBV DNA polymerase, an enzyme that is necessary for the replication of the virus in the body. Entecavir inhibits all three steps in the viral replication process, including inhibiting HBV DNA polymerase, similar to adefovir. Lamivudine blocks the reverse transcriptase of HBV, which the virus needs to make more copies of itself. Ribavirin blocks the ability of HCV to make more copies of itself.

Antiherpes agents prevent HSV from reproducing by interfering with the enzymes the virus needs to replicate the necessary DNA, including inhibiting viral DNA polymerase. Famciclovir is a prodrug, meaning it is not active directly against viruses itself. Rather, famciclovir is converted to penciclovir in the body, and it is the penciclovir that is active against the viruses. Valacyclovir is also a prodrug and is converted to acyclovir in the body.

Amantadine interferes with the viral protein M2, which is needed for the viral particle to become uncoated once it is taken inside the cell and thereby prevents the virus from reproducing. Rimantadine is believed to work similarly to amantadine; however, rimantadine is considered to be more potent than amantadine.

Oseltamivir and zanamivir block the action of neuraminidase, an enzyme that enables influenza virus to spread from infected cells to healthy cells, thereby preventing new viruses from emerging from infected cells.

Approved Uses

Cidofovir and foscarnet are used for the treatment of CMV retinitis, a potentially severe eye infection that can lead to blindness in patients with acquired immune deficiency syndrome (AIDS) who are resistant to ganciclovir. Foscarnet is also approved to treat HSV infections of the skin and mucous membranes in immunocompromised patients whose infections did not improve with acyclovir.

Ganciclovir is approved as both starting and maintenance therapy of CMV retinitis in immunocompromised patients, including AIDS patients, and for prevention of CMV infection in organ transplant patients who are at risk for the disease.

Valganciclovir is approved for the treatment of CMV retinitis in AIDS patients and for the prevention of CMV disease in kidney, heart, and kidney-pancreas transplant patients at high risk.

Adefovir dipivoxil and entecavir are used to treat adults with chronic infections with active hepatitis B virus.

Lamivudine is approved for the treatment of both HBV and HIV infection, with higher doses used for HIV. The lower-dose form of lamivudine is for individuals who have HBV infection only. Patients who have both HBV and HIV infection should not use this lower dose.

Ribavirin is used in combination with interferon alfa-2a or -2b or peginterferon alfa-2a or -2b to treat patients infected with HCV. Ribavirin is also approved in the aerosolized form for the treatment of RSV.

Acyclovir is approved for use in the treatment of herpes simplex infections as well as herpes zoster infections (shingles and chicken pox) caused by varicella-zoster virus. Parenteral acyclovir is approved for severe initial episodes of genital herpes infection, neonatal HSV infection, and herpes simplex encephalitis. It does not cure or prevent herpes infection and does not reduce the risk of passing these viruses to other people.

Famciclovir is used to treat or suppress recurrent episodes of genital herpes, to treat acute shingles, and to treat recurrent herpes simplex infections of the mucous membranes and skin in HIV-infected patients. Famciclovir is also approved for herpes labialis (cold sores).

Penciclovir is used to treat recurring herpes labialis in adults.

Valacyclovir is used to treat herpes zoster, genital herpes, and herpes labialis.

All of the antiinfluenza agents may be effective for influenza A viruses. However, only oseltamivir and zanamivir are effective for treatment and prevention of influenza B viruses. Also, recent evidence indicates that a high proportion of currently circulating influenza A viruses in the United States have developed resistance to amantadine and rimantadine. In June 2007, the Advisory Committee on Immunization Practices recommended that neither amantadine nor rimantadine be used for the treatment or prevention of influenza A in the United States for the 2007–08 influenza season. Because they are not recommended for use, these agents are not included in the sections below.

Antiinfluenza agents are most often used to help control influenza outbreaks in institutions, for example, in nursing homes or in hospital wards, where people at high risk for complications from influenza are in close contact with each other. They also have been used on cruise ships or similar settings to help control influenza outbreaks.

Doctors also can prescribe influenza antiviral medications to people not living in institutional settings, but treatment must begin within two days of the onset of symptoms for the drugs to be effective. Although all antiinfluenza agents lessen symptoms and shorten the duration of illness, only one (oseltamivir) has been shown in a study to reduce lower respiratory tract complications requiring antibiotics. They do not cure influenza outright.

Amantadine is also used as an ANTIPARKINSON AGENT.

Off-Label Uses

Foscarnet is used off-label to treat CMV infections in places other than the eyes, such as the lungs, esophagus, or intestines, and to treat varicella-zoster infection (shingles) that does not respond to treatment with acyclovir in patients with HIV infection.

Ganciclovir is used off-label to treat CMV pneumonia in organ transplant patients, CMV gastroenteritis in patients with irritable bowel disease, and CMV pneumonitis.

The aerosol ribavirin is used off-label to treat influenza A or B viral infection, pneumonia caused by adenovirus, and severe lower respiratory tract infection in adults.

High-dose acyclovir has been used off-label to reduce the risk of CMV infection in certain bone marrow and organ-transplant patients.

Famciclovir is used off-label to manage initial episodes of genital herpes.

Valacyclovir is used off-label for the prevention of CMV in patients who have undergone stem-cell or kidney transplants.

Administration

Cidofovir and foscarnet are administered by intravenous injection. Probenecid as well as IV hydration (with normal saline) must be given with cidofovir. IV hydration is also recommended with foscarnet. Ganciclovir is administered via intravenous injection, oral capsules, or intravitreal implant. Valganciclovir is given orally in the form of tablets. Oral ganciclovir and valganciclovir should be administered with food.

Adefovir dipivoxil is taken orally in tablet form. Entecavir is available as tablets and oral solution and should be taken at least two hours before or after a meal. Lamivudine is available as tablets and as an oral solution and should be taken on an empty stomach. Ribavirin is available as tablets, capsules, and an oral solution. A solution for inhalation is used in hospitals for children with a life-threatening viral infection of the lungs.

Acyclovir comes in capsule, tablet, and suspension form and is taken by mouth. Acyclovir is also available as an intravenous injection and as a topical cream or ointment.

Famciclovir and valacyclovir are taken orally in tablet form. Penciclovir is available as a cream that can be applied to the lips and face.

Oseltamivir is administered orally via capsules and oral suspension. Zanamivir is administered via oral inhalation.

Cautions and Concerns

Uveitis or iritis has been reported in patients receiving cidofovir therapy. Uveitis needs to be considered as a potential complication of cidofovir therapy, particularly in those patients previously treated for CMV retinitis with a high viral load, low CD4 count, and receiving concomitant therapy with HIV protease inhibitors.

Patients taking foscarnet who are dehydrated or have kidney disease may have an increased chance of side effects. Drinking several extra glasses of water every day will help to prevent some unwanted effects foscarnet has on the kidneys (See *Warnings*). Foscarnet may also cause or worsen anemia. Accidental skin and eye contact with foscarnet solution may cause local irritation and burning sensation; the exposed areas should be flushed with water.

Oral doses of ganciclovir and valganciclovir should be taken with a full glass of water and must be taken with food to increase the amount of drug that gets absorbed. As phlebitis or pain may occur at the site of IV infusion, care should be taken that solutions containing ganciclovir be administered only into veins with adequate blood flow to permit rapid dilution and distribution.

Patients taking adefovir dipivoxil along with other drugs that are known to affect kidney function or are excreted via the kidneys need to be closely monitored.

Patients with decreased kidney function may need to take entecavir less than once a day.

Dosage adjustment is recommended when administering acyclovir, valacyclovir, and famciclovir to patients with kidney impairment (see *Warnings*).

Rimantadine and zanamivir require dosage adjustment in kidney dysfunction.

If physicians decide to prescribe zanamivir to patients with underlying chronic respiratory disease after carefully considering potential risks and benefits, the drug should be used with caution under conditions of appropriate monitoring and supportive care. Patients with asthma or chronic obstructive pulmonary disease who use zanamivir are advised to 1) have a fast-acting inhaled bronchodilator available when inhaling zanamivir and 2) stop using zanamivir and contact their physician if they experience difficulty breathing.

Warnings

Renal toxicity, the most significant side effect of cidofovir, can be reduced by administering another drug, probenecid, and by supplemental intravenous saline hydration on days when treatment is given. Some people have had kidney failure after taking only one or two doses of cidofovir.

Renal impairment is the major toxicity of foscarnet. Frequent monitoring of serum creatinine, with dose adjustment for changes in renal function and adequate hydration with administration of Foscavir, is needed. Seizures, related to alterations in plasma minerals and electrolytes, have been associated with Foscavir treatment. Therefore, patients must be carefully monitored for such changes and their potential sequelae (abnormalities). Mineral and electrolyte supplementation may be required.

Serious side effects affecting the blood have been reported with the use of ganciclovir and valganciclovir, including decreased levels of white blood cells, red blood cells, and platelets, leading to life-threatening problems. Because ganciclovir and valganciclovir have caused birth defects and lower sperm counts and fertility problems in animals, women of child-bearing age and men should use an effective form of contraception during treatment and for at least 90 days following treatment with either of these drugs.

Some people who stop taking antihepatitis agents get very serious hepatitis. This usually happens within 12 weeks after stopping the drugs. Patients who stop taking antihepatitis agents need to have regular blood tests to check for liver function and HBV levels. Some people who have taken antihepatitis agents (nucleoside analogs) have developed a serious condition called lactic acidosis (build-up of an acid in the blood). Lactic acidosis is a medical emergency and must be treated in the hospital. Some people who have taken antihepatitis agents and other nucleoside analogs have developed serious liver dysfunction, with liver enlargement (hepatomegaly) and fat in the liver (steatosis). Patients may be more likely to get lactic acidosis or serious liver problems if they are female, very overweight (obese), or have been taking nucleoside analog drugs for a long time.

Adefovir dipivoxil may cause severe kidney dysfunction. It usually happens in people who already have a kidney problem, but it can happen to anyone who uses adefovir dipivoxil; therefore, patients should have regular blood tests to check for kidney function during treatment. If a patient has HIV that is not being treated with drugs, adefovir dipivoxil and entecavir may increase the chances his or her HIV infection becomes resistant to (cannot be helped by) usual HIV medicines. Patients should be tested for HIV before starting therapy with either of these drugs.

Ribavirin monotherapy is not effective for the treatment of chronic HCV infection and should not be used alone for this indication. Ribavirin may cause anemia (a decrease in red blood cells), which may be dangerous in patients who have heart or breathing problems and may make heart or circulatory problems worse. Other significant adverse events caused by combination therapy with ribavirin and interferon or peginterferon therapy include severe depression and thoughts about suicide, suppression of bone marrow function, autoimmune and infectious disorders, pulmonary dysfunction, pancreatitis, and diabetes. Suicidal thoughts or attempts have occurred most frequently among adolescents. Significant birth defects and/or deaths of the fetus have been seen in all animal species exposed to ribavirin. Because ribavirin may remain in the body for as long as six months, at least two reliable forms of effective contraception must be used during therapy and for six months after completion of treatment in both female patients and in female partners of male patients who are taking ribavirin therapy (See also *When Not Advised [Contraindications]*).

Because heart attacks have been reported in patients with anemia caused by ribavirin, patients should be assessed for underlying cardiac disease before beginning this therapy. Patients with preexisting cardiac disease should be appropriately monitored before and during therapy. Dental and periodontal disorders have been reported in patients receiving ribavirin and interferon or peginterferon combination therapy. In addition, dry mouth could have a damaging effect on teeth and mucous membranes of the mouth during long-term treatment with the combination of ribavirin and interferon alfa-2b or peginterferon alfa-2b. Patients should brush their teeth thoroughly twice daily and have regular dental examinations.

Kidney failure, in some cases resulting in death, has been observed with acyclovir and valacyclovir therapy. Also, thrombotic thrombocytopenic purpura/hemolytic uremic syndrome (TTP/HUS), which has resulted in death, has occurred in immunocompromised patients receiving acyclovir therapy.

On November 13, 2006, the FDA approved a labeling supplement for oseltamivir to include a precaution about neuropsychiatric events. The revision is based on postmarketing reports (mostly from Japan) of self-injury and delirium with the use of oseltamivir in patients with influenza. The reports were primarily among pediatric patients. The relative contribution of the drug to these events is not known. However, people with the flu, particularly children, may be at an increased risk of self-injury and confusion shortly after taking oseltamivir and should be closely monitored for signs of unusual behavior. A health-care professional should be contacted immediately if the patient taking oseltamivir shows any signs of unusual behavior.

When Not Advised (Contraindications)

Cidofovir should not be taken along with any other medications that can cause kidney damage, such as amikacin, amphoteracin B, foscarnet, gentamicin, pentamidine, tobramycin, vancomycin, and nonsteroidal anti-inflammatory agents (e.g., Advil, Aleve).

Because of foscarnet's tendency to cause kidney impairment, its use should be avoided in combination with potentially nephrotoxic drugs (e.g., aminoglycosides, cyclosporine, nonsteroidal anti-inflammatory drugs) unless the potential benefits outweigh the risks to the patient.

Ganciclovir and valganciclovir are contraindicated in patients allergic to acyclovir as well as in patients with low neutrophil and platelet counts.

Patients with a history of significant or unstable cardiac disease should not take ribavirin. Ribavirin therapy is contraindicated in women who are pregnant and in the male partners of women who are pregnant (see *Warnings*). Patients with autoimmune hepatitis must not be treated with combination ribavirin/interferon or ribavirin/pegylated interferon therapy because using these medicines can make the hepatitis worse. Patients with sickle-cell anemia should not be treated with ribavirin capsules or oral solution. Ribavirin (when given orally) is contraindicated when the CrCl < 50 ml/min.

Zanamivir is not recommended for treatment of patients with underlying airway disease (see *Cautions and Concerns*).

Side Effects

Cidofovir side effects include decreased white blood cells (which can increase risk of infection), weakness, nausea, vomiting, diarrhea, fever, headache, decreased appetite, and decreased intraocular pressure (low pressure within the eye).

The most common side effects with foscarnet are fever, nausea, anemia, diarrhea, headache, abdominal or stomach pain, anxious feeling, confusion, dizziness, loss of appetite, and unusual tiredness or weakness.

Ganciclovir and valganciclovir may cause black, tarry stools; cough, sore throat, or hoarseness; fever or chills; pain in the lower back or side; painful urination; seeing flashes or sparks of light, floating spots, or a partial veil across vision; neutropenia, thrombocytopenia, and anemia; unusual bleeding or bruising; unusual tiredness or weakness; abdominal pain; changes in behavior; diarrhea; fever; headache; increased sweating; loss of appetite; vomiting; and weight loss.

Adefovir dipivoxil side effects may include headache, abdominal pain, nausea, diarrhea, bloating, indigestion, flatulence, loss of muscle control, unusual tiredness, trouble breathing, dizziness, yellowing of the eyes or skin, dark urine, and lack of appetite.

Entecavir's side effects include headache, unusual tiredness or weakness, dizziness, insomnia, nausea, vomiting, diarrhea, decreased appetite, and skin rash.

Other side effects of ribavirin (see *Warnings*) include chest pain, difficulty breathing, unusual tiredness or weakness, headache, trouble sleeping, loss of appetite, and nausea. Side effects with the use of inhaled ribavirin include skin irritation due to prolonged drug contact and skin rash. Health-care workers who help in the administration of inhaled doses sometimes may have headache and itching, redness, or swelling of the eyes.

Serious side effects of acyclovir include swelling or redness at the intravenous injection site and symptoms of acute kidney failure such as stomach pain, decreased amount of urine, increased thirst, unusual tiredness, and weakness. Other serious side effects include confusion, seizures, tremors, unusual bleeding or bruising, chills, and fever. Less serious side effects include nausea or vomiting, general feeling of sickness, diarrhea, headache, and lightheadedness. Side effects observed with topical acyclovir use include mild pain, burning, and stinging; itching and rash may occur less frequently.

Side effects associated with famciclovir include headache, nausea, diarrhea, and fatigue. Also, confusion (e.g., delirium and disorientation) has been reported in elderly patients taking famciclovir.

The most common side effects of penciclovir are headache and application site reaction.

The most common side effects of valacyclovir are headache, nausea, vomiting, dizziness, and abdominal pain.

The most frequently reported side effects of oseltamivir are nausea, vomiting, and diarrhea.

The most common adverse events reported with zanamivir are diarrhea, nausea, sinusitis, nasal signs and symptoms, bronchitis, cough, headache, dizziness, and ear, nose, and throat infections.

Interactions

Nephrotoxic agents should not be used within at least seven days of cidofovir therapy (see *When Not Advised[Contraindications]*).

The combination of imipenem-cilastatin and ganciclovir increases the risk for seizures. The combination of ziduvidine and ganciclovir increases the risk of neutropenia and anemia. Taking ganciclovir with certain nephrotoxic drugs may increase the chance of kidney impairment, which could subsequently decrease ganciclovir elimination and increase the risk of toxicity. Because valganciclovir is rapidly and extensively converted to ganciclovir, these same interactions can be expected with it.

Because adefovir is eliminated by the kidneys, coadministration of adefovir dipivoxil with other drugs eliminated by the kidneys or with nephrotoxic drugs may cause further toxicity to the kidneys or may increase serum concentrations of either adefovir or the coadministered drugs. Patients should be monitored closely for adverse events when adefovir dipivoxil is coadministered with drugs that are excreted by the kidneys or are known to affect kidney function, such as aminoglycosides, cyclosporin, and nonsteroidal anti-inflammatory drugs. Administration of antihepatitis agents with other nucleoside analogs increases the risk of lactic acidosis and severe hepatomegaly with steatosis (see *Warnings*). Coadministration of these drugs should be suspended in patients who develop symptoms or laboratory findings indicative of hepatic toxicity.

Ribavirin capsules or oral solution should not be given with didanosine because of the potential for fatal liver failure as well as peripheral neuropathy, pancreatitis, and lactic acidosis. Zidovudine combined with ribavirin is associated with higher rates of anemia, suggesting this combination should be avoided when possible.

Sales/Statistics

According to Espicom Business Intelligence, antihepatitis agents constitute the largest segment of the global antiviral market, generating $3 billion in sales in 2005. In the United States, one antihepatitis agent, ribavirin, was listed among the "Top 200 Generic Drugs by Retail Dollars in 2006" (*Drug Topics,* February 19, 2007), ranking #147 with $56,522,000 in sales, a 27.8 percent increase over 2005. One antiherpes agent was on that list: acyclovir (#108, with $85,595,000 in sales). Acyclovir also ranked #87 on the "Top 200 Generic Drugs by Units in 2006" (4,472,000 units). Antivirals on the "Top 200 Brand-Name Drugs by Units in 2006" (*Drug Topics,* March 5, 2007): Valtrex #50 (7,338,000 units), Tamiflu #153 (1,780,000 units), and Zovirax Topical #197 (1,213,000 units). Two antiherpes drugs were on the "Top 200 Brand-Name Drugs by Retail Dollars in 2006": Valtrex #31 ($1,150,247) and Famvir #172 ($160,602).

On the 2010 Top 200 Branded Drugs by Retail Dollars list (*Drug Topics,* June 2011), Valtrex ranked #60 ($533,961,845), Valcyte #164 ($191,160,942), and Zovirax topical #169 ($184,377,339). On the Branded Drugs by Total Prescriptions list, Valtrex ranked #95 (2,180,482) and Zovirax topical #153 (1,075,542). On the 2010 Top 200 Generic Drugs by Retail Dollars list, valacyclovir HCI ranked #10 ($886,255,653), famciclovir #82 ($182,172,076), and acyclovir #145 ($97,124,649). On the 2010 Generic Drugs by Total Prescriptions list, valacyclovir HCI ranked #96 (6,248,479) and acyclovir #113 (4,965,632).

Demographics and Cultural Groups

According to the CDC, in 2002, 50 percent of those infected with HBV were Asian Americans and Pacific Islanders. Black teenagers and young adults become infected with HBV three to four times more often than those who are white, and one study has found that black people have a higher incidence of HCV infection than white people.

In "Health of Minority Women" (2003), the Office on Women's Health reported that of the 45 million Americans ages 12 and over who have genital herpes (HSV-2), almost 46 percent are of African-American descent compared to 18 percent who are white Americans. Also, in the report, African-American women are three times more likely than white women to be infected with HSV-2.

According to the American Lung Association, non-Hispanic blacks were 12 percent more likely to die from influenza than were non-Hispanic whites in 2001. Influenza/pneumonia ranked as the seventh leading cause of death in the African-American population over 65.

Development History

The first experimental antivirals were developed in the 1960s, mostly to deal with herpes viruses, and were found using traditional trial-and-error drug discovery methods. It was a very time-consuming, hit-or-miss procedure. Then, in the 1980s, scientists began to learn more about the structure and replication of viruses and particularly what kinds of molecules were needed to interfere with the viral replication cycle.

Ganciclovir was the first drug approved for use in AIDS patients with CMV retinitis, on June 23, 1989. Foscarnet was then approved by the FDA on September 27, 1991, and cidofovir was approved on June 26, 1996. The ganciclovir intravitreal implant was approved by the FDA on March 5, 1996. Valganciclovir was approved by the FDA on March 29, 2001.

Lamivudine was introduced by GlaxoSmith-Kline in 1998 and was the first FDA-approved oral antiviral for the treatment of chronic hepatitis B.

Ribavirin, a synthetic chemical not found in nature, was first synthesized in 1970. It was approved on December 31, 1985, for the treatment of hospitalized infants and young children with severe lower respiratory tract infections due to respiratory syncytial virus (RSV). The FDA approved the combination of ribavirin and interferon on June 3, 1998, for people with hepatitis C who had previously responded to interferon alone but relapsed (liver enzymes increased again after treatment).

Adefovir dipivoxil was at one time being developed for the treatment of HIV disease, achieving anti-HIV activity at a substantially higher dose than that used to treat HBV. However, kidney toxicity at the higher dose required for HIV therapy led an expert panel to advise the FDA against its approval at these high doses. In December 1999, Gilead Sciences discontinued its development for HIV treatment but continued to develop the drug for HBV, for which it is effective at a much lower dose. FDA approval for use in the treatment of hepatitis B was granted on September 20, 2002.

Entecavir was approved by the FDA on March 30, 2005.

Acyclovir was discovered and marketed by The Wellcome Foundation (now GlaxoSmith-Kline). The original formulation, a topical ointment, was approved by the FDA in 1984. Famciclovir was approved for use by the FDA on June 29, 1994. Penciclovir received its FDA approval in 1996. Valacyclovir was first approved by the FDA in June 1995 for the treatment of shingles. Approvals for other uses followed in 1996 (genital herpes) and 2002 (herpes labialis).

Amantadine was approved by the FDA in 1976 for the treatment of influenza A virus in adults; rimantidine on September 17, 1993. Oseltamivir was the first orally active neuraminidase inhibitor commercially developed. Both zanamivir and oseltamivir were approved in 1999 for treatment of uncomplicated influenza virus infections.

Future Drugs

In a November 2007 report, the Pharmaceutical Research and Manufacturers of America (PhRMA) listed 75 antivirals currently in testing. Among those in Phase III trials:

- emtricitabine (Emtriva), an ANTIRETROVIRAL, is being tested by Gilead Sciences for HBV treatment. (It is currently being used off-label for HBV.)
- taribavirin is an oral synthetic nucleoside analog being developed by Valeant Pharmaceuticals International for the treatment of patients with chronic hepatitis C.

According to LeadDiscovery, Ltd.'s Pipeline Insight, "Current hepatitis B pipeline activity is driven mainly by HBV polymerase inhibitors, raising the possibility of future combination therapy."

Much of the ongoing research to deal with viruses is in the fields of INTERFERONS and VACCINES.

"Medicines In Development For Infectious Diseases 2007." Pharmaceutical Research and Manufacturers of America. Available online. URL: http://www. phrma.org/files/Infectious%20Diseases%202007. pdf. Downloaded on January 31, 2008.
van Regenmortel, Marc H. V., and Brian W. J. Mahy. "Emerging Issues in Virus Taxonomy." *Emerging Infectious Diseases* 10, no. 1 (January 2004): 8–13. Available online. URL: http://www.cdc.gov/ ncidod/EID/vol10no1/03–0279.htm. Downloaded on January 31, 2008.

bronchodilators Drugs that improve bronchial airflow, or the passage of air into the lungs, thereby relieving breathing problems, such as shortness of breath or wheezing and the sensation of chest tightness. Treatment of asthma is the most common application of these drugs. Asthma affects more than 30 million people in the United States—112 people per 1,000—and 4,055 died of the disease in 2003, according to the Centers for Disease Control and Prevention (CDC) National Vital Statistics System. Asthma is also one of the most underdiagnosed diseases in the United States, especially among the elderly. Bronchodilators are also intended to help expand the airways and improve the breathing capacity of patients with chronic obstructive pulmonary disease (COPD) (including emphysema and chronic bronchitis) and pneumonia.

Classes

Bronchodilators are divided into three classes:

- β_2-*adrenergic receptor agonists*—*Examples:* Short-acting: albuterol (ProAir, Proventil, Ventolin, VoSpire), levalbuterol (Xopenex), metaproterenol (Alupent), pirbuterol (Maxair Autohaler), and terbutaline. Long-acting: arformoterol (Brovana), formoterol (Foradil Aerolizer, Performist), and salmeterol (Serevent Diskus).

- *Xanthine derivatives*—*Examples:* aminophylline, dyphylline (Lufyllin), and theophylline (Theo-24, Theochron, Theolair, Uniphyl).

- *Anticholinergics*—*Examples:* ipratropium (Atrovent) and tiotropium (Spiriva).

- *Combinations*—A number of these drugs are available in combination with either an inhaled corticosteroid or an inhaled anticholinergic. *Examples:* Combination with an inhaled corticosteroid: formoterol/budesonide (Symbicort) and salmeterol/fluticasone (Advair); Combination with an inhaled anticholinergic: albuterol/ipratropium (Combivent, DuoNeb).

How They Work

Airways are breathing tubes that carry air in and out of the lungs. These airways can become narrowed due to accumulation of mucus, tightening of the muscle bands that surround these airways (bronchospasm), or inflammation (swelling) of the lining of the airways. When the airways get narrower, less air flows through to the lung tissue, causing wheezing (a whistling sound while breathing), coughing, chest tightness or congestion, and shortness of breath.

Bronchodilators help to relax the smooth muscle bands that tighten around airways. As the airways open, more air comes in and out of the lungs, making breathing easier. Also, as the airways open, mucus from the lungs moves more freely and so can be coughed out more easily.

β_2-agonists stimulate the β_2-adrenergic receptor in the airways, dilating or relaxing the constricted bronchial smooth muscle and thereby resulting in a widening of the airway. Short-acting β_2-agonists act quickly, within minutes, and are taken at the first signs of breathing difficulties; however, they do not work for very long. Long-acting β_2-agonists take a longer time to act but last for a prolonged time period.

Xanthine derivatives relax airway muscles and keep them open to allow more air in, decrease the sensitivity of the lungs to allergens

and other substances that cause inflammation, and increase the contractions of the diaphragm to draw more air into the lungs.

Anticholinergics work by inhibiting a type of acetylcholine receptor in the tissues of the lungs, thereby causing bronchial muscles to relax and reducing the amount of mucus produced.

Approved Uses

β_2-adrenergic receptor agonists are used for the relief of reversible bronchospasm associated with acute and chronic bronchial asthma, exercise-induced bronchospasm, bronchitis, emphysema, bronchiectasis (abnormal dilation of airways in the lungs), or other obstructive pulmonary diseases. Short-acting β_2 agonists are used to relieve acute symptoms and to prevent exercise-induced bronchospasm. Long-acting β_2 agonists are used for long-term control of symptoms, especially while sleeping, and may also be used to prevent exercise-induced bronchospasm.

Xanthine derivatives are used to treat or prevent bronchial asthma and reversible bronchospasm associated with chronic obstructive pulmonary disease (COPD).

Anticholinergics are used as alternatives to short-acting beta-agonists in patients with asthma and for maintenance treatment of bronchospasm associated with COPD. Ipratropium is also used to relieve symptoms of rhinorrhea associated with allergic or nonallergic perennial rhinitis.

Formoterol/budesonide is approved for the long-term maintenance treatment of asthma in patients aged 12 and older. Salmeterol/fluticasone is approved for use in the treatment of COPD associated with chronic bronchitis and is also indicated for the maintenance treatment of asthma in patients at least four years of age. Albuterol/ipratropium is used in patients with COPD who require a second bronchodilator.

Off-Label Uses

Albuterol is used off-label to treat hyperkalemia (elevated potassium levels).

Xanthine derivatives are used off-label as a respiratory stimulant in Cheyne-Stokes respiration and to treat apnea and bradycardia in premature babies.

Administration

Bronchodilators can be taken orally, through injection, or through inhalation.

Albuterol is available as tablets, extended-release tablets, syrup, a metered-dose inhaler, and solution for nebulization. Levalbuterol is available as a metered-dose inhaler and solution for nebulization. Metaproterenol is available as tablets, syrup, nebulizer solution, and a metered-dose inhaler. Pirbuterol is available as a metered-dose inhaler. Terbutaline is administered orally via tablets or by subcutaneous (under the skin) injection. Arformoterol is available as a solution for nebulization. Formoterol is available as a dry powder inhaler or a nebulized solution. Salmeterol is available as a dry powder inhaler.

Aminophylline is administered orally as tablets or liquid and via intravenous injection. Dyphylline is administered orally via tablets and elixir. Theophylline is administered orally via extended-release and controlled-release tablets and capsules and elixir and via intravenous injection.

Ipratropium is available as a metered-dose inhaler, nasal spray, or solution for nebulization. Tiotropium is available as a capsule containing dry powder to be inhaled with an inhalation device.

Formoterol/budesonide is available as a pressurized metered-dose inhaler. Salmeterol/fluticasone is available as a multidose dry powder inhaler or as an aerosol inhaler. Albuterol/ipratropium is available as an aerosol inhaler or a solution for nebulization.

Cautions and Concerns

β_2-agonists should be used with caution in patients with cardiovascular disorders, especially coronary artery disease, cardiac arrhythmias, and hypertension and in patients with seizure

disorders, hyperthyroidism, or diabetes mellitus. Changes in systolic and diastolic blood pressure have been seen in patients after use of β_2-agonists (See *Warnings*).

Xanthine derivatives should be used with caution in patients with cardiac arrhythmias, acute heart attack, congestive heart failure, severe hypertension, severe hypoxemia, kidney or liver disease, hyperthyroidism, or alcoholism as well as in the elderly and neonates.

Anticholinergics may potentially worsen signs and symptoms associated with narrow-angle glaucoma, benign prostatic hyperplasia, or bladder-neck obstruction and should be used with caution in patients with any of these conditions.

Warnings

β_2-agonists can produce paradoxical bronchospasm, which may be life threatening. β_2-agonists can also produce significant cardiovascular effects measured by heart rate, blood pressure, or ECG changes. Large doses of albuterol, levalbuterol, and terbutaline may aggravate preexisting diabetes mellitus and ketoacidosis. Fatalities have been reported following excessive use of β_2-agonist inhalation preparations, and the exact cause is unknown. Cardiac arrest was noted in several cases.

Long-acting β_2-agonists may increase the risk of asthma-related death. Therefore, arformoterol, formoterol, and salmeterol should only be used as additional therapy for asthma patients not adequately controlled on other asthma-controller medications.

Immediate hypersensitivity reactions may occur after administration of β_2-agonists, including anaphylactic reactions, hives, edema, rash, and difficulty swallowing or breathing.

Excessive doses of xanthine derivatives may cause severe toxicity. Serious side effects such as ventricular arrhythmias, seizures, or even death may appear as the first sign of toxicity without any previous warning. Less serious signs of xanthine derivative toxicity (i.e., nausea and restlessness) may occur frequently when initiating therapy but are usually transient.

Immediate hypersensitivity reactions may occur after administration of anticholinergics, including hives, rash, bronchospasm, anaphylaxis, and swelling of the throat. If such a reaction occurs, the drug should be stopped at once and, alternative treatments should be considered.

When Not Advised (Contraindications)

Xanthine derivatives should not be used in patients who have active peptic ulcer disease.

Anticholinergics should not be used by patients with hypersensitivity to atropine or its derivatives. Patients allergic to soya lecithin or related food products such as soybean and peanuts should not use ipratropium by metered-dose inhaler, as the inhaled version of this medication contains soya lecithin. The nebulized and nasal spray formulations of ipratropium do not contain soya lecithin.

Side Effects

Common side effects of β_2-agonists include headache, dizziness, insomnia, tremor, nervousness, tachycardia, palpitations, sweating, nausea, vomiting, diarrhea, and dry mouth.

Common side effects of xanthine derivatives include headache, dizziness, nausea, vomiting, decreased appetite, weight loss, restlessness, tremor, insomnia, and tachycardia.

Common side effects of anticholinergics include dry mouth, cough, headache, nausea, dizziness, and blurred vision.

Interactions

The use of β-blockers (acebutolol, atenolol, labetalol, metoprolol, nadolol, pindolol, propranolol, timolol) may counteract the effects of β_2-agonists and may cause worsening symptoms of asthma or COPD. Over-the-counter (OTC) cough, cold, asthma, allergy, diet, and sinus medications containing sympathomimetic drugs, such as pseudoephedrine or phenylephrine, may increase the side effects of β_2-agonists. β_2-agonists may cause a change in the dosage requirements of insulin or oral antidiabetic drugs. Coadministration of monoamine oxidase

(MAO) inhibitors and β_2-agonists may result in severe headache, severe hypertension, and extremely high fever. Therefore, these drugs should not be administered within two weeks of each other. Caution should be exercised when using β_2-agonists with loop or thiazide diuretics, as hypokalemia may be worsened.

Alcohol, cimetidine, fluoroquinolones, clarithromycin, erythromycin, fluconazole, fluvoxamine, isoniazid, itraconazole, ketoconazole, protease inhibitors, quinidine, and verapamil may increase the blood levels of xanthine derivatives. Aminoglutethimide, carbamazepine, phenobarbital, phenytoin, and rifampin may decrease the blood levels of xanthine derivatives.

The use of other anticholinergic drugs (oral) may worsen the anticholinergic side effects (dry mouth, urinary retention, blurred vision) of anticholinergic bronchodilators.

Sales/Statistics

According to LifeSciencesWorld.com, which monitors the biotechnology, pharmaceutical, medical devices, and life sciences industries, the world market for asthma drugs was expected to exceed $20 billion by 2010, with use in COPD expected to add a further $10 billion. The U.S. market accounts for approximately half of the global total.

However, the market slowed down from 2010 to 2012 due to patent expirations of leading brands. In February 2011, GlobalData, another industry analysis specialist, estimated the global asthma market to be valued at $12.4 billion in 2009 and expected it to grow to $14 billion by 2017.

Albuterol aerosol ranked #11 in the "Top 200 Generic Drugs by Units in 2006" (*Drug Topics*, March 5, 2007), with 31,057,000 prescriptions. It also ranked #17 in the "Top 200 Generic Drugs by Retail Dollars in 2006" (*Drug Topics*, February 19, 2007), with $485,366,000 in sales. Ipratropium ranked #164, with $45,554,000 in sales.

In the "Top 200 Brand-Name Drugs by Retail Dollars in 2006" (*Drug Topics*, March 5, 2006), Advair Diskus ranked #4 ($3,105,780,000 in

sales), Spiriva ranked #59 ($593,334,000), Combivent ranked #70 ($534,477,000), Xopenex ranked #107 ($320,084,000), and DuoNeb ranked #171 ($162,376,000). In the "Top 200 Brand-Name Drugs by Units Sold," Advair Diskus ranked #11 (18,190,000 units), Combivent ranked #61 (5,464,000 units), Spiriva ranked #67 (4,741,000 units), Xopenex ranked #131 (2,205,000 units), and ProAir HFA ranked #167 (1,467,000 units).

The IMS Institute for Healthcare Informatics (the public reporting arm of IMS) listed the following bronchodilators on their "Top 200 Drugs in the U.S. Market by Dispensed Prescriptions 2010" (both branded and generic are on the same listing): Proair HFA ranked #18, Advair Diskus #25, Ventolin HFA #44, Combivent #59, Spiriva Handihaler #86, albuterol #153, Proventil HFA #185, and Combivent #199. On the IMS top 200 drugs by sales in 2010, Advair Diskus ranked #4, with $4,711,436,220. Also on that list were Proventil HFA #25, Symbicort #66, Proair HFA #69, Ventolin HFA #128, and Xopenex #130 (IMS does not include dollars beyond #20).

Demographics and Cultural Groups

Although asthma affects people of all ages, it most often starts in childhood. More boys have asthma than girls, but in adulthood, more women have asthma than men. Although asthma affects people of all races, blacks are more likely than whites to be hospitalized for asthma attacks and to die from asthma. Among all race and ethnicity groups in 2005, according to the National Center for Health Statistics, Puerto Ricans had the highest rate of asthma, and Mexicans had the lowest. Puerto Ricans were 95 percent more likely to have ever been diagnosed with asthma than non-Hispanic white people.

Development History

According to Teresa Hale, the author of *Breathing Free* (Three Rivers Press, 2000), the first bronchodilator (ephedra) was devised 4,000 years ago by a Chinese doctor named Ma Huang. Later, whiskey, caffeine, tobacco, and chloroform were used to treat paroxysms of the bronchial tubes. Early modern-day bronchodilators included ephedrine and epinephrine (adrenaline).

Terbutaline was first approved by the FDA in 1974, followed by pirbuterol in 1986, salmeterol in 1994, levalbuterol in 1999, formoterol in 2001, and arformoterol in 2006.

Theophylline was first extracted from tea leaves around 1888 by the German biologist Albrecht Kossel. The drug was chemically identified in 1896 and eventually synthesized by another German scientist, Wilhelm Traube. Theophylline's first clinical use in asthma treatment came in the 1950s.

The recreational and medicinal properties of atropine, an anticholinergic agent, have been well known to many cultures for many centuries. Atropine, in the form of the leaves and roots of *Datura stramonium*, was introduced into Western medicine in the early 1800s by British military officers who had learned of its use for respiratory disorders in India. Then in recent years, a better understanding of the cholinergic mechanisms that control airway caliber in healthy and disease states has revitalized the interest in anticholinergic bronchodilators. Along with this knowledge, pharmaceutical chemists began to develop synthetic analogs of atropine that were not appreciably absorbed but retained the anticholinergic properties of the atropine. Ipratropium and tiotropium were approved by the FDA in 1986 and 2004, respectively.

Future Drugs

According to LeadDiscovery, Ltd., a pharmaceutical monitoring firm, a number of "moderately successful" drugs to treat asthma, COPD, and allergic rhinitis were expected to launch by 2010, with most of these being new formulations of currently used inhalers or modified versions of available drugs. However, LeadDiscovery stated that companies are still seeking novel combination therapies to create the next generation of blockbuster drugs. LeadDiscovery

reported that 75 drugs to treat these diseases were in the pipeline in 2005. In 2007, Pharmaceutical Research and Manufacturers of America (PhRMA) listed 89 drugs in development to treat asthma. Neither group specified how many of these drugs were bronchodilators.

Flutiform (fluticasone/formoterol), being developed by SkyePharma/KOS Pharmaceuticals, consists of a fixed-dose combination of the long-acting bronchodilator formoterol with the inhaled corticosteroid fluticasone in a proprietary nonchlorofluorocarbon (CFC) metered-dose inhaler. Formoterol provides 12 hours of bronchodilation and has a rapid onset of action (one to three minutes) compared to salmeterol (provides 12 hours of bronchodilation but may take up to 30 minutes to take effect). In 2010, the FDA requested significant new clinical studies. If approved, annual peak sales for Flutiform could reach $1 billion, according to industry experts.

CHF 4226 (carmoterol), being developed by Chiesi Pharmaceuticals for asthma and COPD, is a long-acting bronchodilator supplied as an aerosol spray in a metered-dose inhaler (MDI). While studies have already been conducted in patients with asthma, researchers are seeking to determine the optimal dose of CHF 4226 in patients with COPD.

In 2007, Novartis launched a global Phase III clinical trial to evaluate the efficacy, safety, and tolerability of QAB149 (indacaterol) for the treatment of COPD. QAB149 is a novel, once-daily β_2-agonist combining a fast onset of action with a 24-hour duration of action.

GlaxoSmithKline is developing five new long-acting bronchodilators, either singly or in combination with a corticosteroid; all are in Phase II trials. It is hoped that these ultra-long-acting bronchodilators will offer increased convenience for patients and may have advantages leading to improved adherence and clinical outcomes in patients with asthma and COPD.

central nervous system (CNS) stimulants The U.S. National Library of Medicine defines central nervous system (CNS) stimulants as "a loosely defined group of drugs that tend to increase behavioral alertness, agitation, or excitation. They work by a variety of mechanisms, but usually not by direct excitation of neurons." In more common terms, CNS stimulants increase activity in the brain and spinal cord, producing feelings of alertness. Although most people may equate these drugs with their potential for abuse and misuse (see Appendix V), central nervous system stimulants—commonly referred to as *uppers*—do have medically approved uses.

Historically, according to the National Institute on Drug Abuse (NIDA), stimulants were prescribed to treat asthma and other respiratory problems, obesity, neurological disorders, and a variety of other ailments. As their potential for abuse and addiction became apparent, the prescribing of stimulants by physicians began to wane. Now, stimulants are prescribed for treating only a few health conditions, most notably attention deficit hyperactivity disorder (ADHD), narcolepsy (a sleep disorder that causes excessive daytime sleepiness and sudden attacks of sleep), and, in some instances, depression that has not responded to other treatments.

The Pharmaceutical & Drug Manufacturers Web site adds, "CNS stimulants increase attention, decrease restlessness, and improve physical coordination in people who have ADHD, a condition in which people have unusually high activity levels and short attention spans. The drugs may also curb impulsive and aggressive behavior related to ADHD. Although central nervous system stimulants are effective in treating ADHD, their use is controversial, especially in children. Experts advise that medication is not a cure for ADHD, and should not be used as the only treatment strategy for the condition."

Classes

Central nervous system stimulants can be classified according to chemical structure and further by duration of action.

- *Amphetamines—Examples:* amphetamine salts (dextroamphetamine saccharate)—intermediate-acting (Adderall), long-acting (Adderall XR); dextroamphetamine—short-acting (Dexedrine, Dextrostat), long-acting (Dexedrine Spansule); lisdexamphetamine (Vyvanse); methamphetamine (Desoxyn).

- *Norepinephrine-dopamine reuptake inhibitors (NDRI)—Examples:* methylphenidate—short-acting (Ritalin, Methylin,), intermediate-acting (Daytrana, Ritalin SR, Metadate ER, Methylin ER), long-acting (Concerta, Metadate CR, Ritalin LA); dexmethylphenidate—short-acting (Focalin), long-acting (Focalin XR).

- *Selective norepinephrine reuptake inhibitor (NRI)—Example:* atomoxetine (Strattera). (Technically, atomoxetine is not a stimulant drug. It is included here because of its approval for treating ADHD.)

How They Work

Stimulants have chemical structures that are similar to key brain neurotransmitters called monoamines, including dopamine and norepinephrine. Their therapeutic effect is achieved by slow and steady increases of dopamine that are similar to the natural production of this chemical by the brain. The doses prescribed by physicians start low and increase gradually until a therapeutic effect is reached. However, when taken in doses and routes other than those prescribed, stimulants can increase the brain's dopamine levels in a rapid and highly amplified manner, disrupting normal communication between brain cells, producing euphoria, and increasing the risk of addiction.

The exact mechanism of action for amphetamine is not entirely known; however, as described above, they work by increasing the levels of dopamine, epinephrine, and norepinephrine in the brain, which causes an increase in alertness and attention plus elevated mood. Dextroamphetamine saccharate is a single amphetamine product combining the neutral sulfate salts of dextroamphetamine and amphetamine with the dextro isomer of amphetamine saccharate and d,l-amphetamine aspartate monohydrate. Lisdexamfetamine is a prodrug of dextroamphetamine. After oral administration, lisdexamfetamine is rapidly absorbed from the gastrointestinal tract and converted to dextroamphetamine, which is responsible for the drug's activity.

NDRIs block the action of the norepinephrine transporter and the dopamine transporter, which leads to increased extracellular concentrations of both norepinephrine and dopamine. Dexmethylphenidate is a refined formulation of methylphenidate.

NRIs work by helping to restore the balance of neurotransmitters in the brain. Instead of producing more norepinephrine, they cause the neurons to remain for a longer period of time in the norepinephrine the brain already produces.

Approved Uses

Amphetamines are approved for the treatment of attention deficit hyperactivity disorder (ADHD) and narcolepsy. Because of its history of abuse, only one methamphetamine product,

Desoxyn, is currently marketed—in 5 mg tablets. Desoxyn has very limited use in the treatment of obesity and ADHD. In the treatment of obesity, Desoxyn may be used as a short-term (i.e., a few weeks) adjunct in a regimen of weight reduction based on caloric restriction for patients in whom obesity is refractory to alternative therapy, e.g., repeated diets, group programs, and other drugs.

Methylphenidate and dexmethylphenidate are approved for the treatment of attention deficit disorders and narcolepsy.

Atomoxetine is approved for the treatment of ADHD.

Off-Label Uses

Atomoxetine has been used off-label for weight reduction in women with obesity.

Administration

CNS stimulants are administered orally via tablets, extended release tablets, extended release capsules, and chewable tablets. Methylphenidate is also available as an oral solution and as a transdermal patch.

Cautions and Concerns

The least amount of amphetamine feasible should be prescribed or dispensed at one time in order to minimize the possibility of overdosage. Caution should be exercised in prescribing amphetamines for patients with even mild hypertension. Blood pressure and pulse should be monitored at appropriate intervals in patients taking amphetamine salts, especially patients with hypertension. Sustained increases in blood pressure should be treated with dose reduction and/or appropriate medication.

Amphetamines have been reported to exacerbate motor and phonic tics and Tourette's syndrome. Therefore, clinical evaluation for tics and Tourette's syndrome in children and their families should precede use of stimulant medications.

Aggressive behavior or hostility is often observed in children and adolescents with ADHD and has been reported in clinical trials and the postmarketing experience of some medications indicated for the treatment of ADHD. Although there is no systematic evidence that stimulants cause aggressive behavior or hostility, patients beginning treatment for ADHD should be monitored for the appearance, or worsening, of aggressive behavior or hostility.

Amphetamines have been associated with decreased appetite. Absolute weight increases in treated children over time, but the increases are smaller than expected, based on CDC normative values. These reductions in expected weight attenuate over time and are greatest in the heaviest children.

Difficulties with accommodation and blurring of vision have been reported with stimulant treatment.

Amphetamines may impair the ability of the patient to engage in potentially hazardous activities, such as operating machinery or vehicles.

Methamphetamine should not be used to combat fatigue or to replace rest in normal persons. Prescribing and dispensing of methamphetamine should be limited to the smallest amount that is feasible at one time in order to minimize the possibility of overdosage.

Periodic complete blood count (CBC), differential, and platelet counts are advised during prolonged methylphenidate or dexmethylphenidate therapy.

Prescribers or other health professionals should inform patients, their families, and their caregivers about the benefits and risks associated with treatment with CNS stimulants and should counsel them in the drug's appropriate use. Patient Medication Guides are available for these drugs.

Atomoxetine should be used with caution in patients with hypertension, tachycardia, or cardiovascular or cerebrovascular disease because it can increase blood pressure and heart rate. Pulse and blood pressure should be measured at baseline following atomoxetine dose increases and periodically while on therapy. Although uncommon, allergic reactions, including anaphylactic reactions, angioneurotic edema, urticaria, and rash, have been reported in patients taking ato-

moxetine. In adult ADHD controlled trials, the rates of urinary retention and urinary hesitation were increased among atomoxetine subjects. A complaint of urinary retention or urinary hesitancy should be considered potentially related to atomoxetine. Rare postmarketing cases of priapism (penile erection lasting more than four hours) have been reported for pediatric and adult patients treated with atomoxetine. The erections resolved in cases in which follow-up information was available, some following discontinuation of atomoxetine. Prompt medical attention is required in the event of suspected priapism.

Warnings

Amphetamines have a high potential for abuse. Administration of amphetamines for prolonged periods of time may lead to drug dependence and must be avoided. Particular attention should be paid to the possibility of patients obtaining amphetamines for nontherapeutic use or distribution to others, and the drugs should be prescribed or dispensed sparingly.

Misuse of amphetamines may cause sudden death and serious cardiovascular adverse events. Sudden death has been reported in association with CNS stimulant treatment at usual doses in children and adolescents with structural cardiac abnormalities or other serious heart problems. Although some serious heart problems alone carry an increased risk of sudden death, stimulant products generally should not be used in children or adolescents with known serious structural cardiac abnormalities, cardiomyopathy, serious heart rhythm abnormalities, or other serious cardiac problems that may place them at increased vulnerability to the sympathomimetic effects of a stimulant drug. Although the role of stimulants in these adult cases is also unknown, adults have a greater likelihood than children of having serious structural cardiac abnormalities, cardiomyopathy, serious heart rhythm abnormalities, coronary artery disease, or other serious cardiac problems. Adults with such abnormalities should also generally not be treated with stimulant drugs (see *When Not Advised [Contraindications]*). Administration of CNS stimulants may exacerbate symptoms of behavior disturbance and thought disorder in patients with a preexisting psychotic disorder.

Data are inadequate to determine whether chronic use of stimulants in children, including amphetamine, may be causally associated with suppression of growth. Therefore, growth should be monitored during treatment, and patients who are not growing or gaining weight as expected should have their treatment interrupted.

There is some clinical evidence that stimulants may lower the convulsive threshold in patients with prior history of seizures, in patients with prior EEG abnormalities in absence of seizures, and, very rarely, in patients without a history of seizures and no prior EEG evidence of seizures. In the presence of seizures, the drug should be discontinued.

Methamphetamine has been extensively abused. Tolerance, extreme psychological dependence, and severe social disability have occurred. There are reports of patients who have increased the dosage to many times that recommended. Abrupt cessation following prolonged high dosage administration results in extreme fatigue and mental depression; changes are also noted on the sleep EEG. Manifestations of chronic intoxication with methamphetamine include severe dermatoses, marked insomnia, irritability, hyperactivity, and personality changes. The most severe manifestation of chronic intoxication is psychosis often clinically indistinguishable from schizophrenia. Abuse and/or misuse of methamphetamine have resulted in death. Fatal cardiorespiratory arrest has been reported in the context of abuse and/or misuse of methamphetamine.

Tolerance to the anorectic effect of methamphetamine usually develops within a few weeks. When this occurs, the recommended dose should not be exceeded in an attempt to increase the effect; rather, the drug should be discontinued.

Dexmethylphenidate tablets should be given cautiously to patients with a history of drug dependence or alcoholism. Chronic, abusive use can lead to marked tolerance and psychological dependence with varying degrees of abnormal behavior. Frank psychotic episodes can occur, especially with parenteral abuse. Careful supervision is required during drug withdrawal from abusive use because severe depression may occur. Withdrawal following chronic therapeutic use may unmask symptoms of the underlying disorder that may require follow-up.

Atomoxetine increased the risk of suicidal ideation in short-term studies in children or adolescents with ADHD. Anyone considering the use of atomoxetine in a child or adolescent must balance this risk with the clinical need. Comorbidities occurring with ADHD may be associated with an increase in the risk of suicidal ideation and/or behavior. Patients who are started on therapy should be monitored closely for suicidality (suicidal thinking and behavior), clinical worsening, or unusual changes in behavior. Families and caregivers should be advised of the need for close observation and communication with the prescriber. Postmarketing reports indicate that atomoxetine hydrochloride can cause severe liver injury. Atomoxetine should be discontinued in patients with jaundice or laboratory evidence of liver injury and should not be restarted. Sudden death has been reported in association with atomoxetine treatment at usual doses in children and adolescents with structural cardiac abnormalities or other serious heart problems. Sudden deaths, stroke, and myocardial infarction have been reported in adults taking atomoxetine at usual doses for ADHD. Children, adolescents, or adults who are being considered for treatment with atomoxetine should have a careful history (including assessment for a family history of sudden death or ventricular arrhythmia) and physical exam to assess for the presence of cardiac disease and should receive further cardiac evaluation if findings suggest such disease (e.g., electrocardiogram and echocardiogram). Patients who develop symptoms such as exertional chest pain, unexplained syncope, or other symptoms suggestive of cardiac disease during atomoxetine treatment should undergo a prompt cardiac evaluation.

When Not Advised (Contraindications)

CNS stimulants should not be taken during or within 14 days following the administration of monoamine oxidase inhibitors (MAOI), as hypertensive crises may result. Treatment with an MAOI should not be initiated within two weeks after discontinuing atomoxetine hydrochloride.

Amphetamines are contraindicated for advanced arteriosclerosis, symptomatic cardiovascular disease, moderate to severe hypertension, hyperthyroidism, known hypersensitivity or idiosyncrasy to the sympathomimetic amines, glaucoma, agitated states, and for persons with a history of drug abuse. Amphetamines should not be taken in the late afternoon or evening because they may cause difficulty falling asleep or staying asleep.

Methylphenidate and dexmethylphenidate are contraindicated in patients with marked anxiety, tension, and agitation, as the drugs may aggravate these symptoms. These drugs are also contraindicated in patients with glaucoma, with motor tics, or with a family history or diagnosis of Tourette's syndrome.

In clinical trials, atomoxetine use was associated with an increased risk of mydriasis (reflex dilation of the pupil), and therefore its use is not recommended in patients with narrow angle glaucoma.

Side Effects

Common side effects of amphetamine salts include headache, stomach ache, dry mouth, trouble sleeping, decreased appetite, nervousness, and dizziness. Common side effects of dextroamphetamine include fast heartbeat, decreased appetite, tremors, headache, trouble sleeping, dizziness, stomach upset, weight loss, and dry mouth. Common side effects of lisdexamphetamine include upper belly pain, nausea, dry mouth, dizziness, weight loss, trouble sleeping, irritability, decreased appetite, and vomiting. The most common side effects of prescribed methamphetamine include constipation, diarrhea, dizziness, dry mouth, exaggerated sense of well-being, headache, loss of appetite, mild nervousness, nausea, and upset stomach.

Nervousness and insomnia are the most common adverse reactions reported with methylphenidate or dexmethylphenidate but are usually controlled by reducing dosage and omitting the drug in the afternoon or evening. In children, loss of appetite, abdominal pain, weight loss during prolonged therapy, insomnia, and tachycardia (fast heartbeat) may occur more frequently.

Common side effects with atomoxetine include abdominal pain, vomiting, nausea, decreased appetite, headache, sleepiness, dry mouth, and insomnia.

Interactions

Stimulants should not be mixed with antidepressants, which may enhance the effects of a stimulant, or with OTC cold medicines containing decongestants, which may cause blood pressure to become dangerously high or may lead to irregular heart rhythms. Gastrointestinal acidifying agents (guanethidine, reserpine, glutamic acid HCl, ascorbic acid, fruit juices, etc.) lower absorption of amphetamines. Urinary acidifying agents (e.g., ammonium chloride and sodium acid phosphate) increase the concentration of the ionized species of the amphetamine molecule, thereby increasing urinary excretion and resulting in lowering blood levels and efficacy of amphetamines. Adrenergic blockers are inhibited by amphetamines. Gastrointestinal alkalinizing agents (e.g., sodium bicarbonate) increase absorption of amphetamines. Coadministration of amphetamine salts and gastrointestinal alkalizing agents, such as antacids, should be avoided. Urinary alkalinizing agents (acetazolamide, some thiazides) increase the concentration of the nonionized species of the amphetamine molecule, thereby decreasing urinary excretion and resulting in the increase of blood levels and therefore potentiating the actions of amphetamines. Amphetamines may counteract the sedative effect of antihistamines. Amphetamines may delay intestinal absorption of ethosuximide. Haloperidol blocks dopamine receptors, thus inhibiting the central stimulant effects of amphetamines.

Insulin requirements in diabetes mellitus may be altered in association with the use of methamphetamine and the concomitant dietary regimen. Methamphetamine may decrease the hypotensive effect of guanethidine.

Because of possible effects on blood pressure, methylphenidate should be used cautiously with pressor agents (e.g., dopamine, dobutamine). Methylphenidate may decrease the effectiveness of drugs used to treat hypertension. Human pharmacologic studies have shown that methylphenidate may inhibit the metabolism of coumarin anticoagulants, anticonvulsants (e.g., phenobarbital, phenytoin, primidone), and tricyclic drugs (e.g., imipramine, clomipramine, desipramine). Downward dose adjustments of these drugs may be required when given concomitantly with methylphenidate. It may be necessary to adjust the dosage and monitor plasma drug concentration (or, in case of coumarin, coagulation times) when initiating or discontinuing methylphenidate. These interactions also apply to dexmethylphenidate.

CNS stimulants should not be given concurrently or in close proximity with an MAOI (see *When Not Advised [Contraindications]*). Because of possible effects on blood pressure, atomoxetine should be used cautiously with pressor agents. Atomoxetine should be administered with caution to patients being treated with systemically administered (oral or intravenous) albuterol (or other ß$_2$ agonists) because the action of albuterol on the cardiovascular system can be potentiated, resulting in increases in heart rate and blood pressure.

Sales/Statistics

CNS stimulants were the most commonly used type of prescription drug used by adolescents ages 12 to 19 in the United States during 2007–2008 (6.1 percent of prescriptions in this age group), according to the CDC's National Center for Health Statistics.

IMS Health reported that 14,000 total prescriptions for methamphetamine were dispensed in the United States in 2009.

Demographics and Cultural Groups

Noting that a prior study had shown markedly lower use of stimulant medications by Hispanic children with ADHD compared with non-Hispanic children, Foster et al. wrote, "Our study suggests that this observed difference is likely attributable to the subset of less-acculturated Hispanic children, because more-acculturated children were just as likely as white children to have an ADHD diagnosis and to have used stimulant medications. There is some indication that less-acculturated Hispanic individuals are less inclined to interpret similar symptoms as ADHD. The stark difference in psychiatric medication use according to acculturation in our study and the finding that the mother's citizenship was a significant predictor of use suggest that acculturation may be important in addressing ADHD in the Hispanic population."

Development History

Australia's National Drug Strategy (NDS) history of amphetamines notes, "The use of amphetamine has been documented for centuries in China, where the ma huang plant (*Ephedra vulgaris*) has been used to treat people with asthma. The ma huang plant contains ephedrine which is a central nervous system stimulant first produced by chemical synthesis in 1887 in Germany. Following this discovery, amphetamine came into medical and recreational use in the 1920s primarily through the treatment of colds and asthma. In 1932 the Benzedrine Inhaler was introduced as an over the counter product and became a licit substitute for cocaine, which had been declared illegal by the U.S. federal government in 1914. By 1940, 39 disorders had been identified for which benzedrine—one of the three main kinds of amphetamine—was the recommended treatment, including night blindness, sea sickness and impotence."

The Wikipedia entry on benzedrine continues the story: "In the 1940s and 1950s, reports began to emerge about the recreational use of Benzedrine inhalers, and in 1949, doctors began to move away from prescribing Benzedrine as a bronchodilator and appetite suppressant. In 1959, the Food and Drug Administration (FDA) made it a prescription drug in the United States. Benzedrine and derived amphetamines were used as a stimulant for armed forces in World War II and Vietnam." In 1965, the FDA came to a realization that amphetamine had become an abused drug. It soon became a drug available only through a prescription.

Methamphetamine was originally used in nasal decongestants and bronchial inhalers (the levo isomer of methamphetamine is still utilized for these indications). Later it was available in tablets and injectable formulations and used for weight control, for depression, and to increase alertness and prevent sleep. A broad segment of society used methamphetamine products for stimulant effects.

Lisdexamphetamine was introduced in the United States in July 2007 for the treatment of ADHD in children ages six to 12, approved in April 2008 to treat ADHD in adults, and approved in November 2010 to treat ADHD in adolescents ages 13 to 17.

Methylphenidate was first synthesized in 1944 and was identified as a stimulant in 1954. It began to be used to treat children with ADHD in the 1960s.

Dexmethylphenidate was approved in November 2001.

During development, atomoxetine was initially called tomoxetine; however, because of the similarity between "tomoxetine" and "tamoxifen" (a breast cancer drug—see ANTINEOPLASTICS), the FDA anticipated possible dispensing errors and thus requested a name change. Originally targeted as an antidepressant, atomoxetine did not show any benefit during clinical trials.

Because norepinephrine is believed to play a role in ADHD, atomoxetine was then tested—and subsequently approved in November 2002—as an ADHD treatment.

Future Drugs

The Medco Health Solutions Drug Trend Report for 2011 noted that although few new CNS stimulant drugs were expected in the next few years, several branded drugs were coming off patent. Thus, new generics were expected to help provide cost relief beginning in 2011 and 2012.

"Central Nervous System Stimulants." Pharmaceutical & Drug Manufacturers. Available online. URL: http://www.pharmaceutical-drug-manufacturers.com/pharmaceutical-drugs/central-nervous-system-stimulants.html

Foster, Byron Alexander, Debra Read, and Christina Bethell. "An Analysis of the Association Between Parental Acculturation and Children's Medication Use." Pediatrics 124, no. 4 (October 1, 2009): 1,152–1,161. Available online. URL: http://pediatrics.aappublications.org/content/124/4/1152.full.html

cholinergics   Cholinergic agents enhance (stimulate) the action of the neurotransmitter acetylcholine (ACh) in the central nervous system, the peripheral nervous system, or both. Cholinergics are also known as parasympathomimetics because they produce effects that imitate parasympathetic nerve stimulation. Acetylcholine is the only neurotransmitter used by the parasympathetic nervous system (PSNS). Acetylcholine is found in the brain, spinal cord, and neuromuscular junctions (the points where nerves stimulate the muscles). Acetylcholine and its receptors are involved in many functions, including muscle movement, breathing, heart rate, learning, and memory; thus, cholinergics are used in the treatment of a variety of conditions.

Classes

Cholinergics are classified according to how they stimulate the sympathetic nervous system—directly or indirectly.

Direct-acting cholinergics directly stimulate the muscarinic or nicotinic receptors. Muscarinic receptors are located primarily in the central nervous system and are involved in a large number of functions, including heart rate and force of contraction, contraction of smooth muscles, and the release of neurotransmitters. Nicotinic receptors are located primarily at neuromuscular junctions and are involved in muscular contraction.

- *Choline esters* are structural analogs of acetylcholine—*Examples:* acetylcholine chloride (Miochol-E), bethanechol (Urecholine), carbachol (Isopto Carbachol, Miostat), and cevimeline (Evoxac).
- *Plant alkaloids* are analogs of naturally occurring substances—*Examples:* nicotine (Commit, Nicoderm CQ, Nicorette, Nicotrol) and pilocarpine (Isopto Carpine, Pilopine HS, Salagen).

Indirect acting cholinergics act indirectly by inhibiting the enzyme cholinesterase. When this enzyme, which normally destroys ACh, is inhibited, the concentration of ACh builds up.

- *Reversible cholinesterase inhibitors—Examples:* donepezil (Aricept), edrophonium (Enlon, Reversol, Tensilon), galantamine (Razadyne, [formerly Reminyl]), neostigmine (Prostigmin), physostigmine (Antilirium, Eserine), pyridostigmine (Mestinon, Regonol), rivastigmine (Exelon), and tacrine (Cognex).
- *Irreversible cholinesterase inhibitors—Examples:* echothiophate (Phospholine Iodide) and malathion (Ovide).

How They Work

The synthetic acetylcholine chloride mimics the parasympathomimetic effect of the naturally occurring neurotransmitter ACh. Administered as an ophthalmic solution, this drug stimulates the cholinergic receptors in the sphincter muscle of the iris, causing the pupil to contract and constrict (miosis). Its effect occurs within seconds and lasts for about 10 minutes.

Bethanechol works by stimulating the bladder muscles that are responsible for causing urination. It helps to increase bladder muscle tone and contractility.

Carbachol produces constriction of the iris and ciliary body resulting in miosis and a reduction in eye pressure.

Cevimeline binds to muscarinic receptors, increasing secretion of exocrine glands, such as salivary and sweat glands, and may also increase tone of the smooth muscle in the gastrointestinal (GI) and urinary tracts.

When nicotine gets into the brain, it attaches to acetylcholine receptors and mimics the actions of acetylcholine. Nicotine also activates areas of the brain that are involved in producing feelings of pleasure and reward. Scientists have discovered that nicotine raises the levels of a neurotransmitter called dopamine in the parts of the brain that produce feelings of pleasure and reward. Dopamine, which is sometimes called the pleasure molecule, is the same neurotransmitter that is involved in addictions to other drugs such as cocaine and heroin. Researchers now believe that this change in dopamine may play a key role in all addictions and may help explain why it is so hard for people to stop smoking. As a therapeutic drug, controlled levels of nicotine are given to patients in an effort to wean them off their dependence. The nicotine patch delivers nicotine through the skin and into the bloodstream. Nicotine gum, lozenges, and inhalers deliver nicotine to the blood through the lining of the mouth. Nicotine nasal spray is absorbed through the nasal membranes into veins, transported to the heart, and then sent to the brain.

Pilocarpine acts on a subtype of muscarinic receptor found on the iris sphincter muscle, causing the muscle to tighten and increase the flow of fluid from the eye, thereby decreasing eye pressure. Pilocarpine also stimulates the function of the glands that produce saliva, sweat, tears, and digestive secretions. It also stimulates smooth muscles, such as those found in the bronchus, gallbladder, bile ducts, and intestinal and urinary tracts.

When someone has Alzheimer's disease, nerve cells and vital chemicals in parts of the brain that are key to memory and other mental processes are lost over time. One such chemical is ACh, which helps carry messages from nerve cell to nerve cell in the brain. Alzheimer's disease may impair thinking and memory by disrupting these messages between cells. It is thought that donepezil, galantamine, tacrine, and rivastigmine help reduce the breakdown of ACh. There is no evidence that any of these drugs alter the course of the underlying dementia process.

Edrophonium, neostigmine, physostigmine, and pyridostigmine also prevent destruction of ACh by inhibiting the action of the enzyme acetylcholinesterase, mainly at the neuromuscular junction. This improves the transmission of nerve impulses in muscles so that the muscles are better able to work. These drugs differ in duration of action and in side effects.

Echothiophate reduces pressure in the eye by increasing the amount of fluid that drains from the eye. Echothiophate also causes the pupil to become smaller and reduces its response to light or dark conditions. Because of the very slow rate at which echothiophate is hydrolyzed by cholinesterase, its effects can last a week or more.

Malathion is a pesticide that works by inhibiting cholinesterase activity and disrupting the chemical reactions in the lice's nervous system. This activity is selective to insects because malathion is rapidly hydrolyzed (decomposed in water) and detoxified in mammals.

Approved Uses

Acetylcholine chloride is a miotic cholinergic used during cataract surgery, immediately after delivery of the lens, in order to produce complete miosis (contraction of the sphincter muscle of the iris causing the pupil to become smaller). It is also used in other eye surgery when rapid, complete miosis may be required, such as penetrating keratoplasty (removal of a cloudy/diseased cornea and replacing it with a clear donor cornea), iridectomy (removal of part of the iris), and other anterior segment surgery (in the front third of the eye).

Bethanechol is a urinary cholinergic used to relieve difficulties in urinating due to nerve problems in the bladder or weakness in certain bladder muscles caused by surgery, childbirth, or drugs.

Carbachol is used in the treatment of glaucoma to reduce the pressure in the eye by increasing the amount of fluid that drains from the eye. Carbachol also is used during eye surgery to cause the pupil to become smaller and reduce its response to light or dark conditions.

Cevimeline is used for the treatment of dry mouth symptoms in patients with Sjögren's syndrome.

Nicotine is used as an aid to smoking cessation for the relief of nicotine withdrawal symptoms, including nicotine craving. It is recommended for use as part of a comprehensive behavioral smoking cessation program.

Pilocarpine is used to treat chronic simple glaucoma, especially open-angle glaucoma; to decrease eye pressure prior to surgery; and to treat mydriasis (an excessive dilation of the pupil due to disease or drugs). Pilocarpine is also used to treat dryness of the mouth and throat caused by a decrease in the amount of saliva that may occur after radiation treatment for cancer of the head and neck as well as dry mouth in patients with Sjögren's syndrome.

Donapezil is used for the treatment of mild, moderate, and severe dementia of Alzheimer's disease. Rivastigmine is used to treat mild to moderate dementia associated with Alzheimer's disease or Parkinson's disease. Tacrine is used to treat mild to moderate dementia of Alzheimer's disease.

In myasthenia gravis, the body's immune system destroys many of the muscarinic receptors, so that the muscle becomes less responsive to nervous stimulation. Edrophonium is used to test muscle response and help to diagnose myasthenia gravis, to differentiate myasthenic crisis from cholinergic crisis, and to help evaluate treatment requirements in myasthenia gravis. It can also help reverse the effects of muscle relaxants used during surgery. Because of its brief duration of action (an average of 10 minutes), it is not useful in maintenance therapy.

Neostigmine is used for the symptomatic control of myasthenia gravis when oral therapy is impractical, such as when the patient has difficulty breathing or swallowing. It is also used following surgery to reverse the effects of certain muscle relaxants. It can also be used to prevent or treat urinary retention resulting from general anesthesia when no bladder obstruction exists.

Physostigmine is used to treat the central nervous system effects of atropine overdose and other anticholinergic drug overdoses.

Pyridostigmine is used to decrease muscle weakness resulting from myasthenia gravis. The intravenous form is used to reverse the effects of certain muscle relaxants. Pyridostigmine is also used by U.S. military personnel in combat to increase survival after exposure to Soman, a nerve agent that blocks the cholinesterase enzyme. Soman exposure can cause loss of muscle control and death if the muscles required for breathing are paralyzed.

Echothiophate is used to treat certain types of glaucoma, glaucoma following cataract surgery, and certain eye disorders involving eye focusing, such as crossing of the eyes.

Malathion is used to treat head lice.

Off-Label Uses

Bethanechol has been used off-label in adults for treatment and diagnosis of reflux esophagitis. It has also been used off-label in infants and children for gastroesophageal reflux.

Nicotine has been used off-label along with haloperidol to improve symptoms of Tourette's syndrome.

Galantamine is used off-label to treat vascular dementia.

Neostigmine is used off-label to treat acute colonic pseudo-obstruction (large bowel dilation without bowel obstruction) in patients when conventional therapy has not been effective.

Physostigmine is used off-label to treat delirium tremens (DTs, or acute delirium caused by alcohol poisoning), glaucoma, and Alzheimer's disease.

Companion Drugs

Memantine, a newer agent for Alzheimer's disease, is sometimes used in combination with one of the acetylcholinesterase inhibitors (donepezil, galantamine, rivastigmine), as the response to the two drugs together is considered superior to the acetylcholinesterase inhibitors alone.

Administration

Acetylcholine chloride is administered via injection into the eye.

Bethanechol is available as a tablet to take by mouth. Bethanechol generally should be taken on an empty stomach.

Carbachol is generally administered as an ophthalmic solution (eyedrop). During eye surgery, it is administered via injection.

Cevimeline is available in capsule form and is taken orally.

Nicotine is available as lozenges, inhaler, nasal spray, skin patch, and chewing gum. The inhaler and nasal spray are available by prescription only.

Pilocarpine for eye treatment is available as an ophthalmic solution (eyedrop) or gel. For dry mouth, pilocarpine is taken by mouth via tablets. Pilocarpine eye products should not be taken by mouth.

Donepezil is administered orally via tablets and rapidly disintegrating tablets.

Edrophonium is administered via intravenous (preferred route) or intramuscular injection.

Galantamine is available as a tablet, an extended-release (long-acting) capsule, and a solution to take by mouth.

Neostigmine is administered via intramuscular, intravenous, or subcutaneous injection and is also taken orally via tablets.

Physostigmine is administered via intramuscular, intravenous, and subcutaneous injection.

Pyridostigmine is administered orally via syrup, tablets, and extended-release tablets. It may also be administered via intravenous injection following surgery, during labor or following childbirth, during myasthenic crisis, or when oral therapy is impractical.

Rivastigmine is taken orally via capsules or solution and is also available as a transdermal patch (for dementia associated with Parkinson's disease).

Tacrine is available as a capsule to take by mouth.

Echothiophate is administered an ophthalmic solution (eyedrop).

Malathion is a lotion that is applied to the hair and scalp.

Cautions and Concerns

Direct-acting ophthalmic cholinergics should be used with caution in patients with acute heart failure, bronchial asthma, peptic ulcer disease, hyperthyroidism, gastrointestinal spasm, urinary tract obstruction, Parkinson's disease, recent myocardial infarction, hypertension, or hypotension.

Retinal detachment (separation of the retina from its attachments to the back of the eyeball) has been caused by acetylcholine, carbachol, and pilocarpine in individuals with preexisting retinal disease or in those who are predisposed to retinal tears.

If the sphincter fails to relax as bethanechol contracts the bladder, urine may be forced up the ureter into the kidney pelvis. If there is bacteriuria, this may cause reflux infection.

Corneal clouding, persistent bullous keratopathy (involving decompensation of the cornea), retinal detachment, and postoperative iritis (inflammation of the iris, the colored portion of the eye) following cataract extraction have been reported with carbachol.

Cevimeline and pilocarpine should be administered with caution to patients with a history of kidney stones or gallstones. Contractions of the gallbladder or biliary smooth muscle could lead to complications such as inflammation or obstruction. An increase in the ureteral smooth muscle tone could theoretically precipitate renal colic or ureteral reflux in patients with kidney stones. Patients should be informed that cevimeline and pilocarpine may cause visual disturbances, especially at night, that could impair their ability to drive safely. Patients taking cevimeline or pilocarpine should drink extra water because of the possibility of dehydration caused by excessive sweating.

Smokers should be urged to stop smoking completely when beginning nicotine replacement therapy. If they continue to smoke during therapy, they may experience side effects due to peak nicotine levels higher than those experienced from smoking alone. The risks of nicotine replacement in patients with cardiovascular and peripheral vascular diseases should be weighed against the benefits of including nicotine replacement in a smoking cessation program for them. Nicotine therapy should be used with caution in patients with hyperthyroidism, pheochromocytoma, insulin-dependent diabetes, or peptic ulcer disease.

When given edrophonium, neostigmine, or pyridostigmine, patients may develop anticholinesterase insensitivity for brief or prolonged periods. During these periods, the patients should be carefully monitored and may need respiratory assistance. Dosages of these drugs should be reduced or withheld until patients again become sensitive to them. These drugs should be used with caution in patients with bronchial asthma, epilepsy, bradycardia, recent myocardial infarction, hyperthyroidism, cardiac arrhythmias, or peptic ulcer disease.

Physostigmine contains benzyl alcohol, which has been associated with a fatal "gasping syndrome" in premature infants. It also contains sulfites, which may cause allergic reactions, including anaphylactic symptoms and life-threatening or less severe asthmatic episodes, in certain susceptible people, particularly those with asthma.

Lower doses of pyridostigmine may be required in patients with kidney disease.

Worsening of cognitive function has been reported following abrupt discontinuation of tacrine or after a large reduction in total daily dose.

When echothiophate is used for glaucoma, the patient's eye pressure should be checked at regular intervals. To prevent possible skin absorption, hands should be washed following instillation of echothiophate. Temporary or permanent discontinuation of echothiophate is necessary if cardiac irregularities occur. Echothiophate should be used with great caution, if at all, when there is a prior history of retinal detachment. Temporary discontinuation of echothiophate is necessary if salivation, urinary incontinence, diarrhea, profuse sweating, muscle weakness, or respiratory difficulties occur.

Malathion may cause stinging, especially if the scalp has open sores from scratching. If accidentally placed in the eye, the eye should be flushed immediately with water. Because the potential for absorption of malathion through the skin is not yet known, strict adherence to the dosing instructions regarding its use in children, method of application, duration of exposure, and frequency of application is required.

Warnings

Acetylcholine chloride must be opened under aseptic conditions only.

Because cevimeline and pilocarpine can potentially alter cardiac conduction and/or heart rate, they should be used under close medical supervision in patients with a history of cardiovascular disease, including angina pectoris or myocardial infarction. Because cevimeline and pilocarpine can potentially increase airway resistance, bronchial smooth muscle tone, and bronchial secretions, they should be administered with close medical supervision to patients with controlled asthma, chronic bronchitis, or chronic obstructive pulmonary disease.

Nicotine from any source can be toxic and addictive. Smoking causes lung disease, cancer, and heart disease and may adversely affect pregnant women or the fetus. For any smoker, with or without concomitant disease or pregnancy, the risk of nicotine replacement in a smoking cessation program should be weighed against the hazard of continued smoking and the likelihood of achieving cessation of smoking without nicotine replacement.

Eye formulations of pilocarpine may cause blurred vision, which may result in difficulty seeing, especially at night. Patients should not drive, use machinery, or do anything that requires clear vision until they know how pilocarpine affects them. Pilocarpine may also make the eyes more sensitive to light, necessitating the wearing of dark glasses in bright sun or under any bright lights.

Cholinesterase inhibitors are likely to exaggerate effects of muscle relaxants administered during anesthesia. Cholinesterase inhibitors also have the potential to increase gastric acid secretion. Patients at risk for developing ulcers, including those receiving concurrent nonsteroidal anti-inflammatory drugs (NSAIDs), should be monitored closely for gastrointestinal bleeding. Cholinesterase inhibitors should be prescribed with care to patients with a history of asthma or obstructive pulmonary disease. Also, patients taking cholinesterase inhibitors should be considered at risk for bradycardia and atrioventricular (AV) block.

In clinical trials, fainting episodes have been reported with donepezil.

Whenever edrophonium, neostigmine, or pyridostigmine are used for testing, a syringe containing atropine sulfate should be immediately available to be given intravenously to counteract any severe cholinergic reactions that occur in the hypersensitive individual.

If excessive symptoms of salivation, vomiting, urination, and defecation occur, the use of edrophonium, neostigmine, physostigmine, or pyridostigmine should be terminated. If excessive sweating or nausea occurs, the dosage should be reduced. Rapid administration can cause bradycardia, hypersalivation leading to respiratory difficulties, and seizures.

Rivastigmine can cause serious nausea and vomiting as well as significant loss of appetite and weight loss.

Tacrine may slow the heart rate, which may be particularly important to patients with conduction abnormalities, bradyarrhythmia, or sick sinus syndrome. Tacrine may cause liver damage.

Extreme caution should be observed in treating glaucoma with echothiophate in patients who are at the same time undergoing treatment with systemic anticholinesterase medications for myasthenia gravis because of possible adverse additive effects.

Because malathion is flammable, it should be kept away from heat sources such as hair dryers, electric curlers, cigarettes, or open flames.

When Not Advised (Contraindications)

Direct acting cholinergics should not be used where constriction is undesirable, such as in uveitis, some forms of secondary glaucoma, pupillary block glaucoma (a form of angle closure glaucoma), and acute inflammatory disease of the anterior chamber.

Bethanechol should not be used by anyone who has an overactive thyroid, stomach ulcer, asthma, severe lowering of heart rate or blood pressure, coronary artery disease, epilepsy, Parkinson's disease, had recent urinary bladder surgery, or possible gastrointestinal or bladder obstruction, inflammatory lesions of the GI tract, or peritonitis.

Cevimeline is contraindicated in patients with uncontrolled asthma and when miosis is undesirable, e.g., in acute iritis and in narrow-angle (angle-closure) glaucoma.

Nicotine inhalers generally should not be used in patients during the immediate post–myocardial infarction period, in patients with serious arrhythmias, or in patients with severe or worsening angina.

Pilocarpine should not be taken by people with uncontrolled asthma or such eye problems as inflammation of the iris or angle-closure glaucoma.

Galantamine should not be used in patients with severe kidney or liver impairment.

Edrophonium, neostigmine, and pyridostigmine should not be used in patients with intestinal or urinary tract obstruction.

Neostigmine is contraindicated in patients with peritonitis or with bladder or bowel obstruction.

Physostigmine should not be used in patients who have asthma, gangrene, diabetes, cardiovascular disease, obstruction of the intestine or urogenital tract, or any vagotonic state, nor in patients receiving choline esters and depolarizing neuromuscular blocking agents (succinylcholine).

Echothiophate should not be used if an eye infection is present or if the eye is wounded or injured.

Malathion should not be used on newborns and infants because their scalps are more permeable and may have increased absorption of malathion.

Side Effects

Infrequent cases of corneal edema, corneal clouding, and corneal decompensation have been reported with the use of intraocular acetylcholine. Adverse reactions from systemic absorption have been reported rarely but have included slow heartbeat, low blood pressure, flushing, breathing difficulties, and sweating.

Bethanechol side effects include upset stomach, nausea and vomiting (especially when taken soon after eating), wheezing, sweating, and flushing. Dizziness, lightheadedness, or fainting may occur, especially when getting up from a lying or sitting position.

Side effects such as flushing, sweating, stomach distress, abdominal cramps, tightness in urinary bladder, and headache have been reported with topical or systemic application of carbachol.

The most common side effects reported during cevimeline clinical trials include excessive sweating, headache, nausea, sinusitis, upper respiratory tract infection, rhinitis, and diarrhea.

The most common side effects from wearing a nicotine patch include skin irritation, dizziness, racing heartbeat, sleep problems, headache, nausea, vomiting, and muscle aches and stiffness. The most common side effects of nicotine lozenge use are soreness of the teeth and gums, indigestion, and throat irritation. The most common side effects due to nicotine nasal spray and inhaler are nose and throat irritations. The inhaler may also cause coughing initially, which usually goes away after a while.

The most frequent side effect of pilocarpine is increased sweating; other common side effects include nausea and vomiting, irritated nose, chills, flushing, frequent urination, dizziness, weakness, headache, difficulty with digestion, increased tear production, diarrhea, bloating, abdominal pain, and visual problems.

Common side effects of donepezil include nausea, vomiting, diarrhea, bruising, loss of appetite, abdominal pain, muscle cramps, fatigue, insomnia, and vivid dreams.

Common side effects of edrophonium are abdominal cramps, diarrhea, nausea, vomiting, and increased salivation.

Common side effects of galantamine include bladder pain, bloody or cloudy urine, diarrhea, burning or painful urination, frequent urge to urinate, feeling sad or empty, irritability, loss of appetite, loss of interest or pleasure, lower back or side pain, nausea, tiredness, trouble concentrating, vomiting, and weight loss.

Common side effects of neostigmine include muscle contractions or twitching, excess saliva leading to drooling, abdominal cramps, diarrhea, difficulty speaking, dilation of pupils, dizziness, drowsiness, frequent urination, headache, increased sweating, joint pain, and skin rash.

Side effects of physostigmine include increased sweating, loss of bladder control, muscle weakness, nausea, vomiting, diarrhea or stomach cramps or pain, shortness of breath, tightness in chest or wheezing, slow or irregular heartbeat, unusual tiredness or weakness, watering of mouth, blurred vision or change in near or distant vision, and eye pain.

Pyridostigmine side effects include upset stomach, diarrhea, vomiting, drooling, pale skin, cold sweats, blurred vision, watery eyes, increased urge to urinate, anxiousness and feelings of panic, and muscle weakness.

Rivastigmine side effects include nausea, serious vomiting, loss of appetite, indigestion, weakness or lack of energy, dizziness, diarrhea, headache, and stomach pain.

Common side effects of tacrine include diarrhea, dry mouth, indigestion, loss of appetite, nausea, vomiting, dizziness, headache, behavioral disturbances, abnormal thinking, hostility, tremor, inability to sleep, slow heart rate, changes in blood pressure, urinary difficulties, rash, flushing, aggravation of asthma, and cold-like symptoms.

Common side effects of echothiophate include blurred vision or change in near or distance vision, difficulty in seeing at night or in dim light, headache or browache, twitching of eyelids, and watering of eyes.

Irritation of the skin and scalp may occur with malathion. Accidental contact with the eyes can result in mild conjunctivitis.

Interactions

Although clinical studies with acetylcholine chloride and animal studies with acetylcholine or carbachol revealed no interference, and there is no known pharmacological basis for an interaction, there have been reports that acetylcholine chloride and carbachol have been ineffective when used in patients treated with topical nonsteroidal anti-inflammatory drugs (NSAIDs).

Cholinergics should be used with caution in patients taking ß-blockers due to the possibility of conduction disturbances. Drugs that inhibit CYP2D6 and CYP3A4 will inhibit the metabolism of cevimeline.

Physiological changes resulting from smoking cessation, with or without nicotine replacement, may alter the pharmacokinetics of certain concomitant medications, such as tricyclic antidepressants and theophylline. Doses of these and perhaps other medications may need to be adjusted in patients who successfully quit smoking.

Pilocarpine (when administered orally) is less effective when taken with a meal that is high in fat. Alcohol and antihistamines can cause mouth dryness, which can worsen the condition that oral pilocarpine is being used to treat. ß-blockers and anticholinergics should be used with caution along with pilocarpine.

Cholinergics have the potential to interfere with the activity of anticholinergic medications (e.g., atropine, benztropine, ipratropium).

A synergistic effect may be expected when cholinesterase inhibitors are given concurrently with succinylcholine, similar neuromuscular blocking agents, or direct-acting cholinergic agonists such as bethanechol.

Inducers of CYP2D6 and CYP3A4 (e.g., phenytoin, carbamazepine, dexamethasone, rifampin, and phenobarbital) could increase the rate of elimination of donepezil. Inhibitors of CYP3A4 (e.g., ketoconazole) or CYP2D6 (e.g., quinidine) may increase the concentrations/effects of donepezil.

Care should be given when administering edrophonium to patients with symptoms of myasthenic weakness who are also on other anticholinesterase muscle stimulants. Since symptoms of anticholinesterase overdose (cholinergic crisis) may mimic underdosage (myasthenic weakness), their condition may be worsened by the use of edrophonium.

Drugs that inhibit CYP2D6 or CYP3A4 (e.g., cimetidine, erythromycin, ketoconazole, itraconazole, or paroxetine) may increase the amount of galantamine in the body and increase its effects and toxicities. Taking galantamine with an NSAID may increase stomach irritation and the risk of stomach ulcers.

General anesthetics, procainamide, or quinine derivatives (e.g., quinidine) may decrease the effectiveness of neostigmine.

Propranolol, cimetidine, ciprofloxacin, ketoconazole, fluoxetine, or fluvoxamine may increase some of tacrine's side effects. Carbamazepine, phenobarbital, rifampin, and cigarette smoking may lessen the effects of tacrine. Tacrine may also diminish the effects of levodopa and increase the side effects of theophylline.

Patients receiving echothiophate eye drops who are exposed to carbamate- or organophosphate-type insecticides and pesticides (professional gardeners, farmers, workers in plants manufacturing or formulating such products) should be warned of the additive systemic effects possible from absorption of the pesticide through the respiratory tract or skin. During periods of exposure to such pesticides, the wearing of respiratory masks and frequent washing and clothing changes may be advisable.

Sales/Statistics

Sales of both the branded and generic versions of bethanechol tablets were approximately $33 million in the 12 months ended August 31, 2006, according to Wolters Kluwer Health.

Donepezil is the #1 prescribed Alzheimer's drug—worldwide, more than 3.8 million people had been treated with it through 2007.

Rivastigmine has been used in more than 6 million patients worldwide.

According to the "Top 200 Brand-Name Drugs by Retail Dollars in 2006" (*Drug Topics*, March 5, 2007), Aricept ranked #44 ($799,967,000) and #65 in the "Top 200 Brand-Name Drugs by Units Sold in 2006" (5,036,000 units). Nicotine transdermal patches ranked #182 ($38,767,000) in the "Top 200 Generic Drugs By Retail Dollars." Annual global sales for Razadyne were reported to be $130 million in 2007, a year before its patent expired.

On the lists for 2010 (*Drug Topics*, June 2011), the Exelon Patch ranked #136 in brand dollar sales ($229,601,920) and #158 in brand drug prescriptions dispensed (1,008,200).

Demographics and Cultural Groups

According to the National Institutes of Health (NIH), up to 4.5 million Americans suffer from Alzheimer's disease (AD). The disease usually begins after age 60, and risk goes up with age. While younger people also may get AD, it is much less common. About 5 percent of men and women ages 65 to 74 have AD, and nearly half of those age 85 and older may have the disease.

Development History

Acetylcholine chloride was first approved by the FDA on September 22, 1993.

Bethanechol was approved by the FDA on October 12, 1948.

Carbachol was approved by the FDA on September 28, 1972.

Cevimeline was approved by the FDA on January 11, 2000.

Nicotine, first identified in the early 1800s, is the primary reinforcing component of tobacco that acts on the brain. Nicotine and tobacco's botanical name, *Nicotiana tabacum,* received their name from Jean Nicot, who introduced tobacco into the court of Catherine de Médicis in 1560. Pharmacia was the first pharmaceutical company to manufacture a product for nicotine replacement therapy with nicotine gum in 1971. In 1978, SmithKline Beecham began marketing the gum as Nicorette in Switzerland. Nicorette was approved for sale in the United States in January 1984. In 1996, the FDA approved Nicorette gum for over-the-counter use, making it the first smoking cessation aid for adults available without a prescription. In the early 1980s, Duke University researcher Jed Rose invented and patented the transdermal nicotine patch, which became the basis for SmithKline's Nicoderm, approved by the FDA as a prescription smoking-cessation drug in November 1991. The nicotine nasal spray was approved by the FDA on March 22, 1996, the inhaler on May 2, 1997, and the lozenge on October 31, 2002.

Pilocarpine was originally extracted from the plant *Pilocarpus pennatifoliuis,* which was brought into the United States from South America in 1875 and has been used in the treatment of glaucoma since 1876. It was approved for the treatment of dry mouth on March 22, 1994.

Donepezil was approved for the treatment of mild to moderate Alzheimer's by the FDA in 1996 and for the treatment of severe Alzheimer's in 2006.

Edrophonium was approved by the FDA on May 3, 1951.

Galantamine is a tertiary alkaloid originally extracted from the snowdrop and narcissus bulbs. The active ingredient was discovered accidentally by a Bulgarian pharmacologist in the 1950s. It was first approved by the FDA on February 28, 2001.

Neostigmine was first synthesized in 1931.

Physostigmine was originally obtained from the West African calabar bean. In 1864, researchers isolated physostigmine, and in the 1870s, a German scientist used it successfully to relieve glaucoma. With the synthesis of physostigmine (eserine) by the American chemist Dr. Percy Lavon Julian and his Austrian assistant, Dr. Josef Pikl, in 1935, this carbamate derivative, a reversible inhibitor of cholinesterase, became widely available.

Pyridostigmine was first approved in 1955 to treat myasthenia gravis. In February 2003, the FDA gave approval for military use of pyridostigmine in combat only to prevent death following exposure to the nerve agent Soman.

Rivastigmine was approved by the FDA on February 28, 2001. In 2006, it became the first product approved globally for the treatment of mild to moderate dementia associated with Parkinson's disease.

Tacrine was first synthesized by the University of Sydney's Adrien Albert, a leading authority in the development of medicinal chemistry. Tacrine was the prototypical cholinesterase inhibitor for the treatment of Alzheimer's disease. It was approved by the FDA on September 9, 1993.

Echothiophate was first approved by the FDA on June 27, 1960.

Malathion received FDA approval on August 2, 1982.

corticosteroids Drugs that reduce inflammation and decrease the body's immune response; also called adrenocorticosteroids; sometimes referred to simply as steroids (different from the anabolic steroids sometimes abused by athletes to promote the development of muscle mass). Corticosteroids have many different effects on the body and are used to treat numerous autoimmune and inflammatory conditions, including arthritis, asthma, bursitis, Crohn's disease, skin disorders, systemic lupus erythematosus (SLE), tendinitis, and ulcerative colitis. They are also used to treat severe allergic reactions, in cancer treatment, and to prevent rejection after organ transplant.

Classes

Corticosteroids are divided into the following classes according to their biological activities.

- *Adrenocorticotropin (or adrenocorticotropic) hormone—Examples:* repository corticotropin injection (H.P. Acthar Gel) and cosyntropin (Cortrosyn).

- *Glucocorticoids—Examples:* alclometasone (Aclovate), amcinonide, beclomethasone (Beconase AQ, QVAR), betamethasone (Beta-Val, Celestone, Diprolene, Luxiq), budesonide (Entocort EC, Pulmicort, Rhinocort Aqua), ciclesonide (Alvesco, Omnaris), clobetasol (Clobex, Cormax, Olux, Temovate), clocortolone (Cloderm), cortisone, desonide (Desonate, DesOwen, LoKara, Verdeso), desoximetasone (Topicort), dexamethasone (Dexpak, Maxidex), diflorasone (ApexiCon), difluprednate (Durezol), flunisolide (Aerobid, Aerospan, Nasarel), fluocinolone (Capex, Derma-Smooth/FS, DermOtic, Retisert, Synalar), fluocinonide (Lidex, Vanos), fluorometholone (Flarex, FML), flurandrenolide (Cordran), fluticasone (Cutivate, Flonase, Flovent, Veramyst), halcinonide (Halog), halobetasol (Ultravate), hydrocortisone (Anucort-HC, Cortaid, Cortef, Proctocort, Solu-Cortef), loteprednol (Alrex, Lotemax), methylprednisolone (A-Methapred, Depo-Medrol, Medrol, Solu-Medrol), mometasone (Asmanex, Elocon, Nasonex), prednicarbate (Dermatop), prednisolone (Millipred, Omnipred, Orapred, Pediapred, Pred-Forte, Prelone, Veripred 20), prednisone (Sterapred), rimexolone (Vexol), and triamcinolone (Aristospan, Azmacort, Kenalog, Nasacort AQ, Triderm, Triesence, Trivaris, Zytopic).

- *Mineralocorticoids—Example:* fludrocortisone (Florinef).

How They Work

Corticosteroids are synthetic versions of natural hormones (e.g., cortisol and hydrocortisone) produced in the adrenal cortex—the outer part (cortex) of the adrenal glands, two glands each the size of a pea located in the lower back on top of the kidneys—in response to the release of adrenocorticotropic hormone (ACTH) by the pituitary gland. These hormones help control inflammation, the immune function, and stress due to illness or injury. Corticosteroid drugs mimic the actions of these natural hormones.

Specifically, glucocorticoids bind to the glucocorticoid receptor and exert an anti-inflammatory effect on the body via a number of mechanisms, such as preventing phospholipid release and decreasing eosinophil action, all of which depresses the immune response. Mineralocorticoids work by controlling electrolyte and water levels, mainly by decreasing the amount of sodium that is lost (excreted) in the urine. They bind to the mineralocorticoid receptor, also called the aldosterone receptor.

Approved Uses

Adrenocorticotropin hormone is used for diagnostic testing of adrenocortical function and in the treatment of acute exacerbations of multiple sclerosis.

Glucocorticoids are used widely in the treatment of a variety of medical conditions. Topical glucocorticoids are used to relieve skin inflammation and itching due to several conditions, including contact dermatitis, atopic dermatitis, eczema, insect bite reactions, first- and second-degree burns, and sunburns and as alternative or adjunctive treatment for psoriasis, seborrheic dermatitis, severe diaper rash, and chronic discoid lupus erythematosus. Over-the-counter (OTC) preparations containing hydrocortisone are used for the temporary relief of itching associated with minor skin irritations, inflammation and rashes due to eczema, insect bites, poison ivy, poison oak, poison sumac, soaps, detergents, cosmetics, jewelry, seborrheic dermatitis, psoriasis, and external genital and anal itching.

Oral and injectable glucocorticoids are used to control severe or incapacitating allergic conditions; for exacerbation or maintenance therapy in systemic lupus erythematosus or systemic dermatomyositis; to treat skin diseases such as pemphigus, severe Stevens-Johnson syndrome, mycosis fungoids, severe psoriasis, angioedema, urticaria, and dermatitis; to tide the patient over a critical period of the disease in ulcerative colitis, Crohn's disease, and intractable sprue; to treat autoimmune hemolytic anemia, bronchial asthma, and allergic rhinitis; as short-term adjunctive therapy during acute flare-ups in osteoarthritis, rheumatoid arthritis, bursitis, and gout; and to treat acute exacerbations of multiple sclerosis (MS). Dexamethasone is also indicated for testing of adrenal cortical hyperfunction and cerebral edema associated with brain tumor, craniotomy (surgical opening through the skull), or head injury.

Ophthalmic glucocorticoids are used to treat severe and chronic allergic and inflammatory processes involving the eye, such as allergic conjunctivitis, keratitis, allergic corneal marginal ulcers, herpes zoster ophthalmicus, iritis, diffuse posterior uveitis and choroiditis, optic neuritis, and anterior segment inflammation.

Fludrocortisone acts as a replacement for cortisone when the body does not produce enough. It is used as partial replacement therapy for primary and secondary adrenocortical insufficiency in Addison's disease and for the treatment of salt-losing adrenogenital syndrome.

Off-Label Uses

Adrenocorticotropin hormone is used off-label to treat spasms in infants.

Betamethasone is used off-label to prevent respiratory distress syndrome in premature newborns.

Dexamethasone is used off-label to treat acute mountain sickness and hirsutism (excessive hairiness), to decrease incidence of hearing loss in bacterial meningitis, and as an antiemetic.

Methylprednisolone is used off-label to improve neurologic function in acute spinal cord injury.

Prednisone is used off-label to treat chronic obstructive pulmonary disease (COPD) and to improve strength and function in muscular dystrophy.

Fludrocortisone is used off-label in the management of orthostatic hypotension (a decrease of blood pressure when standing).

Administration

Repository corticotropin injection is administered via intramuscular or subcutaneous injection. Cosyntropin is administered via intramuscular or intravenous injection.

Glucocorticoids are available in various formulations, including oral tablets and liquids, injectables, inhalers, ointments, creams, and ophthalmic solutions.

Fludrocortisone is administered orally via tablets.

Cautions and Concerns

Corticosteroids should be used with caution in patients with congestive heart failure, hypertension, kidney disease, diverticulitis, nonspecific ulcerative colitis if there is a possibility of impending perforation, peptic ulcer disease, osteoporosis, infections (see *Warnings* and *When Not Advised [Contraindications]*), myasthenia gravis, or diabetes. These drugs should also be used with caution in patients with latent tuberculosis, as they may reactivate the disease.

Psychic derangements may appear when corticosteroids are used, ranging from euphoria, insomnia, mood swings, personality changes, and severe depression to psychosis. Also, existing emotional instability or psychotic tendencies may be aggravated.

Some corticosteroid products contain tartrazine, which may cause allergic-type reactions (including bronchial asthma) in susceptible individuals. Tartrazine sensitivity is frequently seen in patients who have aspirin hypersensitivity.

There is an enhanced effect of corticosteroids in patients with hypothyroidism and in those with cirrhosis. Corticosteroids should be used cautiously in patients with ocular herpes simplex because of possible corneal perforation.

Because of the risk of side effects, the lowest possible dose of corticosteroids should be used to control the condition under treatment.

Growth and development of infants and children on prolonged corticosteroid therapy should be carefully observed.

Although controlled clinical trials have shown corticosteroids to be effective in speeding the resolution of acute exacerbations of MS, they do not show that corticosteroids affect the ultimate outcome or natural history of the disease. The studies do show that relatively high doses of corticosteroids are necessary to demonstrate a significant effect.

Persons who are on immunosuppressant doses of corticosteroids should be warned to avoid exposure to chicken pox or measles. Patients should also be advised that if they are exposed, medical advice should be sought without delay.

Adrenocortical insufficiency may result from too rapid withdrawal of corticosteroids and may be minimized by gradual reduction of dosage. This type of relative insufficiency may persist for months after discontinuation of therapy; therefore, in any situation of stress occurring during that period, glucocorticoid therapy should be reinstituted.

Patients taking fludrocortisone should have their blood pressure and electrolytes monitored regularly.

Warnings

Rare instances of serious and rapid allergic reactions have occurred in patients receiving corticosteroid therapy.

Because of an apparent association between use of corticosteroids and left ventricular free wall rupture after a recent myocardial infarction, corticosteroids should be used with great caution in these patients.

Patients who are on corticosteroids are more susceptible to infections than are healthy individuals. Corticosteroids may mask signs of infection, and new infections may occur during their use. These infections may be mild but can be severe and at times fatal. With increasing doses of corticosteroids, the rate of occurrence of infectious complications increases. If an infection occurs during therapy, it should be promptly controlled by suitable antimicrobial therapy (see *When Not Advised [Contraindications]*).

Although advocated for use in chronic active hepatitis, corticosteroids may be harmful in chronic active hepatitis positive for hepatitis B surface antigen.

Prolonged ophthalmic use of corticosteroids may produce cataracts or glaucoma with possible damage to the optic nerves and may encourage secondary eye infections due to fungi or viruses.

Average and large doses of cortisone or hydrocortisone can cause elevation of blood pressure, sodium and water retention, and increased excretion of potassium. These effects are less likely to occur with the synthetic derivatives of these drugs (e.g., prednisone, prednisolone, dexamethasone) except when used in large doses. Dietary salt restriction and potassium supplementation may be necessary. All corticosteroids increase calcium excretion.

Because of its marked effect on sodium retention, the use of fludrocortisone in the treatment of conditions other than those indicated is not advised.

When Not Advised (Contraindications)

Adrenocorticotropin hormone should not be given to patients with scleroderma, osteoporosis, ocular herpes simplex, current or past history of peptic ulcer disease, congestive heart failure, hypertension, or to anyone with reduced function of the adrenal cortex.

The use of methylprednisolone sodium succinate is contraindicated in premature infants because it contains benzyl alcohol, which has been associated with a fatal "gasping syndrome" in these patients.

Corticosteroids should not be used in patients with systemic fungal infections unless they are needed to control life-threatening drug reactions, as they may exacerbate these infections (See *Warnings*).

Live virus vaccines (e.g., smallpox) should not be used during corticosteroid therapy.

Side Effects

Corticosteroid side effects are much more common with high-dose/long-term therapy. Potential side effects include depression, euphoria, headache, convulsions, mood changes, irritability, psychoses, restlessness, insomnia, cataracts, increased eye pressure, high blood pressure, peptic ulcers, heartburn, nausea, vomiting, acne, sodium and water retention, blood clotting, increased blood glucose, increased appetite, weight gain, muscle weakness, osteoporosis, muscle pain, cushingoid appearance (moon face or rounding of the face, buffalo hump), increased facial hair, slow wound healing, skin rashes, and increased susceptibility to infection.

Interactions

Drugs that induce liver enzymes such as phenobarbital, phenytoin, and rifampin may increase the clearance of corticosteroids and may require increases in corticosteroid dose to achieve the desired response. Drugs such as ketoconazole, verapamil, erythromycin, or estrogens may inhibit the metabolism of corticosteroids and thus decrease their clearance. Therefore, the dose of corticosteroid should be titrated to avoid steroid toxicity.

The effect of corticosteroids on warfarin is variable, with reports of enhanced as well as diminished effects of warfarin when given concurrently with corticosteroids. Therefore, coagulation indices should be monitored to maintain the desired anticoagulant effect.

When corticosteroids are administered concomitantly with potassium-depleting agents (e.g., amphotericin B, diuretics), patients should be observed closely for development of hypokalemia.

Concomitant use of anticholinesterase agents and corticosteroids may produce severe weakness in patients with myasthenia gravis. If possible, anticholinesterase agents should be withdrawn at least 24 hours before initiating corticosteroid therapy.

Increased activity of both cyclosporine and corticosteroids may occur when the two are used concurrently. Convulsions have been reported with this concurrent use.

Patients on digitalis glycosides may be at increased risk of arrhythmias due to hypokalemia when taking corticosteroids.

Sales/Statistics

Corticosteroids are among the most widely used drug groups. Listed among the "2008 Top 200 Branded Drugs by Retail Dollars" (*Drug Topics*, May 26, 2009): #42 Nasonex with $904,074,000 in sales, #55 Pulmicort Respules ($651,024,000), #67 Flovent HFA ($553,050,000), #119 Nasacort AQ ($285,359,000), #170 Asmanex ($185,244,000), #171 Rhinocort Aqua ($184,397,000), and #192 Veramyst ($158,347,000).

Corticosteroids listed among the "2008 Top 200 Branded Drugs by Total Prescriptions": #24 Nasonex with 10,463,000 prescriptions, #66 Flovent HFA (4,403,000), #90 Nasacort AQ (3,206,000), #114 Pulmicort Respules (2,413,000), #138 Rhinocort Aqua (1,986,000), #145 Veramyst (1,822,000), #163 Asmanex (1,484,000), and #200 QVAR (1,057,000).

Several corticosteroids also appeared among the "2008 Top 200 Generic Drugs by Retail Dollars": #19 fluticasone nasal with $542,532,000 in sales, #52 prednisone oral ($211,100,000), #90 clobetasol ($127,264,000), #136 desoximetasone ($81,012,000), #148 triamcinolone acetonide topical ($71,678,000), #166 mometasone topical ($60,494,000), and #180 prednisolone sodium phosphate oral ($52,082,000).

Among the "2008 Top 200 Generic Drugs by Total Prescriptions" were #19 prednisone oral with 24,755,000 prescriptions, #36 fluticasone nasal (16,163,000), #54 methylprednisolone tablets (12,141,000), #70 triamcinolone acetonide topical (7,878,000), #124 clobetasol (3,590,000), #143 prednisolone sodium phosphate oral (2,956,000), #152 fluocinonide (2,717,000), #153 hydrocortisone topical (2,702,000), #179 dexamethasone oral (1,995,000), and #183 mometasone topical (1,942,000).

Demographics and Cultural Groups

In a 2007 study of asthma among American Indians, 67.2 percent of participants reported a history of emergency department visits and/or hospitalizations in the previous year, yet only 3 percent were receiving regular inhaled corticosteroids.

Several studies have shown lower inhaled corticosteroid adherence among African-American patients when compared with white patients. A 2007 Michigan study suggests that environmental stressors, such as area crime, influence adherence.

Development History

Corticosteroids have been used as a drug treatment for more than 60 years. Lewis Sarett of Merck & Co. was the first to synthesize cortisone, using a complicated 36-step process that started with deoxycholic acid, which was extracted from ox bile. The low efficiency of converting deoxycholic acid into cortisone led to a cost of $200 per gram. Russell Marker at Syntex discovered a much cheaper and more convenient starting material, diosgenin from wild Mexican yams. His conversion of diosgenin into progesterone by a four-step process now known as Marker degradation was an important step in mass production of all steroidal hormones, including cortisone and chemicals used in hormonal contraception. During this time, the research chemist Percy Julian also contributed to progress in producing cortisone.

In 1952, D. H. Peterson and H. C. Murray of Upjohn Co. developed a process that used *Rhizopus* mold to oxidize progesterone into a compound that was readily converted to cortisone. The ability to cheaply synthesize large quantities of cortisone from the diosgenin in yams resulted in a rapid drop in price to $6 per gram, falling to 46 cents per gram by 1980.

According to Saklatvala, the anti-inflammatory action of glucocorticoid hormones was discovered by the American biochemist Philip Showalter Hench and his Mayo Foundation colleagues more than 50 years ago. "Hench had noted that the symptoms of rheumatoid arthritis were often improved in pregnancy and when a patient had jaundice, both situations in which, he reasoned, there was an increase in steroids in the body. The active substances of the adrenal cortex had then recently been isolated by Reichstein and Kendall and shown to be steroids. It seemed possible that these might alleviate inflammatory symptoms. Hench and his co-workers found that small doses of cortisone dramatically improved the symptoms of patients with rheumatoid arthritis. Hench, Kendall, and Reichstein were jointly awarded the Nobel Prize in physiology and medicine in 1950. Powerful synthetic glucocorticoids were then developed."

Prednisone was invented in the early 1950s, when Arthur Nobile at Schering demonstrated that the side effects of cortisone, such as water retention, high blood pressure, and muscle weakness could be removed by oxidization of the drug through exposure to microbes. The drug was approved on June 21, 1955. Methylprednisolone sodium succinate was approved on May 18, 1959.

Saklatvala, Jeremy. "Glucocorticoids: Do We Know How They Work?" *Arthritis Research* 4, no. 3 (2002): 146–150. Available online. URL: http://www.pubmedcentral.nih.gov/articlerender.fcgi?artid=128923. Accessed November 6, 2011.

decongestants Drugs used to relieve sinus and nasal congestion (stuffy nose) caused by swollen, expanded, or dilated blood vessels in the membranes of the nose and air passages and to reduce eye congestion and thereby relieve redness in the eyes. Nasal congestion has many causes and can range from a mild annoyance to a life-threatening condition. Most commonly, nasal congestion is caused by allergic rhinitis, vasomotor (nonallergenic) rhinitis (oversensitive or excessive blood vessels in the nasal membrane), chronic sinusitis, and upper respiratory viral infections (common colds). Nasal congestion can lead to other conditions, such as otitis media (inflammation of the middle ear) and the onset or worsening of mild to severe sleep disturbances, including obstructive sleep apnea. Decongestants are most often used to treat congestion due to colds and other respiratory infections, especially in people who easily develop middle ear or sinus infections. Decongestants are available over the counter (OTC).

Classes

Decongestants are divided into two classes:

- *Sympathomimetic amines*—Mimic the chemical behavior of the nervous system hormones epinephrine (adrenaline) and norepinephrine (noradrenaline). *Examples:* phenylephrine (Neo-Synephrine, Sudafed PE, Vicks Sinex Nasal Spray) and pseudoephedrine (Sudafed).

- *Imidazolines*—Derivatives of sympathomimetic amines, these drugs act by adrenergic stimulation (stimulating the adrenergic nerves directly by mimicking the action of epineph-

rine and norepinephrine). *Examples:* naphazoline (Naphcon, Privine), oxymetazoline (Afrin Original, Vicks Sinex 12 Hours, Visine LR), and tetrahydrozoline (Murine Tears Plus, Tyzine, Visine).

How They Work

Generally, decongestants work by constricting, or tightening, blood vessels in the mucous membranes, forcing much of the blood out of the membranes so that they shrink, thus reopening the air passages and improving the stuffy feeling.

Approved Uses

Phenylephrine is used for prompt and temporary relief of nasal congestion due to the common cold, sinusitis, hay fever, or other upper respiratory allergies. It is also used to provide relief of minor eye irritation, to dilate the pupil during eye exams, prior to surgery, and in open-angle glaucoma. Phenylephrine is also sometimes used as a vasopressor to increase the blood pressure in unstable patients with seriously low blood pressure.

Pseudoephedrine is used for nasal or sinus congestion.

The imidazolines are used for the temporary relief of nasal congestion due to the common cold, sinusitis, hay fever, allergies, or sinusitis. These drugs are also used to relieve redness, burning, irritation, and dryness of the eye caused by wind, sun, and other minor irritants.

Off-Label Uses

Pseudoephedrine is used to relieve priapism, a condition in which the penis is continually erect without sexual or psychological stimulation. It has also been used off-label to treat urinary stress incontinence by increasing the muscle pressure of the bladder neck and the urethra, which helps retain the urine within the bladder.

Naphazoline nasal drops are used off-label to relieve "plugged ears" and to reduce swelling in the nose before certain surgeries or procedures.

Administration

Phenylephrine used as a nasal decongestant is available OTC in tablet form, quick-dissolve strips, and as a nasal spray. It is also available OTC as eye drops. When used as a vasopressor, it is administered via injection in a hospital setting.

Pseudoephedrine is available OTC as a regular tablet, a chewable tablet, a 12-hour extended-release (long-acting) tablet, a 24-hour extended-release tablet, and a liquid solution.

Naphazoline and tetrahydrozoline are available OTC as nasal drops and spray and as eye drops.

Oxymetazoline nasal is available OTC as a nasal spray and as eye drops.

Cautions and Concerns

Decongestants administered intranasally should be used sparingly and not longer than three days because of the potential for rebound congestion. Longer use could damage the nasal tissue and lead to chronic congestion.

Some decongestant products contain sulfites that may cause allergic-type reactions in certain susceptible persons.

Decongestants should be used with caution in elderly patients or in patients with hypertension, diabetes, hyperthyroidism, or cardiovascular disease.

Decongestants have a hyperglycemic effect and cause an elevation in blood glucose; therefore, blood glucose should be closely monitored in patients with diabetes.

A mild, temporary stinging sensation may occur after use of topical decongestants.

Because decongestant eye drops may cause temporary blurred vision, caution should be used while driving or performing other hazardous tasks.

People with bipolar disorder should use care when taking decongestants, as they can cause insomnia and thus trigger a manic episode.

Chronic use of ophthalmic decongestants may damage the blood vessels in the eyes.

Warnings

Rarely, decongestant tablets may cause bowel obstruction or blockage; thus, patients who have had obstruction or narrowing of the bowel need to consult their physicians before taking oral tablet products.

Patients with high blood pressure should use decongestants only with medical advice.

If nervousness, dizziness, or sleeplessness occurs, patients should discontinue use and consult a physician.

Rebound congestion may occur with frequent or extended nasal or ophthalmic use of decongestants. Patients who increase the amount of drug and frequency of use may produce toxicity and perpetuate the rebound congestion. If completely withdrawing the topical nasal drug is too uncomfortable, initially discontinuing the drug in one nostril, followed by total withdrawal, may be more acceptable. Substituting an oral decongestant for a topical one may also be useful.

When Not Advised (Contraindications)

Decongestants are contraindicated in patients with narrow-angle glaucoma.

Decongestants should not be used in patients taking monoamine oxidase inhibitor (MAOI) therapy.

Side Effects

Side effects related to decongestants include jittery or nervous feeling, palpitations, headache, lightheadedness, difficulty going to sleep, elevated blood pressure and heart rate, difficulty with urination, nausea, gastric irritation, and rash.

Ophthalmic decongestants may also cause burning, stinging, pain, or increased redness of the eye and tearing or blurred vision.

Nasal decongestants may cause burning, stinging, or irritation inside the nose, sneezing, and nasal dryness.

Interactions

MAOIs taken with decongestants may result in severe headaches, hypertension, and extremely high fever, possibly resulting in hypertensive crisis (see *When Not Advised[Contraindications]*).

Tricyclic antidepressants facilitate and increase the sympathomimetic response of decongestants. Increased cardiovascular effects can lead to arrhythmias, tachycardia, and hypertensive crisis.

Decongestants may decrease the effects of sulfonylureas, which may lead to an increase in blood glucose levels.

Diet pills that contain decongestants should not be taken along with decongestants to treat congestion because the additive effect may cause excessive stimulating effects, including insomnia.

Decongestants reduce the blood pressure–lowering effects of high blood pressure drugs. These drugs can increase the central nervous system side effects of stimulants (including caffeine-containing beverages), such as anxiety, restlessness, and insomnia.

ß-blockers may increase the effects of ophthalmic decongestants, causing systemic side effects to occur more readily.

Sales/Statistics

According to a 2006 article in the *New York Times,* the nasal decongestant spray market is around $210 million in the United States. Other reports show the combined U.S. annual market for decongestants at around $1 billion.

Development History

The term *sympathomimetic amines* was coined in 1910 by the British pharmacologists George Barger and Henry Hallett Dale.

Decongestants have been approved drugs since the 1970s and are now available without prescriptions.

The Combat Methamphetamine Epidemic Act of 2005 banned OTC sales of cold medicines that contain pseudoephedrine, which is commonly used to make methamphetamine. Effective September 30, 2006, the sale of cold medicines containing pseudoephedrine became limited to behind the counter. The amount of pseudoephedrine that an individual can purchase each month is limited, and individuals are required to present photo identification to purchase products containing pseudoephedrine. In addition, stores are required to keep personal information about purchasers for at least two years.

Future Drugs

In November 2007, the Pharmaceutical Research and Manufacturers of America (PhRMA) database showed no decongestants in development. Also, according to *Express Scripts Drug Trend Report 2004,* "The pipeline offers no new drugs that appear better than currently-available products."

disease-modifying antirheumatic drugs (DMARDs)

Drugs that not only treat symptoms but also slow down or alter disease progression. First used in the treatment of rheumatoid arthritis (RA), thus their name, they are now used for other diseases, such as Crohn's disease (CD), ulcerative colitis (UC), systemic lupus erythematosus (SLE), idiopathic thrombocytopenic purpura (ITP), ankylosing spondylitis, psoriatic arthritis, and myasthenia gravis. DMARDs also have anti-inflammatory effects, and some have been used to treat other diseases, such as cancer and malaria. A patient may be prescribed several DMARDs over the course of his or her disease.

Classes

DMARDs are divided into the following classes:

- *Antimalarials—Example:* hydroxychloroquine (Plaquenil).
- *Cytotoxic agents—Example:* methotrexate (Rheumatrex, Trexall) (see also ANTINEOPLASTICS).

- *Immunosuppressants—Examples:* azathioprine (Azasan, Imuran) and cyclosporine (Gengraf, Neoral, Sandimmune) (see also IMMUNOSUPPRESSIVES).

- *Gold compounds* (or gold salts)—*Examples:* auranofin (Ridaura) and gold sodium thiomalate (Myochrysine).

- *Biologics—Examples:* abatacept (Orencia), adalimumab (Humira), anakinra (Kineret), etanercept (Enbrel), infliximab (Remicade), and rituximab (Rituxan).

- *Miscellaneous*—leflunomide (Arava), minocycline (Dynacin, Minocin), penicillamine (Cuprimine, Depen), and sulfasalazine (Azulfidine).

How They Work

Exactly how DMARDs work to modify disease progression is still unknown, but they are believed to suppress the body's overactive immune and/or inflammatory systems and thereby slow down progressive joint destruction seen in certain autoimmune diseases. In RA, for example, the immune system attacks and destroys joints, leading to painful inflammation in the affected joints. DMARDs work to prevent that autoimmune response and also help lessen the inflammation.

It is believed that hydroxychloroquine interferes with communication of cells in the immune system.

Cytotoxic agents restrain the overactive immune system by blocking the production of some immune cells and curbing the action of others. By interfering with the DNA in cells, they prevent the cells from dividing, leading to cell death. Some of the cells affected are immune cells, which are involved in the development of autoimmune diseases such as RA, SLE, scleroderma, and vasculitis. A folic acid derivative, methotrexate acts by inhibiting the metabolism of folic acid (a folate antagonist) during DNA synthesis, which interferes with cellular repair and reproduction, particularly on rapidly dividing cancerous cells. Its mechanism of action in autoimmune disorders is thought to be different, with the lower doses inhibiting T cell activation. T cells, or T-lymphocytes, are small white blood cells that orchestrate and/or directly participate in the immune defenses. T cells are involved in attacking joint tissue and contributing to the inflammation associated with autoimmune diseases such as RA and SLE.

Azathioprine inhibits the synthesis necessary for the proliferation of cells, especially leukocytes and lymphocytes. Cyclosporine is believed to inhibit T cells.

Exactly how gold compounds work is not well understood, but it is believed that they interrupt the actions of white blood cells that are involved in inflammation of the joint lining.

Biologics, or biologic response modifiers, inhibit or inactivate signaling pathways involved in inflammation. Abatacept blocks a signal that activates the immune system's T cells. Adalimumab, etanercept, and infliximab bind to and inhibit tumor necrosis factor (TNF), a cytokine that acts to increase inflammation. Cytokines are messenger molecules made by many of the body's cells that act to excite other immune system cells. Anakinra inhibits another cytokine, interleukin (IL)-1. TNF and IL-1 are made in large amounts in persons with RA, thus amplifying and worsening inflammation and joint damage. Rituximab works by depleting B cells, a type of white blood cell associated with inflammation. B cells are believed to play a role in the development of RA, including through production of rheumatoid factor (RF) (an antibody found in about 85 percent of people with RA), T cell activation, and/or proinflammatory cytokine production. Biologics often work rapidly, having an effect within two weeks; however, it may take up to three months for these drugs to begin to work

Leflunomide inhibits production of inflammatory cells to reduce inflammation.

Minocycline is a member of the tetracycline group of ANTIBACTERIALS. Although RA is not an infection, there is evidence that minocycline may slow the progression of joint damage. When used to treat RA, minocycline works by decreasing the production of substances causing inflammation, such as prostaglandins and leukotrienes, while increasing production of IL-10, which reduces inflammation.

Penicillamine works by reducing the number of T cells, inhibiting macrophages (immune cells), decreasing IL-1, decreasing RF, and preventing collagen from cross-linking. Collagen is the main protein found in cartilage, connective tissue, tendons, bones, muscle, and skin. It is crucial to joint health and function. Strands of collagen bond together through chemical cross-linking to form collagen fibers. The more cross-linking, the stiffer the collagen fiber.

Sulfasalazine works by reducing inflammation inside the body, although its exact mode of action is still under investigation.

Approved Uses

Hydroxychloroquine is approved to prevent and treat malaria. It is also approved to treat RA, SLE, and discoid lupus erythematosus.

Methotrexate is used to treat some types of cancer (see ANTINEOPLASTICS), severe psoriasis, RA, and juvenile RA.

Azathioprine is approved to prevent organ transplant rejection and for the management of severe, active RA unresponsive to conventional treatment.

Cyclosporine, used originally to prevent the rejection of transplanted kidneys, continues to be used for a variety of organ transplants. It is also approved for the treatment of RA that has not responded well to other medications as well as severe forms of psoriasis.

Gold compounds are used in the treatment of RA; gold sodium thiomalate is also approved to treat juvenile RA.

Biologics are approved to treat adult patients with RA. Adalimumab, etanercept, and infliximab are also used to treat ankylosing spondylitis, psoriatic arthritis, and plaque psoriasis. Etanercept is also approved to treat juvenile RA. Adalimumab and infliximab are both approved to treat CD, while infliximab is approved to treat UC. Rituximab is used in combination with methotrexate for patients with moderate to severe RA who have not responded to anti-TNF therapies. Rituximab is also approved for treatment of non-Hodgkin's lymphoma.

Leflunomide is approved for the treatment of RA.

Minocycline has been used extensively for decades as an antibiotic and is approved to treat a number of infections (see ANTIBACTERIALS).

Penicillamine is approved to treat Wilson's disease (too much copper in the body), to treat severe RA unresponsive to other therapy, and to prevent kidney stones caused by a condition known as cystinuria.

Sulfasalazine is used in the treatment of RA and juvenile RA when the disease has not responded well to other medications and for UC.

Off-Label Uses

Methotrexate has been used off-label to terminate ectopic pregnancies (the life-threatening condition in which fertilized eggs grow outside the uterus) and to relieve symptoms of pain, swelling, and stiffness in autoimmune diseases such as multiple sclerosis, dermatomyositis, polymyositis, juvenile dermatomyositis, and psoriatic arthritis. Low-dose methotrexate has been used off-label to treat patients with moderate to severe CD.

Azathioprine is also used to treat uveitis (inflammation in the eyes), the progression of Behçet's disease (a rare and chronic autoimmune disorder that involves inflammation of blood vessels throughout the body), psoriasis, reactive arthritis, polymyositis, SLE, CD, and UC.

Intravenous cyclosporine has also been used to treat patients with severe UC or CD who do not respond to treatment with steroids.

Gold compounds are used off-label as an alternative to or along with CORTICOSTEROIDS to treat pemphigus (a group of rare chronic autoimmune skin diseases characterized by blister formations in the outer layer of the skin and the mucous membranes). These drugs are also used to treat psoriatic arthritis in patients who do not tolerate or respond to nonsteroidal anti-inflammatory drugs (NSAIDs).

Adalimumab has been used effectively in psoriasis as an off-label indication. Anakinra is used off-label for the treatment of uveitis and juvenile RA. The off-label uses for etanercept include Behçet's disease, Churg Strauss vasculitis (an autoimmune disorder accompanied by abnormal clustering of certain white blood cells and inflammation of blood vessels), giant cell arteritis (a group of diseases whose typical feature is inflammation of blood vessels), dermatomyositis (a group of muscle diseases characterized by rash and muscle weakness), antiphospholipid antibody syndrome (also referred to as "sticky blood," an immune disorder in which the body appears to recognize certain fatty molecules as foreign substances and produces antibodies against them), and pemphigus. Infliximab's off-label uses include Behçet's disease, Wegener's granulomatosis (an uncommon autoimmune disease characterized by inflammation of the blood vessels), Churg Strauss vasculitis, and giant cell arteritis. Rituximab is increasingly used off label for a number of difficult-to-treat autoimmune diseases such as pemphigus, SLE, and Wegener's granulomatosis.

Leflunomide has been used off-label to treat psoriatic arthritis, SLE, polyoma BK virus (a common dormant DNA virus that reactivates in kidney transplant recipients), and uveitis.

Minocycline is used off-label in the treatment of RA.

Penicillamine is used off-label to treat scleroderma, Felty's syndrome (a rare disorder that involves RA, a swollen spleen, decreased white blood cell count, and repeated infections), mercury and lead poisoning, primary biliary cirrhosis, and rheumatoid vasculitis.

Sulfasalazine is used off-label for CD and psoriatic arthritis.

Companion Drugs

Because DMARDs take effect over weeks or months, they do not give immediate relief of symptoms and so are often prescribed in combination with NSAIDs or steroids for faster relief of ongoing symptoms.

Biologics may be used in combination with other DMARDs. When used for RA, infliximab and rituximab must be used with methotrexate. In addition, abatacept should not be used in combination with anakinra.

Administration

Hydroxychloroquine is taken orally in tablet form. It may be administered with food or milk to minimize gastrointestinal (GI) upset.

Methotrexate is usually taken once per week as a tablet or injection. The injectable form may be given intravenously, intramuscularly, subcutaneously (under the skin), or intrathecally (directly into the spinal fluid).

Azathioprine is available as tablets to be taken orally. It may be administered after meals to minimize GI upset.

Cyclosporine is available as an intravenous solution, an oral solution, and an oral capsule.

Auranofin is taken orally in capsule form. Gold sodium thiomalate is administered via intramuscular injection.

All biologics must be injected. Adalimumab, anakinra, and etanercept are injected subcutaneously by the patient, a family member, or nurse. Intravenous infusion is necessary for abatacept, infliximab, and rituximab, which is typically done in a doctor's office or clinic. Patients receiving infliximab need to be premedicated prior to receiving the infusion to prevent infusion-related reactions. Patients usually receive an antihistamine, acetaminophen, and/or a corticosteroid. Premedication with acetaminophen and an antihistamine is also recommended with rituximab.

Leflunomide is available in tablet form.

Minocycline is available in capsule form.

Penicillamine is available in capsule or tablet form. It must be taken on an empty stomach, at least one hour before meals and at least one hour apart from any other drug, food, or milk.

Sulfasalazine is available as regular and delayed-release tablets. It may be administered with meals to minimize GI upset.

Cautions and Concerns

Long-term treatment with DMARDs may be limited by diminished therapeutic response over time and/or onset of serious adverse events. For example, they may increase risk of infection, hair loss, and kidney or liver damage.

A complete blood cell count (CBC) should be obtained if patients are given prolonged hydroxychloroquine therapy. If any severe blood disorder appears that is not attributable to the disease under treatment, discontinuation of the drug should be considered. This drug should be administered with caution to patients having G6PD (glucose-6 phosphate dehydrogenase) deficiency, liver disease, alcoholism, or damaged hearing.

Methotrexate has the potential for serious toxicity (see *Warnings*). Because toxic effects can occur at any time during therapy, it is necessary to follow patients on methotrexate closely. Most adverse reactions are reversible if detected early. Patients should be informed of the early signs and symptoms of toxicity, of the need to see their physician promptly if they occur, and of the need for close follow-up, including periodic laboratory tests to monitor toxicity. Methotrexate has not been well studied in older individuals. Due to diminished liver and kidney function as well as decreased folate stores in this population, relatively low doses should be considered, and these patients should be closely monitored for early signs of toxicity.

A GI reaction characterized by severe nausea and vomiting has been reported by 10 to 15 percent of RA patients taking azathioprine. These symptoms may also be accompanied by diarrhea, rash, fever, malaise, muscle pain, elevated liver enzymes, and low blood pressure. Symptoms of GI toxicity most often develop within the first several weeks of therapy and are reversible upon discontinuation of the drug. Taking the medication twice daily instead of all at once or taking it after eating may help avoid these problems. Azathioprine should be avoided during pregnancy, as potential complications for the baby include lower birth weights, prematurity, jaundice, and respiratory distress syndrome. Men who take azathioprine should stop taking it three months before their partner tries to conceive.

Approximately 25 percent of patients taking cyclosporine for RA develop mild to moderate high blood pressure. Approximately half of the patients taking this medication develop mild kidney problems and may need to adjust their dosage or discontinue the medication. Kidney function usually improves after stopping the medication. Cyclosporine can also cause gout in some individuals or worsen underlying gout in others.

Beneficial effects of gold compounds may not occur until after three to six months of treatment. Gold compounds may cause increased sensitivity to sunlight in some people. These patients may break out in a rash after being in the sun or exposed to sunlamps, or a skin rash that is already present may worsen. Gold compounds should be used with caution in patients with history of blood or blood vessel disease, colitis, previous kidney or liver disease, Sjögren's syndrome, or skin rash. Gold injections may cause immediate dizziness, flushing or redness of the face, nausea or vomiting, increased sweating, or unusual weakness, all of which will usually go away after the patient lies down for a few minutes. Joint pain may occur for one or two days after receiving an injection of gold sodium thiomalate, but this effect usually disappears after the first few injections.

Live vaccines should not be given concurrently with biologics or within three months of the biologic's discontinuation, as the resulting immunosuppression from the biologic and the underlying disease state may increase the risk of infection. In addition, some biologics may blunt the effectiveness of these immunizations.

Physicians should exercise caution when considering the use of abatacept in patients with a history of recurrent infections, underlying conditions that may predispose them to infections, or chronic, latent, or localized infections. Patients who develop a new infection while undergoing treatment with abatacept should be monitored closely (see *Warnings*). Because there were two cases of anaphylaxis or anaphylactoid reactions in abatacept clinical trials, appropriate medical support measures for the treatment of hypersensitivity reactions should be available for immediate use in the event of a reaction. Abatacept should be used with caution in patients with chronic obstructive pulmonary disease (COPD), as these individuals may be at greater risk for developing adverse events, including COPD exacerbations, cough, and breathing difficulties. Abatacept can cause falsely elevated blood glucose readings on the day of infusion.

Use of the TNF blocking agents (adalimumab, etanercept, and infliximab) has been associated with rare cases of new onset or worsening of clinical symptoms and/or radiographic evidence of demyelinating disease. Caution should be used in considering the use of these agents in patients with preexisting or recent-onset central nervous system demyelinating disorders. Treatment with etanercept or infliximab may result in the formation of autoantibodies and, rarely, in the development of a lupuslike syndrome or autoimmune hepatitis. If a patient develops symptoms suggestive of these syndromes following treatment with either of these agents, treatment should be discontinued. Adalimumab, etanercept, and infliximab may increase the risk of reactivation of hepatitis B virus (HBV) in patients who are chronic carriers of this virus. A CBC should be obtained at regular intervals during rituximab therapy and more frequently in patients who develop blood disorders. The duration of blood disorders caused by rituximab can extend well beyond the treatment period.

The risk of toxic reactions to anakinra may be greater in patients with impaired kidney function. Patients receiving anakinra may experience a decrease in neutrophil counts.

Leflunomide is eliminated slowly from the blood. In instances of any serious toxicity from this drug, including hypersensitivity, use of a drug elimination procedure (e.g., cholestyramine and/or activated charcoal) is highly recommended to reduce the drug concentration more rapidly after stopping therapy. (Cholestyramine and activated charcoal bind some drugs in the intestine, preventing their absorption and hastening their elimination.) Interstitial lung disease (an inflammation of lung tissue) has been reported during treatment with leflunomide; thus, new-onset or worsening pulmonary symptoms, such as cough and difficulty breathing with or without associated fever, may be a reason for discontinuation of the therapy. Vaccination with live vaccines is not recommended during leflunomide therapy. Leflunomide should be used with caution in patients who have liver disease, including hepatitis B or hepatitis C (see *Warnings*), kidney problems, severe immune system disorders, bone marrow disorders, or uncontrolled infection.

Some women who take minocycline develop vaginal yeast infections, which is believed to be caused by the drug's killing bacteria normally present in the body that protect against yeast infections. Minocycline may increase sensitivity to sunlight, resulting in more frequent sunburns or the development of rashes following sun exposure. Patients should apply sunscreen (SPF 15 or greater) before outdoor activities or avoid prolonged exposure to the sun while taking minocycline (see ANTIBACTERIALS for other precautions with tetracyclines).

Some patients taking penicillamine may experience drug fever, usually in the second to third week following initiation of therapy. In the case of drug fever in RA patients, penicillamine should be discontinued and another DMARD tried, as experience indicates that the fever reaction will recur in a very high percentage of patients upon readministration of penicillamine. Because both early and late rashes have occurred with penicillamine, the skin and mucous membranes should be observed for allergic reactions. Patients with RA whose nutrition is impaired should also be given a daily supplement of pyridoxine. All patients with Wilson's disease or cystinuria should receive a pyridoxine supplement. Iron deficiency may develop, especially in pediatric patients and in menstruating women.

Sulfasalazine should be given with caution to patients with severe allergies or bronchial asthma. Adequate fluid intake must be maintained in order to prevent kidney stone formation. Patients with G6PD deficiency should be observed closely for signs of hemolytic anemia. Because sulfasalazine inhibits absorption and metabolism of folic acid, patients on chronic sulfasalazine therapy may need to increase their dietary folate intake and to take a folic acid supplement if they have any other condition that could also contribute to deficiency.

Warnings

None of the DMARDs used in the treatment of RA is absolutely safe during pregnancy. Thus, the decision to use DMARDs should be made after careful assessment of the risks and benefits. Patients may need a reminder about the importance of using contraception while on DMARDs, especially methotrexate, leflunomide, azathioprine, and cyclosporine (see individual drugs below).

Irreversible damage to the retina of the eye has been observed in some patients who have received long-term or high-dosage hydroxychloroquine therapy. All patients on long-term therapy with hydroxychloroquine should have ophthalmic checkups performed every year. Also, patients on long-term therapy with hydroxychloroquine should be examined periodically for any evidence of muscular weakness. If weakness occurs, this drug should be discontinued. Hydroxychloroquine may also worsen psoriasis or porphyria.

Methotrexate should be used only by physicians who have knowledge of and experience with this drug. Because of the possibility of serious toxic reactions (which can be fatal), methotrexate should be used only in life-threatening neoplastic diseases or in patients with psoriasis or RA with severe, recalcitrant, disabling disease which is not adequately responsive to other forms of therapy. Patients should be closely monitored for bone marrow, liver, lung, and kidney toxicities. CBC and renal and liver function tests should be performed every month for the first six months of therapy and then every one to two months thereafter. Patients should be informed by their physicians of the risks involved and should be under a physician's care throughout therapy.

Because methotrexate elimination is reduced in patients with impaired kidney function, these patients require careful monitoring for toxicity as well as dose reduction; in some cases, the methotrexate may need to be discontinued in these patients. Unexpectedly severe (sometimes fatal) bone marrow suppression, aplastic anemia, and GI toxicity have been reported with concomitant administration of methotrexate (usually in high dosage) and some NSAIDs.

Methotrexate causes liver damage, fibrosis, and cirrhosis, but generally only after prolonged use. Acutely, liver enzyme elevations are frequently seen but are usually transient and not predictive of subsequent liver disease. Liver biopsy after sustained use often shows histologic changes, and fibrosis and cirrhosis have been reported; these latter lesions may not be preceded by symptoms or abnormal liver function tests in patients with psoriasis. For this reason, periodic liver biopsies are usually recommended for psoriatic patients who are under long-term treatment. Routine liver biopsies are not recommended in RA patients. Persistent abnormalities in liver function tests may precede appearance of fibrosis or cirrhosis in patients with RA.

Methotrexate-induced lung disease is potentially dangerous, may occur acutely at any time during therapy, and has been reported at doses as low as 7.5 mg/week. It is not always fully reversible. Pulmonary symptoms (especially a dry, nonproductive cough) may require interruption of treatment and careful investigation.

Diarrhea and ulcerative stomatitis require interruption of methotrexate therapy; otherwise, hemorrhagic enteritis and death from intestinal perforation may occur. Potentially fatal opportunistic infections, especially *Pneumocystis carinii* pneumonia, may also occur with methotrexate therapy. Severe, occasionally fatal, skin reactions have been reported following single or multiple doses of methotrexate. Reactions have occurred within days of oral, intramuscular, intravenous, or intrathecal methotrexate administration. Recovery has been reported with discontinuation of therapy.

Azathioprine has been associated with liver test abnormalities, hepatitis, pancreatitis, and an allergic reaction that may include a flulike syndrome (see *Cautions and Concerns*).

Azathioprine also can lower infection-fighting white blood cells, although the incidence of infection in transplant patients is 30 to 60 times higher than that observed in patients with RA. A CBC should be performed one to two weeks after the initiation of therapy or after changing the dose and then every one to three months thereafter. Long-term use of azathioprine in combination with other immune-suppressing medications in transplant patients has been associated with a slightly elevated risk of cancer. It is not clear whether patients with RA face a similar risk.

Cyclosporine may increase the risk of some kinds of infections and may be toxic to the kidneys and liver. Patients receiving cyclosporine are at increased risk for development of lymphomas and other malignancies, particularly those of the skin. Patients taking cyclosporine should be warned to avoid excessive ultraviolet light exposure. Cyclosporine can cause serious complications during pregnancy such as preeclampsia (the development of high blood pressure and fluid retention), also called toxemia of pregnancy, and preterm labor.

Because gold compounds can cause gold toxicity, the results of recommended laboratory work (CBC with differential, platelet count, urinalysis, and renal and liver function tests) should be performed prior to initial therapy to establish a baseline and to identify any preexisting conditions. In patients receiving gold injections, a CBC and urinalysis should be monitored every one to two weeks for the first 20 weeks of therapy and then with every injection. For those patients receiving oral gold therapy, these tests should be performed every one to three months. Kidney disorders, particularly proteinuria and hematuria, have occurred in patients taking gold compounds.

Because biologics modify the response of the immune system, the risk of infection is potentially increased. Serious infections, sepsis, tuberculosis, and cases of opportunistic infections, including fatalities, have been reported with the use of TNF antagonists (adalimumab, etanercept, and infliximab). In controlled clinical trials, patients receiving concomitant therapy with TNF antagonists and either abatacept or anakinra experienced more infections and a greater number of serious infections compared to patients treated with only TNF antagonists. Consequently, abatacept and anakinra should not be used with TNF antagonists. A purified protein derivative (PPD) test needs to be performed at baseline to rule out latent tuberculosis infection in patients receiving the TNF antagonists and abatacept.

Rituximab has been associated with cases of a rare and deadly brain infection called progressive multifocal leukoencephalopathy (PML). The Food and Drug Administration (FDA) has reported the death of two patients who were treated with rituximab off-label for SLE. Even though rituximab is not approved for the treatment of SLE, the FDA reported that approximately 10,000 patients with SLE have been treated with this drug. Rituximab also may cause HBV reactivation, viral infections, and heart problems such as arrhythmias and angina. In addition, deaths within 24 hours of receiving a rituximab infusion have been reported following development of an infusion reaction. Approximately 80 percent of fatal infusion reactions occurred with the first infusion. In addition, urticaria, hypotension, angioedema, hypoxia, bronchospasm, pulmonary infiltrates, acute respiratory distress syndrome, myocardial infarction, ventricular fibrillation, and cardiogenic shock can occur during the infusion.

As a precaution, patients using cytotoxics, immunosuppressants, or biologics should avoid contact with people who have existing infections, should not have dental work done while on these medications, and should not touch their eyes or inside of their nose unless they have just washed their hands.

A higher incidence of malignancies (lymphoma and nonmelanoma skin cancer) has been observed in patients receiving adalimumab, etanercept, and infliximab. More cases of lung cancer were observed in abatacept-treated patients than placebo-treated patients in clinical trials.

Severe hepatic reactions, including acute liver failure, jaundice, hepatitis, and cholestasis, have been reported rarely in patients receiving infliximab. Infliximab has been associated with adverse outcomes in patients with heart failure and should be used in these patients only after consideration of other treatment options. Cases of leukopenia, neutropenia, thrombocytopenia, and pancytopenia, some with a fatal outcome, have been reported in patients receiving infliximab.

Leflunomide is not considered safe for use during pregnancy. Based on animal studies, leflunomide may increase the risk of fetal death or birth defects. Upon discontinuing leflunomide, all women of childbearing age should undergo a drug elimination procedure. Rare cases of severe liver injury, including cases with fatal outcome, have been reported during treatment with leflunomide. Most cases of severe liver injury occur within six months of therapy and in a setting of multiple risk factors for liver disease or use of other hepatotoxic agents. Patients receiving leflunomide should have a CBC and their renal and liver function monitored every month for the first six months of therapy and then every one to two months thereafter. Rare cases of Stevens-Johnson syndrome and toxic epidermal necrolysis have been reported in patients taking leflunomide.

Minocycline can cause birth defects when administered to a pregnant woman. Central nervous system side effects, including dizziness, or vertigo, have been reported with minocycline therapy. Patients who experience these symptoms should be cautioned about driving vehicles or using hazardous machinery while on minocycline therapy. Rarely, minocycline can affect the kidneys or liver, so doctors may recommend periodic blood tests for long-term users. In equally rare cases, minocycline can induce a lupuslike condition, but this disorder usually improves after stopping the medication (see ANTIBACTERIALS for other warnings with tetracyclines).

Penicillamine may be more toxic than other DMARDs and should be used only under the supervision of a rheumatologist who is familiar with its side effects. Penicillamine use may lead to serious infection, low blood counts, inflammation in the pancreas, serious skin rash, excessive bleeding or bruising, muscle weakness (due to myasthenia gravis or myositis), or protein loss in the kidney; some of these reactions may be fatal. Penicillamine may also cause birth defects. Because of the potential for serious hematological and renal adverse reactions to occur at any time, a urinalysis and CBC must be performed every two weeks until the dose is stabilized and then every one to three months thereafter. In addition, the patient's skin, lymph nodes, and body temperature should be regularly monitored during the course of therapy. Patients should be instructed to report promptly the development of signs and symptoms of granulocytopenia and/or thrombocytopenia such as fever, sore throat, chills, bruising, or bleeding. Laboratory studies should then be promptly repeated.

Only after critical appraisal should sulfasalazine be given to patients with liver or kidney damage or blood abnormalities. Deaths associated with the administration of sulfasalazine have been reported from hypersensitivity reactions, agranulocytosis, aplastic anemia, other blood dyscrasias, kidney and liver damage, irreversible neuromuscular and central nervous system changes, and fibrosing alveolitis (inflammation and scarring of the alveoli [the tiny air sacs of the lungs] and lung tissue). The presence of sore throat, fever, pallor, purpura, or jaundice may be indications of serious blood disorders. A CBC should be performed every two to four weeks for the first three months of therapy and then every three months thereafter in patients receiving sulfasalazine. A urinalysis and renal function tests should also be done frequently in these patients. Low sperm count and infertility have been observed in men treated with sulfasalazine; however, withdrawal of the drug appears to reverse these effects.

When Not Advised (Contraindications)

DMARDS generally should not be used in pregnant women or in women trying to become pregnant (see *Warnings*).

Hydroxychloroquine should not be used in patients who develop retinal or visual field changes (blurring of vision and difficulty of focusing) attributable to the use of either this drug or chloroquine.

Because of the potential for serious adverse reactions from methotrexate in breast-fed infants, it is contraindicated in nursing mothers. Patients with psoriasis or RA with alcoholism, alcoholic liver disease, chronic liver disease, evidence of immunodeficiency syndromes, or preexisting blood abnormalities (e.g., bone marrow hypoplasia, leukopenia, thrombocytopenia, or significant anemia) should not receive methotrexate.

Patients with high blood pressure, kidney problems, or cancer should not take cyclosporine.

Auranofin is contraindicated in patients with a history of any of the following gold-induced disorders: anaphylactic reactions, necrotizing enterocolitis, pulmonary fibrosis, exfoliative dermatitis, bone marrow aplasia, or other severe blood disorders. Gold sodium thiomalate should not be given to patients who have had severe toxicity resulting from previous exposure to gold or other heavy metals or who have SLE.

Anakinra is contraindicated in patients with known hypersensitivity to *E. coli*–derived proteins.

Etanercept should not be administered to patients with sepsis.

Infliximab at doses greater than 5 mg/kg should not be administered to patients with moderate to severe heart failure (see *Warnings*).

Minocycline is not recommended for children under nine years of age because of the potential for permanent tooth discoloration.

Mothers taking penicillamine should not nurse their infants. Patients with a history of penicillamine-related aplastic anemia or agranulocytosis should not be restarted on penicillamine (see *Warnings*). Because of its potential for causing kidney damage, penicillamine should not be administered to patients with RA who have a history or evidence of renal insufficiency.

Sulfasalazine is contraindicated in patients with intestinal or urinary obstruction, porphyria (a genetic abnormality of metabolism causing abdominal pains and mental confusion), or an allergy to sulfa drugs or salicylates.

Side Effects

Hydroxychloroquine may cause diarrhea, loss of appetite, nausea, vomiting, headache, muscle weakness, or skin rash.

Common side effects with methotrexate include nausea, mouth sores, fatigue, chills, and dizziness. Methotrexate can interfere with the bone marrow's production of blood cells, and low blood cell counts can cause fever, infections, and susceptibility to bruising and bleeding. Liver or lung damage can occur, even with low doses, and therefore requires monitoring (see *Warnings*).

In addition to GI (see *Cautions and Concerns*) and hematologic (see *Warnings*) adverse events, additional side effects reported with azathioprine include skin rash, hair loss, fever, joint pain, diarrhea, and loss of appetite.

In addition to high blood pressure and kidney problems (see *Cautions and Concerns*), common side effects with cyclosporine include headache, nausea, vomiting, abdominal pain, swelling of the hands or feet, tremors, increased hair growth, muscle cramps, and neuropathy (numbness and tingling of the hands or feet).

Side effects of gold compounds include diarrhea, nausea, vomiting, rash, itching, mouth ulcers, anemia, low white blood cell count, and liver and kidney problems (see *Warnings*). The most common side effects of abatacept are headache, dizziness, upper respiratory tract infection, cough, back pain, and nausea. The most serious side effects are serious infections and malignancies (see *Warnings*). Infusion-related reactions have occurred in patients receiving abatacept with the most frequently reported being dizziness, headache, and hypertension.

The most common side effects of adalimumab are injection site reaction (characterized by skin redness, bruising, inflammation, or pain), upper respiratory tract infections (cold, sinusitis, bronchitis), flu syndrome, nausea, headache, rash, back pain, and urinary tract infection. The most serious side effects are serious infections, neurologic reactions, and malignancies (see *Warnings* and *Cautions and Concerns*).

The most common side effects with anakinra are injection-site reactions. Other common side effects include a worsening of RA, upper respiratory tract infections, and headache. The most serious side effects are serious infections (see *Warnings*) and neutropenia (see *Cautions and Concerns*), particularly when used in combination with TNF blocking agents.

Common side effects with etanercept include injection site reactions, upper respiratory tract infections, headache, nausea, rhinitis, dizziness, and rash. The most serious side effects are malignancies, neurologic reactions, and infections (see *Warnings* and *Cautions and Concerns*).

The most common side effects with infliximab include infusion-related reactions (flushing, headache, and rash), infections, and delayed hypersensitivity reactions (joint and/or muscle pain with fever and/or rash occurring within two weeks after repeat infusion). Other common side effects include nausea, abdominal pain, diarrhea, heartburn, cough, and headache. The most serious side effects are heart failure, serious infections, neurologic reactions, and malignancies (see *Warnings* and *Cautions and Concerns*).

In addition to serious infusion reactions (see *Warnings*), other common side effects with rituximab include fever, chills, infection, headache, abdominal pain, back pain, hypotension, nausea, diarrhea, vomiting, lymphopenia, leukopenia, dizziness, cough, muscle pain, joint pain, night sweats, and rash.

Common side effects with leflunomide include rash, temporary hair loss, liver damage (see *Cautions and Concerns* and *Warnings*), elevated liver enzymes, nausea, diarrhea, weight loss, mouth sores, and fatigue.

Common side effects from minocycline include nausea, vomiting, diarrhea, dizziness (see *Warnings*), rash, sensitivity to sunlight, skin discoloration with long-term use, and headache.

Common side effects from penicillamine include fever; joint pain; lesions on the face, neck, scalp, and/or trunk; rash, hives, or itching; swollen and/or painful glands; and ulcers, sores, or white spots on lips or in mouth (see *Warnings*). Less serious but common side effects include diarrhea, lessening or loss of sense of taste, loss of appetite, nausea, or vomiting.

Common side effects of sulfasalazine include low blood counts, nausea, vomiting, sensitivity to sunlight, rash, and headache. People who are allergic to sulfa drugs may have a cross reaction to sulfasalazine (see *When Not Advised [Contraindications]*). Sulfasalazine may cause an orange discoloration of body fluids (urine, tears) which may stain clothing and contact lenses.

Interactions

Antacids can reduce absorption of hydroxychloroquine. Cimetidine may inhibit the metabolism of hydroxychloroquine, increasing its blood level.

Concomitant administration of some NSAIDs or high-dose salicylates with high-dose methotrexate therapy has been reported to increase methotrexate levels, resulting in deaths from severe liver and GI toxicity (see *Warnings*). Because penicillins may reduce the renal clearance of methotrexate, concomitant use of these drugs should be carefully monitored. Vitamin preparations containing folic acid or its derivatives may decrease responses to methotrexate.

Allopurinol may increase the action and side effects of azathioprine. The use of angiotensin-converting enzyme (ACE) inhibitors in patients receiving azathioprine has been reported to induce severe leukopenia. Sulfasalazine, mesalamine, or olsalazine may increase the side effects of azathioprine. Azathioprine may decrease the effects of warfarin.

Because cyclosporine interacts with a large number of other drugs, patients need to inform their physician about each and every drug they are taking. Drugs that may make cyclosporine less effective include carbamazepine, phenobarbital, phenytoin, and rifampin. Drugs that may increase cyclosporine's toxicity include amiodarone; clarithromycin; erythromycin; some antifungals, including fluconazole, itraconazole, and ketoconazole; protease inhibitors; and calcium channel blockers. Cyclosporine can also increase the effects of a number of drugs including benzodiazepines, calcium channel blockers, simvastatin, atorvastatin, lovastatin, sildenafil, tadalafil, and vardenafil. During treatment with cyclosporine, vaccination may be less effective, and the use of live vaccines should be avoided. Because cyclosporine may cause hyperkalemia, potassium-sparing diuretics should not be used. The use of cyclosporine along with other drugs that are toxic to the kidneys must be closely monitored. Grapefruit juice can increase cyclosporine levels and should be avoided in patients taking this drug.

Auranofin may increase phenytoin blood levels. The potential for increasing gold toxicity is great when gold compounds are used along with penicillamine, aminoglycosides, amphotericin B, penicillins, phenytoin, sulfonamides, acyclovir, and alcohol.

Concurrent administration of abatacept or anakinra with a TNF antagonist has been associated with an increased risk of serious infections and no significant additional efficacy over use of the TNF antagonists alone. Therefore, concurrent therapy with either abatacept or anakinra and TNF antagonists is not recommended.

No formal drug interaction studies have been performed with rituximab.

Increased side effects may occur when leflunomide is given along with hepatotoxic substances. Rifampin may raise levels of leflunomide.

Minocycline may decrease the effectiveness of birth control pills and may increase tendency to bleed in patients on warfarin. Absorption of minocycline may be impaired by products containing calcium, magnesium, iron, or aluminum.

Penicillamine may decrease the effects of digoxin. Antacids and products containing iron can decrease the absorption of penicillamine. No other prescription or over-the-counter drugs or supplements should be taken within one hour of a penicillamine dose.

Sulfasalazine may increase the effects of oral hypoglycemic agents or warfarin and may decrease the absorption of folic acid and digoxin.

Sales/Statistics

According to analysts, the worldwide pharmaceutical market for TNF antagonists was worth more than $6 billion in 2005. It was estimated that abatacept sales could reach $1 billion by 2009/2010.

In the United States, among the "Top 200 Generic Drugs by Retail Dollars in 2006" (*Drug Topics*, February 19, 2007), minocycline ranked #46 with $210,309,000 in sales (includes usage as an antibiotic), methotrexate #91 ($101,927,000—includes usage for other disease states, such as malignancies), hydroxychloroquine #115 ($76,765,000), azathioprine #143 ($58,872,000—primarily used in transplant patients as an immunosuppressant), leflunomide #166 ($45,230,000), and cyclosporine #185 ($38,070,000—primarily used in transplant patients as an immunosuppressant).

Among the "Top 200 Brand Drugs by Retail Dollars in 2006," Enbrel ranked #36 with $1,084,243,000 in sales, and Humira ranked #79 ($505,566,000).

Among the "Top 200 Generic Drugs by Units in 2007" (*Drug Topics*, March 10, 2008), methotrexate ranked #97 with 4,385,000 units, minocycline #103 (4,249,000 units, which includes usage as an antibiotic), and hydroxychloroquine #132 (3,093,000 units).

On the Top 200 lists for 2010 (*Drug Topics*, June 2011), those rankings had changed: On the generic sales list, minocycline ranked #133 ($108,018,438), methotrexate #162 ($81,603,353), and hydroxychloroquine #190 ($65,986,315). On generic prescriptions, methotrexate ranked #115 (4,824,399), hydroxychloroquine #148 (3,499,968), and minocycline #151 (3,473,461). On the branded drug sales, Enbrel ranked #59 ($546,814,765), Enbrel Sureclick #75 ($474,602,259), Humira Pen #63 ($514,735,868), and Humira #96 ($358,012,620).

Interestingly, the IMS Institute for Healthcare Informatics ranked Remicade #11 in sales in 2010 ($3,301,801,836), Enbrel #12 ($3,288,832,959), Humira #18 ($2,925,455,932), and Rituxan #20 ($2,760,661,034).

Demographics and Cultural Groups

In a 2002 multiuniversity Texas study funded by the National Institutes of Health (NIH), the Arthritis Foundation, and the American Heart Association, compared with non-Hispanic whites, Hispanics had significantly more tender joints, more swollen joints, and more frequent RF yet had taken a lower number of DMARDs (1.9 versus 2.5).

Development History

Hydroxychloroquine, originally developed as a treatment for malaria, was later found to improve symptoms of arthritis. It was first approved by the FDA in April 1955.

Azathioprine was first introduced into clinical practice by Sir Roy Calne, a British pioneer in organ transplantation. In March 1968, the FDA approved azathioprine for use in organ transplantation. Azathioprine was first used in the treatment of RA in the 1950s.

The immunosuppressive effect of cyclosporine, which was initially isolated from a fungus, was discovered on January 31, 1972, by employees of Sandoz (now Novartis) in Basel, Switzer-

land. The success of cyclosporine in preventing organ rejection was shown in liver transplants performed at the University of Pittsburgh hospital in 1980. Cyclosporine was subsequently approved for use in 1983.

In 1890, a German doctor named Robert Koch found that gold effectively killed the bacteria that caused tuberculosis. In 1929, based on a widely held belief at the time of a connection between tuberculosis and RA, a French doctor, Jacques Forestier, pioneered the use of gold for the treatment of RA. Subsequent controlled studies confirmed its effectiveness.

With better appreciation of the concept of inflammatory processes and mediators involved in the pathogenesis of RA, scientists began working on the development of biological agents during the 1980s in an attempt to modify the disease process. Because biologics affect a specific component of the immune system and not the entire immune system, the belief was that they would have fewer side effects. Infliximab was the first biologic approved by the FDA, on August 24, 1998. Etanercept received approval on November 2, 1998; anakinra on November 14, 2001; adalimumab on December 31, 2002; and abatacept on December 23, 2005.

Unlike other DMARDs, which had been used for other diseases prior to RA, leflunomide was developed specifically for RA, having been initially discovered by observing its effect in a living arthritis rat model. Leflunomide was approved by the FDA on September 10, 1998.

In the 1940s, Sidney Farber at Harvard's Children's Hospital began testing the effects of folic acid on leukemia. This inspired chemists at the drug company Lederle to start looking for antimetabolites resembling folate. The result was methotrexate, which was developed in 1948 by Yellapragada Subbarao from Lederle. Methotrexate gained FDA approval as a leukemia drug in 1953. By the 1950s, antimetabolites were being used to treat RA, and methotrexate was first used off-label for the treatment of RA in 1951. By chance, RA patients who also had psoriasis noticed that their skin improved. Methotrexate was eventually approved for this use by the FDA in the 1970s. By the mid-1980s, four randomized clinical trials had proven beyond doubt the beneficial effects of methotrexate when administered to patients with established RA disease who had failed to respond to other compounds such as gold salts and penicillamine. Subsequently, the drug was approved for use in RA in 1987.

Dr. Thomas McPherson Brown, a world renowned rheumatologist who pioneered antibiotic treatments, first reported the beneficial effects of tetracyclines for RA in 1949 at the Seventh International Congress on Rheumatic Diseases. Two weeks after Dr. Brown's death in 1989, the NIH requested grant applications for the controlled clinical trials of tetracycline therapy for RA, which he had been seeking. The preliminary results of the clinical trials, known now as MIRA, or Minocycline in Rheumatoid Arthritis, reported in 1993, were promising, and the NIH requested grant applications for studies of mycoplasma and other infectious agents as causes for rheumatoid diseases in 1993 and a pilot study for intravenous antibiotics for RA in 1994. In the January 15, 1995, issue of the *Annals of Internal Medicine,* investigators reported the final results of the MIRA study. However, the Arthritis Foundation was reported to be unimpressed even after antibiotic therapy was deemed safe and effective. The foundation's medical director reportedly said he did not view the treatment as a breakthrough and that more study of dosages and long-term use of minocycline would be needed. The Road Back Foundation, an advocacy group for antibiotic treatment for rheumatic diseases, notes, "Modern trials have provided sufficient evidence of the effectiveness and safety of tetracycline derivatives that should allow an almost certain approval by the FDA for the use of minocycline in the treatment of RA if a formal application were submitted to the agency. Unfortunately, the oldness and generic availability of tetracyclines make it commercially non-viable for drug companies to pursue this FDA track." Thus, minocycline

continues to be used off-label in the treatment of RA.

Dr. John Walshe of the University of Cambridge in England first described the use of penicillamine in Wilson's disease in 1956; it was approved by the FDA for this use in 1963. Sulfasalazine was developed specifically for the treatment of RA. Following the discovery of sulfonamides as antibacterial agents, they were used in numerous nonbacterial inflammatory disease with little success. In the late 1930s, Nana Svartz, Sweden's first female professor of medicine, designed a compound that contained both a salicylate and a sulfa component and in early 1942 reported its positive therapeutic benefits in RA. Sulfasalazine was approved by the FDA in 1950.

Future Drugs

Tacrolimus (Prograf) is an IMMUNOSUPPRESSIVE that blocks the action of T cells. It is already approved for people who have received liver or kidney transplants to keep their bodies from attacking their new organs. Researchers hope tacrolimus can help people with RA by stopping T cells from causing inflammation. Thus far, its side effects and comparative efficacy to biologics are major drawbacks.

Iguratimod (T-614), a novel DMARD expected to be a useful treatment for patients with RA, has potent anti-inflammatory, analgesic, and antipyretic activity. A Phase III study presented in 2004 showed that iguratimod had comparable efficacy and safety to sulfasalazine. Iguratimod was also effective among patients with an insufficient response to other DMARDs. It is expected that iguratimod will have a broad application as a first-line agent and for patients who have not responded to other DMARDs. The drug is a selective inhibitor of cyclo-oxygenase-2 (COX-2) and inhibits the production of IL-1, IL-6, IL-8, and TNF. Its broad action has raised side effect concerns. Iguratimod is being codeveloped by Toyama Chemical Co., Ltd. and Eisai Co., Ltd. in Japan.

Tocilizumab (Actemra) inhibits IL-6. Specifically, there is substantial evidence that IL-6 is a major mediator of systemic juvenile idiopathic arthritis (SJIA), an autoimmune disease that affects children who are less than 16 years old. In a preliminary open-label study of 11 children in Japan with severe SJIA unresponsive to high-dose steroids, 10 patients had rapid and dramatic improvement within two weeks after receiving tocilizumab, with resolution of fever and normalization of C-reactive protein (CRP) in the blood (elevated CRP is an indicator of certain disorders including SJIA). A controlled study is currently under way. Tocilizumab is being codeveloped by Chugai Pharmaceutical Co., Ltd., Japan, and F. Hoffmann-La Roche, Ltd., Switzerland.

expectorants Drugs that loosen secretions (phlegm, mucus, or other matter) from the respiratory tract in order to promote a productive cough (see also ANTITUSSIVES, which suppress nonproductive coughing). Expectorants are available as prescription and over-the-counter (OTC) products.

Classes

Two types of expectorants are in use:

- *guaifenesin* (Guiatuss, Humibid, Mucinex, Organidin, Robitussin)
- *potassium iodide* (Pima, SSKI)

How They Work

Expectorants work by increasing fluids in the respiratory tract, loosening phlegm (mucus), and reducing the thickness of bronchial secretions (called sputum). Thinner sputum flows better and is easier to cough out, thus relieving the cough indirectly.

Approved Uses

Guaifenesin is indicated for the temporary relief of symptoms associated with respiratory tract infections and related conditions such as sinusitis, pharyngitis, bronchitis, and allergies when these conditions are complicated by tenacious mucus and/or mucous plugs and excess secretions.

Potassium iodide is approved to use as an expectorant to treat chronic pulmonary (lung) diseases when tenacious mucus complicates the problem, including bronchial asthma, chronic bronchitis, and pulmonary emphysema. It is also used as adjunctive treatment in respiratory tract conditions such as cystic fibrosis and chronic sinusitis. That said, potassium iodide is rarely used as an expectorant because of the potential for adverse events; therefore, guaifenesin is usually preferred for this purpose. Potassium iodide is also used to protect the thyroid gland from radiation injury before and following administration of radioactive iodide (e.g., for diagnostic purposes) and in radiation emergencies (e.g., accidental exposure to radiation).

Off-Label Uses

Guaifenesin also has neurological properties, including an analgesic effect related to its action as a muscle relaxant, and is used in veterinary medicine to anesthetize horses being prepared for surgery.

Opera singers use guaifenesin to improve the state of their vocal folds in very humid or very dry weather locations, after flying long distances, and during mild allergies. Guaifenesin has the ability to promote secondary mucosal secretion, a thinner, lubricating mucus that occurs on the vocal cords naturally when they are healthy and well hydrated.

Companion Drugs

According to the Food and Drug Administration (FDA), thousands of products intended to relieve symptoms associated with cough, colds, allergies, and similar conditions are marketed that contain guaifenesin in combination with other active ingredients, such as ANTITUSSIVES (for instance, dextromethorphan or hydrocodone), DECONGESTANTS (for instance, pseudoephedrine or phenylephrine), and ANALGESICS (for instance,

294

acetaminophen). These products are marketed both OTC and by prescription and in immediate- and timed-release dosage forms. Guaifenesin products are also available that contain guaifenesin only.

Administration

Guaifenesin is taken orally as tablets, capsules, or liquid. Potassium iodide is available as a solution to be diluted in water and as a syrup.

Cautions and Concerns

Vomiting may result when taking guaifenesin doses larger than those required for expectorant action. To preserve the long-acting effect of guaifenesin, tablets must not be crushed or chewed prior to taking.

In some patients, prolonged use of potassium iodide can lead to hypothyroidism, a glandular disorder resulting from insufficient production of thyroid hormones. Potassium iodide may cause a flare-up of adolescent acne. Potassium iodide should be used with caution in patients having tuberculosis, Addison's disease, cardiac disease, hyperthyroidism (overactive thyroid gland), or kidney impairment, and children with cystic fibrosis appear to have an exaggerated effect from it.

Warnings

Reports in the literature have suggested that consumption of large quantities of guaifenesin-containing medications may be associated with an increased risk of drug-induced kidney stone formation.

When Not Advised (Contraindications)

Guaifenesin should not be used for a persistent cough such as occurs with smoking, asthma, chronic bronchitis, or emphysema or when coughing is accompanied by excessive secretions. A persistent cough may indicate a serious condition.

Patients with a history of thyroid disease should avoid taking potassium iodide.

Because iodide crosses the placenta and may cause hypothyroidism and goiter in the fetus/newborn, use of potassium iodide as an expectorant during pregnancy is contraindicated.

Side Effects

Guaifenesin is well tolerated, with side effects being generally mild and infrequent. Nausea and vomiting are the most common but still infrequent. Dizziness, headache, rash, and hives have been reported. Patients may notice a sense of dry mouth when taking this medication; thus, water consumption is important, not only to help with dry mouth but also to improve the effectiveness of the drug.

Potassium iodide side effects include irregular heartbeat, confusion, tiredness, fever, skin rash, goiter, salivary gland swelling/tenderness, swelling of neck/throat, hyper-/hypothyroidism, diarrhea, gastrointestinal bleeding, metallic taste, nausea, stomach pain, stomach upset, vomiting, numbness, tingling, weakness, and joint pain.

Interactions

Guaifenesin and potassium iodide may interfere with certain urine laboratory tests; thus, these agents should not be taken during the 48 hours prior to the collection of urinary specimens for such tests.

Potassium iodide taken with angiotensin-converting enzyme (ACE) inhibitors, potassium-sparing diuretics, or potassium-containing products may lead to hyperkalemia, cardiac arrhythmias, or cardiac arrest. Potassium iodide taken with lithium may cause additive hypothyroid effects.

Sales/Statistics

Americans spend $3.5 billion annually on OTC cough remedies. Expectorants constitute 20 percent of all cough and cold remedies.

Development History

Medicines similar to guaifenesin, derived from the guaiac tree, were in use as a general remedy by Native Americans when explorers reached North America in the 1500s, but guaifenesin was first approved by the FDA in 1952.

In 1978, the FDA found potassium iodide to be safe and effective for use in radiologic emergencies and approved its over-the-counter sale. In November 2001, the FDA approved potassium iodide as a thyroid-blocking agent in radiation emergencies.

Future Drugs

In November 2007, the Pharmaceutical Research and Manufacturers of America (PhRMA) database showed no expectorants in development.

hematopoietic agents Drugs that act on the blood or hemotopoietic system. They improve the quality of the blood, increasing the hemoglobin level and the number of erythrocytes (red blood cells), neutrophils (a type of white blood cell), or thrombocytes (platelets). A deficiency of red blood cells and/or hemoglobin is called anemia, which can result in a reduced ability of blood to transfer oxygen to tissues in the body. Hemoglobin (the oxygen-carrying protein in the red blood cells) has to be present to ensure adequate oxygenation of all body tissues and organs. When the body as a whole or a region of the body is deprived of sufficient oxygen, it is called hypoxia. Because all human cells depend on oxygen for survival, varying degrees of anemia can have a wide range of clinical consequences. Anemia may be due to several causes including iron, folate, or vitamin B_{12} deficiency, cancer chemotherapy, diseases that break down red blood cells faster than bone marrow can produce them, chronic diseases, failure of the bone marrow to properly develop blood cells, inherited abnormalities that cause the body to manufacture defective hemoglobin, and excessive bleeding.

A lower than normal white blood cell count is referred to as neutropenia, which can place an individual at risk for infection. Neutropenia may be inherited, result from autoimmune disease, or be drug-induced, such as from cancer chemotherapy.

Another hematologic abnormality, thrombocytopenia (lower than normal number of platelets in the blood), makes bleeding more likely. Platelets are colorless blood cells produced in the bone marrow that stop blood loss by helping the blood to clot. Thrombocytopenia may result from a separate disorder, such as leukemia or an immune system malfunction, may be drug-induced, or may be inherited.

According to a 1996 National Center for Health Statistics (NCHS) survey, 3.4 million people in the United States have anemia, but the actual number is believed to be much higher. The NCHS 2005 mortality report showed 4,624 deaths from anemia (1.6 per 100,000 population). The incidence of severe chronic neutropenia is not known, but estimates have been 3.4 cases per million persons per year. Cyclic neutropenia (a rare disorder in which the number of white blood cells drops dramatically in a cyclical pattern—usually about every 21 days) and drug-induced neutropenia are believed to each have an incidence of one case per million persons per year. Congenital (present at birth but not necessarily inherited) and idiopathic (no known cause) neutropenia have an estimated frequency of five per million of the population. Thrombocytopenia is a common finding in the critically ill and has been reported to occur in up to 50 percent of patients at some point during their stay in medical and surgical intensive care units. However, Wester wrote in the journal *Critical Care*, "Most often, the thrombocytopenia is a transient phenomenon, and recovery of the platelet count often reflects clinical improvement. On the other hand, a persistent low platelet count or relapse of thrombocytopenia often portends clinical deterioration and death."

Classes

Hematopoietic agents are divided into 4 classes:

- *Recombinant human erythropoietin—Examples:* darbepoetin alfa (Aranesp) and epoetin alfa (Epogen, Procrit).

- *Colony-stimulating factors—Examples:* filgrastim (Neupogen), pegfilgrastim (Neulasta), and sargramostim (Leukine).

- *Interleukins—Example:* oprelvekin (Neumega).

- *Thrombopoeitin (TPO) receptor agonists—Examples:* eltrombopag (Promacta) and romiplostim (Nplate).

How They Work

Recombinant human erythropoietin is a biologically engineered (man-made, or synthetic) protein that emulates the body's natural erythropoietin (a hormone that is normally made by the kidneys) to stimulate the bone marrow to make new red blood cells. Darbepoetin alfa contains two additional sialic acid–containing carbohydrate chains compared with epoetin alfa, resulting in an approximately threefold longer half-life, which affords the benefit of extended dosing intervals (fewer injections).

Filgrastim binds to stem cells in the bone marrow, stimulating the production of a type of white blood cells known as neutrophils. Filgrastim is a synthetic copy of the body's own growth factor to make more neutrophils. Pegfilgrastim is a long-acting, or pegylated, form of filgrastim, which affords the benefit of extended dosing intervals (fewer injections). Sargramostim stimulates the production of both neutrophils and macrophages. A macrophage is an immune cell that devours invading pathogens and other intruders.

Oprelvekin is a synthetic version of the naturally occurring interleukin-11, a growth factor produced by bone marrow cells, which stimulates the formation of platelets. Oprelvekin acts like that same growth factor and similarly stimulates stem cells to proliferate, thereby resulting in an increase in the amount of platelets.

Thrombopoeitin receptor agonists work by stimulating cells in the bone marrow (megakaryocytes) to produce more platelets.

Approved Uses

Recombinant human erythropoietin is used when the body does not make enough erythropoietin, causing anemia. Darbepoetin alfa is approved for treatment of anemia in patients with chronic kidney disease (CKD) or those receiving cancer chemotherapy for nonmyeloid cancers (cancer not involving myeloid cells [white blood cells that include neutrophils]). Epoetin alfa is approved to treat anemia in patients with CKD, patients receiving cancer chemotherapy for nonmyeloid cancers, human immunodeficiency virus (HIV)–infected patients being treated with zidovudine, and patients undergoing elective, noncardiac, nonvascular surgery to reduce the need for blood transfusions.

Filgrastim is approved to treat neutropenia and to prevent infections in patients undergoing chemotherapy for nonmyeloid cancers (although it has been approved for use in one type of myeloid cancer called acute myelogenous leukemia [AML]), in cancer patients receiving bone marrow transplants, to aid in the collection of stem cells for use in stem cell transplantation, and to treat patients with severe chronic neutropenia. Pegfilgrastim is approved to decrease the incidence of infections in people undergoing chemotherapy for nonmyeloid cancers. Sargramostim has been approved for use following the first cycle of chemotherapy in patients 55 years and older with AML to shorten time to neutrophil recovery and to reduce the incidence of severe and life-threatening infections. Sargramostim is also used in multiple stem cell transplantation settings.

Oprelvekin is approved for the prevention of severe thrombocytopenia and the reduction of the need for platelet transfusions following myelosuppressive chemotherapy in patients with nonmyeloid malignancies who are at high risk of severe thrombocytopenia.

Eltrombopag and romiplostim are used to increase the number of platelets in order to decrease the risk of bleeding in people who have chronic idiopathic thrombocytopenic purpura (ITP), an ongoing condition that may cause easy bruising or bleeding due to an abnormally low number of platelets in the blood. The drugs should only be used in people who cannot be treated or have had an insufficient response to corticosteroids, immunoglobulins, or a splenectomy (surgery to remove the spleen).

Off-Label Uses

Epoetin alfa is used off-label to treat anemia in premature infants, to treat chronic inflammatory disorders such as rheumatoid arthritis and ribavirin-treated hepatitis C, and to prevent anemia associated with frequent blood donation.

Filgrastim is used off-label to treat neutropenia caused by nonchemotherapy drugs and aplastic anemia (a severe form of anemia that affects white blood cells, red blood cells, and platelets).

Pegfilgrastim is used off-label for treating neutropenia due to causes other than chemotherapy and to aid in collecting stem cells for transplantation.

Sargramostim is used off-label to treat Crohn's disease and melanoma and in wound healing.

Oprelvekin is used off-label to treat Crohn's disease.

Companion Drugs

Most patients taking erythropoietin therapy need to take iron supplements; a few may also need vitamin B_{12} and folic acid supplements.

Administration

Epoetin alfa and darbepoetin alfa can be administered via intravenous or subcutaneous (under the skin) injection.

Filgrastim is administered intravenously or subcutaneously. Pegfilgrastim is administered subcutaneously.

Sargramostim is administered intravenously or subcutaneously.

Oprelvekin is administered via subcutaneous injection.

Eltrombopag is administered orally via tablets. Romiplostin is administered via subcutaneous injection.

Cautions and Concerns

The safety and efficacy of erythropoietin therapy have not been established in patients with underlying hematologic diseases (e.g., hemolytic anemia, sickle-cell anemia). If the patient fails to respond to erythropoietin therapy or to maintain a response to doses within the recommended dosing range, the possible causes should be considered and evaluated (e.g., iron, folic acid, or vitamin B_{12} deficiency, underlying infection, aluminum intoxication). Recombinant human erythropoietin has been used by athletes to increase their performance by increasing hemoglobin, resulting in several deaths.

The needle cover of the prefilled darbepoetin alfa syringe contains dry natural rubber (a derivative of latex), which may cause allergic reactions in individuals sensitive to latex. There have been rare reports of potentially serious, recurring allergic reactions, including skin rash and urticaria, associated with darbepoetin alfa. If a serious allergic or anaphylactic reaction occurs, darbepoetin alfa should be immediately and permanently discontinued, and appropriate therapy should be administered. Therapy with darbepoetin alfa or epoetin alfa results in an increase in red blood cells and a decrease in plasma volume, which could reduce dialysis efficiency; patients who are marginally dialyzed may require adjustments in their dialysis prescription. Patients with CKD not yet requiring dialysis may require lower maintenance doses of darbepoetin alfa or epoetin alfa compared to patients receiving dialysis. Sufficient time should be allowed to determine a patient's responsiveness to a dosage of darbepoetin alfa or epoetin alfa before adjusting the dose. An interval of two to six weeks may occur between the time of a dose adjustment (initiation, increase, decrease, or discontinuation) and a significant change in hemoglobin.

In some female patients, menses have resumed following epoetin alfa therapy; the possibility of pregnancy should be discussed and the need for contraception evaluated. Epoetin alfa should be used with caution in patients with known porphyria (a group of disorders caused by abnormalities in the chemical steps leading to the production of heme [a substance found in the blood, bone marrow, liver, and other tissues]).

A complete blood count (CBC) to obtain the hemoglobin and hematocrit should be performed regularly with epoetin alfa and darbepoetin alfa to make sure the drug is working.

A CBC should be obtained regularly during colony-stimulating factor therapy to make sure the drug is working and to ensure neutrophil levels do not get too high. While colony-stimulating factors are growth factors that primarily stimulate neutrophils, the possibility that these drugs can act as a growth factor for any tumor type cannot be excluded. Precaution should be exercised when using these drugs in any malignancy with myeloid characteristics.

Filgrastim and sargramostim should not be given within 24 hours before or after administration of chemotherapy because of the potential sensitivity of rapidly dividing myeloid cells to cytotoxic chemotherapy. Pegfilgrastim should not be administered in the period between 14 days before and 24 hours after administration of chemotherapy. The safety and efficacy of filgrastim and pegfilgrastim have not been evaluated in patients undergoing radiation treatments. Thus, concurrent use should be avoided. Moderate or severe cutaneous vasculitis (inflammation of the blood vessels of the skin) has been reported in patients treated with filgrastim, usually involving patients with severe chronic neutropenia receiving long-term filgrastim therapy. Serious allergic or anaphylactic reactions have been reported with sargramostim therapy.

Administration of oprelvekin should begin six to 24 hours following the completion of chemotherapy, as its safety and efficacy when given immediately prior to or concurrently with chemotherapy have not been established. Oprelvekin has been administered safely using the recommended dosage schedule for up to six cycles following chemotherapy; safety and efficacy of chronic oprelvekin administration have not been established. Because oprelvekin

has been associated with the development of arrhythmias, it should be used with caution in patients with a history of atrial arrhythmias and only after consideration of the potential risks in relation to anticipated benefit (see *Warnings*).

CBCs, including platelet counts and peripheral blood smears, should be performed prior to initiation, throughout, and following discontinuation of therapy with TPO receptor agonists. Caution should be used when administering these drugs to patients with known risk factors for thromboembolism.

Warnings

Erythropoietin drugs increase the risk of cardiovascular problems, including cardiac arrest, seizures, arrhythmia, stroke, hypertension, hypertensive encephalopathy, congestive heart failure, vascular thrombosis or ischemia, myocardial infarction, and edema. All of these issues in various cancer patients were associated with dosing these agents to a hemoglobin to 12 g/dl or higher.

In studies, erythropoietin drugs shortened the time to tumor progression in patients with advanced head and neck cancer receiving radiation therapy. These drugs also shortened survival in patients with metastatic breast cancer and cervical cancer and in patients with lymphoid malignancy receiving chemotherapy. In addition, they shortened survival in patients with non-small-cell lung cancer and in patients with various malignancies who were not receiving chemotherapy or radiotherapy. In March 2008, the FDA released a Public Health Advisory recommending use of these agents in cancer patients who are receiving chemotherapy. They should be discontinued following completion of the chemotherapy treatment regimen and should be dosed to maintain a hemoglobin < 12 g/dl.

Seizures have occurred in patients with CKD participating in clinical trials of erythropoietin drugs. Patients with CKD are at increased risk for mortality and cardiovascular events with these agents (when a hemoglobin > 12 g/dl was targeted). Therefore, a target hemoglobin of 10–12 g/dl is recommended for this population. Cases of pure red cell aplasia and of severe anemia have been reported in patients treated with erythropoietin agents. This has been reported predominantly in patients with CKD receiving erythropoietin by subcutaneous administration. Epoetin alfa has increased the rate of deep venous thromboses in patients not receiving prophylactic anticoagulation. Physicians should consider deep venous thrombosis prophylaxis.

Epoetin alfa contains albumin, a derivative of human blood. Based on effective donor screening and product-manufacturing processes, it carries an extremely remote risk for transmission of viral diseases. A theoretical risk for transmission of Creutzfeldt-Jakob disease also is considered extremely remote. Darbepoetin alfa is supplied in two formulations, one containing albumin.

Special care should be taken to closely monitor and aggressively control blood pressure in CKD patients treated with erythropoietin agents, as blood pressure may rise during therapy. During the early phase of treatment with epoetin alfa when the hematocrit is increasing, approximately 25 percent of patients on dialysis may require initiation of or increases in antihypertensive therapy. In darbepoetin alfa clinical trials, approximately 40 percent of patients with CKD required initiation or intensification of antihypertensive therapy during the early phase of treatment when the hematocrit was increasing. Hypertensive encephalopathy and seizures have been observed in patients with CKD treated with these agents. Patients should be advised as to the importance of compliance with antihypertensive therapy and dietary restrictions.

Very rarely, filgrastim and pegfilgrastim may cause enlargement and rupture of the spleen, which is located in the upper left side of the abdomen just under the ribs. Symptoms of an enlarged spleen include upper abdominal or shoulder pain. Allergic-type reactions, both skin and respiratory, have been reported with filgrastim and pegfilgrastim, occurring on initial or subsequent treatment. Acute respiratory distress syndrome has been reported in patients receiving filgrastim and pegfilgrastim and is assumed to be secondary to an influx of neutrophils to sites of inflammation in the lungs. Severe sickle-cell crises, resulting in death in some cases, have been associated with the use of filgrastim and pegfilgrastim in patients with sickle-cell disorders. Only physicians qualified by specialized training or experience in the treatment of patients with sickle-cell disorders should prescribe these drugs for such patients and only after careful consideration of the potential risks and benefits.

Fluid retention, shortness of breath, supraventricular tachycardia, and laboratory abnormalities (increases in creatinine, bilirubin, and liver enzymes) have been reported in patients after sargramostim administration.

Oprelvekin has caused allergic or hypersensitivity reactions, including anaphylaxis. The administration of oprelvekin should be attended by appropriate precautions in case allergic reactions occur. In addition, patients should be counseled about the symptoms for which they should seek medical attention, including swelling of the face, tongue, or throat, shortness of breath, wheezing, chest pain, hypotension (including shock), speech difficulty, loss of consciousness, mental status changes, rash, hives, flushing, and fever. Oprelvekin is also known to cause serious fluid retention that can result in peripheral edema, shortness of breath on exertion, pulmonary edema, atrial arrhythmias, and exacerbation of preexisting pleural effusions. Severe fluid retention, in some cases resulting in death, was reported following recent bone marrow transplantation in patients who have received oprelvekin.

Eltrombopag may cause liver damage. Increases in serum aminotransferase levels and bilirubin were observed. Liver chemistries must be measured before the initiation of treatment and regularly during treatment. Because of the risk for hepatotoxicity and other risks, eltrombopag is available only through a restricted distribution program.

Romiplostim is available only through a restricted distribution program called the Nplate NEXUS (Network of Experts Understanding and Supporting Nplate and Patients) Program. Under the Nplate NEXUS Program, only prescribers and patients registered with the program are able to prescribe, administer, and receive the product.

TPO-receptor agonists increase the risk for development or progression of reticulin fiber deposition within the bone marrow. Physicians must monitor peripheral blood for signs of marrow fibrosis. Discontinuation of TPO-receptor agonists may result in worsened thrombocytopenia than was present prior to TPO-receptor agonist therapy. CBCs, including platelet counts, should be monitored for at least two weeks following discontinuation of a TPO-receptor agonist. TPO-receptor agonists may increase the risk for hematological malignancies, especially in patients with myelodysplastic syndrome.

When Not Advised (Contraindications)

Recombinant human erythropoietin drugs are contraindicated in patients with uncontrolled hypertension and with known hypersensitivity to mammalian cell–derived products or albumin.

Filgrastim and pegfilgrastim are contraindicated in patients with known hypersensitivity to E. coli–derived proteins.

Sargramostim is contraindicated in patients with excessive leukemic myeloid blasts in the bone marrow or peripheral blood and in patients with known hypersensitivity to yeast-derived products.

Side Effects

Common side effects associated with darbepoetin alfa and epoetin alfa include edema, hypertension, hypotension, arrhythmias, fever, headache, diarrhea, vomiting, nausea, abdominal pain, myalgia, arthralgia, limb pain, infection (including sepsis, pneumonia, peritonitis, and abscess), upper respiratory infection, rash, fatigue, shortness of breath, and cough.

The most common side effect with filgrastim and pegfilgrastim is bone pain due to the pressure of the increasing new cells in the bone marrow pushing on the inside of the bones. Other common side effects with these drugs include nausea, nosebleeds, vomiting, hypertension, muscle pain, headaches, joint pain, constipation, weakness, and swelling or water retention in the ankles or feet.

Bone pain is also a common side effect with sargramostim. Other common side effects of this drug include fever (with no infection), infection, weight loss, chills, allergic reaction, nausea, diarrhea, vomiting, stomach pain, skin rash, edema, bleeding, hypertension, and hypotension.

The most common side effects with oprelvekin are slight water weight gain, some numbness in the arms and/or legs, shortness of breath when walking or moving around, red eyes, rash, and weakness. For most people, the water weight gain will go away a few days after the last injection of oprelvekin. More serious side effects that should be related to the patient's healthcare provider include rapid or irregular heartbeat, swelling of the feet and legs, blurred vision, heart palpitations, and swelling or bruising that does not go away in the injection location.

The most common side effects of eltrombopag are nausea, diarrhea, upper respiratory tract infection, vomiting, myalgia, urinary tract infection, oropharyngeal (back of the mouth) pain, pharyngitis (sore throat), back pain, influenza, paresthesia (abnormal skin sensations, such as tingling, tickling, itching, or burning), and rash. The most common side effects with romiplostim are arthralgia (joint pain), dizziness, insomnia, myalgia, pain in extremity, abdominal pain, shoulder pain, dyspepsia (heartburn or indigestion), and paresthesia.

Interactions

No drug interactions have been found or studied for either epoetin alfa or darbepoietin alfa.

Interactions between colony-stimulating factors and other drugs have not been fully evaluated. Drugs that may increase the release of neutrophils such as lithium should be used with caution, and patients receiving these drugs concomitantly should have more frequent monitoring of neutrophil counts. Drugs that may increase the myeloproliferative effects (proliferation of the bone marrow cells) of sargramostim, such as lithium and corticosteroids, should be used with caution.

Drug interactions between oprelvekin and other drugs have not been fully evaluated.

Polyvalent cations (e.g., iron, calcium, aluminum, magnesium, selenium, and zinc) significantly reduce the absorption of eltrombopag. Thus, eltrombopag must not be taken within four hours of having taken any medications or products containing polyvalent cations, such as antacids, dairy products, and mineral supplements. Eltrombopag is an inhibitor of OATP1B1 and BCRP transporters. Patients should be monitored closely for signs and symptoms of excessive exposure to the drugs that are substrates of OATP1B1 and BCRP (e.g., rosuvastatin) and consider reduction of the dose of these drugs.

No formal drug interaction studies of romiplostim have been performed.

Sales/Statistics

According to one industry report, Epogen and Aranesp had more than $6 billion in combined sales globally in 2006, while Procrit sales were about $3.2 billion.

In the United States, two hematopoietic agents appeared on the "Top Brand Drugs by Retail Dollars in 2007" (*Drug Topics,* March 10, 2008): #105 Procrit with $353,189,000 in sales, and #189 Neupogen with $150,110,000 in sales. Only Procrit was on their 2010 list, ranking #174 with $174,622,884 in sales.

Demographics and Cultural Groups

Anemia occurs in all age groups and in all racial and ethnic groups. Both men and women can have anemia; however, women of childbearing age are more at risk for anemia than men. Women in this age range lose blood from menstruation and childbirth.

According to Hsieh et al., in the United States, neutrophil counts are lower in black persons than in white persons, and neutropenia is more prevalent in black persons. Neutrophil counts are slightly higher in Mexican-American persons than in white persons, and neutropenia is uncommon in both groups. Neutropenia occurs more commonly in females than in males, and elderly individuals have a higher incidence rate than younger individuals.

Development History

Amgen Inc., a biotechnology company, revolutionized anemia treatment with the discovery of recombinant human erythropoietin in 1984, which led to the development of epoetin alfa— approved by the FDA on June 1, 1989. Building on this success, Amgen next created darbepoetin alfa to simplify anemia management, and this drug received FDA approval on September 18, 2001. Epoetin alfa and filgrastim were the first biologically derived human therapeutics.

Colony-stimulating factors were discovered accidentally by the Australian professor and researcher Donald Metcalf, whose research focused on understanding how the body generates blood cells. In 1965, Metcalf and his team found they could grow blood-forming cells as colonies if they added a colony-stimulating factor to the medium. His subsequent work on colony-stimulating factors led to the discovery that they are the proteins that control white blood cell formation and therefore are responsible for the body's resistance to infection. His collaborators then documented the effectiveness of colony-stimulating factors when injected into patients. Amgen eventually received approval for filgrastim in February 1991, then pegfilgrastim in January 31, 2002. Sargramostim was developed by Immunex and received FDA approval in March 1991.

Genetics Institute, Inc., St. Davids, Pennsylvania, developed and launched oprelvekin, which was approved by the FDA on November 25, 1997. It is marketed by Wyeth.

Designated an orphan drug in the United States and European Union (EU), eltrombopag was discovered as a result of research collaboration between GlaxoSmithKline (GSK) and

Ligand Pharmaceuticals. It was developed and is manufactured and marketed by GSK (marketed as Revolade in the EU) and was approved by the FDA on November 20, 2008. Romiplostim was developed by Amgen and approved on August 22, 2008.

Future Drugs

Maxygen, Inc., a biopharmaceutical company focused on developing improved versions of protein drugs, is developing MAXY-G34 for the treatment of chemotherapy-induced neutropenia. MAXY-G34 is a pegylated granulocyte colony-stimulating factor shown in early studies to have novel and potentially superior properties compared to current colony-stimulating factors. In Phase I studies, the drug exhibited a median half-life approximately 2.3 times that of pegfilgrastim. MAXY-G34 entered into a Phase IIa trial in summer 2007.

Minneapolis-based MGI is testing AKR-501, a small-molecule thrombopoietin mimetic, in three indications. The drug was originated by the Japanese firm Astellas Pharma, which may be acquired by MGI if the drug reaches expectations. AKR-501, a full agonist targeting the c-Mpl receptor to stimulate platelet production, has shown promising results in Phase I studies, with researchers observing significant increases in platelet count relative to baseline values. The drug is in ongoing trials in idiopathic thrombocytopenic purpura (ITP), and MGI intends to pursue Phase II testing in hepatitis C–related thrombocytopenia and in chemotherapy-induced thrombocytopenia. Other indications could follow, such as thrombocytopenia associated with myelodysplastic syndromes.

Another company developing a thrombocytopenia drug is Protalex, Inc., of New Hope, Pennsylvania, which is in Phase I testing with PRTX-100, a purified form of Protein A, a staphylococcal bacterial protein, for potential application in ITP and other autoimmune diseases.

In early 2007, South San Francisco–based Rigel Pharmaceuticals, Inc. started an exploratory Phase II study of R788, an oral syk kinase inhibitor, in ITP patients; and San Diego–based Ligand Pharmaceuticals, Inc. is in Phase I trials with its ITP drug, LGD 4665.

Hsieh, Matthew M., James E. Everhart, Danita D. Byrd-Holt, John F. Tisdale, and Griffin P. Rodgers. "Prevalence of Neutropenia in the U.S. Population: Age, Sex, Smoking Status, and Ethnic Differences." *Annals of Internal Medicine* 146, no. 7 (April 3, 2007): 486–492.

News-Medical Net. "Novel Drug Romiplostim Significantly Improves Treatment of Dangerous Blood Disorder." *Medical Studies/Trials.* Available online. URL: http://www.news-medical.net/?id=34920. Published on February 5, 2008.

Wester, Joseph P. "A Rare Disease." *Critical Care* 11, no. 1 (January 2007): 102.

immunosuppressives These drugs, also referred to as immunosuppressants, are used to slow or halt the activity of the immune system. Clinically, they are used to prevent the immune system's rejection of transplanted organs and tissues (e.g., bone marrow, heart, kidney, liver) and in treatment of autoimmune diseases or diseases that are most likely of autoimmune origin (e.g., rheumatoid arthritis [RA], myasthenia gravis, Crohn's disease, and ulcerative colitis).

Classes

Immunosuppressive drugs can be divided into six classes.

- *Glucocorticoids* are given in much higher doses (called pharmacologic doses) in immunosuppressive therapy. (Doses that provide approximately the same glucocorticoid effects as normal cortisol production are referred to as physiologic, replacement, or maintenance dosing; see CORTICOSTEROIDS.) *Examples:* methylprednisolone sodium succinate (Solu-Medrol) and prednisone (Sterapred).

- *Calcineurin inhibitors—Examples:* cyclosporine (Gengraf, Neoral, Restasis, Sandimmune) and tacrolimus (Prograf, Protopic).

- *mTOR (mammalian target of rapamycin) inhibitors—Example:* sirolimus (Rapamune).

- *Antimetabolites—Examples:* azathioprine (Azasan, Imuran), methotrexate (Rheumatrex, Trexall), mycophenolate mofetil (CellCept), and mycophenolate sodium (Myfortic).

- *Alkylating agent—Example:* cyclophosphamide.

- Antibodies can be further subdivided as *monoclonal antibodies* and *polyclonal antibodies.*

Examples: Monoclonal: adalimumab (Humira), alefacept (Amevive), basiliximab (Simulect), daclizumab (Zenapax), infliximab (Remicade), muromonab-CD3 (Orthoclone OKT3), and rituximab (Rituxan). Polyclonal: antithymocyte globulin (horses) (Atgam) and antithymocyte globulin (rabbit) (Thymoglobulin).

How They Work

A basic concept of immunosuppression is to prevent production of antibodies. An antibody is a protein molecule compound (also called an immunoglobulin) produced by B cells that has the purpose of controlling the immune response to a specific and unique antigen. An antigen is a substance that induces an immune response. The antigen can be foreign material from the environment (e.g., viruses or bacteria) or formed within the cells of one's own body. Antigens on the body's own cells are called autoantigens. Antigens on all other cells are called foreign antigens. When the antibody binds to the antigen, this forms an antigen-antibody complex. This complex may make the antigen harmless or may trigger an inflammatory response.

At first, an antibody is bound to a B cell, but when it encounters its specific antigen, the antibody-antigen complex stimulates the B cell to produce copies of the antibody—all of which are designed to recognize the infecting antigen. Then the new group of antibodies bind to the infecting antigen, leading to its control or destruction.

Thus, in instances of autoimmune diseases, when the antibodies are erroneously attacking the body's own organs and tissues (called autoantibodies), and in transplantations, when

305

the antibodies attack (reject) the new "foreign" tissue or organ, it is helpful to suppress this antibody formation.

In addition to suppressing the production of antibodies, glucocorticoids decrease inflammation (swelling) by preventing infection-fighting white blood cells (polymorphonuclear leukocytes) from traveling to the area of swelling. Although this makes the patient more prone to infection, it reduces the heat, redness, swelling, and pain associated with inflammation.

Calcineurin inhibitors are believed to inhibit T lymphocytes, which are small white blood cells that orchestrate and/or directly participate in the immune defenses. T cells are the major cells involved in immunosuppression. Calcineurin inhibitors inhibit T cell activation in the early stages of the immune response. Cyclosporine binds to cyclophilin protein, while tacrolimus binds to tacrolimus-binding protein. Cyclosporine emulsion (eye drops) is believed to inhibit the activation of T cells that cause inflammation and disrupt the normal production of tears in the lacrimal glands. Improving the lacrimal glands' function is believed to result in increased tear production.

Sirolimus acts by binding the TOR protein kinases, which in turn prevents cell cycle progression by blocking the ability of T cells to proliferate in response to interleukin (IL)-2 stimulus.

Antimetabolites work by blocking metabolic steps within immune cells and then interfering with immune function. For azathioprine and methotrexate, see DISEASE-MODIFYING ANTIRHEUMATIC DRUGS (DMARDs).

Cyclophosphamide works in immunosuppressive therapy by suppressing B cell activity and antibody formation. B cells are affected more by cyclophosphamide than are T cells because their rate of recovery from an alkylating agent is slower.

Antibody drugs work by depleting or inactivating T cells. Polyclonal antibodies target all lymphocytes, producing a generalized immunosuppression. Monoclonal antibodies are directed toward exactly defined antigens on the receptors of specific cells. Adalimumab and infliximab specifically are tumor necrosis factor (TNF) inhibitors.

Approved Uses

At pharmacologic doses, glucocorticoids are used to suppress various allergic (e.g., bronchial asthma, contact dermatitis, atopic dermatitis, allergic rhinitis), inflammatory (e.g., bursitis, gout, ulcerative colitis), and autoimmune (e.g., ankylosing spondylitis, multiple sclerosis [MS], RA, and systemic lupus erythematosus [SLE; often referred to simply as lupus]) disorders. Glucocorticoids are also administered prior to and following transplantation to prevent acute transplant rejection and graft-versus-host disease.

Calcineurin inhibitors are used to prevent organ rejection in kidney, liver, and heart allogeneic transplants. (Allogeneic refers to cells or tissues from individuals belonging to the same species but genetically dissimilar and thus immunologically incompatible.) Cyclosporine is also approved for the treatment of RA that has not responded well to methotrexate alone as well as severe forms of plaque psoriasis that are not responsive to conventional treatments. Cyclosporine ophthalmic emulsion is used to increase tear production in patients whose tear production is presumed to be suppressed due to ocular inflammation associated with keratoconjunctivitis sicca. Tacrolimus ointment is used to treat moderate to severe atopic dermatitis (eczema) when other topical treatments have failed to respond adequately.

Sirolimus is approved for the prevention of organ rejection in patients receiving kidney transplants.

Azathioprine is approved to prevent kidney transplant rejection and for the management of severe, active RA unresponsive to conventional treatment. Methotrexate is approved to treat some types of cancer (see ANTINEOPLASTICS), severe psoriasis, RA, and juvenile rheumatoid arthritis (JRA). Mycophenolate is approved for the prevention of organ rejection in patients receiving kidney, cardiac, or liver transplants.

For cyclophosphamide, see ANTINEOPLASTICS.

Antibodies are used in immunosuppressive therapy to prevent acute rejection reaction. Antibodies are also used to treat cancer and various autoimmune diseases (see ANTINEOPLASTICS and DMARDs). Specifically, adalimumab is used to treat moderate to severe RA or active psoriatic arthritis, JRA, Crohn's disease, and plaque psoriasis. Alefacept is used to treat plaque psoriasis. Basiliximab and daclizumab are approved for the prevention of organ rejection in patients receiving kidney transplants. Infliximab is used to treat moderate to severe RA (with methotrexate), psoriatic arthritis, ankylosing spondylitis, Crohn's disease, plaque psoriasis, and ulcerative colitis (not responsive to conventional therapy). Muromonab-CD3 is used to prevent acute rejection in kidney or liver transplant patients. Rituximab is used to treat certain types of B cell non-Hodgkin's lymphoma. It is also used with methotrexate to treat RA. Both formulations of antithymocyte globulin (horse and rabbit) are used to prevent acute rejection in renal transplant patients. The horse formulation is also used to treat aplastic anemia in patients unsuited to undergo bone marrow transplantation.

Off-Label Uses

Cyclosporine has been used off-label to treat Crohn's disease and ulcerative colitis. Tacrolimus is used off-label to treat RA, SLE, inflammatory bowel disease, and severe recalcitrant psoriasis.

Sirolimus is used off-label to treat psoriasis and to prevent organ rejection in heart transplant patients.

Azathioprine is used off-label to treat uveitis (inflammation in the eyes), chronic ulcerative colitis, psoriasis, SLE, and Crohn's disease.

Methotrexate has been used off-label to terminate ectopic pregnancies (the life-threatening condition in which fertilized eggs grow outside the uterus) and to relieve symptoms of pain, swelling, and stiffness in autoimmune diseases such as MS, dermatomyositis, polymyositis, and psoriatic arthritis. Low-dose methotrexate has been used off-label to treat patients with moderate to severe Crohn's disease.

Cyclophosphamide is used off-label to treat severe rheumatologic diseases such as Wegener's granulomatosis, progressive RA, and SLE. Cyclophosphamide has also been used to halt the progression of or decrease the frequence and duration of episodes of MS.

Infliximab is used off-label to treat juvenile RA.

Rituximab is used off-label to treat a number of autoimmune disorders, such as SLE, pemphigus, thrombocytopenic purpura, hemolytic autoimmune anemia, cold agglutinin disease, and cryoglobulinemia.

Antithymocyte globulin (horse) is used off-label to treat MS, myasthenia gravis, pure red-cell aplasia, and scleroderma.

Administration

Methylprednisolone sodium succinate is administered via intravenous or intramuscular injection. Prednisone is administered orally via tablets.

Cyclosporine is administered via intravenous injection, orally via a solution (which can be diluted with room-temperature orange juice) or a capsule, and as eye drops. Tacrolimus is administered orally via capsule, via intravenous injection, and topically via ointment.

Sirolimus is taken by mouth via tablets or solution.

Azathioprine is administered orally via tablets and via intravenous injection.

Methotrexate is administered via tablet or injection. The injectable form may be given intravenously or intramuscularly.

Mycophenolate is administered orally via capsules, tablets, or oral suspension. It may be administered via intravenous injection for patients unable to take it orally.

Cyclophosphamide is administered orally via tablets or via intravenous injection.

Antibodies are administered via injection. Adalimumab is injected subcutaneously (under the skin) by the patient, a family member, or a nurse. Alefacept is administered via intramuscular injection. Other antibodies need to be administered by intravenous infusion, which is typically done in a doctor's office or clinic.

Cautions and Concerns

For glucocorticoids *Cautions and Concerns,* see CORTICOSTEROIDS.

Calcineurin inhibitors often lead to hypertension, with mild or moderate hypertension more frequent than severe hypertension. Antihypertensive therapy may be required in these patients. (See DMARDs for additional cyclosporine *Cautions and Concerns.*) Cyclosporine eye drops should not be administered while wearing contact lenses. The eye drops from a single-use vial must be used immediately after opening for administration to one or both eyes and the remaining contents discarded immediately after administration. Tacrolimus ointment should be avoided on premalignant and malignant skin conditions; some malignant skin conditions, such as cutaneous T cell lymphoma, may mimic atopic dermatitis. Before beginning treatment with tacrolimus ointment, cutaneous bacterial or viral infections at treatment sites should be resolved.

Sirolimus has been associated with the development of angioedema. The concomitant use of sirolimus with other drugs known to cause angioedema, such as angiotensin-converting enzyme inhibitors, may increase this risk. There have been reports of impaired or delayed wound healing in patients receiving sirolimus.

For azathioprine and methotrexate *Cautions and Concerns,* see DMARDs. Mycophenolate mofetil and mycophenolate sodium dosage forms should not be interchanged. Gastrointestinal bleeding requiring hospitalization has been observed in various transplant patients treated with mycophenolate. Because mycophenolate has been associated with an increased incidence of digestive system adverse events, including infrequent cases of gastrointestinal tract ulceration, hemorrhage, and perforation, this drug should be administered with caution in patients with active serious digestive system disease.

Because mycophenolate may cause anemia, complete blood counts should be monitored weekly during the first month of treatment, twice monthly for the second and third months, then monthly through the first year.

For cyclophosphamide *Cautions and Concerns,* see ANTINEOPLASTICS.

For adalimumab, infliximab, and rituximab *Cautions and Concerns,* see DMARDs.

Caution should be exercised when considering the use of alefacept in patients at high risk for malignancy (see *Warnings*). Urticaria and angioedema have been associated with the administration of alefacept. If an anaphylactic reaction or other serious allergic reaction occurs, administration of alefacept should be discontinued immediately and appropriate therapy initiated. Because there have been postmarketing reports of liver injury with alefacept, and even though the exact relationship of these occurrences with the use of alefacept has not been established, patients with signs or symptoms of liver injury should be fully evaluated before starting therapy with this drug. Alefacept should be discontinued in patients who develop significant clinical signs of liver injury.

It is not known whether the immune response to vaccines, infection, and other antigens first encountered during basiliximab or daclizumab therapy is impaired or whether such response will remain impaired after treatment with these drugs.

Muromonab-CD3 commonly causes chest pain, dizziness, fever and chills, shortness of breath, stomach upset, and trembling within a few hours after the first dose. These effects are usually less after the second dose.

Patients treated with antithymocyte globulin should be watched carefully for signs of leukopenia, thrombocytopenia, or concurrent infection.

Warnings

Increased susceptibility to infection, including opportunistic infections and sepsis, and the possible development of lymphomas and other malignancies, particularly of the skin, may result from immunosuppression. The risk appears to be related to the intensity and duration of immunosuppression rather than to the use of any specific agent. Exposure to sunlight and ultraviolet light should be limited by wearing protective clothing and using a sunscreen with a high protection factor.

Only physicians experienced in immunosuppressive therapy and management of organ transplant patients should prescribe calcineurin inhibitors. Calcineurin inhibitors can cause neurotoxicity and nephrotoxicity, particularly when used in high doses. Rare cases of malignancy (e.g., skin and lymphoma) have been reported in patients treated with topical calcineurin inhibitors, including tacrolimus ointment. Therefore, continuous long-term use of topical tacrolimus should be avoided and application limited to areas of involvement with atopic dermatitis.

Sandimmune soft gelatin capsules and Sandimmune oral solution have decreased bioavailability in comparison to Neoral soft gelatin capsules and Neoral oral solution. Because Sandimmune and Neoral are not bioequivalent, they cannot be used interchangeably without physician supervision. (See also DMARDs for additional cyclosporine *Warnings*.)

New-onset insulin-dependent post-transplant diabetes mellitus (PTDM) has been reported in tacrolimus-treated kidney transplant patients. This condition may be reversible with time following the transplant. African-American and Hispanic kidney transplant patients are at an increased risk of developing diabetes with the use of tacrolimus following transplantation.

A few patients receiving intravenous cyclosporine or tacrolimus injections have experienced anaphylactic reactions. Although the exact cause of these reactions is not known, other drugs with castor oil derivatives in the formulation have been associated with anaphylaxis in a small percentage of patients. Because of this potential risk of anaphylaxis, intravenous administration of these drugs should be reserved for patients who are unable to take these drugs orally. Patients receiving the drugs via intra-venous injection should be under continuous observation for at least the first 30 minutes following the start of the infusion and at frequent intervals thereafter. If signs or symptoms of anaphylaxis occur, the infusion should be stopped. Epinephrine should be available at the bedside as well as oxygen.

Increased serum cholesterol and triglycerides requiring treatment occurred more frequently in patients treated with sirolimus compared with azathioprine or placebo controls in studies. The risk/benefit should be carefully considered in patients with established hyperlipidemia before initiating an immunosuppressive regimen including sirolimus. Any patient who is administered sirolimus should be monitored for hyperlipidemia. If detected, interventions such as diet, exercise, and lipid-lowering agents should be initiated.

Cases of interstitial lung disease (including pneumonitis, bronchiolitis obliterans organizing pneumonia, and pulmonary fibrosis), some fatal, with no identified infectious etiology have occurred in patients receiving immunosuppressive regimens including sirolimus. In some cases, the interstitial lung disease has resolved upon discontinuation or dose reduction of sirolimus.

For azathioprine and methotrexate *Warnings,* see DMARDs.

Female users of childbearing potential must use contraception during mycophenolate treatment. Use of this drug during pregnancy is associated with an increased risk of spontaneous abortions and birth defects. Cases of progressive multifocal leukoencephalopathy (PML), a rare and potentially fatal disease caused by the reactivation of a common virus in the central nervous system of immune-compromised individuals, have been reported in patients treated with mycophenolate.

For cyclophosphamide *Warnings,* see ANTINEOPLASTICS.

For adalimumab, infliximab, and rituximab *Warnings,* see DMARDs.

Alefacept reduces CD4+ and CD8+ T lymphocyte counts; therefore, alefacept therapy should not be initiated in patients with a CD4+ T cell count below normal. The CD4+ T cell counts of patients receiving alefacept should be monitored every two weeks during the 12-week treatment course. Retreatment with an additional 12-week course may be initiated after a minimum of 12 weeks off treatment, provided CD4+ T cell counts are within the normal range.

Only physicians experienced in immunosuppression therapy and management of organ transplantation patients should prescribe basiliximab, daclizumab, or muromonab-CD3. Severe acute (onset within 24 hours) hypersensitivity reactions including anaphylaxis have been observed both on initial exposure to these drugs and/or following reexposure after several months. These reactions may include hypotension, tachycardia, cardiac failure, difficulty breathing, wheezing, bronchospasm, pulmonary edema, respiratory failure, urticaria, rash, pruritus, and/or sneezing. If a severe hypersensitivity reaction occurs, therapy should be permanently discontinued. Medications for the treatment of severe hypersensitivity reactions should be available for immediate use. Patients previously administered these drugs should only be reexposed to a subsequent course of therapy with extreme caution. The potential risks of such readministration, specifically those associated with immunosuppression, are not known.

The use of daclizumab as part of an immunosuppressive regimen including cyclosporine, mycophenolate, and corticosteroids may be associated with an increase in mortality.

Seizures, encephalopathy (brain disease), cerebral edema, aseptic meningitis, and headache have been reported, even following the first dose, with muromonab-CD3.

Only physicians experienced in immunosuppressive therapy and the management of renal transplant or aplastic anemia patients should use antithymocyte globulin. Precise methods of determining the potency of antithymocyte globulin have not been established; thus, activity may potentially vary from lot to lot. Treatment with antithymocyte globulin should be discontinued if symptoms of anaphylaxis, severe and unremitting thrombocytopenia, or leucopenia occur. Antithymocyte globulin may carry a risk of transmitting infectious agents, such as viruses, and theoretically, the Creutzfeldt-Jakob disease agent.

When Not Advised (Contraindications)

For glucocorticoid *Contraindications*, see CORTICOSTEROIDS.

Calcineurin inhibitor injection is contraindicated in patients with a hypersensitivity to polyoxyethylated castor oil (see *Warnings*). Patients with RA or psoriasis who also have high blood pressure, kidney problems, or cancer should not take cyclosporine. Cyclosporine eye drops are contraindicated in patients with active eye infections.

For methotrexate, infliximab, and rituximab *Contraindications*, see DMARDs.

Allergic reactions to mycophenolate have been observed; therefore, mycophenolate is contraindicated in patients with a hypersensitivity to mycophenolic acid or any component of the drug product. Mycophenolate injection is contraindicated in patients who are allergic to Polysorbate 80 (Tween).

For cyclophosphamide *Contraindications*, see ANTINEOPLASTICS.

For adalimumab and infliximab *Contraindications*, see DMARDs.

Alefacept is contraindicated in patients with a history of systemic malignancy (see *Warnings*) or with a serious infection (requiring hospitalization) and in patients receiving other immunosuppressive agents or phototherapy because of the possibility of excessive immunosuppression.

Muromonab-CD3 should not be given to patients who have antimouse antibody titers >/=1:1000; are in uncompensated heart failure or in fluid overload, as evidenced by chest X-ray or a greater than 3 percent weight gain within the week prior to treatment; have uncontrolled hypertension; or have a history of or are predisposed to seizures.

Side Effects

All immunosuppressives lower a person's resistance to infection and can make infections more difficult to treat.

The most common side effect for cyclosporine eye drops is a temporary burning sensation in the eyes. For other cyclosporine *Side Effects*, see DMARDs.

The most common side effects with tacrolimus are tremor, headache, diarrhea, hypertension, nausea, and renal dysfunction. These occur with both oral and IV administration and may respond to a reduction in dosing. Diarrhea has sometimes been associated with other gastrointestinal complaints such as nausea and vomiting. Topical tacrolimus may cause a skin-burning sensation, stinging, soreness, or itching, especially during the first few days of use.

The most common side effects with sirolimus include peripheral edema, hypertriglyceridemia, hypertension, hypercholesterolemia, renal dysfunction, constipation, abdominal pain, diarrhea, headache, fever, anemia, nausea, arthralgia, pain, and thrombocytopenia.

For azathioprine and methotrexate *Side Effects*, see DMARDs.

The most common side effects associated with mycophenolate include diarrhea, leukopenia, sepsis, and vomiting.

For cyclophosphamide *Side Effects*, see ANTINEOPLASTICS.

For adalimumab, infliximab, and rituximab *Side Effects*, see DMARDs.

Common side effects with alefacept include sore throat, dizziness, cough, nausea, itching, muscle pain, chills, injection site pain, and injection site inflammation.

Common side effects with basiliximab include constipation, nausea, abdominal pain, vomiting, diarrhea, indigestion, pain, peripheral edema, fever, hyperkalemia, hypokalemia, hyperglycemia, hypercholesterolemia, hypophosphatemia, hyperuricemia, difficulty breathing, surgical wound complications, acne, hypertension, headache, tremor, insomnia, and anemia.

Common side effects with daclizumab include constipation, nausea, diarrhea, vomiting, abdominal pain, heartburn, indigestion, abdominal distention, edema, tremor, headache, dizziness, decreased or painful urination, posttraumatic pain (pain after surgery), chest pain, fever, pain, fatigue, hypertension, hypotension, difficulty breathing, pulmonary edema, cough, impaired wound healing, acne, insomnia, musculoskeletal pain, tachycardia, thrombosis, and bleeding.

Common side effects with muromonab-CD3 include nausea, vomiting, diarrhea, dizziness, fever, chills, general feeling of discomfort or illness, headache, and muscle or joint pain.

Common side effects with antithymocyte globulin include fever, chills, leukopenia, thrombocytopenia, dermatologic reactions (e.g., rash, itching, hives, welts, and flare), headache, joint or muscle pain, and nausea.

Interactions

Immunosuppressants may affect response to vaccination. In particular, immunosuppressants may enhance the adverse/toxic effect of live vaccines, and infections from the vaccines may develop. Immunosuppressants may also decrease the therapeutic response to vaccines.

For glucocorticoid *Interactions*, see CORTICOSTEROIDS.

For cyclosporine and methotrexate *Interactions*, see DMARDs.

Due to the potential for additive or synergistic impairment of kidney function, care should be taken when administering tacrolimus with drugs that may be associated with kidney dysfunction. These include but are not limited to aminoglycosides, amphotericin B, and cisplatin. Patients switched from cyclosporine to tacrolimus should receive the first tacrolimus dose no sooner than 24 hours after the last cyclosporine dose. Dosing may be further delayed in the presence of elevated cyclosporine levels.

Since tacrolimus is metabolized mainly by the CYP3A enzyme systems, substances known to inhibit these enzymes may decrease the metabolism or increase bioavailability of tacrolimus as indicated by increased whole blood or plasma concentrations (increased risk of toxicity). Drugs known to induce these enzyme systems may result in an increased metabolism of tacrolimus or decreased bioavailability as indicated by decreased whole blood or plasma concentrations (increased risk of organ rejection). Monitoring of blood concentrations and appropriate dosage adjustments are essential when such drugs are used concomitantly.

Drugs that may increase tacrolimus blood concentrations include calcium channel blockers (diltiazem, nicardipine, nifedipine, verapamil), antifungal agents (fluconazole, itraconazole, ketoconazole, voriconazole), macrolide antibiotics (clarithromycin, erythromycin), gastrointestinal prokinetic agents (cisapride, metoclopramide), and protease inhibitors.

Drugs that may decrease tacrolimus blood concentrations include anticonvulsants (carbamazepine, phenobarbital, phenytoin), antimicrobials (rifabutin, caspofungin, rifampin), and herbal preparations (Saint-John's-wort).

Sirolimus should not be used with strong inducers (e.g., rifampin, rifabutin) and strong inhibitors (e.g., ketoconazole, voriconazole, itraconazole, erythromycin, telithromycin, clarithromycin) of CYP3A4 and P-gp. Because grapefruit juice inhibits the CYP3A4-mediated metabolism of sirolimus, it must not be taken with or be used for dilution of this drug.

For azathioprine and rituximab *Interactions,* see DMARDs.

The potential exists for mycophenolate and acyclovir (or valacyclovir) to compete for tubular secretion, further increasing the concentrations of both drugs. Mycophenolate must be separated from antacids containing magnesium and aluminum hydroxides.

For cyclophosphamide *Interactions,* see ANTINEOPLASTICS.

The use of muromonab-CD3 with indomethacin (a nonsteroidal anti-inflammatory drug [NSAID]) may increase the risk of encephalopathy and other central nervous system (CNS) effects.

Sales/Statistics

According to a Kalorama Information market research report (December 1, 2007), the number of organ transplants performed worldwide is approximately 70,000 annually. Some 30,000 kidney transplants were performed in 2005, with that number expected to increase to 43,000 by 2015. The market for immunosuppressants used in transplantation is set to grow to $4.3 billion by 2015.

In the United States, several immunosuppressives were listed on the "2008 Top 200 Branded Drugs by Retail Dollars" list (*Drug Topics,* May 26, 2009): #50 CellCept ($711,530,000 in sales), #62 Prograf ($584,703,000), #85 Humira ($455,911,000), and #107 Restasis ($339,110,000). On the "2008 Top 200 Branded Drugs by Total Prescriptions," Restasis ranked #107 with 339,110,000 prescriptions and CellCept #199 (1,075,000 prescriptions). On the "2008 Top 200 Generic Drugs by Retail Dollars" list, prednisone ranked #52 ($211,100,000 in sales), methotrexate #117 ($96,809,000 in sales), cyclosporine #173 ($55,977,000 in sales), and azathioprine #178 ($53,428,000 in sales). Listed on the "2008 Top 200 Generic Drugs by Total Prescriptions" were #19 prednisone (24,755,000 prescriptions) and #104 methotrexate (4,623,000 prescriptions).

According to a report from the IMS Institute for Healthcare Informatics (the public reporting arm of IMS, a pharmaceutical market intelligence firm), drugs used to treat autoimmune diseases, which would largely include immunosuppressives, were the eighth-largest therapeutic class in drug spending in the United States in 2010, with $10.6 billion in sales. That was up from $7 billion in 2006.

Demographics and Cultural Groups

In clinical trials, black and Hispanic kidney transplant patients were at an increased risk of development of PTDM when treated with tacrolimus.

Development History

The use of glucocorticoids in transplantation was first discovered in the 1950s with experiments demonstrating the ability of these agents to enhance survival of rabbit skin grafts. These observations led to the clinical use of glucocorticoids to reverse severe kidney transplant rejection. The combined administration of glucocorticoids and azathioprine was subsequently introduced as maintenance immunosuppressive therapy. Significant benefits with this regimen helped transform transplantation from an experimental, infrequently used procedure to a widespread, extremely successful clinical option. For more on the development of glucocorticoids, see CORTICOSTEROIDS *Development History.*

In 1959, cyclophosphamide was shown to suppress the formation of antibodies and was used for bone marrow transplantation.

In the 1960s, azathioprine was found to delay organ graft rejection and was used to suppress rejection of transplanted kidneys. In 1969, methotrexate was shown to inhibit antibody formation and the development of delayed hypersensitivity in guinea pigs. For more on the development history of azathioprine and methotrexate, see DMARDs. Mycophenolate was approved on May 9, 1995.

The T cell–inhibiting properties of cyclosporine were discovered in 1976. In 1979, U.S. trials of cyclosporine in cadaver kidney transplants began at the Peter Bent Brigham Hospital in Boston and at the University of Colorado. The results showed that cyclosporine combined with steroids controlled rejection better than any drug therapy had in the past. In 1983, the FDA approved cyclosporine for general use in the United States, heralding a new era for kidney, liver, and heart transplantation.

Tacrolimus was shown to inhibit IL-2 production and lymphocyte proliferation in 1987 and was approved on April 8, 1994.

Interest in the antibiotic sirolimus was renewed in the 1980s when it was shown to prevent allograft rejection. Sirolimus was approved on September 15, 1999.

In the early 1980s, Dr. A. Benedict Cosimi and his associates at Massachusetts General Hospital began clinical trials using monoclonal antibodies against mature T lymphocytes. Soon afterward, other studies demonstrated that intractable rejection of renal grafts could be reversed with monoclonal antibodies. In 1986, muromonab-CD3 was approved by the FDA. Approval of other monoclonal antibodies followed: rituximab (November 26, 1997), daclizumab (December 10, 1997), basiliximab (May 12, 1998), infliximab (August 24, 1998), adalimumab (December 31, 2002), and alefacept (January 30, 2003).

Antithymocyte globulin (horse) gained FDA approval in 1981 and antithymocyte globulin (rabbit) on December 30, 1998.

Future Drugs

In 2008, the Pharmaceutical Research and Manufacturers of America (PhRMA) listed two drugs in development for immunosuppression:

Pfizer is developing a janus kinase 3 (JAK-3) inhibitor, CP-690550, which is selective for JAK-3 and no other form of JAK and thus should cause fewer adverse events than previous immunosuppressives. JAK-3 is one of the many cytokines that is required for immune cell development and homeostasis. It has the additional advantage of being a pill. Trials have been carried out in a number of conditions, including kidney transplantation, RA, and chronic plaque psoriasis. Pfizer announced in March 2011 that CP-690550 (tofacitinib; formerly tasocitinib) met its goals in its second Phase III clinical trial for moderate to severe RA.

Daiichi Sankyo Company, Tokyo, is in Phase I studies with CS 0777, an immunosuppressant in tablet form being tested for MS treatment.

interferons Interferons are natural proteins produced by the cells of the immune system in response to challenges by foreign agents such as viruses, parasites, and tumor cells. They belong to a large class of glycoproteins known as cytokines. The name *interferon* comes from the fact that they literally interfere with a virus's ability to reproduce and proliferate. Through recombinant DNA technology, various interferons have been genetically engineered (copied) for use in the medical treatment of disease. Interferons affect the immune system in a number of ways. Some of these agents increase the cell-killing activity of the immune system, making tumor cells more vulnerable to immune attack by increasing antigens and blocking the formation of new blood vessels by tumors. They also slow tumor cell replication by inhibiting DNA and protein synthesis. Some interferons regulate the immune system and are used to treat various autoimmune diseases.

Classes

Interferons are classified according to their chemical structures, biologic activities, and other criteria. Currently known classes of interferons:

- *Alfa-interferons—Examples:* interferon alfa-2b, recombinant (Intron A), interferon alfa-n3 (Alferon N), interferon alfacon-1 (Infergen), peginterferon alfa-2a (Pegasys), and peginterferon alfa-2b (Peg-Intron).
- *Beta-interferons—Examples:* interferon beta-1a (Avonex, Rebif) and interferon beta-1b (Betaseron).
- *Gamma-interferons—Example:* interferon gamma-1b (Actimmune).

How They Work

The mechanism by which interferons act against tumors or viruses is not clearly understood. Generally, interferons exert their cellular activities by binding to specific membrane receptors on the cell surface. Interferons initiate a complex sequence of intracellular events when they are bound to the cell membrane. Researchers believe that some interferons may also help the immune system work more effectively against cells that are not normal.

It is believed that alfa-interferons work in certain conditions by reducing the amount of virus in the body, slowing the growth of cancer cells or shutting off their ability to make new cancer cells (replicate), destroying cells that may be harmful to the body, and keeping the body from producing too many of certain blood cells.

Peginterferon alfa-2a and peginterferon alfa-2b are long-acting interferons. The Body (http://www.thebody.com) explains, "Pegylation is the process by which a molecule of polyethylene glycol (PEG) is attached to a molecule of interferon. The resulting 'pegylated' compound has a longer half-life and duration of action. As a result, the pegylated interferon preparation only has to be injected once a week, and since it provides continued therapeutic levels of interferon in blood, it has a more potent antiviral action."

It is believed that beta-interferons achieve their beneficial effect on multiple sclerosis (MS) progression by reducing the number of inflammatory T cells (small white blood cells) that are transported from the blood stream to the central nervous system while at the same time allowing the cells that reduce inflammation to dominate the central nervous system. By obstructing the damaging white cells, beta-interferons reduce the number of attacks (flare-ups or flares) and severity of MS symptoms in patients. Studies have also determined that beta-interferon improves the integrity of the blood-brain barrier (BBB), which generally breaks down in patients with MS, making it possible for unwanted cells to invade and break down nerves. This strengthening of the BBB may be a contributing factor to beta-interferon's beneficial effects.

Interferon gamma-1b is a bioengineered form of interferon gamma, a protein in the body that acts as a biologic response modifier through stimulation of the human immune system. Exactly how interferon gamma-1b works is not fully understood, but it is thought to help the immune system work better by enhancing the action of cells the body uses in defense against certain diseases.

Approved Uses

Interferon alfa-2b is approved for the treatment of hairy cell leukemia, malignant melanoma, non-Hodgkin's lymphoma, acquired immune deficiency syndrome (AIDS)–related Kaposi's sarcoma, and genital warts in patients 18 years of age or older. It is also approved to treat chronic hepatitis B virus (HBV) in patients at least one year of age and chronic hepatitis C virus (HCV) in patients three years of age and older.

Interferon alfa-n3 is approved to treat refractory (resistant to other treatment) or recurring external genital warts in patients 18 years of age or older.

Interferon alfacon-1 is approved for the treatment of chronic HCV infection in patients 18 years of age or older with compensated liver disease who have anti-HCV serum antibodies and/ or the presence of HCV RNA.

Peginterferon alfa-2a is approved for the treatment of adults with chronic HCV infection who have compensated liver disease and histological evidence of cirrhosis. Peginterferon alfa-2a may also be used in patients who are infected with both chronic HCV and the human immunodeficiency virus (HIV). Peginterferon alfa-2a is also approved for the treatment of adult patients with HBeAg positive and HBeAg negative chronic HBV who have compensated liver disease and evidence of viral replication and liver inflammation.

Peginterferon alfa-2b is approved for the treatment of adults with chronic HCV infection and compensated liver disease who have not previously been treated with alfa-interferons. For the treatment of chronic HCV, either peginterferon alfa-2a or -2b may be used alone or in combination with ribavirin.

Beta-interferons are approved to treat relapsing forms of MS to reduce the frequency of flares.

Interferon gamma-1b is approved for reducing the number and severity of infections associated with chronic granulomatous disease (CGD), an inherited disorder in which white blood cells lose their ability to destroy certain bacteria and fungi. It is also used to delay the progression of severe, malignant osteopetrosis, a congenital disorder in which the bones become overly dense.

Off-Label Uses

Interferon alfa-2b is used off-label to treat chronic myelogenous leukemia, multiple myeloma, renal cell carcinoma, and various skin cancers.

Peginterferon alfa-2a and peginterferon alfa-2b are used off-label to treat renal cell carcinoma. Peginterferon alfa-2b is also used off-label to treat advanced melanomas.

Companion Drugs

Interferon alfa-2b is approved to treat HCV in combination with ribavirin tablets. A combination product that contains both of these drugs in a package, Rebetron, is available. Peginterferon alfa-2a and peginterferon alfa-2b are also used in combination with ribavirin to treat HCV.

Administration

Depending on the indication, interferon alfa-2b may be administered subcutaneously, intramuscularly, intravenously, or intralesionally (into the base of the wart). Interferon alfacon-1, peginterferon alfa-2a, peginterferon alfa-2b, beta-interferons, and interferon gamma-1b are administered via subcutaneous injection. Interferon alfa-n3 is injected directly into the base of the wart.

Cautions and Concerns

Variations in dosage and adverse reactions exist among different brands of interferon. Therefore, different brands of interferon should not be used in a single treatment regimen.

Infrequently, severe kidney toxicities, sometimes requiring dialysis, have been reported with alfa-interferon therapy alone or in combination with interleukin-2. In patients with impaired kidney function, signs and symptoms of interferon toxicity should be closely monitored.

Transplantation patients or other chronically immunosuppressed patients should receive alfa-interferon therapy with caution.

Interferon may impair fertility. Therefore, fertile women should not receive interferon therapy unless they are using effective contraception during the therapy period. Interferon therapy should also be used with caution in fertile men.

Because of fever and other flulike symptoms associated with interferon alfa-n3, it should be used with caution in patients with debilitating medical conditions, such as cardiovascular disease (e.g., unstable angina and uncontrolled congestive heart failure), severe pulmonary disease (e.g., chronic obstructive pulmonary disease), or diabetes mellitus with ketoacidosis (see *Warnings*). Also, use this agent cautiously in patients with coagulation disorders (e.g., thrombophlebitis, pulmonary embolism, and hemophilia), severe myelosuppression, or seizure disorders. Because interferon alfa-n3 is made from human blood, it may carry a risk of transmitting infectious agents such as viruses.

While fever may be related to the flulike symptoms reported in patients treated with interferon alfacon-1, when fever occurs, other possible causes of persistent fever should be ruled out. Interferon alfacon-1 should be used cautiously in patients with abnormally low peripheral blood cell counts or who are receiving agents that are known to cause myelosuppression. Interferon alfacon-1 should be administered with caution to patients with preexisting cardiac disease, as hypertension, tachycardia, palpitations, and arrhythmias have been reported.

The safety and efficacy of peginterferon alfa-2a or peginterferon alfa-2b has not been established in patients who have failed alfa-interferon treatment with or without ribavirin, in liver or other organ transplant recipients, in patients with HBV who are coinfected with HCV or HIV, or in patients with HCV who are coinfected with HBV or HIV.

Caution should be exercised in initiating peginterferon alfa-2a treatment in any patient with risk of severe anemia (e.g., spherocytosis [a disease of the blood characterized by the production of sphere-shaped red blood cells] or a history of gastrointestinal [GI] bleeding). In patients with impaired kidney function, signs and symptoms of peginterferon alfa-2a toxicity should be closely monitored. Peginterferon alfa-2a should be used with caution in patients with creatinine clearance <50 mL/min.

The safety and efficacy of beta-interferons in chronic-progressive MS have not been evaluated.

Patients should be instructed in injection techniques to assure the safe self-administration of beta-interferons (see *Warnings*). Patients with cardiac disease, such as angina, congestive heart failure, or arrhythmia, should be closely monitored for worsening of their clinical condition during initiation and continued treatment with beta-interferons. While beta-interferons do not have any known direct-acting cardiac toxicity, during the postmarketing period infrequent cases of cardiomyopathy have been reported in patients without known predisposition to these events and without other known causes being established. Autoimmune disorders of multiple target organs have been reported with beta-interferons in postmarketing reports, including idiopathic thrombocytopenia, hyper- and hypothyroidism, and rare cases of autoimmune hepatitis. Patients should be monitored for signs of these disorders and appropriate treatment implemented when observed.

Caution should be exercised when administering interferon beta-1a to patients with preexisting seizure disorders. Seizures have been reported in clinical trials in patients receiving interferon beta-1a with no prior history of seizures. It is not known whether these events were related to the effects of MS alone, to interferon beta-1a, or to a combination of both. The effect of interferon beta-1a administration on the medical management of patients with seizure disorder is unknown.

Isolated cases of acute serious hypersensitivity reactions have been observed in patients receiving interferon gamma-1b. If such an acute reaction develops, the drug should be discontinued immediately and appropriate medical therapy instituted. Transient skin rashes have occurred in some patients following injection but have rarely necessitated treatment interruption.

In addition to those tests normally required for monitoring patients with CGD and osteopetrosis, the following laboratory tests are recommended for all patients on interferon gamma-1b therapy prior to the beginning of and at three month intervals during treatment: complete blood counts (with differential), platelet counts, kidney and liver function tests, and urinalysis (see *Warnings*).

Warnings

Alfa-interferons cause or aggravate fatal or life-threatening neuropsychiatric, autoimmune, and infectious disorders and ischemic heart disease. Patients being administered alfa-interferons should be monitored closely with periodic clinical and laboratory evaluations. Patients with persistently severe or worsening signs or symptoms of these conditions should be withdrawn from therapy. In many, but not all, cases these disorders resolve after stopping therapy.

Baseline eye exams should be performed in all patients, with periodic reassessment in patients with abnormalities. Patients with thyroid abnormalities should be monitored by having thyroid hormone levels measured at baseline and every three months during therapy.

In those patients being treated for chronic HCV, liver enzymes should be monitored at baseline, after the initial two weeks of therapy, and then monthly thereafter. In these patients, HCV-RNA levels should also be monitored, particularly in first three months of therapy.

In those patients being treated for chronic myelogenous leukemia or hairy cell leukemia, hematologic monitoring should be performed on a monthly basis.

Interferon alfa-2b should be used cautiously in patients with a history of cardiovascular disease. Those patients with a history of myocardial infarction or arrhythmias who require interferon alfa-2b therapy should be closely monitored.

Development or exacerbation of autoimmune diseases including idiopathic thrombocytopenic purpura, vasculitis, Raynaud's syndrome, rheumatoid arthritis, psoriasis, interstitial nephritis, thyroiditis, systemic lupus erythematosus, hepatitis, myositis, rhabdomyolysis, and sarcoidosis have been observed in patients treated with alfa-interferons. Any patient developing an autoimmune disorder during treatment should be closely monitored, and, if appropriate, treatment should be discontinued.

Depression and suicidal behavior have been reported in association with treatment with alfa- or beta-interferons in patients with and without previous psychiatric illness. These agents should be used with extreme caution in patients who report a history of depression or other mood disorders. Patients should be informed that depression and suicidal ideation may be side effects of treatment and should be advised to report these side effects immediately to the prescribing physician. Patients receiving this therapy should receive close monitoring for symptoms of depression. Psychiatric intervention and/or cessation of treatment should be considered for patients experiencing depression. Although dose reduction or stopping treatment may resolve its symptoms, depression may persist, and suicides have occurred after withdrawing therapy.

Serious, acute hypersensitivity reactions (e.g., urticaria, angioedema, bronchoconstriction, and anaphylaxis) as well as skin rashes have been rarely observed during alfa-interferon therapy. Development of a serious reaction requires discontinuation of treatment and immediate appropriate medical therapy. Transient rashes do not necessitate interruption of treatment.

Severe liver damage, including rare cases of liver failure requiring liver transplantation and also of fatality, has been observed in patients treated with alfa-interferons or interferon beta-1a. Symptoms of liver dysfunction have begun from one to six months following the initiation of therapy. Any patient developing liver function abnormalities during treatment should be monitored closely, and if appropriate, treatment should be discontinued. In patients with chronic HCV, initiation of alfa-interferon therapy has been reported to cause transient liver abnormalities, which in patients with poorly compensated liver disease can result in increased fluid accumulation, liver failure, or death. Patients with chronic HCV or HBC and concomitant decompensated liver disease, autoimmune hepatitis, a history of autoimmune disease, and those who are immunosuppressed transplant recipients should not be treated with interferon alfa-2b. Worsening liver disease including jaundice, hepatic encephalopathy, liver failure, and death following interferon alfa-2b therapy have been reported in such patients. If jaundice or other symptoms of liver dysfunction appear, treatment with interferon beta-1a should be discontinued immediately due to the potential for rapid progression to liver failure.

Infrequently, severe or fatal gastrointestinal hemorrhage has been reported in association with alfa-interferon therapy. Ulcerative and hemorrhagic/ischemic colitis, sometimes fatal, have been observed within 12 weeks of starting alfa-interferon treatment. The alfa-interferon should be discontinued immediately if symptoms (abdominal pain, bloody diarrhea, and fever) develop. The colitis usually resolves within one to three weeks of discontinuation of alfa-interferon.

While fever may be associated with the flulike syndrome reported commonly during interferon therapy, other causes of high or persistent fever must be ruled out, particularly in patients with neutropenia. Severe infections (bacterial, viral, fungal), some fatal, have been reported during treatment with alfa-interferons. Appropriate anti-infective therapy should be started immediately, and discontinuation of interferon therapy should be considered.

Alfa-interferons suppress bone marrow function and may result in severe cytopenias (e.g., leukopenia, thrombocytopenia) and anemia, including very rare events of aplastic anemia. Cytopenias can lead to an increased risk of infections or hemorrhage. A complete blood count should be obtained pretreatment and monitored routinely during therapy. Alfa-interferon therapy should be discontinued in patients who develop severe decreases in neutrophil ($<0.5 \times 10^9$/L) or platelet counts ($<25 \times 10^9$/L).

Shortness of breath, pneumonia, bronchiolitis obliterans (an inflammation of the bronchioles and surrounding tissue in the lungs), interstitial pneumonitis, and sarcoidosis, sometimes resulting in respiratory failure and/or death, may be induced or aggravated by alfa-interferon therapy. Patients who develop persistent or unexplained pulmonary infiltrates or pulmonary function impairment should discontinue treatment with alfa-interferons.

Decrease or loss of vision, retinopathy including macular edema, retinal artery or vein thrombosis, retinal hemorrhages, optic neuritis, and papilledema may be induced or aggravated by treatment with alfa-interferons. All patients should receive an eye examination at baseline. Patients with preexisting ophthalmologic disorders (e.g., diabetic or hypertensive retinopathy) should receive periodic ophthalmologic exams during alfa-interferon treatment. Any patient who develops ocular symptoms should receive a prompt and complete eye examination. Interferon treatment should be discontinued in patients who develop new or worsening ophthalmologic disorders.

Pancreatitis has been observed in patients receiving alfa-interferon treatment, including those who developed elevated triglyceride levels. In some cases, fatalities have been observed. Although a causal relationship to interferon therapy has not been established, marked triglyceride elevation is a risk factor for development of pancreatitis. Interferon therapy should be suspended if signs or symptoms suggestive of pancreatitis are observed. In patients diagnosed with pancreatitis, discontinuation of therapy with interferon treatment should be considered.

Caution should be exercised when administering interferon alfa-2b to patients with myelosuppression or when these drugs are used in combination with other agents that are known to cause myelosuppression. Also, patients receiving interferon alfa-2b along with zidovudine may have an increased incidence of neutropenia.

Supraventricular arrhythmias, chest pain, and myocardial infarction have been associated with alfa-interferon therapies. Cases of cardiomyopathy have also been observed on rare occasions in patients treated with alfa-interferons.

Infrequently, patients receiving alfa-interferon therapy develop thyroid abnormalities, including hypothyroidism or hyperthyroidism. Patients developing symptoms consistent with possible thyroid dysfunction during the course of interferon therapy should have their thyroid function evaluated and appropriate treatment instituted. Discontinuation of interferon therapy has not always reversed thyroid dysfunction occurring during treatment. Diabetes mellitus has been observed in patients treated with alfa-interferons. Patients with these conditions who cannot be effectively treated by medication should not begin interferon therapy. Patients who develop these conditions during treatment and cannot be controlled with medication should not continue interferon therapy. Patients with diabetes mellitus may require adjustment of their diabetes medications.

Use of interferon alfa-2b with ribavirin may cause birth defects and/or death of an unborn child. This combination therapy should not be started until a report of a negative pregnancy test has been obtained immediately prior to planned initiation of therapy. Women of childbearing potential should not receive interferon alfa-2b with ribavirin unless they are using two reliable forms of contraception during the therapy period. In addition, effective contraception should be utilized for six months after therapy is completed. Female patients should also have monthly pregnancy tests. Male patients and their female partners must practice two reliable forms of contraception during treatment with this combination.

Use of interferon alfa-2b with ribavirin has also been associated with hemolytic anemia (the abnormal breakdown of red blood cells). Anemia occurred within one to two weeks of initiation of ribavirin therapy. Because of this initial acute drop in hemoglobin, complete blood counts should be obtained before treatment is initiated and at week two and week four of therapy or more frequently if clinically indicated.

Anaphylaxis has been reported as a rare complication of interferon beta-1a use. Other allergic reactions have included skin rash and urticaria and have ranged from mild to severe without a clear relationship to dose or duration of exposure. Several allergic reactions, some severe, have occurred after prolonged use.

Some interferon beta-1a products contain albumin, a derivative of human blood. Based on effective donor screening and product manufacturing processes, these products carry an extremely remote risk for transmission of viral diseases.

Acute and transient flulike symptoms such as fever and chills induced by interferon gamma-1b higher than recommended doses may exacerbate preexisting cardiac conditions. Interferon gamma-1b should be used with caution in patients with preexisting cardiac conditions, including ischemia, congestive heart failure, or arrhythmia.

Decreased mental status, gait disturbance, and dizziness have been observed, particularly in patients receiving interferon gamma-1b greater than recommended doses. Most of these abnormalities were mild and reversible within a few days upon dose reduction or discontinuation of therapy. Caution should be exercised when administering interferon gamma-1b to patients with seizure disorders or compromised central nervous system function.

Reversible neutropenia and thrombocytopenia that can be severe and may be dose-related have been observed during interferon gamma-1b therapy. Caution should be exercised when administering interferon gamma-1b to patients with myelosuppression.

Elevated liver enzymes have been observed during interferon gamma-1b therapy. The incidence appeared to be higher in patients less than one year of age compared to older children. Patients begun on this agent before age one year should receive monthly assessments of liver function. If severe liver enzyme elevations develop, dosage should be modified.

When Not Advised (Contraindications)

Peginterferon alfa-2a should not be used in patients with known hypersensitivity to *E. coli*–derived products, autoimmune hepatitis, or hepatic decompensation (Child-Pugh class B and C) before or during treatment. This agent is also contraindicated in newborns and infants because it contains benzyl alcohol. Benzyl alcohol is associated with an increased incidence of sometimes fatal neurologic and other complications in these patients.

Interferon alfa-2b, interferon alfacon-1, and peginterferon alfa-2b should not be used in patients with autoimmune hepatitis or decompensated liver disease.

Combination therapy containing interferon alfa-2b, peginterferon alfa-2a, or peginterferon alfa-2b with ribavirin is contraindicated in women who are pregnant, men whose female partners are pregnant, patients with hemoglobinopathies (e.g., thalassemia major, sickle-cell anemia), and patients with creatinine clearance <50 mL/min (see *Warnings*).

Interferon alfa-n3 is contraindicated in patients who have anaphylactic sensitivity to mouse immunoglobulin, egg protein, or neomycin.

Interferon beta-1b and interferon gamma-1b should not be used in patients with known hypersensitivity to *E. coli*–derived products.

Side Effects

Depression and suicidal behavior have been reported in association with the use of alfa-interferon products (see *Warnings*).

Other common side effects with peginterferon alfa-2a include headache, dizziness, injection site reaction, skin rash, nausea, vomiting, loss of appetite, diarrhea, flulike symptoms (e.g., fever, chills, sweating, muscle aches, and tiredness), and joint or bone pain.

The most frequently reported side effects with interferon alfa-2b are flulike symptoms such as fever, headache, chills, myalgia (muscle pain), and fatigue.

Nearly one-third of patients receiving interferon alfa-n3 therapy in clinical trials reported flulike symptoms, which in most cases were mild and transient (see *Cautions and Concerns* and *Warnings*). In addition to these symptoms and the depression reported with alfa-interferons, other common side effects with interferon alfa-n3 include fatigue, nausea, lack of appetite, vomiting, and diarrhea.

In addition to flulike symptoms and depression (see *Warnings*), common side effects with interferon alfacon-1 therapy include amnesia, dizziness, insomnia, alopecia, itching, rash, abdominal pain, loss of appetite, diarrhea, nausea, vomiting, back and limb pain, anxiety, nervousness, cough, sinusitis, upper respiratory tract congestion, noncardiac chest pain, and hot flushes.

In clinical trials, peginterferon alfa-2b induced fatigue or headache in approximately two-thirds of patients and induced fever or rigors in approximately half of the patients. The severity of these side effects tends to decrease as treatment continues. Other common side effects with peginterferon alfa-2b therapy include insomnia, alopecia, abdominal pain, loss of appetite, nausea, and musculoskeletal pain.

In addition to depression and suicidal ideation (see *Warnings*), the most common side effects with beta-interferons include flulike symptoms, loss of strength, nausea, sinusitis, and headache.

The most common side effects from interferon gamma-1b are flulike symptoms that include fever, headache, chills, muscle pain, and fatigue (see *Warnings*). Other common side effects include rash, injection site tenderness, diarrhea, vomiting, and nausea.

Interactions

Coadministration of interferons with other agents known to induce liver damage may increase the risk of liver injury (see *Warnings*).

Concomitant use of alfa-interferon and theophylline decreases theophylline clearance resulting in a 100 percent increase in serum theophylline levels. Interactions between alfa-interferons and other drugs have not been fully evaluated. Caution should be exercised when administering alfa-interferons in combination with other potentially myelosuppressive agents.

No drug interactions with interferon alfa-n3 have been reported.

Peginterferon alfa-2a and peginterferon alfa-2b may increase concentrations of methadone; thus, it may be appropriate to monitor for signs and symptoms of increased narcotic effect during coadministration of these drugs.

No formal drug interaction studies have been conducted with beta- or gamma-interferons. Due to its potential to cause neutropenia and lymphopenia, proper monitoring of patients is required if interferon beta-1a is given in combination with myelosuppressive agents. Caution should also be exercised when administering interferon gamma-1b in combination with other potentially myelosuppressive agents.

Sales/Statistics

Global sales for interferons are reported to be U.S. $5 billion, with the market for interferons in HCV a little more than $2 billion. But that number only scratches the surface of what is possible, according to a pharmaceutical executive, because only about 40 percent of people who are diagnosed with HCV in the United States and in other developed countries are actually treated.

In the United States, two interferons appeared on the "2008 Top 200 Branded Drugs by Retail Dollars" (*Drug Topics,* May 26, 2009): #123, Avonex, with sales of $273,303,000, and #164, Pegasys, with $164,472,000 in sales.

Three interferons were on the 2010 list (*Drug Topics,* June 2011): Avonex ranked #109 ($303,147,918 in sales), Betaseron #192 ($155,952,005), and Pegasys #195 ($153,101,276).

Demographics and Cultural Groups

Black patients with chronic HCV have lower response rates than white patients to both interferon monotherapy and combination therapy of interferon plus ribavirin. In one analysis of two multicenter trials involving combination therapy, sustained response was highest among Asians (61 percent), followed by whites (39 percent), Hispanics (23 percent), and blacks (14 percent). The factors responsible for these differences are unknown.

Development History

Interferon was discovered by the British virologist Alick Isaacs and the Swiss researcher Jean Lindenmann at the National Institute for Medical Research in London. They noticed an interference effect caused by heat-inactivated influenza virus on the growth of live influenza virus in chicken egg membranes in a nutritive (providing nourishment) solution chorioallantoic membrane (the membrane in hens' eggs that helps chicken embryos get enough oxygen and calcium for development) and published their results in 1957. In this paper, they coined the term *interferon.*

Marcus wrote 50 years later, "That seminal finding launched a new era in our understanding of viral interference, and what was to become a new class of potent biological response modifiers." Interferon was scarce and expensive until 1980, when the interferon gene was inserted into bacteria using recombinant DNA technology, allowing mass cultivation and purification from bacterial cultures. Approvals for the current interferon agents: interferon alfa-n3 in 1989, interferon gamma-1b in 1990, interferon alfa-2b in 1991, interferon beta-1b in 1993, interferon beta-1a in 1996, interferon alfacon-1 in 1997, peginterferon alfa-2b in 2001, and peginterferon alfa-2a in 2002.

Future Drugs

PEG-interferon lambda (IL-29) is a novel interferon being developed by ZymoGenetics as a potential treatment for patients infected with HCV. PEG-interferon lambda is generated in response to viral infection, signals through a receptor with a more restricted expression pattern than that used by alfa- or beta-interferons, and has broad antiviral activity. Researchers have completed a Phase Ia study in healthy volunteers showing that this drug has the potential to be an effective antiviral agent without the toxicities of other interferons. Even if it is later confirmed that interferon lambda is not as effective at attacking the hepatitis virus as interferon alfa, it is possible that it could become a treatment option at some level because it may cause fewer side effects.

OctoPlus, a Netherlands biopharmaceutical company, is in Phase II clinical trials with Locteron, a sustained-release formulation of interferon alfa for the treatment of chronic HCV. The developers hope that Locteron will induce fewer side effects, improve patient compliance, and provide a more convenient dosing schedule compared with current therapies.

Amarillo Biosciences, in partnership with Hayashibara Group, has been testing an oral interferon alfa for several indications, including thrombocytosis, Sjögren's syndrome, pulmonary fibrosis, polycythemia vera, human papillomavirus infections, and fibromyalgia.

Much of the current interferon research involves new indications for current drugs. For example, Hemispherx Biopharma, Inc. has interferon alfa-n3 in clinical development for treating West Nile virus, MS, influenza virus infections, HIV infections, HCV, human papillomavirus infections, and coronavirus infections. Also, Genentech and InterMune are studying interferon gamma-1b for possible treatment of HCV and cystic fibrosis.

Isaacs, Alick, and Jean Lindenmann. "Virus Interference. I. The interferon." *Proceedings of the Royal Society of London. Series B, Biological Sciences* 147, no. 927 (September 12, 1957): 258–267.

Marcus, Philip I. "Celebrating the 50th Anniversary of the Discovery of Interferon." *Journal of Interferon & Cytokine Research* 27, no. 2 (February 1, 2007): 87–90.

laxatives Drugs used to stimulate a person's bowels for defecation, or the expulsion of feces; also known as cathartics and purgatives. Laxatives are most often taken to treat constipation, which is one of the most common gastrointestinal (GI) complaints in the United States. More than 4 million Americans have frequent constipation, accounting for 2.5 million physician visits a year, according to the National Institute of Diabetes and Digestive and Kidney Diseases (NIDDK). Those reporting constipation most often are women and adults ages 65 and older. Pregnant women may have constipation, and it is a common problem following childbirth or surgery. Some laxatives are used to empty the colon for rectal and bowel examinations. Most laxatives are available over the counter (OTC); a few only by prescription.

Classes

Laxatives are divided into several types according to how they function.

- *Bulk-forming—Examples:* methylcellulose (Citrucel), polycarbophil (Equalactin, Fiber-Con, Fiber-Lax, Konsyl Fiber), and psyllium (Fiberall, Konsyl-D, Metamucil).
- *Lubricants—Example:* mineral oil (Fleet Mineral Oil Enema, Kondremul).
- *Osmotic laxatives—Examples:* glycerin (Colace Suppositories, Fleet Babylax), lactulose (Constulose, Enulose, Generlac, Kristalose), sorbitol, polyethylene glycol 3350 (GlycoLax, MiraLAX), and polyethylene glycol-electrolyte solution (Colyte, GoLytely, MoviPrep, NuLytely, Trilyte).

- *Saline laxatives—Examples:* magnesium citrate (Citroma), magnesium hydroxide (Phillips' Milk of Magnesia), magnesium sulfate, and sodium phosphates (Fleet Enema, Fleet Phospho-Soda, OsmoPrep, Visicol).
- *Stimulants—Examples:* bisacodyl (Correctol, Doxidan, Dulcolax, Fleet Bisacodyl), cascara sagrada, castor oil, and senna (Ex-Lax, Senokot, SenoSol).
- *Stool softeners* (also called surfactants and emollients)—*Example:* docusate (Colace, Genasoft, Surfak).

How They Work

Bulk-forming laxatives are taken with water. They absorb the water, making the stool softer and more bulky in the intestine. This stimulates the normal forward movement of the intestines (peristalsis), resulting in a bowel movement within 12 to 24 hours.

Lubricants grease the stool, enabling it to move through the intestine more easily.

Osmotic laxatives cause fluids to flow in a special way through the colon, resulting in bowel distention.

Saline laxatives act like a sponge to draw water into the colon for easier passage of stool.

Stimulants cause rhythmic muscle contractions in the intestines, increasing motility. They also increase water secretion and decrease reabsorption.

Stool softeners moisten the stool and prevent dehydration. They decrease surface tension, increase water secretion, and limit its reabsorption by the intestinal wall.

Approved Uses

All laxatives are approved to treat constipation.

Polycarbophil and psyllium are also used to slow down diarrhea associated with conditions such as irritable bowel syndrome (IBS) and diverticulosis.

Lubricants and stool softeners are used in patients who should not strain during defecation, such as following anorectal surgery. Mineral oil enema is used for relief of fecal impaction.

Osmotic laxatives are useful for people with idiopathic constipation (no known cause). In patients with a history of chronic constipation, lactulose therapy increases the number of bowel movements per day and the number of days on which bowel movements occur. Polyethylene glycol-electrolyte solution is used for bowel cleansing prior to colonoscopy or barium enema X-ray examination. Lactulose is also used for the prevention and treatment of portal-systemic encephalopathy (a major neuropsychiatric complication of chronic liver disease), including the stages of hepatic pre-coma and coma.

Saline laxatives are used to treat acute constipation if there is no indication of bowel obstruction.

Stool softeners are used to prevent dry, hard stools. They are often recommended after childbirth or surgery.

Off-Label Uses

Psyllium is used off-label to reduce cholesterol levels as an adjunct to diet.

Polyethylene glycol 3350 is used off-label in the management of acute iron overdose in children.

Administration

Laxatives are taken by mouth and are available in liquid, tablet, powder, and granule forms.

Mineral oil, bisacodyl, and sodium phosphates are also given as enemas.

Glycerin and bisacodyl are also available as rectal suppositories.

Cautions and Concerns

Rectal bleeding or failure to respond to laxative therapy may indicate a serious condition that may require further medical attention.

Some laxative products contain tartrazine, which may cause allergic-type reactions (including bronchial asthma) in susceptible individuals, particularly those who have aspirin hypersensitivity.

Blockage of the intestine or the esophagus may be caused by bulk-forming agents in patients with narrowing of the digestive tract (including esophageal stricture, intestinal stricture, or severe adhesions). It is important that plenty of fluid be taken with these agents.

In the overall management of portal-systemic encephalopathy, there is serious underlying liver disease with complications such as electrolyte disturbance (e.g., hypokalemia), which may require other specific therapy. Elderly, debilitated patients who receive lactulose longer than six months should have serum electrolytes (potassium, chloride) and carbon dioxide measured periodically. Because lactulose syrup contains galactose and lactose, it should be used with caution in these individuals.

Laxative products containing sodium (e.g., sodium phosphates) should be used cautiously by individuals on a sodium-restricted diet and in the presence of edema, chronic heart failure (CHF), kidney failure, or borderline hypertension (see *When Not Advised [Contraindications]*).

Patients with impaired gag reflex, unconscious or semiconscious patients, and patients prone to regurgitation or aspiration should be observed during the administration of polyethylene glycol-electrolyte solution, especially if it is administered via nasogastric tube (a tube passing through the nose and into the stomach).

Warnings

Laxatives should be restricted for short-term therapy of constipation; chronic use of laxatives (particularly stimulants) may lead to dependence.

Excessive laxative use may lead to significant fluid and electrolyte imbalance. Cathartic colon, a poorly functioning colon, results from chronic abuse of stimulant laxatives.

Prescription oral sodium-phosphate products carry a risk of acute phosphate nephropathy (a type of acute kidney injury) when used to cleanse the bowel before a colonoscopy (colon examination) and other medical procedures. The available data do not show a risk of acute kidney injury when over-the-counter oral sodium phosphate products are used at the lower doses for laxative use. However, when used for bowel cleansing, these products have the same risks as prescription products. Oral sodium-phosphate prescription products should be used with caution for bowel cleansing by the following at risk groups: people over 55 years of age; people who suffer from dehydration, kidney disease, acute colitis, or delayed bowel emptying; and people taking drugs that affect kidney function (e.g., diuretics, angiotensin-converting enzyme inhibitors [used to treat high blood pressure, heart disease, or kidney failure], angiotensin receptor blockers [used to treat high blood pressure, heart disease, or kidney failure], and nonsteroidal anti-inflammatory drugs).

No additional ingredients (e.g., flavorings) should be added to the polyethylene glycol-electrolyte solution. Polyethylene glycol-electrolyte solution should be used with caution in patients with severe ulcerative colitis.

When Not Advised (Contraindications)

Laxatives should not be taken by patients who are experiencing nausea, vomiting, or other symptoms of appendicitis, fecal impaction, intestinal obstruction, or undiagnosed abdominal pain.

Polyethylene glycol-electrolyte solution should not be used in patients with ileus, gastric retention, gastrointestinal obstruction, bowel perforation, toxic colitis, and toxic megacolon.

Sodium phosphates should not be used in patients with bowel obstruction or CHF, as dehydration may occur.

Patients who require a low galactose diet should not take lactulose.

Side Effects

Common side effects of laxatives include diarrhea, nausea, vomiting, fainting, bloating, flatulence, and cramps.

When bulk-forming laxatives are taken without adequate fluids or in patients with intestinal stenosis (narrowing), obstruction of the esophagus, stomach, small intestine, or colon may occur (see *Cautions and Concerns*).

Large doses of mineral oil may cause anal seepage, resulting in rectal inflammation, itching, and discomfort.

Interactions

Mineral oil and docusate should not be used in combination, as docusate will increase the absorption of mineral oil. Absorption of lipid-soluble vitamins may decrease during prolonged use of mineral oil.

Lactulose decreases the effects of neomycin and antacids.

Polyethylene glycol 3500, polyethylene glycol-electrolyte solution, polycarbophil, and psyllium may decrease absorption of oral medications, thereby reducing effectiveness. These laxatives should be spaced apart from other drug therapies by at least two hours.

Bisacodyl tablets are enteric coated and should not be used in combination with antacids. The antacids may cause the enteric coating to dissolve, resulting in gastric lining irritation or heartburn.

Sales/Statistics

Around $725 million is spent on laxative products each year in America, according to NIDDK.

Among the prescription laxatives, polyethylene glycol ranked #104 on *Drug Topics* "2010 Top 200 Generic Drugs by Retail Dollars," with $136,775,971 in sales, and #111 on the "2010 Top 200 Generic Drugs by Total Prescriptions," with 5,058,545 units sold (*Drug Topics,* June 2011).

Demographics and Cultural Groups

Constipation with no known organic cause (no medical explanation) is more prevalent in females than in males. However, there are no significant differences in the way laxatives function in males and females.

Development History

Laxative use goes back at least to the Egyptians, with these agents appearing to "have dominated their pharmaceuticals," according to a *Discovery News* report, with bulk laxatives, such as figs, bran, and dates in common use.

Polyethylene glycol 3350 first became available after receiving FDA approval in 1999 as a prescription drug and later, in 2006, as an OTC medicine.

According to the FDA, one of the first brand names of lactulose (Chronulac, which is no longer available) was approved in 1979.

Future Drugs

Linaclotide is a first-in-class compound in Phase II trials for the treatment of IBS, chronic constipation, and other GI disorders. Linaclotide is an agonist of guanylate cyclase type-C, a receptor found on the lining of the intestine. In preclinical testing, linaclotide was shown to decrease visceral pain, increase fluid secretion into the intestine, and accelerate intestinal transit. Linaclotide is being developed by Ironwood Pharmaceuticals, Inc. and Forest Laboratories, Inc.

Callisto Pharmaceuticals, Inc. filed an IND (Investigational New Drug application) on April 2, 2008, with the FDA for SP-304 (guanilib) for the treatment of chronic constipation and constipation-predominant irritable bowel syndrome. SP-304 is an analog of uroguanylin, a natural hormone produced in the GI tract that is a key regulator of intestinal function. SP-304 works by activating a unique receptor, the GC-C receptor, on intestinal epithelial cells, promoting fluid and ion transport. The drug is administered orally.

Theravance, Inc. is developing a new GI motility drug, TD-5018, designed to treat chronic constipation and other disorders related to reduced GI motility. In early clinical trials, low doses of TD-5108 were well tolerated with a low incidence of adverse events.

leukotriene modifiers (LTMs) The first new classification of drugs approved for specific treatment of asthma since inhaled corticosteroids were introduced in 1972. According to the National Heart, Lung, and Blood Institute's (NHLBI) National Asthma Education and Prevention Program (NAEPP), leukotriene modifiers are an alternative medication for use in children with mild persistent asthma, particularly for children unable to comply with inhaled corticosteroids. They are considered to be an additional medication for the step-up approach, or combination therapy, recommended by the NAEPP for moderate and severe persistent asthma not controlled with inhaled corticosteroids alone. They have been shown to be effective in long-term symptom control in patients with asthma and allergic rhinitis (sneezing, stuffy nose, runny nose, and itching of the nose). NAEPP found these drugs to provide only a modest improvement in lung function and generally to be less effective than inhaled corticosteroids.

According to the National Quality Measures Clearinghouse (Agency for Healthcare Research and Quality) in 2011, "Asthma is one of the nation's most costly and high-impact diseases. It has become increasingly common over the past two decades. Approximately 34.1 million Americans have been diagnosed with asthma and each year nearly 5,000 Americans die of it. Many asthma-related deaths, hospitalizations, emergency room visits and missed work and school days could be avoided if patients had appropriate medications and medical management."

Classes

The three approved leukotriene modifiers are divided into two classes:

• Leukotriene-receptor antagonists (LTRAs, also known as cysteinyl leukotriene receptor antagonists, prevent leukotriene binding. *Examples:* montelukast (Singulair) and zafirlukast (Accolate).

- Leukotriene-receptor inhibitors focus on synthesis inhibition. *Example:* zileuton (Zyflo) and zileuton ER (Zyflo CR).

How They Work

Leukotrienes are chemicals released by mast cells in the airways that act as a trigger for an asthma attack. Overproduction of leukotrienes in response to allergens, exercise, or other irritants is a major cause of inflammation in asthma and allergic rhinitis. Blocking the actions of leukotrienes helps prevent these attacks from occurring.

LTRAs are antagonists of cysteinyl leukotriene and exert their biological effect by binding to receptors located on airway smooth muscles. By blocking the interaction between leukotrienes and their respective receptors, it is believed that they inhibit the inflammatory effects.

Zileuton blocks the synthesis of 5-lipoxygenase from arachidonic acid and thus inhibits leukotriene formation.

In common terms, leukotriene modifiers reduce and prevent swelling inside the airways, stop mucus from forming, and relax smooth muscles around the airways. Leukotriene modifiers do not show immediate results but work slowly over time. They do not stop an asthma episode once it has started.

Approved Uses

Montelukast is used for prevention and chronic treatment of asthma in patients 12 months of age and older, for acute prevention of exercise-induced bronchoconstriction (EIB) in patients 15 years of age and older, and for relief of symptoms of allergic rhinitis (AR) (seasonal allergic rhinitis [SAR] in patients two years of age and older and perennial allergic rhinitis [PAR] in patients six months of age and older).

Zafirlukast is used for the chronic treatment of asthma in adults and children five years of age and older.

Zileuton is used for the prevention and chronic treatment of asthma in adults and children 12 years of age and older.

Off-Label Uses

Leukotriene modifiers are used off-label to treat sinusitis and nasal polyps, particularly in patients who cannot take aspirin.

Companion Drugs

Leukotriene modifiers are often used along with intranasal corticosteroids and/or antihistamines.

Administration

Montelukast is taken once a day (in the evening for asthma and at least two hours before exercise for prevention of exercise-induced bronchoconstriction) and is available as tablets, chewable tablets, and oral granules.

Zafirlukast is a tablet taken twice a day on an empty stomach (one hour before eating or two hours after eating).

Zileuton is a tablet taken four times a day with or without food. Zileuton extended release tablets are taken twice daily within one hour after morning and evening meals.

Cautions and Concerns

Neuropsychiatric events have been reported in some patients taking leukotriene modifiers. The reported neuropsychiatric events include postmarket cases of agitation, aggression, anxiousness, dream abnormalities and hallucinations, depression, insomnia, irritability, restlessness, suicidal thinking and behavior (including suicide), and tremor.

Zafirlukast and zileuton affect theophylline and warfarin levels, requiring frequent monitoring of theophylline level and prothrombin time in those individuals taking these medications.

The dose of zafirlukast may need to be reduced in patients over 65 years of age due to reduced clearance in urine.

Systemic eosinophilia, sometimes presenting with clinical features of vasculitis consistent with Churg-Strauss syndrome, has been reported with monteluskat. These events usually, but not always, have been associated with the reduction of oral corticosteroid therapy. Physicians should be alert to eosinophilia, vasculitic rash, worsening pulmonary symptoms, cardiac complications, and/or neuropathy presenting in their patients. A causal association between montelukast and these underlying conditions has not been established.

Patients with known aspirin sensitivity should continue to avoid aspirin or nonsteroidal anti-inflammatory agents (NSAIDs) while taking montelukast.

Due to the effect that zileuton has on the hepatic system, zileuton should be used with caution in patients who consume substantial quantities of alcohol and/or have a past history of liver disease.

Warnings

Zileuton can cause liver injury, and its use requires pretreatment baseline and periodic liver function monitoring for patient safety. Patients will need to have blood tests every month for the first three months, then every two to three months for the next nine months, and then periodically while taking zileuton.

Because elevated liver transaminases have been noted in individuals taking leukotriene modifiers, the FDA advises that liver function be tested monthly for three months, then quarterly for the next year, followed by intermittent testing.

When Not Advised (Contraindications)

Zafirlukast is contraindicated in patients with liver impairment, including cirrhosis.

Zileuton ER is contraindicated in patients with active liver disease or persistent alanine aminotransferase (ALT) elevations of three times or more the upper limit of normal.

Side Effects

Side effects of leukotriene modifiers include upper respiratory infection, headache, dental pain, stomachache, nausea, diarrhea, and flulike symptoms

Interactions

Zileuton has been shown to increase the blood levels or effects of theophylline, propranolol, and warfarin (see *Cautions and Concerns*). The avoidance of alcohol is recommended, owing to increased risk of central nervous system depression as well as an increased risk of liver toxicity. In addition, the herbal supplement Saint-John's-wort may decrease blood levels of zileuton

Sales/Statistics

According to a report from the IMS Institute for Healthcare Informatics (the public reporting arm of IMS, a pharmaceutical market intelligence firm), Singulair was the seventh-highest U.S. pharmaceutical product by spending in 2010, accounting for $4,072,796,545 in sales. Singulair ranked tenth in number of prescriptions dispensed (28,479,750).

Demographics and Cultural Groups

See BRONCHODILATORS for asthma demographics and cultural groups.

Development History

Zafirlukast was the first oral leukotriene-receptor antagonist approved by the FDA, with approval coming on September 26, 1996. Approval of montelukast tablets and chewable tablets followed on February 20, 1998. The montelukast oral gruanules formulation was approved on July 26, 2002.

Although a new formulation was launched in 2005, zileuton was originally approved on December 9, 1996. A sustained-release formulation was approved on May 30, 2007.

Future Drugs

According to an article in *Nature Medicine,* "Asthma affects an estimated 235 million people globally, and as that number grows, so does the demand for drugs to cope with the illness. GlobalData, a London-based research firm, says the global asthma market will expand from around $12.4 billion in 2009 to $14 billion by 2017. GlobalData identified no fewer than 229 molecules in the pharmaceutical pipeline in development against asthma. Many of those drugs will be inhalers, but because tablets offer more likelihood of compliance, experts expect research and development to continue in the leukotriene modifier classes.

May, Mike. "Drug Companies Hope to Breathe Life into Asthma Pipeline." *Nature Medicine* 17, no. 6 (June 2011): 642–643.

muscle relaxants Drugs used to treat pain, stiffness, and other discomfort caused by strains, spasms, spasticity, or injuries to muscles that control the skeleton (striated muscles). A spasm occurs when a muscle suddenly tightens uncontrollably. Spasticity is an abnormal increase in involuntary muscle tone caused by damage to the central nervous system. It is characterized by muscle stiffness and rigidity and is often accompanied by painful muscle spasms. In addition to easing pain from strain injuries, muscle relaxants are used in neuromuscular diseases such as multiple sclerosis as well as for spinal cord injury and stroke.

Classes

Muscle relaxants are divided into two classes according to their mechanism of action:

- *Centrally acting*—Act on the central nervous system (CNS). *Examples:* baclofen (Kemstro, Lioresal), carisoprodol (Soma), chlorzoxazone (Parafon Forte DSC), cyclobenzaprine (Flexeril), diazepam (Valium), metaxalone (Skelaxin), methocarbamol (Robaxin), orphenadrine (Norflex), and tizanidine (Zanaflex).
- *Peripherally (direct) acting*—Act directly on the muscle itself. *Example:* dantrolene (Dantrium).

How They Work

Precisely how muscle relaxants work is not known, but centrally acting muscle relaxants appear to work by blocking nerve impulses (or pain sensations) that are sent to the brain. They do not heal the muscle but relax tension in the muscle, reducing pain that might be caused by that tension. It is also believed that they help mask the pain, helping the patient put less tension on the muscle and thereby allowing the muscle time to heal itself.

Baclofen's beneficial effects result from actions in the spinal cord, the main connection between the brain and the rest of the body.

The skeletal muscle relaxant action of carisoprodol, chlorzoxazone, metaxalone, and methocarbamol may be related to their sedative properties.

Cyclobenzaprine is thought to act within the CNS primarily at the brain stem rather than spinal cord levels, although its action on the latter may contribute to some of its therapeutic effect on skeletal muscle relaxant activity.

Diazepam works by focusing on gamma-aminobutyric acid (GABA) receptors in the brain, helping to release the neurotransmitter chemical called GABA, which is used as a calming agent by the brain. The drug acts on muscle contractions by relaxing them. Diazepam serves both to relieve muscle spasms and to relieve anxiety about these spasms.

While the precise mode of orphenadrine's therapeutic action has not been clearly identified, it may be related to its analgesic properties.

Tizanidine is believed to reduce spasticity by increasing presynaptic inhibition of motor neurons—in effect, slowing action in the brain and CNS to allow the muscles to relax.

Peripherally (direct) acting muscle relaxants act directly on the muscle itself. Dantrolene has a direct effect at the level of the nerve-muscle connection, affecting the ability of the muscles to contract (stiffen).

Approved Uses

Baclofen is approved for the treatment of spasticity resulting from spinal cord injury/disease and multiple sclerosis.

Carisoprodol, chlorzoxazone, cyclobenzaprine, metaxalone, methocarbamol, and orphenadrine are used primarily as an adjunct to rest and physical therapy to relieve pain and stiffness associated with acute musculoskeletal conditions such as muscle spasms associated with sprains and strains. Methocarbamol is also used to control the muscle symptoms of tetanus (a potentially life-threatening bacterial disease that leads to stiffness of the jaw [lockjaw] and other muscles).

Diazepam is used for the relief of muscle spasm resulting from inflammation of the muscles or joints or secondary to trauma; spasticity caused by upper motor neuron disorders (such as cerebral palsy and paraplegia); athetosis (involuntary writhing movements particularly of the arms and hands); and stiff-man syndrome (a rare, severe autoimmune disease involving the CNS and characterized by a progressive rigidity or stiffness of the neck, shoulders, trunk, arm, and leg muscles). Injectable diazepam is used in the treatment of tetanus. Diazepam is also indicated as an adjunct treatment for convulsive disorders (see ANTICONVULSANTS) and the management of anxiety disorders (see ANTIANXIETY AGENTS).

Tizanidine is approved for the management of spasticity and is often used in the treatment of multiple sclerosis. Because it is effective for only a short duration, treatment with tizanidine should be reserved for those daily activities and times when relief of spasticity is most important.

Dantrolene is used to treat muscle spasticity caused by conditions such as spinal cord injury, stroke, cerebral palsy, or multiple sclerosis. It is also approved to prevent the development of malignant hyperthermia (a rapid rise in body temperature) and stiff muscles caused by anesthesia during or after surgery.

Off-Label Uses

Baclofen is used off-label to treat hiccups; to reduce rigidity in patients with parkinsonism syndrome; to reduce spasticity in patients with cerebral lesions, cerebral palsy, stroke, or rheumatic disorders; to reduce the number of gastroesophageal reflux episodes; to treat Tourette's syndrome in children; for neuropathic pain; and to prevent migraine.

Cyclobenzaprine is used off-label in the management of fibromyalgia.

Diazepam is used off-label for panic disorders, preoperative sedation, light anesthesia, and amnesia.

Orphenadrine is used off-label at bedtime in the treatment of quinine-resistant leg cramps.

Tizanidine is used off-label to treat tension headaches, seizures, low back pain, and fibromyalgia.

Dantrolene is used off-label to treat exercise-induced muscle pain, neuroleptic malignant syndrome, and heat stroke.

Administration

All centrally acting muscle relaxants are available as tablets. Baclofen may also be administered intrathecally (directly into the fluid around the spinal cord). Diazepam is also available as an injection and oral solution (see also ANTICONVULSANTS). Methocarbamol and orphenadrine are also administered via injection. Tizanidine is also available as capsules, which may be opened and sprinkled on soft foods such as applesauce (see *Warnings*).

Dantrolene is administered orally in capsule form and as an intravenous injection.

Cautions and Concerns

Muscle relaxants may impair the mental and/or physical abilities required for the performance of potentially hazardous tasks such as driving a motor vehicle or operating machinery.

Baclofen should be used with caution when spasticity is utilized to sustain upright posture and balance in locomotion or whenever spasticity is utilized to obtain increased function. In patients with seizure disorders, the clinical state and electroencephalogram (EEG) should be monitored at regular intervals, since deterioration in seizure control and EEG have been reported occasionally in patients taking baclofen. Ovarian cysts have been found in about 4 percent of the multiple sclerosis patients treated with baclofen for up to one year. In most cases, these cysts disappeared spontaneously while patients continued to receive the drug. Patients should be infection-free prior to the screening trial with baclofen intrathecal because the presence of a systemic infection may interfere with an assessment of the patient's response to the drug.

To reduce the chance of carisoprodol dependence, withdrawal, or abuse (see *Warnings*), carisoprodol should be used with caution in addiction-prone patients and in patients taking other CNS depressants including alcohol, and carisoprodol should not be used more than two to three weeks for the relief of acute musculoskeletal discomfort. There have been post-marketing reports of seizures in patients taking carisoprodol. Most of these cases have occurred in the setting of multiple drug overdoses (including drugs of abuse, illegal drugs, and alcohol). Since carisoprodol is metabolized in the liver and excreted by the kidney, caution should be exercised if it is administered to patients with impaired liver or kidney function.

Because chlorzoxazone has caused allergic-type skin rashes, it should be used with caution in patients with known allergies or a history of allergic drug reactions. If a sensitivity reaction occurs such as hives, redness, or itching of the skin, the drug should be stopped.

Because of its atropinelike action, cyclobenzaprine should be used with caution in patients with a history of urinary retention, angle-closure glaucoma, or increased intraocular pressure and in patients taking anticholinergic medications. Cyclobenzaprine should be used with caution in patients with mild liver impairment and is not recommended for patients with moderate to severe liver impairment. Cyclobenzaprine should be used in the elderly only if clearly needed, as plasma concentrations of cyclobenzaprine are increased in this population.

For diazepam *Cautions and Concerns,* see ANTI-ANXIETY AGENTS and ANTICONVULSANTS.

Taking metaxalone with food may increase the risk of drowsiness or dizziness.

Careful supervision of dose and rate of methocarbamol injection should be observed. Caution should be observed in using the injectable form in patients with suspected or known seizure disorders.

Orphenadrine should be used with caution in conditions that are affected by its anticholinergic and antihistaminic effects, which include gastroesophageal reflux disease (GERD), asthma, and glaucoma. Orphenadrine should also be used with caution in older patients who do not tolerate anticholinergics well. Additionally, caution should be taken when administering to patients with tachycardia, cardiac decompensation, coronary insufficiency, or cardiac arrhythmias. Safety of continuous long-term therapy with orphenadrine has not been established. Therefore, if orphenadrine is prescribed for prolonged use, periodic monitoring of blood, renal, and liver function values is recommended. Orphenadrine has been chronically abused for its euphoric effects. The mood-elevating effects may occur at therapeutic doses of orphenadrine.

Reductions in blood pressure and pulse rate have occurred with all doses of tizanidine. Caution is advised when tizanidine is to be used in patients receiving concurrent antihypertensive therapy. Tizanidine should be used with caution in patients with kidney insufficiency, as clearance is reduced by more than 50 percent. These patients should be monitored closely for the onset or increase in severity of the common side effects as indicators of potential overdose.

Dantrolene should be used with caution in patients with impaired pulmonary function, particularly those with obstructive pulmonary disease, and in patients with severely impaired cardiac function due to myocardial disease. It should also be used with caution in patients with a history of previous liver disease (see *Warnings*). Caution should be exercised in the concomitant administration of tranquilizing agents. Dantrolene might possibly evoke a photosensitivity reaction; patients should be cautioned about exposure to sunlight while taking it. Diarrhea (see *Side Effects*) may be severe and may necessitate temporary withdrawal of dantrolene therapy. If diarrhea recurs upon readministration of dantrolene, therapy should probably be withdrawn permanently.

Warnings

Hallucinations and seizures have occurred on abrupt withdrawal of oral baclofen. Therefore, except for serious adverse reactions, the dose should be reduced slowly when the drug is discontinued. Abrupt discontinuation of intrathecal baclofen has resulted in high fever, altered mental status, exaggerated rebound spasticity, and muscle rigidity that in rare cases has advanced to rhabdomyolysis (the breakdown of muscle fibers resulting in the release of muscle fiber contents [myoglobin] into the bloodstream), multiple organ-system failure, and death. Prevention of abrupt discontinuation of intrathecal baclofen requires careful attention to programming and monitoring of the infusion system, refill scheduling and procedures, and pump alarms. Patients and caregivers should be advised of the importance of keeping scheduled refill visits and should be educated on the early symptoms of baclofen withdrawal. Because of the possibility of potentially life-threatening CNS depression, cardiovascular collapse, and/or respiratory failure, physicians must be adequately trained and educated in chronic intrathecal infusion therapy. Because baclofen is primarily excreted unchanged by the kidneys, it should be given with caution, and it may be necessary to reduce the dosage in patients with impaired kidney function.

One of the metabolites of carisoprodol, meprobamate (a controlled substance), may cause dependence. In the postmarketing experience with carisoprodol, cases of dependence, withdrawal, and abuse have been reported with prolonged use. Most of these cases occurred in patients who have had a history of addiction or who used carisoprodol in combination with other drugs with abuse potential. Withdrawal symptoms have been reported following abrupt cessation after prolonged use. The first dose of carisoprodol has been followed very rarely by idiosyncratic (unique to each individual) symptoms that appear within minutes or hours, including extreme weakness, transient quadriplegia, dizziness, involuntary muscle movement, temporary loss of vision, double vision, speech defect, agitation, euphoria, confusion, and disorientation. Although these effects usually subside over the course of several hours, supportive and symptomatic therapy (including hospitalization) may be necessary. Occasionally, within the period of the first to fourth dose of carisoprodol, allergic reactions have occurred in patients who have had no previous contact with the drug. Symptoms have included skin rash or redness, itching, and fixed drug eruption (a type of allergic reaction to a particular drug, usually recurring in the same site or sites each time that drug is administered); severe reactions have manifested as asthmatic episodes, fever, weakness, dizziness, smarting eyes, low blood pressure, and anaphylactoid shock. Carisoprodol should be discontinued in patients with allergic or idiosyncratic reactions and appropriate therapy initiated. This may include use of epinephrine, antihistamines, and (in severe cases) corticosteroids.

Serious (including fatal) liver toxicity has been reported rarely in patients receiving chlorzoxazone. The mechanism is unknown but appears to be idiosyncratic and unpredictable. Factors predisposing patients to this rare event are not known. Patients should be instructed to report early signs and/or symptoms of liver toxicity such as fever, rash, anorexia, nausea, vomiting, fatigue, right upper quadrant pain, dark urine, or jaundice. Chlorzoxazone should be discontinued immediately and a physician consulted if any of these signs or symptoms develop. Chlorzoxazone use should also be discontinued if a patient develops abnormal liver enzymes (e.g., AST, ALT, alkaline phosphatase, and bilirubin).

Cyclobenzaprine is closely related to tricyclic antidepressants (e.g., amitriptyline and imipramine), which have been reported to produce arrhythmias, sinus tachycardia, prolongation of the conduction time leading to myocardial infarction, and stroke.

For diazepam *Warnings,* see ANTIANXIETY AGENTS and ANTICONVULSANTS.

Metaxalone should be administered with great care to patients with preexisting liver damage. Serial liver function studies should be performed in these patients.

Orphenadrine injection contains a sulfite that may cause allergic-type reactions including anaphylactic symptoms and life-threatening or less severe asthmatic episodes in certain susceptible people. Sulfite sensitivity is seen more frequently in asthmatic than nonasthmatic people.

Tizanidine capsules are not bioequivalent (when two different dosage forms of the same drug possess similar bioavailability and produce the same clinical effect) to tizanidine tablets in the fed state, meaning they are absorbed differently by the body when the patient has taken food within the previous 12 to 15 hours, so one product cannot be easily substituted for the other. Tizanidine capsules and tablets are bioequivalent when the patient has fasted for 12 to 15 hours prior to taking the drug. Tizanidine is an alpha$_2$-adrenergic agonist (like clonidine) and can produce hypotension. Rising from a sitting or lying position, climbing stairs, or engaging in activities requiring quick movements may increase the risk for hypotension and orthostatic effects (dizziness or fainting on changing position). Tizanidine occasionally causes liver injury. Because of the potential toxic hepatic effect of tizanidine, the drug should be avoided or used with extreme caution in patients with impaired liver function. Tizanidine use has been associated with hallucinations. In multiple dose, controlled clinical studies, nearly half of patients receiving any dose of tizanidine reported sedation as an adverse event. In 10 percent of these cases, the sedation was rated as severe. Sedation may interfere with everyday activity. If tizanidine therapy needs to be discontinued, particularly in patients who have been receiving high doses for long periods, the dose should be decreased slowly to minimize the risk of withdrawal and rebound hypertension, tachycardia, and hypertonia (a condition marked by an abnormal increase in muscle tension and a reduced ability of muscle to stretch).

Fatal and nonfatal liver disorders of an idiosyncratic or hypersensitivity type may occur with dantrolene therapy. At the start of dantrolene therapy, it is desirable to do liver function studies (AST, ALT, alkaline phosphatase, total bilirubin) at baseline to establish whether there is preexisting liver disease. If baseline liver abnormalities exist and are confirmed, there is a clear possibility that the potential for dantrolene hepatotoxicity could be enhanced. Liver function studies should be performed at appropriate intervals during dantrolene therapy. If such studies reveal abnormal values, therapy should generally be discontinued. Only when benefits of the drug have been of major importance to the patient should reinitiation or continuation of therapy be considered. Some patients have revealed a return to normal laboratory values in the face of continued therapy, while others have not. If symptoms compatible with hepatitis, accompanied by abnormalities in liver function tests or jaundice, appear, dantrolene should be discontinued. Dantrolene should be used with particular caution in females and in patients over 35 years of age in view of apparent greater likelihood of drug-induced, potentially fatal, hepatotoxicity in these groups.

The use of intravenous dantrolene in the management of malignant hyperthermia crisis is not a substitute for previously known supportive measures. These measures must be individualized, but it will usually be necessary to discontinue the suspect triggering agents, attend to increased oxygen requirements, manage the metabolic acidosis, institute cooling when necessary, monitor urinary output, and monitor for electrolyte imbalance. Since the effect of disease state and other drugs on dantrolene-related skeletal muscle weakness, including possible respiratory depression, cannot be predicted, patients who receive intravenous dantrolene preoperatively should have vital signs monitored.

When Not Advised (Contraindications)

Carisoprodol is contraindicated in patients with acute intermittent porphyria (a genetic abnormality of metabolism) and those who are allergic to or who have had idiosyncratic reactions to meprobamate-related compounds (see *Warnings*).

Chlorzoxazone is not advised for patients with impaired liver function.

Cyclobenzaprine should not be used along with monoamine oxidase (MAO) inhibitors or within 14 days after their discontinuation. Hyperpyretic (extremely high fever) crises, seizures, and deaths have occurred in patients receiving cyclobenzaprine (or structurally similar tricyclic antidepressants) concomitantly with MAO inhibitor drugs. Cyclobenzaprine is also contraindicated in the acute recovery phase of myocardial infarction and in patients with arrhythmias, heart block or conduction disturbances, congestive heart failure, or hyperthyroidism.

For diazepam *Contraindications,* see ANTIANXIETY AGENTS and ANTICONVULSANTS.

Metaxalone is contraindicated in patients with a known tendency to drug-induced, hemolytic, or other anemias; also in patients with significantly impaired kidney or liver function.

Methocarbamol injectable should not be administered to patients with known or suspected kidney impairment due to the presence of polyethylene glycol 300 in the vehicle.

Orphenadrine is contraindicated in patients with glaucoma, pyloric or duodenal obstruction, peptic ulcer disease, enlarged prostate or bladder obstruction, megaesophagus, or myasthenia gravis.

Tizanidine should not be used concomitantly with either of two CYP1A2 inhibitors: fluvoxamine, which is used to treat depression and anxiety disorders, or the antibiotic ciprofloxacin (see *Interactions*).

Dantrolene is contraindicated in patients with active liver disease, such as hepatitis and cirrhosis (see *Warnings*) and also when spasticity is utilized to sustain upright posture and balance in locomotion or whenever spasticity is utilized to obtain or maintain increased function.

Side Effects

The most common side effect with baclofen is temporary drowsiness. Other common side effects include dizziness, weakness, and fatigue. In addition to these, common side effects with baclofen intrathecal include nausea, low blood pressure, headache, convulsions, and decreased muscle tone.

The most common side effects with carisoprodol are drowsiness, dizziness, and headache.

Chlorzoxazone is well tolerated and seldom produces undesirable side effects. Occasionally, chlorzoxazone may be associated with drowsiness, dizziness, lightheadedness, malaise, or overstimulation. It may also cause urine discoloration, which is clinically insignificant.

The most common side effects with cyclobenzaprine include drowsiness, dizziness, dry mouth, fatigue, and headache.

For diazepam side effects, see ANTIANXIETY AGENTS and ANTICONVULSANTS.

Common side effects with metaxalone are drowsiness, dizziness, headache, nervousness, nausea, vomiting, rash, leukopenia (a condition in which the number of white blood cells drops to a dangerously low level), hemolytic anemia, and jaundice.

Common side effects with methocarbamol include fainting, flushing, low blood pressure, dizziness, drowsiness, itching, rash, nausea, nasal congestion, and pain at injection site.

The most common side effects with orphenadrine are dry mouth, drowsiness, dizziness, and blurred vision.

The most common side effects with tizanidine are dry mouth, somnolence/sedation, tiredness, dizziness, and urinary tract infection.

The most frequently occurring side effects of dantrolene have been drowsiness, dizziness, weakness, general malaise, fatigue, and diarrhea (see *Cautions and Concerns*).

Interactions

The CNS depressant effects of muscle relaxants may be additive to those of alcohol and other CNS depressants (e.g., benzodiazepines, opioids, tricyclic antidepressants).

Coadministration of CYP2C19 inhibitors, such as omeprazole or fluvoxamine, with carisoprodol could result in increased exposure of carisoprodol and decreased exposure of meprobamate. Coadministration of CYP2C19 inducers, such as rifampin or Saint-John's-wort, with carisoprodol could result in decreased exposure of carisoprodol and increased exposure of meprobamate.

CYP2E1 inhibitors, such as disulfiram, isoniazid, and miconazole, may increase the levels/effects of chlorzoxazone. Disulfiram and isoniazid may increase chlorzoxazone concentration.

Cyclobenzaprine may have life-threatening interactions with MAO inhibitors (see *When Not Advised [Contraindications]*).

For diazepam interactions, see ANTIANXIETY AGENTS and ANTICONVULSANTS.

Methocarbamol may inhibit the effect of pyridostigmine bromide. Therefore, methocarbamol should be used with caution in patients with myasthenia gravis receiving anticholinesterase agents.

Confusion, anxiety, and tremors have been reported in a few patients receiving propoxyphene and orphenadrine concomitantly. As these symptoms may be simply due to an additive effect, reduction of dosage and/or discontinuation of one or both agents is recommended in such cases. Therapeutic effects of levodopa and phenothiazines (e.g., chlorpromazine, fluphenazine, thioridazine) may be decreased by orphenadrine.

Taking either fluvoxamine or ciprofloxacin together with tizanidine (see *When Not Advised [Contraindications]*) can cause dangerously elevated blood levels of tizanidine, which can lead to severe hypotension and sedation (see *Warnings*). Other CYP1A2 inhibitors may also lead to substantial increases in tizanidine blood concentrations, although there have been no clinical studies to substantiate this. Therefore, using tizanidine with other CYP1A2 inhibitors should ordinarily be avoided. These drugs include zileuton, other fluoroquinolones, antiarrhythmics (amiodarone, lidocaine, mexiletine, and propafenone), cimetidine, oral contraceptives, acyclovir, and ticlopidine.

While a definite drug interaction with estrogen therapy and dantrolene has not yet been established, caution should be observed if the two drugs are to be given concomitantly. Hepatotoxicity has occurred more often in women over 35 years of age receiving concomitant estrogen therapy. The combination of dantrolene and calcium channel blockers is not recommended during the management of malignant hyperthermia, as it may produce life-threatening hyperkalemia and myocardial depression. Administration of dantrolene may potentiate vecuronium-induced neuromuscular block.

Sales/Statistics

One muscle relaxant was listed on the "2008 Top 200 Branded Drugs by Retail Dollars" (*Drug Topics,* May 26, 2009): #80 Skelaxin, $501,310,000. Skelaxin ranked #89 among the "2008 Top 200 Branded Drugs by Total Prescriptions," with 3,218,000 prescriptions. As it came off patent in 2010, Skelaxin sales dropped precipitously—from $102 million in the second quarter of 2009 to $5 million in the second quarter of 2010, according to a King Pharmaceuticals (its manufacturer) financial report. The 2010 *Drug Topics* lists ranked Skelaxin #191 in sales for the year ($156,372,879) and #191 in brand prescriptions, with 759,046.

Several muscle relaxants appeared among the "2008 Top 200 Generic Drugs by Retail Dollars" (*Drug Topics,* May, 26, 2009): #54 cyclobenzaprine ($208,738,000 in sales), #57 carisoprodol ($204,236,000), #97 diazepam ($119,556,000) (but used for other indications in addition to muscle relaxant), #102 tizanidine ($115,382,000), #141 baclofen ($77,558,000), and #181 methocarbamol ($52,013,000). Their rankings by total prescriptions in 2008: #33 cyclobenzaprine (19,874,000 units), #41 diazepam (13,870,000), #52 carisoprodol (12,245,000), #118 tizanidine (3,818,000), #120 methocarbamol (3,722,000), and #136 baclofen (3,221,000).

On the "2010 Top 200 Generic Drugs by Retail Dollars" list, metaxalone ranked #65 ($226,373,763), cyclobenzaprine #68 ($223,823,780), carisoprodol #77 ($196,949,818), diazepam #109 ($135,729,840), tizanidine #144 ($98,132,116), and baclofen #196 ($62,082,676). On the "2010 Top 200 Generic Drugs by Total Prescriptions" list, cyclobenzaprine ranked #30 (22,240,071), diazepam #44 (14,584,147), tizanidine #123 (4,456,271), methocarbamol #129 (4,312,914), carisoprodol #56 (12,392,709), and baclofen #139 (3,926,533). Both lists appeared in the June 2011 issue of *Drug Topics*.

Development History

Baclofen was originally designed to be a drug for epilepsy in the 1920s. Although its effect on epilepsy was disappointing, investigators discovered that spasticity decreased in some patients taking it. Baclofen was first approved by the FDA on November 22, 1977. How baclofen came to be used intrathecally is not clear, but it received approval for that usage on June 17, 1992.

Carisoprodol was developed by a psychiatrist/pharmacologist, Dr. Frank M. Berger, at Wallace Laboratories in Cranbury, New Jersey. Dr. Berger had earlier developed the tranquilizer meprobamate, and he developed carisoprodol in the hope that it would have better muscle relaxing properties, less potential for abuse, and less risk of overdose than meprobamate. Carisoprodol received FDA approval on April 9, 1959.

Chlorzoxazone received FDA approval on August 15, 1958.

Cyclobenzaprine was developed in the Merck Frosst Canada laboratories in the 1960s and 1970s. It arose out of the discovery that the original compound, synthesized a decade earlier by Merck scientists in the United States in their search for a psychiatric medication, was exceptionally effective in relieving muscle spasms despite its ineffectiveness at the psychiatric level. Cyclobenzaprine was approved by the FDA on August 26, 1977.

Diazepam was invented by the chemist Leo Sternbach of Hoffmann-La Roche, Nutley, New Jersey, and was approved for use on November 15, 1963. Valium became the first "blockbuster" brand-name drug, initially used as a tranquilizer, and was the most prescribed drug in the United States from 1969 to 1982.

Metaxalone received FDA approval on August 13, 1962.

Methocarbamol received FDA approval on July 16, 1957.

Orphenadrine was first synthesized in the late 1940s in Europe and then patented in the United States by Parke-Davis in July 1951. It received FDA approval on November 4, 1959.

Tizanidine received FDA approval on November 27, 1996.

Dantrolene was discovered by Keith Ellis, M.D., working at Norwich Eaton Pharmaceuticals in Norwich, New York, during the early 1970s. Dantrolene was approved by the FDA on January 15, 1974.

Future Drugs

Avigen, Inc., an Alameda, California, biopharmaceutical company, has partnered with Sanochemia Pharmazeutika, AG, an Austrian-based pharmaceutical company, to develop tolperisone (AV650), a neuroactive drug to treat disabling neuromuscular spasm and spasticity resulting from muscle injuries and serious neurological diseases. The compound is a leading treatment in Europe for painful muscle spasm but has never been submitted for approval in the United States. Tolperisone is an oral centrally acting neuromuscular compound, exerting its action at three levels: peripheral, spinal, and brainstem levels of the nervous system.

respiratory inhalants Drugs used to treat the symptoms of diseases affecting the lungs and nasal passages that make it difficult to breathe. Among these diseases are asthma; chronic obstructive pulmonary disease (COPD), which includes emphysema and chronic bronchitis; and cystic fibrosis (CF). Certain classes treat allergic rhinitis, a disorder characterized by inflammation of the mucous membranes lining the nasal passages that is caused by an allergic reaction. (BRONCHODILATORS, also used to treat breathing problems, open narrowed airways, whereas respiratory inhalants reduce airway inflammation, swelling, and mucus.) In 2007, the Centers for Disease Control and Prevention (CDC) reported 23 million Americans, including 6.7 million children under age 18, as having asthma. Asthma is the leading cause of hospitalization and school absenteeism among children under the age of 15. COPD is the fourth leading cause of death in America, claiming the lives of 122,283 Americans in 2003, according to the American Lung Association. In 2004, 11.4 million U.S. adults were estimated to have COPD. Some 20 to 40 million Americans are affected by allergic rhinitis, making it the sixth most prevalent chronic illness.

Classes

Respiratory inhalants are divided into four classes:

- *Oral inhalation corticosteroids*—Reduce airway inflammation (swelling). *Examples:* beclomethasone (QVAR), budesonide (Pulmicort), ciclesonide (Alvesco), flunisolide (AeroBid, Aerospan), fluticasone (Flovent), mometa-sone (Asmanex), and triamcinolone acetonide (Azmacort).

- *Intranasal corticosteroids*—Reduce swelling and secretions in the nose. *Examples:* beclomethasone (Beconase AQ), budesonide (Rhinocort Aqua), ciclesonide (Omnaris), flunisolide (Nasarel), fluticasone (Flonase, Veramyst), mometasone (Nasonex), and triamcinolone acetonide (Nasacort AQ).

- *Mucolytics*—Reduce the stickiness of mucus in the airways. *Examples:* acetylcysteine (Mucomyst) and dornase alpha (Pulmozyme).

- *Mast cell stabilizers*—Reduce airway inflammation (swelling). *Example:* cromolyn sodium (Nasalcrom [intranasal]).

How They Work

Exactly how inhaled corticosteroids work to prevent asthma attacks is still not fully understood, but they are known to reduce and prevent inflammation and mucus in the airways. Airway inflammation, in both large and small airways, is known to be an important component in the development of asthma. Corticosteroids have multiple anti-inflammatory effects, inhibiting both inflammatory cells (e.g., mast cells, eosinophils, neutrophils, macrophages, and lymphocytes) and release of inflammatory mediators (substances the body produces that trigger inflammation, such as histamine, eicosanoids, leukotrienes, and cytokines). By reducing airway inflammation, inhaled corticosteroids help control symptoms and improve lung function in asthma.

Intranasal corticosteroids reduce swelling and nasal congestion by decreasing the number of mediators (histamine and prostaglandins) in the nose, which blocks inflammation.

Mucolytics dissolve or "thin" thickened mucus in the lungs, making it less sticky so that it is easier to cough out of one's airways. Acetylcysteine does this by reducing disulfide bonds between protein molecules present in the mucus (mucoproteins); the more of these bonds, the stickier the mucus. Dornase alfa thins the mucus by hydrolyzing (decomposing by reacting with water) the DNA in sputum (phlegm) of cystic fibrosis patients.

Mast cell stabilizers prevent a type of white blood cell called mast cells from releasing histamine and related substances that cause inflammation. When mast cells, which collect in tissues including the lungs, are activated by irritants, they degranulate (break down), releasing histamine and other proinflammatory substances. By stabilizing these cells and preventing them from breaking down, the histamine and other inflammatory mediators do not get released into the airways.

Approved Uses

Inhaled corticosteroids are used in the maintenance treatment of asthma as preventive therapy in adults and children (various age limits, depending on product). They are also indicated for asthma patients who require systemic corticosteroid administration, when adding an inhaled corticosteroid may reduce or eliminate the need for the systemic corticosteroids. Budesonide nebulizer is also indicated for the maintenance treatment of asthma and as preventive therapy in children 12 months to eight years of age.

Intranasal corticosteroids are approved for the relief of the symptoms of seasonal or perennial allergic rhinitis. Beclomethasone and fluticasone are also used in the treatment of nonallergic (vasomotor) rhinitis. Beclomethasone is also approved for the prevention of recurrence of nasal polyps following surgical removal. Mometasone is also approved for the treatment of nasal polyps in adults.

Inhaled acetylcysteine is indicated as adjuvant therapy for patients with abnormal, sticky, or thickened mucous secretions in such conditions as chronic bronchopulmonary disease (chronic emphysema, emphysema with bronchitis, chronic asthmatic bronchitis, tuberculosis, bronchiectasis [abnormal dilation of airways in the lungs], and primary amyloidosis of the lung), acute bronchopulmonary disease (pneumonia, bronchitis, tracheobronchitis), pulmonary complications of CF, tracheostomy care, pulmonary complications associated with surgery, use during anesthesia, posttraumatic chest conditions, lung collapse due to mucous obstruction, and diagnostic bronchial studies (bronchograms, bronchospirometry, and bronchial wedge catheterization).

Dornase alfa is indicated in the management of CF to improve pulmonary function. In certain patients, daily administration of this drug has also been shown to reduce the risk of respiratory tract infections requiring parenteral antibiotics.

As oral inhalers, mast cell stabilizers are approved to prevent and manage bronchial asthma and to prevent acute bronchospasm induced by exercise or environmental pollutants. As a nasal spray, cromolyn is approved to prevent and treat hay fever (allergic rhinitis) and other nasal allergies (runny/itchy nose, sneezing, allergic stuffy nose).

Off-Label Uses

Budesonide and fluticasone are used off-label in the treatment of nasal polyps. Budesonide, fluticasone, and mometasone are used off-label in the treatment of recurrent chronic sinusitis.

Acetylcysteine is used off-label as an ophthalmic solution to treat dry eye. It is also used off-label orally to prevent contrast-induced nephropathy (acute kidney failure associated with radiographic contrast media).

Cromolyn has been used off-label as an alternative therapy in chronic uticaria/angioedema (hives and swelling) that does not respond to usual treatment.

Administration

Inhaled corticosteroids are available in a metered-dose inhaler, a dry powder, and a nebulizer form.

Intranasal corticosteroids are sprayed into the nose.

Mucolytics are available as solutions for inhalation. Dornase alfa is administered by inhalation of an aerosol mist produced by a compressed air–driven nebulizer system.

Cromolyn is available as a solution for oral inhalation and as a nasal spray.

Cautions and Concerns

During withdrawal from oral corticosteroids, some patients may experience symptoms of systemically active corticosteroid withdrawal (e.g., joint and/or muscular pain, lassitude, and depression) despite maintenance or even improvement of respiratory function. Because of the possibility of systemic absorption of inhaled corticosteroids, patients treated with these drugs should be observed carefully for any evidence of systemic corticosteroid effect. It is possible that systemic corticosteroid effects, such as hypercorticism (excessive production of adrenocortical hormones) and suppression of hypothalamic-pituitary-adrenal (HPA) function, may appear in a small number of patients, particularly at higher doses. If such changes occur, the inhaled corticosteroid should be reduced slowly, consistent with accepted procedures for management of asthma symptoms and for tapering of systemic corticosteroids. Inhaled corticosteroids may slow growth when administered to pediatric patients. In studies, the average reduction in growth velocity was approximately 1 centimeter (about 1/3 of an inch) per year. It appears that the reduction is related to dose and how long the child takes the drug. Rare instances of glaucoma, increased intraocular pressure, and cataracts have been reported following the inhaled administration of corticosteroids. The long-term and systemic effects of oral inhalation corticosteroids are still not fully known. Inhaled corticosteroids should be used with caution, if at all, in patients with tuberculosis; untreated systemic

fungal, bacterial, parasitic, or viral infections; or ocular herpes simplex.

Rarely, immediate or delayed hypersensitivity reactions (e.g., bronchospasm, rash, itching) may occur after the intranasal administration of corticosteroids. In clinical studies with intranasal corticosteroids, infections of the nose and pharynx with *Candida albicans* have occurred only rarely. When such an infection develops, it may require treatment with appropriate local therapy and discontinuation of treatment with the nasal spray. Use of excessive doses of intranasal corticosteroids may suppress HPA function (see *Warnings*). As with any long-term treatment, patients using intranasal corticosteroids over several months or longer should be examined periodically for possible changes in the nasal mucous membrane. Because of the inhibitory effect of corticosteroids on wound healing, patients who have experienced recent nasal septal ulcers, nasal surgery, or nasal trauma should not use a nasal corticosteroid until healing has occurred.

For beclomethasone to be effective in the treatment of nasal polyps, the spray must be able to enter the nose. Therefore, treatment of nasal polyps with beclomethasone should be considered adjunctive therapy to surgical removal and/or the use of other medications that will permit effective penetration of beclomethasone into the nose. Nasal polyps may recur after any form of treatment.

Administration of acetylcysteine may initially produce a slight disagreeable odor, which soon disappears. With a face mask there may be stickiness on the face after nebulization. This is easily removed by washing with water. Under certain conditions, a color change may occur in acetylcysteine in the opened bottle. The light purple color is the result of a chemical reaction and does not significantly affect the safety or mucolytic effectiveness of acetylcysteine. Continued nebulization of acetylcysteine solution with a dry gas will result in an increased concentration of the drug in the nebulizer because of evaporation of the solvent. Extreme concentration may impede nebulization and efficient delivery of the drug. Dilution of the nebulizing solution with appropriate amounts of Sterile Water for Injection, USP, as concentration occurs, will obviate this problem.

Occasionally, patients may experience cough and/or bronchospasm following cromolyn sodium inhalation. At times, patients who develop bronchospasm may not be able to continue administration despite prior bronchodilator administration. Rarely, very severe bronchospasm has been encountered. Some patients may experience transient nasal stinging and/or sneezing immediately following instillation of cromolyn sodium nasal solution.

Warnings

Deaths due to adrenal insufficiency have occurred in asthmatic patients during and after transfer from systemic corticosteroids to inhaled or intranasal corticosteroids. After withdrawal from systemic corticosteroids, several months are required for recovery of HPA function. Patients who have been previously maintained on 20 mg or more per day of prednisone (or its equivalent) may be most susceptible, particularly when their systemic corticosteroids have been almost completely withdrawn. During periods of stress or a severe asthmatic attack, patients who have been withdrawn from systemic corticosteroids should be instructed to resume oral corticosteroids (in large doses) immediately and to contact their physician for further instruction. These patients should also be instructed to carry a warning card indicating that they may need supplementary systemic corticosteroids during periods of stress or a severe asthma attack. Transfer of patients from systemic to oral inhalation corticosteroid therapy may unmask allergic conditions previously suppressed by systemic therapy, such as rhinitis, conjunctivitis, and eczema.

If recommended doses of inhaled or intranasal corticosteroids are exceeded or if individuals are particularly sensitive or predisposed by virtue of recent systemic corticosteroid therapy, symptoms of hypercorticism may occur, includ-

ing very rare cases of menstrual irregularities, acneiform lesions, cataracts, and cushingoid features. If such changes occur, the inhaled or intranasal corticosteroid should be discontinued slowly, consistent with accepted procedures for discontinuing therapy. Doses greater than recommended should be avoided.

Persons who are on drugs that suppress the immune system, such as corticosteroids, are more susceptible to infections than healthy individuals. Chicken pox and measles, for example, can have a more serious or even fatal course in children or adults on corticosteroids who have not had these diseases or been properly immunized. Therefore, particular care should be taken to avoid exposure.

Bronchospasm, with an immediate increase in wheezing, may occur after use of an oral inhalation corticosteroid. If bronchospasm does occur, it should be treated immediately with a short-acting inhaled bronchodilator, and the inhaled corticosteroid should be discontinued. Nasal septal perforations have been reported in rare instances with the use of nasally inhaled corticosteroids. Also, temporary or permanent loss of the senses of smell and taste has been reported with flunisolide use.

After proper administration of acetylcysteine, an increased volume of liquified bronchial secretions may occur. When cough is inadequate, the airway must be maintained open by mechanical suction if necessary. When there is a mechanical block due to foreign body or local accumulation, the airway should be cleared by endotracheal aspiration, with or without bronchoscopy. Asthmatics under treatment with acetylcysteine should be watched carefully. Most patients with bronchospasm are quickly relieved by the use of a bronchodilator given by nebulization. If bronchospasm progresses, the medication should be discontinued immediately.

Severe anaphylactic reactions can occur after cromolyn sodium administration. In view of the biliary and renal routes of excretion for cromolyn sodium, consideration should be given to decreasing the dosage or discontinuing the administration of the drug in patients with impaired kidney or liver function. Cromolyn should be discontinued if the patient develops eosinophilic pneumonia (or pulmonary infiltrates with eosinophilia). Because of the propellants in this preparation, it should be used with caution in patients with coronary artery disease or a history of cardiac arrhythmias.

When Not Advised (Contraindications)

Respiratory inhalants have no role in the treatment of an acute attack of asthma, especially status asthmaticus, and are contraindicated for the rapid relief of acute bronchospasm and in the primary treatment of status asthmaticus or other acute episodes of asthma when intensive measures are required.

Dornase alfa is contraindicated in patients with known hypersensitivity to Chinese hamster ovary cell products.

Side Effects

Common side effects with oral inhalation corticosteroids include headache, sore throat, upper respiratory tract infection, fungal infection (see *Warnings*), and rhinitis (nasal inflammation).

Common side effects with intranasal corticosteroids include burning, dryness, or other irritation inside the nose, increased sneezing, nosebleeds, and irritation of the throat. Fluticasone and mometasome also commonly cause headache.

Common side effects with acetylcysteine include inflammation of the mucous membrane of the mouth, nausea, vomiting, fever, watery mucus discharge from the nose, drowsiness, clamminess, chest tightness, and bronchoconstriction.

The most common side effects with dornase alfa include voice alteration, sore throat, laryngitis, rash, chest pain, and conjunctivitis.

The most common side effects with cromolyn sodium oral inhalation are throat irritation or dryness, bad taste, cough, wheeze, and nausea. With cromolyn sodium nasal solution, the most common are nasal stinging, nasal burning, and nasal irritation.

Interactions

All corticosteroids are CYP3A4 substrates and need to be used with caution with potent CYP3A4 inhibitors (e.g., ketoconazole, erythromycin, clarithromycin).

Ritonavir, an ANTIRETROVIRAL, can significantly increase blood levels of fluticasone, resulting in systemic corticosteroid effects, including Cushing's syndrome and adrenal suppression. Therefore, coadministration of fluticasone and ritonavir is not recommended unless the potential benefit to the patient outweighs the risk of systemic corticosteroid side effects.

No formal drug interaction studies have been performed with dornase alfa or with mast cell stabilizers.

Sales/Statistics

A number of respiratory inhalants are listed each year on the top drug sales lists. On the "2008 Top 200 Branded Drugs by Retail Dollars" (*Drug Topics*, May 26, 2009), Nasonex ranked #42 with $904,074,000 in sales. Others listed and their rankings: #55 Pulmicort Respules ($651,024,000), #67 Flovent HFA ($553,050,000), #119 Nasacort AQ ($285,359,000), #170 Asmanex ($185,244,000), #171 Rhinocort Aqua ($184,397,000), and #192 Veramyst ($158,347,000).

On the "2008 Top 200 Branded Drugs by Total Prescriptions" (*Drug Topics*, May 26, 2009), Nasonex ranked #24 with 10,463,000 prescriptions. Others listed and their rankings: #66 Flovent HFA (4,403,000 prescriptions), #90 Nasacort AQ (3,206,000 prescriptions), #114 Pulmicort Respules (2,413,000 units), #138 Rhinocort Aqua (1,986,000 prescriptions), and #145 Veramyst (1,822,000 prescriptions).

Fluticasone nasal ranked #19 among the "2008 Top 200 Generic Drugs by Retail Dollars" (*Drug Topics*, May 26, 2009), with $728,916,000 in sales, and #36 among the "2008 Top 200 Generic Drugs by Total Prescriptions" with 16,163,000 prescriptions.

According to a report from the IMS Institute for Healthcare Informatics (the public reporting arm of IMS, a pharmaceutical market intelligence firm), respiratory agents were the second-largest therapeutic class by spending in the United States in 2010, with $19.3 billion in sales, up from $13.1 billion in 2006. IMS ranked respiratory agents the seventh-largest therapeutic class by prescriptions in 2010, with 153.3 million prescriptions dispensed. That was up from 139.8 million in 2006. In addition to respiratory inhalants, respiratory agents typically include antihistamines, antitussives, bronchodilators, certain corticosteroids, decongestants, and leukotriene modifiers.

Demographics and Cultural Groups

Although asthma affects people of all ages, it most often starts in childhood. More boys have asthma than girls, but in adulthood, more women have asthma than men. Asthma is particularly common among urban Hispanics (affecting about 11 percent) and among blacks (7 percent). A study released in June 2008 looked at the prevalence of asthma among 10 racial and ethnic groups in New York City and how housing and neighborhood conditions can contribute to a disparity in prevalence. Researchers found that Puerto Rican Americans, other Hispanics, and blacks had the highest levels of asthma, while Mexican Americans, Chinese Americans and Asian/Indians had the lowest levels. They also found that reducing minorities' exposure to deteriorated housing conditions and increasing levels of community unity as well as making improvements in other household factors reduced asthma rates among blacks and Puerto Rican Americans. However, even after such interventions, asthma rates among those two groups still remain significantly higher than those among whites.

In past years, COPD was exclusively a disease of elderly white men, but since 2000, more women than men have died of COPD in the United States. In a 1987 survey, the COPD breakdown was 61 percent male and 39 percent female. In 2001, that had reversed to 40 percent male and 60 percent female. Among the reasons given for this is the increase in women smoking; in one study, 84 percent of men and 80 percent of women with COPD smoked.

Although CF affects all races and ethnic groups, it is most common in whites of northern European ancestry.

Development History

Inhaled corticosteroids have been available in the United States for the treatment of asthma since 1976. Hara describes their development: "The clinical value of the glucocorticoids as anti-inflammatory agents was generally known after a report that the Mayo Clinic in the United States had successfully used cortisone, one of the glucocorticoids, for the treatment of rheumatoid arthritis in 1948 to 1949. The application of cortisone for the treatment of asthma was reported as early as 1950. However, the problem of how to reduce systemic side effects prevented its use for the long-term treatment of asthma except in severe cases. Inhalation of corticoids had been tried since 1951 but these trials did not bring good results."

According to Hara, Britain's Glaxo Laboratories (now GlaxoSmithKline) had had many years' experience in manufacturing cortisone and its analogs, plus had conducted research on glucocorticoid, when they synthesized a new glucocortoid called beclomethasone dipropionate in 1964. "These experiences and the consequent knowledge, skills, facilities and other material resources possessed, individually and collectively, by the organization, probably played a significant role in connecting the needs of anti-inflammatory agents in asthma treatment with the idea of using topical glucocorticoids by inhalation."

Beclomethasone was approved for use in the United States on May 12, 1976. Triamcinolone acetonide's approval followed on April 23, 1982; flunisolide on August 17, 1984; budesonide on February 14, 1994; fluticasone on March 27, 1996; and mometasone on March 31, 2005.

Beclomethasone received FDA approval for intranasal use on July 27, 1987. Budesonide approval followed on February 21, 1994; fluticasone on October 19, 1994; flunisolide on March 8, 1995; triamcinolone acetonide on May 20, 1996; and mometasone on October 1, 1997.

Mucolytic and related agents have been in use since prehistoric times. Acetylcysteine was approved as a mucolytic agent for chronic pulmonary diseases on September 14, 1963. Dornase alfa was the first drug approved specifically for cystic fibrosis, on December 30, 1993.

Cromolyn was the first drug licensed as a mast cell stabilizer, receiving FDA approval on May 28, 1982.

Future Drugs

Aerovance, Inc., Berkeley, California, is developing pitrakinra, an inhibitor of interleukins-4 and -13 in the lungs. Scientists have long believed that these cytokines play a vital role in the onset and development of asthma, although no scientific evidence has proven this to be so. In Phase II clinical trials reported in the October 20–26, 2007, *Lancet,* pitrakinra by subcutaneous injection and pitrakinra by nebulization were both successful in reducing asthma symptoms.

MOLI 1901, an aerosol inhalant, is being developed by MoliChem Medicines, Inc., Chapel Hill, North Carolina. This is a long-term drug that allows cells to release water to hydrate and break down the thick, sticky mucus inherent in CF.

(See also future drugs in BRONCHODILATORS.)

Hara, Takuji. *Innovation in the Pharmaceutical Industry: The Process of Drug Discovery.* Cheltenham, U.K.: Edward Elgar, 2003.

sex hormones Drugs that mimic the effects of hormones naturally produced by the sex glands and to a smaller degree secreted by the adrenal glands. Female sex hormones are used to treat menstrual and menopausal disorders, to prevent pregnancy, and to treat infertility. Of the 62 million women aged 15 to 44 who are currently using at least one form of birth control, 30.6 percent are reported to be using a contraceptive drug. Male sex hormones are given to compensate for hormonal deficiency in hypopituitarism (a deficiency of one or more hormones of the pituitary gland), for delayed male puberty, or for disorders of the testes. Low testosterone, also known as hypogonadism, affects approximately 4 to 5 million American men. Sex hormones may also be used to treat breast cancer, prostate cancer, and endometriosis.

Classes

Sex hormones are divided into several classes.

- *Estrogens—Examples:* estradiol (tablet: Femtrace, Estrace; topical emulsion: Estrasorb; topical gel: Divigel, Elestrin, EstroGel; topical solution: Evamist; transdermal system: Alora, Climara, Estraderm, Menostar, Vivelle, Vivelle-Dot; vaginal cream: Estrace; vaginal ring: Estring, Femring; vaginal tablet: Vagifem), estradiol cypionate injection in oil (Depo-Estradiol), estradiol valerate injection in oil (Delestrogen), estrogens conjugated equine (Premarin), estrogens esterified (Menest), estropipate (Ogen, Ortho-Est), estrogens conjugated synthetic A (Cenestin), and estrogens conjugated synthetic B (Enjuvia).

- *Selective estrogen receptor modulator—Example:* raloxifene (Evista).

- *Progestins—Examples:* medroxyprogesterone (Depo-Provera, Provera), megestrol (Megace), norethindrone acetate (Aygestin), and progesterone (capsule: Prometrium; vaginal gel: Crinone, Endometrin; vaginal tablet: Proachieve).

- *Combinations—Examples:* estrogen/progestin (Femhrt, Premphase, Prempro) and estrogen/androgen (Covaryx, Estratest).

- *Contraceptives*—Oral contraceptives contain either a combination of a synthetic estrogen (mestranol or ethinyl estradiol) and a synthetic progestin (e.g., desogestrel, drosperinone, ethynodiol diacetate, levonorgestrol, norethindrone, norelgestromin, norgestimate, norgestrel) or a progestin alone. Given the extensive number of combination oral contraceptives on the market, it is impossible to list all the various combinations with the respective brand names. Therefore, only the brand names are presented for the contraceptive products that contain progestin only or those that are available for other routes of administration than tablets (e.g., transdermal, ring). *Examples:* progestin only (Camila, Errin, Jolivette, Micronor, Nor-QD), emergency oral contraceptive (Plan B [contains levonorgestrol]), injection (Depo-Provera [contains medroxyprogesterone]), intrauterine devices (Mirena [contains levonorgestrel], Paragard [contains copper]), subdermal implant (Implanon [contains etonogestrel]), transdermal (OrthoEvra [contains ethinyl estradiol/norelgestromin]), and vaginal ring (NuvaRing [contains ethinyl estradiol/etonogestrel]).

- *Ovulation stimulants—Examples:* choriogonado-tropin alfa (Ovidrel), chorionic gonadotro-pin (Novarel, Pregnyl), clomiphene citrate (Clomid, Milophene, Serophene), follitropin alfa (Gonal-f), follitropin beta (Follistim AQ), lutropin alfa (Luveris), menotropins (Meno-pur, Repronex), and urofollitropin (Bravelle).

- *Gonadotropin-releasing agonists—Examples:* gosere-lin acetate (Zoladex), histrelin acetate (Suppre-lin LA, Vantas), and nafarelin acetate (Synarel).

- *Gonadotropin-releasing hormone antagonists—Examples:* ganirelix acetate (Antagon) and cetrorelix acetate (Cetrotide).

- *Androgens—Examples:* danazol, fluoxymester-one (Androxy), methyltestosterone (Android, Testred, Virilon), testosterone (buccal: Stri-ant; subcutaneous pellet: Testopel; topical gel: AndroGel, Testim; transdermal system: Androderm), testosterone cypionate injection in oil (Depo-Testosterone), testosterone enan-thate injection in oil (Delatestryl), and testos-terone propionate injection in oil.

- *Anabolic steroids—Examples:* nandrolone, oxan-drolone (Oxandrin), and oxymetholone (Anadrol).

How They Work

All estrogen- and progestin-containing drug products work in similar ways—basically, they correct the overproduction or underproduction of the body's natural sex hormones.

Selective estrogen receptor modulators work like the hormone estrogen in some parts of the body and not in other parts.

Contraceptives work by preventing ovulation (release of an egg), altering the cervical mucus, and changing the lining of the uterus.

Ovulation stimulants work by triggering secre-tion of hormones that women need to get preg-nant. This leads to ovarian stimulation, ovarian follicle maturation, and corpus luteum develop-ment. Corpus luteum is yellow endocrine tissue that forms following the release of an ovum (female reproductive cell); it degenerates after a few days unless pregnancy has begun.

The ovulation stimulant human chorionic gonadotropin (HCG) stimulates production of gonadal steroid hormones by stimulating the interstitial cells (Leydig cells) of the testes to produce androgens and the corpus luteum of the ovary to produce progesterone. Androgen stimu-lation in the male leads to the development of secondary sex characteristics and may stimulate testicular descent when no anatomical impedi-ment to descent is present. This descent is usually reversible when HCG is discontinued. During the normal menstrual cycle, luteinizing hormone (LH) participates with follicle-stimulating hor-mone (FSH) in the development and maturation of the normal ovarian follicle, and the mid-cycle LH surge triggers ovulation. HCG can substitute for LH in this function. During a normal preg-nancy, HCG secreted by the placenta maintains the corpus luteum after LH secretion decreases, supporting continued secretion of estrogen and progesterone and preventing menstruation.

Gonadotropin-releasing agonists overstimu-late the pituitary gland, triggering production of more LH and FSH than normal, which makes the pituitary gland temporarily shut down. The "disabled" pituitary gland then stops producing LH and FSH, which in turn stops the monthly menstrual hormonal cycle and results in a condi-tion similar to menopause.

Gonadotropin-releasing hormone antagonists also stop the pituitary from making LH and FSH, but they do so almost immediately, within a couple of hours, and thus do not have to be used for as many days as gonadotropin-releasing agonists do.

Androgens are hormones produced in males (although the female body also produces small amounts of androgens), primarily in the testes, that play a major role in the development and maintenance of masculine sexual characteris-tics plus influence male hair growth and voice change during puberty and adolescence. Andro-gen drugs work by mimicking the effects of these natural hormones.

Anabolic steroids are derived from or are closely related to the natural androgen, testosterone. They work by promoting body tissue–building processes while reversing tissue-depleting processes.

Approved Uses

Estrogens and progestins are used as components of contraceptives, in hormone replacement therapy (HRT) for postmenopausal women, and to treat menstrual disorders. Estrogens may also be used as palliative therapy (alleviating pain without curing) of cancer of the breast or prostate.

In menopausal women, estrogens are used to treat moderate to severe vasomotor symptoms (e.g., night sweats and hot flashes) and to decrease the risk of osteoporosis. (A progestin should be used with estrogen therapy in women who have an intact uterus.) Topical vaginal estrogens are used to treat symptoms of vulvar and vaginal atrophy. Estrogens are also used to treat female hypoestrogenism caused by hypogonadism, castration, and primary ovarian failure.

Progestins are also used to treat amenorrhea (absence or suppression of normal menstrual flow), abnormal uterine bleeding, and endometriosis. Progestins are also used as palliative treatment of endometrial cancer, renal cell carcinoma, breast cancer, and prostate cancer. High-dose megestrol acetate is used to treat anorexia, cachexia, and acquired immune deficiency syndrome (AIDS)–related wasting syndrome. Progesterone gel is used as part of infertility treatment in women with progesterone deficiency.

Raloxifene is used to treat and prevent osteoporosis in postmenopausal women, to reduce the risk of invasive breast cancer in postmenopausal women with osteoporosis, and to reduce the risk of invasive breast cancer in postmenopausal women at high risk of invasive breast cancer.

Contraceptives are used to prevent pregnancy.

Choriogonadotropin alfa is indicated for the induction of final follicular maturation and early luteinization in infertile women who have undergone pituitary desensitization and who have been appropriately pretreated with follicle-stimulating hormones as part of an Assisted Reproductive Technology (ART) program such as in vitro fertilization and embryo transfer. Choriogonadotropin alfa is also used to induce ovulation and pregnancy in anovulatory infertile patients (women who menstruate without ovulating) in whom the cause of infertility is not due to primary ovarian failure.

Chorionic gonadotropin is used to induce testicular descent in situations when descent would have occurred at puberty. Although, in some cases, descent following HCG administration is permanent, in most cases, the response is temporary. Therapy is usually instituted in children between the ages of four and nine. It is also used to treat hypogonadism secondary to pituitary deficiency in males and to induce ovulation and pregnancy in the anovulatory, infertile woman in whom the cause of anovulation is secondary and not due to primary ovarian failure and who has been appropriately pretreated with human menotropins.

Clomiphene citrate is used for the treatment of ovulatory failure in women desiring pregnancy whose partners are fertile and potent.

Follitropins are used to induce ovulation and pregnancy in women when the cause of infertility is not due to primary ovarian failure. They are also used for the development of multiple follicles in the ovulatory patient participating in an ART program. Follitropin alfa is also indicated for the induction of spermatogenesis in men with primary and secondary hypogonadotropic hypogonadism in whom the cause of infertility is not due to primary testicular failure.

Lutropin alfa, a gonadotropin, is administered along with follitropin alfa for stimulation of follicular development in infertile hypogonadotropic hypogonadal (HH) women with profound LH deficiency. (HH is absent or decreased function of the male testes or the female ovaries.) Women with HH are unable to produce the hormones needed for full development of follicles in the ovaries.

Menotropins, a combination of two hormones, FSH and LH, is given sequentially with

HCG to cause ovulation. It also stimulates sperm production in men with certain types of infertility.

Goserelin acetate is used primarily as palliative treatment for prostate cancer in men and advanced breast cancer in women. It is also approved for management of endometriosis, uterine fibroids, and endometrial thinning.

Nafarelin acetate and histrelin acetate (Supprelin LA) are used to treat central precocious puberty (CPP) (gonadotropin-dependent precocious puberty) in children of both sexes. CPP is suspected when premature development of secondary sexual characteristics occurs at or before the age of eight years in girls and nine years in boys and is accompanied by significant advancement of bone age and/or a poor adult height prediction. Nafarelin acetate is also used for management of endometriosis, including pain relief and reduction of endometriotic lesions. Histrelin acetate (Vantas) is used for palliative treatment of advanced prostate cancer.

Gonadotropin-releasing hormone antagonists are used to prevent the premature LH surges during ovarian stimulation for in vitro fertilization and may improve the patient's response to lower doses of gonadotropins.

Androgens are given to compensate for hormonal deficiency in hypopituitarism or disorders of the testes. They are prescribed for men when testosterone is not naturally produced by the body or to correct natural hormone deficiencies, for male children to make undescended testes descend or to bring about male puberty when it is seriously delayed, and for women with some forms of breast cancer. Methyltestosterone and fluoxymesterone are synthetic versions of testosterone. Danazol is indicated for the treatment of endometriosis amenable to hormonal management, management of severe fibrocystic breast disease, and the prevention of attacks of hereditary angioedema (swelling that occurs in the tissue just below the surface of the skin).

Oxymetholone is indicated in the treatment of anemias caused by deficient red cell production. Acquired aplastic anemia, congenital aplastic anemia, myelofibrosis, and the hypoplastic anemias due to the administration of myelotoxic drugs often respond to oxymetholone therapy.

Oxandrolone is indicated to offset the protein catabolism (breakdown) associated with prolonged administration of corticosteroids, for the relief of the bone pain frequently accompanying osteoporosis, and to aid weight gain after weight loss following extensive surgery, chronic infections, or severe trauma.

Nandrolone decanoate is indicated for the treatment of metastatic breast cancer and the management of the anemia of renal insufficiency.

Off-Label Uses

In the treatment of Turner syndrome (ovarian dysgenesis [infertility]), estrogen therapy replicates the events of puberty.

Medroxyprogesterone has been used off-label in the treatment of menopausal symptoms. Progesterone suppositories (rectal or vaginal), compounded by individual pharmacists, have been used in premenstrual syndrome (PMS).

Clomiphene citrate has been used off-label to treat male infertility.

Danazol has been used off-label to treat precocious puberty, gynecomastia (excessive development of the breasts in males), and menorrhagia (abnormally heavy or prolonged menstruation).

Testosterone is used off-label for the treatment of AIDS-wasting syndrome and to increase muscle mass and decrease body fat in patients with human immunodeficiency virus (HIV).

Oxandrolone is used off-label to treat alcoholic hepatitis.

Administration

Estrogens are available in oral versions, transdermal preparations, injections, vaginal creams, and vaginal rings (see *Classes*).

Progesterone is available as capsules, injections, vaginal gels, and vaginal tablets. Medroxyprogesterone, norethindrone acetate, and megestrol are available in tablet form. Medroxyprogesterone is also available as an injection. Megestrol is also available as a suspension.

Raloxifene is available as tablets.

Contraceptives are available as tablets, transdermal patches, vaginal rings, intrauterine rings, and injections.

Ovulation stimulants are administered via injection except for clomiphene citrate, which is taken orally via tablets.

Goserelin acetate is implanted under the skin.

Nafarelin acetate is available as an intranasal spray.

Histrelin acetate is implanted under the skin.

Gonadotropin-releasing hormone antagonists are administered via injection.

Androgens are available as tablets, capsules (danazol), buccal system (adheres to the gum or inner cheek), patch, gel, and injection (see *Classes*).

Oxymetholone and oxandrolone are taken orally via tablets; nandrolone decanoate is injected into the muscle (preferably the gluteal muscle).

Cautions and Concerns

In a small number of case reports, substantial increases in blood pressure have been attributed to idiosyncratic reactions to estrogens. In a large, randomized, placebo-controlled clinical trial, a generalized effect of estrogens on blood pressure was not seen. However, blood pressure should be monitored at regular intervals with estrogen use.

Because estrogens may cause some degree of fluid retention, patients with conditions that might be influenced by this factor (e.g., heart failure or kidney dysfunction) warrant careful observation when estrogens are prescribed.

In patients with preexisting hypertriglyceridemia, estrogen therapy may be associated with elevations of plasma triglycerides leading to pancreatitis and other complications.

Estrogens may be poorly metabolized in patients with impaired liver function. For patients with a history of cholestatic jaundice associated with past estrogen use or with pregnancy, caution should be exercised, and, in the case of recurrence, medication should be discontinued.

Estrogen administration leads to increased thyroid-binding globulin (TBG) levels. Patients with normal thyroid function can compensate for the increased TBG by making more thyroid hormone, thus maintaining free T4 and T3 serum concentrations in the normal range. Patients dependent on thyroid hormone replacement therapy who are also receiving estrogens may require increased doses of their thyroid replacement therapy. These patients should have their thyroid function monitored in order to maintain their free thyroid hormone levels in an acceptable range.

Endometriosis may be exacerbated with administration of estrogens. A few cases of malignant transformation of residual endometrial implants have been reported in women treated posthysterectomy with estrogen alone therapy. For patients known to have residual endometriosis posthysterectomy, the addition of progestin should be considered.

Estrogens may cause an exacerbation of asthma, diabetes mellitus, seizure disorders, migraine, and systemic lupus erythematosus (SLE) and should be used with caution in women with these conditions. Estrogens should also be used with caution in individuals with severe hypocalcemia.

Safety of raloxifene in premenopausal women has not been established, and its use in this population is not recommended. Raloxifene should be used with caution in patients with liver or kidney impairment, as its safety and efficacy have not been established in these patients. Raloxifene has also not been adequately studied in women with a prior history of breast cancer or in men; therefore, its use in either of these populations is not recommended.

The physical examination prior to progestin therapy should include special reference to breasts, abdomen, and pelvic organs as well as a Pap smear.

Because progestins may cause some degree of fluid retention, conditions that might be influenced by this factor, such as heart failure or kidney dysfunction, require careful observation.

Patients taking progestins who have a history of clinical depression should be carefully observed and the drug discontinued if the depression recurs to a serious degree.

A decrease in glucose tolerance has been observed in a small percentage of patients on estrogen-progestin combination drugs. The mechanism of this decrease is not known. For this reason, diabetic patients should be carefully observed while receiving any progestin therapy.

Transient dizziness may occur in some patients taking progestins; therefore, patients should use caution when driving a motor vehicle or operating machinery. A small percentage of women may experience the following symptoms upon initial therapy: extreme dizziness and/or drowsiness, blurred vision, slurred speech, difficulty walking, loss of consciousness, vertigo, confusion, disorientation, feeling drunk, and shortness of breath. For these women, consultation with their health-care provider regarding their treatment is advised. Bedtime dosing may alleviate these symptoms.

Treatment with progestins may mask the onset of menopause.

Contraceptives generally carry the same *Cautions and Concerns* as estrogens and progestins above.

Patients with a history of jaundice during pregnancy have an increased risk of recurrence of jaundice when taking oral contraceptives. Several cases of oral contraceptive failures have been reported due to malabsorption resulting from vomiting or diarrhea. If significant gastrointestinal disturbance occurs, a backup method of contraception for the remainder of the cycle is recommended. Oral contraceptives do not protect against HIV infection and other sexually transmitted diseases. Some oral contraceptive products contain tartrazine, which may cause allergic-type reactions (including bronchial asthma) in susceptible individuals.

Before treatment with ovulation stimulants is begun, a thorough gynecologic and endocrinologic evaluation, including an assessment of pelvic anatomy, must be performed. Patients with tubal obstruction should receive ovulation stimulants only if enrolled in an in vitro fertilization program. Primary ovarian failure should be excluded by the determination of gonadotropin levels. Appropriate evaluation should be performed to exclude pregnancy. Patients in later reproductive life have a greater predisposition to endometrial carcinoma as well as a higher incidence of anovulatory disorders. A thorough diagnostic evaluation should always be performed in patients who demonstrate abnormal uterine bleeding or other signs of endometrial abnormalities before starting FSH and ovulation stimulation therapy. Evaluation of the partner's fertility potential should be included in the initial evaluation.

Because chorionic gonadotropin may cause fluid retention, it should be used with caution in patients with cardiac or kidney disease, seizure disorders, migraine, or asthma.

Pelvic examination is necessary prior to clomiphene citrate treatment and before each subsequent course. Clomiphene citrate should not be administered in the presence of an ovarian cyst, as further enlargement may occur (see *Warnings*).

Careful attention should be given to the diagnosis of infertility in candidates for ovulation stimulation therapy.

For goserelin acetate precautions, see ANTINEOPLASTICS.

LH, FSH, and either estradiol (in females) or testosterone (in males) should be monitored at the one month point following histrelin acetate (Supprelin LA) implantation, then every six months thereafter. Additionally, height (for calculation of height velocity or rate of growth) and bone age should be assessed every six to 12 months. In their article, "Bone Age Assessment of Children Using a Digital Hand Atlas," Gertych et al. explain, "Bone age assessment is a common radiological examination used in pediatrics to determine any discrepancy between a child's skeletal age (the developmental age of their bones) and their chronological age (in years, taken from birth date). A difference between chronological age and skeletal age may suggest abnormalities in skeletal development. Assessment of skeletal age is helpful in the monitoring of growth hormone therapy and diagnosis of endocrine disorders."

In adult women with endometriosis, ovarian cysts have been reported to occur in the first two months of therapy with nafarelin acetate. Many, but not all, of these events occurred in women with polycystic ovarian disease. These cystic enlargements may resolve spontaneously, generally by about four to six weeks of therapy, but in some cases may require discontinuation of the drug and/or surgical intervention. The relevance, if any, of such events in children is unknown.

Since menstruation should stop with effective doses of nafarelin, the patient should notify her physician if regular menstruation persists. The cause of vaginal spotting, bleeding, or menstruation could be noncompliance with the treatment regimen, or it could be that a higher dose of the drug is required to achieve amenorrhea. Patients missing successive doses may experience breakthrough bleeding.

Nafarelin leads to a small loss in bone density over the course of treatment, some of which may not be reversible. During one six-month treatment period, this bone loss should not be important. In patients with major risk factors for decreased bone mineral content such as chronic alcohol and/or tobacco use, strong family history of osteoporosis, or chronic use of drugs that can reduce bone mass such as anticonvulsants or corticosteroids, therapy with nafarelin may pose an additional risk. In these patients, the risks and benefits must be weighed carefully before therapy with nafarelin is instituted. Repeated courses of treatment with gonadotropin-releasing hormone analogs are not advisable in patients with major risk factors for loss of bone mineral content.

Patients who also have rhinitis should consult their physician for the use of a topical nasal decongestant. If the use of a topical nasal decongestant is required during treatment with nafarelin, the decongestant should not be used until at least two hours following dosing with nafarelin. Sneezing during or immediately after dosing with nafarelin should be avoided, if possible, as this may impair drug absorption.

Retreatment with nafarelin cannot be recommended because safety data beyond six months are not available.

The packaging of ganirelix acetate contains natural rubber latex, which may cause allergic reactions.

Cases of hypersensitivity reactions, including anaphylactoid reactions with the first dose, have been reported during postmarketing surveillance with cetrorelix acetate. A severe anaphylactic reaction associated with cough, rash, and hypotension was observed in one patient after seven months of treatment in a study for an indication unrelated to infertility. Special care should be taken in women with signs and symptoms of active allergic conditions or known history of allergic predisposition. Treatment with cetrorelix acetate is not advised in women with severe allergic conditions.

Because danazol may cause some degree of fluid retention, conditions that might be influenced by this factor, such as as seizure disorders, migraine, heart failure, or kidney dysfunction, require careful observation. In patients receiving long-term therapy, liver function must be monitored on a periodic basis.

Women on androgen or anabolic steroid therapy should be observed for signs of virilization (e.g., deepening of the voice, hirsutism, acne, menstrual irregularities). Discontinuation of drug therapy at the time of evidence of mild virilism is necessary to prevent irreversible virilization. Such virilization is usual following androgen or anabolic steroid use at high doses and is not prevented by concomitant use of estrogens. A decision may be made by the patient and the physician that some virilization will be tolerated during treatment for breast cancer. Menstrual irregularities, including amenorrhea, may also occur.

Because androgens may alter blood cholesterol concentration, caution should be used when administering these drugs to patients with a history of coronary artery disease.

Androgen therapy should be used cautiously in healthy males with delayed puberty. The effect on bone maturation should be monitored by assessing bone age of the wrist and hand every six months. In children, androgen treatment may accelerate bone maturation without producing compensatory gain in linear growth. This adverse effect may result in compromised adult stature. The younger the child, the greater the risk of compromising final mature height. When androgens are used in high doses in males, they interfere with the production of sperm. This effect is usually temporary and happens only while taking the medicine.

Patients using the brand name Androgel should wait five or six hours after applying the gel before showering or swimming. The gel contains alcohol, which is flammable; fire, flame, or smoking should be avoided until the gel is dried.

Concurrent dosing of an anabolic steroid and warfarin may result in unexpectedly large increases in the international normalized ratio (INR). When an anabolic steroid is prescribed to a patient being treated with warfarin, doses of warfarin may need to be decreased significantly to maintain the desirable INR level and diminish the risk of potentially serious bleeding.

The insulin or oral hypoglycemic dosage may need adjustment in diabetic patients who receive anabolic steroids.

Warnings

Cigarette smoking increases the risk of serious cardiovascular side effects from estrogens, progestins, and contraceptives, including myocardial infarction. This risk increases with age and with heavy smoking and is quite marked in women over 35 years of age. Women who use oral contraceptives should not smoke.

The use of unopposed estrogens (without a counterbalance of a progestin) in women who have a uterus is associated with an increased risk of endometrial cancer.

Using estrogens with or without progestins may increase chances of getting heart attacks, strokes, breast cancer, and blood clots. Use of estrogens with a progestin may increase the risk of breast cancer and dementia compared to estrogen alone. Estrogens increase the chances of getting uterine cancer. Vaginal bleeding after menopause may be a warning sign of uterine cancer.

A twofold to fourfold increase in the risk of gallbladder disease requiring surgery in postmenopausal women receiving estrogens has been reported.

Estrogen administration may lead to severe hypercalcemia (abnormally high levels of calcium in the blood) in patients with breast cancer and bone metastases. If hypercalcemia occurs, use of the drug should be stopped and appropriate measures taken to reduce the serum calcium level.

In clinical trials, raloxifene-treated women had an increased risk of deep vein thrombosis and pulmonary embolism, with the greatest risk occurring during the first four months of treatment. The drug should be discontinued at least 72 hours prior to and during prolonged immobilization (e.g., postsurgical recovery, prolonged bed rest) and should be resumed only after the patient is fully ambulatory. In addition, women taking raloxifene should move about periodically during prolonged travel. In a clinical trial of postmenopausal women with documented coronary heart disease or at increased risk for coronary events, an increased risk of death due to stroke was observed after treatment with raloxifene.

Thrombotic disorders occasionally occur in patients taking progestins. If early manifestations of the disease occur or are suspected, the drug should be withdrawn immediately.

Medroxyprogesterone at high doses is an antifertility drug. High doses would be expected to impair fertility until the cessation of treatment.

Benign tumors of the liver appear to be associated with the use of contraceptives. Although benign and rare, these may rupture and may cause death through intra-abdominal hemorrhage. Such lesions should be considered in estrogen users having abdominal pain and tenderness, abdominal mass, or hypovolemic shock. Liver cancer has also been reported in women taking estrogen-containing oral contraceptives. The relationship of this malignancy to these drugs is not known at this time.

Women with a history of hypertension or hypertension-related diseases or kidney disease should be encouraged to use a birth control method other than an estrogen- or progestin-containing contraceptive.

The onset or worsening of migraine or development of headache with a new pattern that is recurrent, persistent, or severe requires discontinuation of hormonal contraceptives and evaluation of the cause.

Breakthrough bleeding and spotting are sometimes encountered in patients on contraceptives, especially during the first three months of use. Nonhormonal causes should be considered and adequate diagnostic measures taken to rule out malignancy or pregnancy in the event of breakthrough bleeding, as in the case of any abnormal vaginal bleeding. In the event of amenorrhea, pregnancy should be ruled out. Some women may encounter postpill amenorrhea or oligomenorrhea (abnormally light or infrequent menstruation), especially when such a condition was preexistent.

Ectopic (outside the womb) as well as intrauterine pregnancy may occur in contraceptive failures.

An increased risk of pelvic inflammatory disease (PID) has been reported with intrauterine (IUD) contraceptive use. Partial penetration or lodging of an IUD in the endometrium can result in difficult removal, which in some cases may necessitate surgical removal. Partial or total perforation of the uterine wall or cervix may occur with IUD use.

Ovulation stimulants should be used only by physicians who are thoroughly familiar with infertility problems and their management. These drugs are capable of causing ovarian hyperstimulation syndrome (OHSS) (excessive stimulation of the ovaries causing them to become swollen and painful) in women with or without pulmonary or vascular complications. Ovulation stimulation therapy requires a certain time commitment by physicians and supportive health professionals and requires the availability of appropriate monitoring facilities. Reports of multiple births have been associated with ovulation stimulant therapy. The patient should be advised of the potential risk of multiple births before starting treatment. A potential for the occurrence of arterial thromboembolism exists with choriogonadotropin alfa.

Blurring or other visual symptoms such as spots or flashes may occasionally occur during therapy with clomiphene citrate. These visual symptoms increase in incidence with increasing total dose or therapy duration and generally disappear within a few days or weeks after clomiphene citrate is discontinued. These visual symptoms may render such activities as driving a car or operating machinery more hazardous than usual, particularly under conditions of variable lighting.

To minimize the hazard associated with occasional abnormal ovarian enlargement associated with clomiphene citrate therapy, the lowest dose consistent with expected clinical results should be used. Maximal enlargement of the ovary, whether physiologic or abnormal, may not occur until several days after discontinuation of the recommended dose of clomiphene citrate. Some patients with polycystic ovary syndrome who are unusually sensitive to gonadotropin may have an exaggerated response to usual doses of clomiphene citrate. Therefore, patients with polycystic ovary syndrome should be started on the lowest recommended dose and shortest treatment duration for the first course of therapy. If enlargement of the ovary occurs, additional clomiphene citrate therapy should not be given until the ovaries have returned to pretreatment size, and the dosage or duration of the next course should be reduced. Ovarian enlargement and cyst formation associated with clomiphene citrate therapy usually regresses spontaneously within a few days or weeks after discontinuing treatment. The potential benefit of subsequent clomiphene citrate therapy in these cases should exceed the risk. Because a correlation between ovarian cancer and infertility and age has been suggested, if ovarian cysts do not regress spontaneously, a thorough evaluation should be performed to rule out the presence of ovarian tumor growth.

Serious pulmonary conditions have been reported with follitropins and gonadotropins. In addition, thromboembolic events both in association with and separate from OHSS have been reported. Intravascular thrombosis and embolism can result in reduced blood flow to critical organs or the extremities. These conditions have led to venous thrombophlebitis, pulmonary embolism, pulmonary infarction, cerebral vascular occlusion (stroke), and arterial occlusion resulting in loss of limb. In rare cases, pulmonary complications and/or thromboembolic events have resulted in death.

Mild to moderate uncomplicated ovarian enlargement that may be accompanied by abdominal distension and/or abdominal pain may occur in patients treated with gonadotropins. These conditions generally regress without treatment within two or three weeks. Careful monitoring of ovarian response can further minimize the risk of overstimulation. If the ovaries are abnormally enlarged on the last day of therapy with lutropin alfa and follitropin alfa, human chorionic gonadotropin should not be administered in this course of therapy. This will reduce the risk of development of OHSS.

For goserelin acetate warnings, see ANTINEOPLASTICS.

Histrelin acetate (Supprelin LA) insertion is a surgical procedure, and it is important that the insertion instructions are followed to avoid potential complications. On occasion, localizing and/or removal of the implant has been difficult, and imaging techniques have been used, including ultrasound, CT, or MRI. Histrelin acetate causes a temporary increase in blood levels of estradiol in females and testosterone in both sexes during the first week of treatment. Patients may experience worsening of symptoms or onset of new symptoms during this period. However, within four weeks of histrelin therapy, suppression of gonadal steroids occurs, and manifestations of puberty decrease.

The diagnosis of CPP must be established before treatment with nafarelin is initiated. Regular monitoring of patients with CPP is needed to assess patient response as well as compliance. This is particularly important during the first six to eight weeks of treatment to assure that suppression of pituitary-gonadal function is rapid.

Gonadotropin-releasing agonists should be prescribed by physicians who are experienced in infertility treatment.

A sensitive test capable of determining early pregnancy is recommended immediately prior to start of danazol therapy. Additionally, a nonhormonal method of contraception should be used while taking this drug. If a patient becomes pregnant while taking danazol, administration of the drug should be discontinued and the patient should be apprised of the potential risk to the fetus (see *When Not Advised [Contraindications]*).

Thrombotic events, including life-threatening or fatal strokes, have been reported with danazol therapy. Danazol has been associated with several cases of benign intracranial hypertension. Early signs and symptoms of benign intracranial hypertension include papilledema (swelling near the optic nerve), headache, nausea and vomiting, and visual disturbances. Patients with these symptoms should be screened for papilledema, and, if present, the patients should be advised to discontinue danazol immediately and be referred to a neurologist for further diagnosis and care.

Before initiating therapy of fibrocystic breast disease with danazol, breast cancer should be excluded.

In patients with breast cancer and in immobilized patients, androgen and anabolic steroid therapy may cause hypercalcemia by stimulating osteolysis. In patients with cancer, hypercalcemia may indicate progression of bony metastasis.

If hypercalcemia occurs, the drug should be discontinued and appropriate measures instituted.

Prolonged use of high doses of androgens and use of anabolic steroids has been associated with the development of peliosis hepatis (a form of liver disease). Peliosis hepatis can be a life-threatening or fatal complication. Liver cell tumors are also reported with androgen and anabolic steroid therapy. Most often these tumors are benign and androgen-dependent, but fatal malignant tumors have been reported. Withdrawal of the drug often results in regression or cessation of progression of the tumor. However, liver tumors associated with androgens or anabolic steroids are much more vascular than other hepatic tumors and may be silent until life-threatening intra-abdominal hemorrhage develops.

Blood lipid changes that are known to be associated with increased risk of atherosclerosis are seen in patients treated with androgens and anabolic steroids. These changes include decreased high-density lipoprotein cholesterol and sometimes increased low-density lipoprotein cholesterol. The changes may be very marked and could have a serious impact on the risk of atherosclerosis and coronary artery disease.

Androgens can stimulate existing prostate cancer in men who have not yet been diagnosed. Also, the prostate may become enlarged. Enlargement of the prostate does not mean that cancer will develop. Geriatric patients in particular treated with androgens or anabolic steroids are at increased risk for the development of enlarged prostate and prostate cancer.

Androgens and anabolic steroids have been abused for athletic enhancement purposes; however, these drugs have not been shown to enhance athletic ability. In addition, these drugs are not safe and effective for this use and have a potential of serious side effects. An addiction syndrome is now being recognized with the chronic use of these drugs.

When Not Advised (Contraindications)

Estrogens and progestins (including contraceptives) should not be used in women with any of the following conditions: undiagnosed abnormal genital bleeding; known, suspected, or history of breast cancer except in appropriately selected patients being treated for metastatic disease; known or suspected estrogen-dependent neoplasia; active deep vein thrombosis, pulmonary embolism, or a history of these conditions; active or recent (e.g., within the past year) arterial thromboembolic disease (e.g., stroke, myocardial infarction); and liver dysfunction or disease.

Raloxifene is contraindicated in women with an active or past history of venous thromboembolism (VTE), including deep vein thrombosis, pulmonary embolism, and retinal vein thrombosis (see *Warnings*).

Progesterone capsules contain peanut oil and should never be used by patients allergic to peanuts.

Choriogonadotropin alfa injection is contraindicated in women who exhibit primary ovarian failure, uncontrolled thyroid or adrenal dysfunction, an uncontrolled organic intracranial lesion such as a pituitary tumor, abnormal uterine bleeding of undetermined origin, ovarian cyst or enlargement of undetermined origin, sex hormone–dependent tumors of the reproductive tract and accessory organs, or pregnancy.

Chorionic gonadotropin should not be used in patients with precocious puberty, prostate cancer, or other androgen-dependent tumor.

Clomiphene citrate should not be administered during pregnancy or in patients with liver disease or a history of liver dysfunction, abnormal uterine bleeding of undetermined origin, ovarian cysts or enlargement not due to polycystic ovarian syndrome, uncontrolled thyroid or adrenal dysfunction, or in the presence of an organic intracranial lesion such as pituitary tumor.

Follitropins and gonadotropins are contraindicated in women and men who exhibit high levels of FSH indicating primary gonadal failure, uncontrolled thyroid or adrenal dysfunction, sex hormone–dependent tumors of the reproductive tract and accessory organs, or an organic intracranial lesion such as a pituitary tumor and in women who exhibit abnormal uterine bleeding of undetermined origin, ovarian cyst or enlargement of undetermined origin, or pregnancy. Menotropins is contraindicated in men with normal gonadotropin levels indicating normal pituitary function and with infertility disorders other than hypogonadotropic hypogonadism.

For goserelin acetate contraindications, see ANTINEOPLASTICS.

Histrelin acetate (Supprelin LA) is contraindicated in females who are or may become pregnant while receiving the drug, as it may cause fetal harm when administered to pregnant patients.

Nafarelin acetate should not be used in patients with undiagnosed abnormal vaginal bleeding, during pregnancy or in women who may become pregnant while receiving the drug, or in women who are breast-feeding.

Gonadotropin-releasing agonists are contraindicated for known or suspected pregnancy.

Cetrorelix acetate should not be used in patients with severe kidney impairment.

Danazol should not be administered to patients with undiagnosed abnormal genital bleeding or markedly impaired liver, kidney, or cardiac function; who are pregnant (see *Warnings*); who are breast-feeding; or with porphyria (a genetic abnormality of metabolism causing abdominal pains and mental confusion).

Androgens and anabolic steroids are contraindicated in men with breast cancer or with known or suspected prostate cancer and in women who are or may become pregnant. When administered to pregnant women, androgens cause masculinization of the external genitalia of the female fetus. The degree of masculinization is related to the amount of drug given and the age of the fetus and is most likely to occur when the drugs are given in the first trimester.

Anabolic steroids are contraindicated with breast cancer in females with hypercalcemia as they may stimulate osteolytic bone resorption. They are also contraindicated in patients with nephrosis (a syndrome characterized by edema and large amounts of protein in the urine and usually increased blood cholesterol) or the nephrotic phase of nephritis (an inflammation of the kidney). Oxymetholone is contraindicated for patients with severe liver dysfunction.

Side Effects

Common side effects with estrogens and/or progestin therapy, including contraceptives, include breast pain or tenderness, dizziness or lightheadedness, headache, swelling of feet and lower legs, rapid weight gain, and vaginal bleeding.

Common side effects with choriogonadotropin alfa include injection site pain or bruising and abdominal pain.

Common side effects with raloxifene include flulike symptoms, hot flashes, headache, and joint pain.

Common side effects with chorionic gonadotropin include headache, irritability, restlessness, depression, fatigue, edema, precocious puberty, breast development in males, and pain at the site of injection.

Side effects with clomiphene citrate at recommended dosages are usually mild and transient, disappearing promptly after treatment is discontinued. The most common of these is menopausal-like "hot flushes."

Common side effects with follitropins include headache, ovarian cyst, nausea, and upper respiratory tract infection.

Common side effects with lutropin alfa include headache, nausea, breast pain, and abdominal pain.

Common side effects with menotropins include abdominal pain, back pain, chills, dizziness, fever, flulike symptoms, flushing, general body discomfort, headache, menstrual changes in women, muscle or joint pain, pain or rash at the injection site, and breast enlargement in men.

For goserelin acetate side effects, see ANTINEOPLASTICS.

The most common side effects with histrelin acetate (Supprelin LA) involve implant site reactions such as bruising, pain, soreness, redness, and swelling.

Common side effects with nafarelin include acne, transient breast enlargement, and vaginal bleeding.

Common side effects with gonadotropin-releasing agonists include abdominal pain, headache, OHSS, and vaginal bleeding.

Common side effects with danazol include acne, oily skin, and unwanted hair growth.

The most common side effects of androgen and anabolic steroid therapy for women are menstrual irregularities, decreased breast size, acne or oily skin, hoarseness or deepening of the voice, increased size of female genitals, unnatural hair growth, and male pattern baldness. For men, common side effects include breast soreness or enlargement, gynecomastia, frequent urge to urinate, and excessive frequency and duration of penile erections. Insufficient spermatozoa in the semen may occur at high dosages. Common side effects of topical androgens also include male pattern baldness and acne, and of the patch, blistering or itching of the skin under the patch. For prepubertal boys, common side effects include acne, early growth of pubic hair, enlargement of penis, and frequent or continuing erections.

In both sexes, anabolic steroids may cause increased or decreased libido.

Interactions

Estrogens are metabolized partially by cytochrome P450 3A4 (CYP3A4). Therefore, inducers or inhibitors of CYP3A4 may affect estrogen drug metabolism. Inducers of CYP3A4 such as Saint-John's-wort preparations (Hypericum perforatum), phenobarbital, carbamazepine, and rifampin may reduce plasma concentrations of estrogens, possibly resulting in a decrease in therapeutic effects and/or changes in the uterine bleeding profile. Inhibitors of CYP3A4 such as erythromycin, clarithromycin, ketoconazole, itraconazole, ritonavir, and grapefruit juice may increase plasma concentrations of estrogens and may result in side effects. Oral contraceptives may significantly intensify the effects of alcohol.

Use of cholestyramine with raloxifene is not recommended as it reduces the absorption of raloxifene. Also, raloxifene should be used with caution with certain other highly protein-bound drugs such as diazepam, diazoxide, and lidocaine.

Rifampin may decrease the effectiveness of norethindrone acetate.

No drug-drug interaction studies have been conducted for choriogonadotropin alfa.

No drug-drug interaction information is provided for chorionic gonadotropin.

Drug interactions with clomiphene citrate have not been documented.

No drug-drug interaction studies have been performed with follitropins.

No drug-drug interaction studies have been conducted with lutropin alfa.

Ganirelix can suppress the secretion of menotropins.

For goserelin acetate interactions, see ANTINEOPLASTICS.

No formal drug-drug, drug-food, or drug-herb interaction studies have been performed with histrelin acetate (Supprelin LA).

No drug-drug interaction studies have been conducted with nafarelin.

No formal drug-drug interaction studies have been performed with gonadotropin-releasing agonists.

Prolongation of prothrombin time may occur in patients stabilized on warfarin who take danazol. Danazol may cause an increase in carbamazepine and cyclosporine levels.

In diabetic patients, the metabolic effects of androgens may decrease oral hypoglycemic and insulin requirements.

Anabolic steroids may interfere with warfarin (see *Cautions and Concerns*) and sulfonylureas.

Sales/Statistics

According to IMS Health, a pharmaceutical market research firm, U.S. sales of prescription testosterone soared to $568 million in 2006, nearly double what they were in 2002. Decision Resources, Inc., another health data company, reported that in 2007 the market for women's reproductive drugs exceeded $23 billion worldwide. Sales of hormone replacement drugs topped $2 billion in 2007 in the United States alone, according to IMS Health. The U.S. estrogen therapy market is estimated at approximately $1.4 billion in annual sales, of which the transdermal segment, mostly patches, is about $260 million.

According to a report from the IMS Institute for Healthcare Informatics (the public reporting arm of IMS Health), hormonal contraceptives were the 18th largest therapeutic class by spending in the United States in 2010, with $4.8 billion in sales, up from $3.9 billion in 2006. IMS ranked hormonal contraceptives the 15th-largest therapeutic class by prescriptions in 2010, with 92.3 million prescriptions dispensed. That was down from 94.3 million in 2006.

Development History

Fuller Albright, a clinical researcher in the 1930s, observed that most of his patients with osteoporosis were postmenopausal women. Given this, Albright proposed that estrogen triggers a buildup of calcium reserves in bone during adolescence to provide for later reproductive needs (pregnancy and lactation) and that bone is lost after menopause when estrogen levels decrease. Many subsequent observations have confirmed the theory that "replacing" estrogen in postmenopausal women prevents bone loss, and thus this approach naturally seemed to be an effective way to stave off the effects of menopause on bone.

The FDA approved estrogen in 1942 in the form of conjugated equine estrogens, derived from the urine of pregnant horses, for the relief of menopausal symptoms. (The name Premarin came from PREgnant MARe's urINe.) The use of hormone therapy by postmenopausal women increased dramatically during the 1960s, and, in 1972, FDA approval was extended to postmenopausal osteoporosis. This latter approval was based on evidence from trials that evaluated the impact of estrogen therapy on bone mass, not on fracture reduction. However, by the early 1970s, it also became clear that estrogen alone (with-

out progestin) was associated with an increased risk of endometrial (uterine) cancer. Since this time, only women who have had their uterus removed by hysterectomy are prescribed estrogen alone; others receive estrogen combined with some form of progesterone, another hormone, to protect the uterus.

The recognition of progesterone's ability to suppress ovulation during pregnancy led to a search for a similar hormone that could bypass the problems associated with administering progesterone (low bioavailability when administered orally and local irritation and pain when continually administered parenterally) and, at the same time, serve the purpose of controlling ovulation. The many synthetic hormones that resulted became known as progestins.

The first orally active progestin, ethisterone, was synthesized in 1938 by scientists at Schering, AG in Berlin; it was marketed in Germany in 1939 as Proluton C and by Schering in the United States in 1945 as Pranone. Ethisterone was also marketed in the United States from the 1950s into the 1960s under a variety of trade names.

A more potent oral progestin, norethisterone, was synthesized in 1951 by scientists at Syntex in Mexico City and marketed by Parke-Davis in the United States in 1957 as Norlutin for use in menstrual disorders. It was used as the progestin in some of the first oral contraceptives (e.g., Ortho-Novum, Norinyl) in the early 1960s.

Norethynodrel, an isomer of norethisterone, was synthesized in 1952 by Frank B. Colton at Searle in Skokie, Illinois, and used as the progestin in Enovid, which was marketed in the United States in 1957 for menstrual disorders and infertility, then approved as the first oral contraceptive in 1960.

The first successful induction of ovulation and pregnancy in the human was described in 1958 utilizing FSH derived from human pituitary glands removed at autopsy. The real breakthrough came, though, only when an easy source of gonadotropins became available in the form of human menopausal gonadotropin (hMG) derived from the urine of postmeno-pausal women.

Among the ovulation stimulants, clomiphene citrate was approved in 1967, followed by chorionic gonadotropin (1973), menotropins (1975), urofollitropin (1996), follitropin alfa and beta (1997), choriogonadotropin alfa (2000), and lutropin alfa (2004).

Among the gonadotropin-releasing drugs, goserelin acetate was approved on December 29, 1989, followed by nafarelin acetate (February 13, 1990) and histrelin acetate (December 24, 1991). Ganirelix acetate was approved on July 29, 1999, and cetrorelix acetate on August 11, 2000.

Danazol was approved by the FDA as the first drug to specifically treat endometriosis in the early 1970s.

Testosterone therapy has been used for more than 60 years, beginning with the treatment of male hypogonadism. A Netherlands group was the first to isolate the testosterone hormone, which they identified and named in May 1935. The term *testosterone* was derived from the stems of testicle, sterol, and ketone. The chemical synthesis of testosterone was achieved in August 1935. The period from the 1930s to the 1950s has been called the "Golden Age of Steroid Chemistry," as research on testosterone and its many derivatives (androgens and anabolic steroids) proved it to have potent virilizing and anabolic effects.

More recently, the FDA approved histrelin acetate subcutaneous implant on May 3, 2007, for the treatment of CPP.

Future Drugs

The Pill-Plus is an oral contraceptive currently in development by Illinois's BioSante Pharmaceuticals and Pantarhei Bioscience, B.V. of The Netherlands. The Pill-Plus is a triple-hormone formulation, which adds an androgen to the typical contraceptive combination of estrogen and progestin. This triple-hormone formulation was developed in order to increase the sex drive of contraceptive users, which is usually diminished with the typical estrogen-progestin combination. Along with it, The Pill-Plus Transdermal is being developed as a once-daily transdermal contraceptive.

Many of the contraceptive products under development by the Population Council, an international, nonprofit, nongovernmental organization, employ nestorone, a new versatile synthetic progestin similar to the natural hormone progesterone. Nestorone, appropriate for breast-feeding women, can be delivered transdermally not only through a patch but also through a spray or gel. Phase I clinical trials of the Nestorone Metered Dose Transdermal System, a daily progestin-only spray-on contraceptive, began in Australia in 2004. The spray-on approach is a new technique for transferring a preset dose of fast-drying hormones onto the skin. The spray is absorbed almost instantaneously, so there is no risk of washing it off. The hormone collects as a reservoir within the skin, from which it then slowly diffuses into the bloodstream. In a clinical trial, a nestorone gel applied to the skin daily for three months suppressed ovulation in 83 percent of participants applying 1.2 mg per day.

Lasofoxifene tartrate (Fablyn, formerly, Oporia) is a selective estrogen receptor modulator being developed by Pfizer. The drug would give women an alternative to other osteoporosis treatments, some of which have multiple side effects, and would most benefit postmenopausal women at high risk of fractures.

Gertych, Arkadiusz, Aifeng Zhang, James Sayre, Sylwia Pospiech-Kurkowska, and H. K. Huang. "Bone Age Assessment of Children Using a Digital Hand Atlas." *Computerized Medical Imaging and Graphics* 31, no. 4 (2007): 322–331. Available online. URL: http://www.pubmedcentral.nih.gov/articlerender.fcgi?artid=1978493. Published online March 26, 2007.

thrombolytics Drugs used to break up blood clots (thrombi) that block blood flow; also called clot busters. Blood clots lodged in the coronary arteries cause most heart attacks. When clots reduce blood flow to the brain, they can cause a stroke. A blood clot that suddenly blocks the blood vessels in the lung is called a pulmonary embolus. Thrombolytics can be used to break up blood clots that are blocking blood flow to the heart (during a heart attack), brain (during an ischemic stroke), or lungs (during a pulmonary embolus). By breaking up a clot and returning normal blood flow through the blood vessel, the disease process can be arrested, damage limited, or the complications reduced. While ANTICOAGU-LANTS decrease the growth of a clot, thrombolytic agents actively reduce the size of the clot.

Classes

Thrombolytic drugs are divided into two classes:

- *Fibrin-specific agents—Examples:* Tissue plasminogen activators (alteplase [Activase, Cathflo Activase], reteplase [Retavase], and tenecteplase [TNKase]).

- *Fibrin-nonspecific agents—Examples:* streptokinase (Streptase) and urokinase (Abbokinase).

How They Work

Fibrin-specific agents work by targeting fibrin (the substance that causes blood to clot), dissolving the blood clot, and restoring flow to the area where the blockage occurred. Specifically, they convert clot-bound plasminogen to plasmin, an enzyme that dissolves the fibrin of blood clots.

Because alteplase binds more tightly to fibrin and the clot surface, its penetration into the clot is decreased. Reteplase is about six times more potent than alteplase and has an improved ability to penetrate into clots. Tenecteplase has a higher fibrin specificity and causes less disturbance of the body's natural clotting system.

Fibrin-nonspecific agents work by activating plasminogen, leading to extra production of plasmin, which triggers a natural body proteolysis cascade to break down unwanted blood clots. These drugs activate both clot-bound and free (circulating) plasminogen, which leads to systemic lysis of fibrin.

Approved Uses

Alteplase is approved to dissolve blood clots that have formed in the blood vessels in the heart, brain, or lungs. It is used immediately after symptoms of a heart attack (i.e., ST-segment elevation myocardial infarction [MI]) occur, following symptoms of a stroke, and to treat blood clots in the lungs (i.e., pulmonary embolism). Alteplase is also used to dissolve blood clots in tubes (catheters) that are placed in large blood vessels (central venous access devices) for the infusion of intravenous fluids or medicines.

Both reteplase and tenecteplase are approved for the treatment of ST-segment elevation MI.

Streptokinase is used to dissolve blood clots that form in the heart, lungs, or blood vessels (i.e., deep vein thrombosis [DVT] or arterial thrombosis). It is also used to dissolve blood clots that form in intravenous catheters.

Urokinase is used to dissolve blood clots that form in the lungs.

Off-Label Uses

Reteplase has been used off-label to dissolve blood clots in patients with acute and chronic deep venous thrombosis (DVT).

Companion Drugs

Thrombolytics may be administered along with or prior to heparin, an anticoagulant.

Administration

Thrombolytics are administered via intravenous injection.

Cautions and Concerns

Standard management of MI or pulmonary embolism should be implemented concurrently with thrombolytic treatment. Arterial and venous punctures should be minimized. In the event of serious bleeding, thrombolytic and concurrent heparin therapy should be discontinued immediately.

Because there has been little experience with patients receiving repeat courses of therapy with fibrin-specific agents, if an anaphylactoid reaction occurs, the infusion should be discontinued immediately, appropriate therapy initiated, and readministration undertaken with extreme caution.

Because of the increased likelihood of resistance due to antistreptokinase antibody, streptokinase may not be effective if administered between five days and 12 months of prior streptokinase administration or streptococcal infections, such as streptococcal pharyngitis, acute rheumatic fever, or acute glomerulonephritis secondary to a streptococcal infection.

Urokinase should be used in hospitals where the recommended diagnostic and monitoring techniques are available. The clinical response and vital signs should be observed frequently during and following urokinase infusion. Blood pressure should not be taken in the lower extremities to avoid dislodgement of possible deep vein thrombi.

Warnings

Cholesterol embolism has been reported rarely in patients treated with all types of thrombolytic agents; the true incidence is unknown. This serious condition, which can be lethal, is also associated with invasive vascular procedures (e.g., cardiac catheterization, angiography, vascular surgery) and/or anticoagulant therapy. Clinical features of cholesterol embolism may include "purple toe" syndrome, acute kidney failure, gangrene, hypertension, pancreatitis, MI, stroke, spinal cord infarction, retinal artery occlusion, bowel infarction, and rhabdomyolysis (breakdown of skeletal muscle).

The most common complication encountered with fibrin-specific agents is bleeding. The type of bleeding associated with thrombolytic therapy can be divided into two broad categories: internal bleeding (e.g., intracranial, gastrointestinal, genitourinary, respiratory tract) and superficial or surface bleeding (e.g., arterial punctures, sites of recent surgical intervention). Thrombolytic therapy requires careful attention to all potential bleeding sites, including catheter insertion sites, arterial and venous puncture sites, cutdown sites (small incisions to locate a vein or artery), and needle puncture sites. The concomitant use of heparin may contribute to bleeding. In clinical trials, some of the hemorrhage episodes occurred one or more days after the effects of the thrombolytic had dissipated but while heparin therapy was continuing. Should serious bleeding (not controlled by local pressure) occur, any concomitant anticoagulant (e.g., heparin) or antiplatelet agent (e.g., aspirin, clopidogrel) should be discontinued immediately.

To minimize the risk of bleeding, intramuscular injections and nonessential handling of the patient must be avoided during treatment with thrombolytic agents. Venipunctures should be performed as infrequently as possible and with care. Should an arterial puncture be necessary, upper extremity vessels are preferable. Direct pressure should be applied for at least 30 minutes, a pressure dressing applied, and the puncture site checked frequently for evidence of bleeding.

In the following conditions, the risk of bleeding may be increased and should be weighed against the anticipated benefits of thrombolytic therapy: recent (within 10 days) major surgery, obstetrical delivery, organ biopsy, previous puncture of noncompressible vessels, recent (within 10 days) serious gastrointestinal bleeding, high likelihood of a left heart thrombus (blood clot), subacute bacterial endocarditis, hemostatic defects including those secondary to severe hepatic or renal disease, pregnancy, cerebrovascular disease, diabetic hemorrhagic retinopathy, and any other condition in which bleeding might constitute a significant hazard or be particularly difficult to manage because of its location.

After administration of thrombolytic therapy for the treatment of an MI, cardiac arrhythmias may develop and are believed to be associated with restoration of blood flow. Antiarrhythmic drugs should be available in case treatment for these rhythm disturbances becomes warranted.

In acute ischemic stroke, neither the incidence of intracranial hemorrhage nor the benefits of therapy are known in patients treated with alteplase more than three hours after the onset of symptoms. Therefore, treatment of patients with acute ischemic stroke more than three hours after symptom onset is not recommended.

Streptokinase and urokinase contain albumin, a derivative of human blood. Based on effective donor screening and product manufacturing processes, they carry an extremely remote risk for transmission of viral diseases and Creutzfeldt-Jakob disease.

Postmarketing reports of hypersensitivity reactions with urokinase have included anaphylaxis (with rare reports of fatal anaphylaxis), bronchospasm, edema of the mouth, and hives.

When Not Advised (Contraindications)

Because thrombolytic therapy increases the risk of bleeding, it is contraindicated in the following situations: active internal bleeding, history of hemorrhagic stroke, ischemic stroke within the previous three months, recent intracranial or intraspinal surgery or trauma, intracranial tumor, arteriovenous malformation (a congenital disorder of blood vessels in the brain, brainstem, or spinal cord), aneurysm (dilatation of an artery, vein, or the heart), known bleeding tendency, or severe uncontrolled hypertension. For use in the acute treatment of stroke, thrombolysis is also contraindicated if the patient had major surgery within the past 14 days.

Side Effects

Bleeding is the most frequent adverse reaction associated with thrombolytics and can be fatal (see *Warnings*).

Fever and shivering are the most commonly reported allergic reactions with intravenous use of streptokinase.

Bronchospasm, edema of the mouth, hives, skin rash, and itching have been reported with urokinase therapy. The most serious side effects reported with urokinase administration include fatal hemorrhage and anaphylaxis (see *Warnings*).

Interactions

Use of anticoagulants (e.g., heparin, warfarin, direct thrombin inhibitors) and/or antiplatelet drugs (e.g., aspirin, clopidogrel, glycoprotein IIb/IIIa receptor blockers) may increase the risk of bleeding if administered prior to, during, or after thrombolytic therapy.

Sales/Statistics

Thrombolytic sales in the United States were $67 million in the third quarter of 2007, a 12 percent increase over the same quarter the previous year.

Demographics and Cultural Groups

According to Diane Hayes and Wendy L. Schneider, writing in *Health Management Technology* (September 1, 2006), "Use of thrombolytics for patients following a heart attack, while underused by all, has been markedly underused for African American Medicare beneficiaries."

Development History

Streptokinase is produced by streptococcal bacteria. According to Sikri and Bardia, "A serendipitous discovery by William Smith Tillett in 1933, followed by many years of work with his student Sol Sherry, laid a sound foundation for the use of streptokinase as a thrombolytic agent. The drug found initial clinical application in combating fibrinous pleural exudates, hemothorax, and tuberculous meningitis. In 1958, Sherry and others started using streptokinase in patients with acute myocardial infarction and changed the focus of treatment from palliation to 'cure.' Initial trials that used streptokinase infusion produced conflicting results. An innovative approach of intracoronary streptokinase infusion was initiated by Rentrop and colleagues in 1979." Streptokinase was approved by the FDA in 1982.

While Sherry and his team were working with streptokinase, other researchers (as well as Sherry's group) were forging ahead with another naturally occurring thrombolytic, urokinase, which is produced by kidney cells. Urokinase had been isolated first by MacFarlane and Pilings in 1946 and subsequently by Williams in 1951. Urokinase was approved by the FDA in 1978. In 1999, the FDA withdrew urokinase from the marketplace because of concerns over potential viral contamination. After these concerns were addressed and with new manufacturing and purification processes in place, urokinase was reapproved in October 2002.

Alteplase is a genetically engineered copy of a protein produced naturally by the body. According to Carey, "In 1979, scientists in Belgium first purified alteplase and showed that it could dissolve clots in laboratory animals. But the amount produced in the body, or from most human cells in culture, is so minute that large-scale production would be impractical. So, in 1981, Genentech Inc., of South San Francisco, Calif., began using recombinant DNA technology to produce enough alteplase to be tested in heart attack victims. Genetically engineered alteplase is made by introducing the human gene that holds the instructions for producing the protein into cells originally derived from the ovaries of Chinese hamsters. The inserted gene programs the cells to consistently produce large quantities of alteplase. Clinical trials of alteplase began in 1984." On February 23, 1989, alteplase received FDA approval.

Retavase was developed by Boehringer Mannheim Pharmaceuticals Corporation in Penzberg, Germany. It is produced by recombinant DNA technology in the bacterium *Escherichia coli*. Reteplase was approved by the FDA on October 30, 1996.

Tenecteplase was also developed by Genentech and is produced by recombinant DNA technology using an established mammalian cell line (Chinese hamster ovary cells). Tenecteplase was approved by the FDA on June 2, 2000.

Future Drugs

Saruplase, generated by genetically transformed *E. coli* and closely related to urokinase, is being studied in Europe. Grünenthal, GmbH, Aachen, Germany, is the manufacturer of saruplase.

Prourokinase is currently undergoing clinical trials by Abbott for a variety of indications including ischemic stroke and peripheral arterial occlusive disease. It is a relatively inactive precursor of urokinase that must be converted to urokinase before it becomes active in vivo. Thus far, the use of prourokinase has been limited to catheter delivery because of the risk of hemorrhage.

Staphylokinase, a bacterial plasminogen activator protein produced by *Staphylococcus aureus*, is being investigated for potential use as a thrombolytic by the Belgian biopharmaceutical company ThromboGenics.

The Danish pharmaceutical company Lundbeck A/S and PAION, a biopharmaceutical company based in Aachen, Germany, entered into an agreement in December 2007 to develop desmoteplase, which has the potential to treat patients with acute ischemic stroke up to nine hours after onset of symptoms. Desmoteplase, the most fibrin-specific plasminogen activator known today according to a company news release, is a genetically engineered version of a clot-dissolving protein found in the saliva of the vampire bat *Desmodus rotundus*. It has received fast-track designation from the FDA for the indication of acute ischemic stroke.

Carey, Catherine. "Clot-busting Drugs to Turn off Heart Attacks." *FDA Consumer,* February 1, 1988.
Sikri, Nikhil, and Amit Bardia. "A History of Streptokinase Use in Acute Myocardial Infarction." *Texas Heart Institute Journal* 34, no. 3 (2007): 318–327.

V

vaccines   Drugs used to produce active immunity to diseases caused by bacteria and viruses. The process of administering vaccines is referred to as vaccination. Vaccines contain antigens, which stimulate an immune response, especially the production of antibodies, which prevent or ameliorate the effects of infection by any natural strain of the organism. Vaccines take advantage of the body's natural ability to learn how to combat many disease-causing germs, or microbes, that attack it. They expose people safely to germs so that they can become protected from a disease but not come down with the disease.

The term *vaccine* derives from Edward Jenner's use of cowpox (*vacca* means cow in Latin), which, when administered to humans, provided them protection against smallpox. Vaccines may be living, weakened strains of viruses or bacteria, or they may be killed or inactivated organisms or purified products derived from them. Historically, vaccines have proven to be the most effective weapon in the fight against infectious diseases such as smallpox, polio, measles, and yellow fever.

Classes

Vaccines are divided into three classes:

- *Bacterial vaccines*—Stimulate the immune reaction in an individual to prevent him or her from being infected with certain bacterial diseases. *Examples:* anthrax vaccine adsorbed (Biothrax), BCG vaccine (Mycobax, TICE BCG), *Haemophilus* b conjugate vaccine (ActHIB, PedvaxHIB), *Haemophilus* b conjugate with hepatitis B vaccine (Comvax), meningococcal polysaccharide vaccine (Groups A, C, Y, and W-135 combined) (Menomune-A/C/Y/W-135), diphtheria toxoid conjugate vaccine (Menactra), pneumococcal vaccine polyvalent (Pneumovax 23), pneumococcal 7-valent conjugate vaccine (Prevnar), typhoid vaccine live oral Ty21a (Vivotif), and typhoid Vi polysaccharide vaccine (TYPHIM Vi).

- *Viral vaccines*—Stimulate the immune reaction in an individual to prevent him or her from being infected with certain viruses. *Examples:* hepatitis A vaccine inactivated (Havrix, Vaqta), hepatitis B vaccine recombinant (Engerix-B, Recombivax HB), hepatitis A inactivated and hepatitis B recombinant vaccine (Twinrix), human papillomavirus (Types 6, 11, 16, 18) recombinant vaccine (Gardasil), influenza virus vaccine trivalent inactivated (Afluria, Fluarix, FluLaval, Fluvirin, Fluzone), influenza virus vaccine live intranasal (FluMist), Japanese encephalitis (JE) virus vaccine inactivated (Ixiaro, JE-Vax), measles virus vaccine live (Attenuvax), mumps virus vaccine live (Mumpsvax), measles and mumps virus vaccine live (M-M-Vax), measles, mumps and rubella virus vaccine live (M-M-R II), measles, mumps, rubella, and varicella virus vaccine live (ProQuad), poliovirus vaccine inactivated (IPOL, Poliovax), rabies vaccine (Imovax, RabAvert), rotavirus vaccine live oral (Rotarix), rotavirus vaccine live oral pentavalent (RotaTeq), rubella virus vaccine live (Meruvax II), smallpox vaccine live (ACAM 2000), varicella virus vaccine live (Varivax), yellow fever vaccine (YF-Vax), and zoster vaccine live (Zostavax).

- *Toxoids*—By-products derived from bacterial organisms that cause disease by producing toxins that invade the bloodstream. *Examples:* tetanus toxoid adsorbed; diphtheria and tetanus toxoids adsorbed (DECAVAC); diphtheria and tetanus toxoids and acellular pertussis vaccine adsorbed (Adacel, Boostrix, Daptacel, Infanrix, Tripedia); diphtheria and tetanus toxoids and acellular pertussis and *Haemophilus influenzae* type b conjugate vaccines (TriHIBit); diphtheria and tetanus toxoids and acellular pertussis vaccine adsorbed, hepatitis B (recombinant), and inactivated poliovirus vaccine combined (Pediarix); diphtheria and tetanus toxoids and acellular pertussis adsorbed, inactivated poliovirus vaccine, and *Haemophilus* b conjugate (tetanus toxoid conjugate) vaccine (Pentacel); and diphtheria and tetanus toxoids and acellular pertussis and inactivated poliovirus vaccine (Kinrix).

How They Work

A vaccine contains a killed or weakened part of a germ that is responsible for infection. Because the germ has been killed or weakened before it is used to make the vaccine, it cannot make the person sick. When a person receives a vaccine, the body reacts by making protective substances called antibodies. Antibodies are the body's defenders and help to kill off the germs, or microbes, that enter the body. In addition, the body "remembers" how to protect itself from the microbes it has encountered before. Collectively, the parts of the body that remember and repel microbes are called the immune system. Vaccines teach the immune system by mimicking a natural infection. Later, if the body encounters the real disease, it remembers the antibodies that it made earlier and easily fights off the illness.

Approved Uses

Because vaccine guidelines and immunization schedules change from year to year, it is important to refer to the Centers for Disease Control and Prevention (CDC) Web site for the latest immunization schedule and patient populations for vaccines currently in use:

Recommendations and Guidelines http://www. cdc.gov/vaccines/recs/default.htm
Immunization Schedules for Various Age Groups http://www.cdc.gov/vaccines/recs/ schedules/
Vaccinations and Travel http://wwwnc.cdc.gov/ travel/content/vaccinations.aspx

The following is general approved usage information.

Anthrax vaccine protects against anthrax disease. Based on limited but convincing evidence, the vaccine protects against both cutaneous (skin) and inhalational anthrax. Anthrax vaccine is approved for and available only to people potentially exposed to large amounts of *Bacillus anthracis* bacteria on the job, such as laboratory workers, and for military personnel in areas where there may be an increased risk of anthrax exposure. Routine immunization with the anthrax vaccine is not recommended.

BCG, or Bacillus Calmette-Guérin, is used for the prevention of tuberculosis (TB) in people not previously infected with *Mycobacterium tuberculosis* who are at high risk for exposure. People at risk for exposure to TB include those who share the same household of persons known or suspected to have TB, persons infected with human immunodeficiency virus (HIV), persons who inject illicit drugs, residents and employees of high-risk residential settings (e.g., correctional institutions, nursing homes, mental institutions, and shelters for the homeless), healthcare workers who serve high-risk clients, and foreign-born persons recently arrived (within five years) from countries that have a high TB incidence or prevalence. TB is spread through the air when a person with untreated pulmonary TB coughs or sneezes. BCG is also used to treat bladder cancer.

Haemophilus b conjugate vaccine is used to prevent *Haemophilus influenzae* type b (Hib) disease, which can cause bacterial meningitis, an infection of the brain and spinal cord coverings that can lead to lasting brain damage and deafness. Hib bacteria are spread through contact with mucus or droplets from the nose and throat of an infected person when they cough or sneeze. The vaccine is usually given to children between the ages of two months and 18 months old.

Haemophilus b conjugate with hepatitis B vaccine is used for the routine vaccination against invasive disease caused by Hib and against infection caused by all known subtypes of hepatitis B virus (HBV). The vaccine is given to infants six weeks to 15 months of age born of hepatitis B surface antigen (HBsAg) negative mothers.

Meningococcal vaccines are used to prevent meningococcal disease, a leading cause of bacterial meningitis (an inflammation of the membranes that cover the brain and spinal cord [meninges]). This vaccine is recommended for individuals two to 55 years of age who are at increased risk for the disease. For example, people who travel to parts of the world where the disease is very common are at risk, as are military recruits who live in close quarters. Children and adults with damaged or removed spleens are at higher risk. People who live in college dormitories are also at greater risk of infection. Meningococcal disease is spread through the exchange of respiratory and throat secretions, such as through kissing or coughing.

Pneumococcal vaccine polyvalent is used to protect against pneumococcal disease, which can lead to serious infections of the lungs (pneumonia), the blood (bacteremia), and the covering of the brain or spinal cord (meningitis). This vaccine protects against 23 types of *Streptococcus pneumoniae*. It is recommended for use in all adults who are older than 65 years of age and for persons who are two years and older and at high risk for disease (e.g., sickle-cell disease, HIV infection, or other immunocompromising conditions). Pneumococcal disease is spread by close contact with persons who carry the bacteria in their nose or throat.

Pneumococcal 7-valent conjugate vaccine protects against seven strains of *Streptococcus pneumoniae*. These seven strains are responsible for the most severe pneumococcal infections among children. This vaccine is routinely given to children between two months and 15 months of age.

Typhoid vaccines are used to prevent typhoid, a serious disease caused by the *Salmonella typhi* bacteria. Typhoid causes a high fever, weakness, stomach pains, headache, loss of appetite, and sometimes a rash. If it is not treated, it can kill up to 30 percent of people who get it. Some people who get typhoid become carriers who can then spread the disease to others. Typhoid vaccine is recommended for travelers to parts of the world where typhoid is common, people in close contact with a typhoid carrier, and laboratory workers who work with *Salmonella typhi* bacteria.

Hepatitis A vaccine inactivated is used to prevent hepatitis A, a serious liver disease caused by the hepatitis A virus (HAV). HAV is usually spread by close personal contact and sometimes by eating food or drinking water containing the HAV. Hepatitis A vaccination is recommended for all children starting at age one year, travelers to countries with high rates of hepatitis A, and people at risk. Those at risk for hepatitis A include men who have sex with other men, people who share needles or syringes, those with long-term liver disease, people receiving blood products to help their blood clot, and people who work with HAV in a research setting.

Hepatitis B vaccine recombinant is used for protection against infection caused by all known subtypes of the HBV, a serious disease that affects the liver and can cause liver cancer and cirrhosis. HBV is spread by direct contact with the blood or body fluids of an infected person. Hepatitis B vaccination is recommended for all infants, older children and adolescents who were not vaccinated previously, and adults at risk for HBV infection. Those at risk include people whose sex partners have HBV, people who have multiple sex partners, people who are being treated for sexually transmitted diseases, men who have sexual contact with other men, people who share needles or syringes, people who have close contact with someone infected with HBV, health-care and public safety workers at risk for exposure to blood or blood-contaminated fluids on the job, people undergoing kidney dialysis, people with chronic liver disease, and people with HIV infection.

Human papillomavirus (Types 6, 11, 16, 18) recombinant vaccine is indicated for females nine to 26 years of age for the prevention of diseases caused by human papillomavirus (HPV) types 6, 11, 16, and 18, including cervical, vulvar, and vaginal cancer as well as genital warts and precancerous lesions. This vaccine is also indicated in males nine through 26 years of age for the prevention of genital warts caused by HPV types 6 and 11. HPV can be spread through all types of sexual contact.

Influenza virus vaccine trivalent inactivated and influenza virus vaccine live intranasal are used to protect against the specific influenza (flu) strains contained in the formulation. Influenza viruses are always changing. Because of this, influenza vaccines are updated every year, and an annual vaccination is recommended. The optimal time for flu vaccination is during October or November, but getting vaccinated in December or even later will still be beneficial in most years. Influenza can occur any time from November through May, but it most often peaks in January or February. Influenza is spread through contact with mucus or droplets from the nose and throat of an infected person when they cough or sneeze.

JE virus vaccine inactivated protects against JE, a serious infection caused by a virus that occurs in certain rural parts of Asia and leads to swelling of the brain. JE spreads through the bite of infected mosquitoes. It cannot spread directly from one person to another. People who live or travel in certain rural parts of Asia and laboratory workers at risk of exposure to JE virus should get the vaccine.

Measles virus vaccine live is used for vaccination against measles (rubeola). The measles virus is spread through the air or by direct contact with nose or throat discharges from someone who is infected. This vaccine is given to children who are 12 months through 12 years old.

Mumps virus vaccine live is used for vaccination against the mumps virus, which causes fever, headache, and swollen glands. Mumps can lead to deafness, meningitis, painful swelling of the testicles or ovaries, and, rarely, death. Mumps is spread by mucus or droplets from the nose or throat of an infected person, usually when a person coughs or sneezes. Mumps vaccine is given to children between 12 months and six years of age, usually as part of the measles, mumps, and rubella virus vaccine.

Measles, mumps, and rubella virus vaccine live is used for simultaneous vaccination against measles, mumps, and rubella (German measles) in individuals 12 months of age or older. This is the preferred vaccine for most children and adults, rather than using the individual vaccines.

Measles, mumps, rubella, and varicella virus vaccine live is used for simultaneous vaccination against measles, mumps, rubella, and varicella (chicken pox).

Poliovirus vaccine inactivated is used to prevent poliomyelitis caused by poliovirus Types 1, 2, and 3. Once very common in the United States, polio paralyzed and killed thousands of people each year before a vaccine became available. Polio is primarily spread from the feces (stool) of an infected person to the mouth of another person from contaminated hands or such objects as eating utensils. Poliovirus vaccine is given to children between two months and six years of age.

Rabies vaccine is used to prevent rabies both prior to and after exposure. Rabies is mainly a disease of animals caused by a virus. Humans get rabies when they are bitten by infected animals. Human rabies is rare in the United States, with only 39 cases diagnosed between 1990 and 2006, according to the CDC. An average of two to three deaths occur each year from rabies. However, between 16,000 and 39,000 people are treated each year for possible exposure to rabies after animal bites. Also, rabies is far more common in other parts of the world, with 40,000 to 70,000 rabies-related deaths each year. Rabies vaccine is given to people at high risk of rabies (e.g., veterinarians, animal handlers, cave explorers, rabies laboratory workers, rabies biologics production workers, and travelers to parts of the world where rabies is common) to protect them if they are exposed. The vaccine can also prevent the disease if it is given to a person after they have been exposed.

Rotavirus vaccine live oral pentavalent is used to prevent rotavirus, a virus that causes severe diarrhea, often accompanied by vomiting and fever, mostly in infants and young children. Rotavirus is not the only cause of severe diarrhea in this patient population, but it is one of the most serious. Each year in the United States, rotavirus is responsible for more than 200,000 emergency room visits, 55,000 to 70,000 hospitalizations, and 20 to 60 deaths. Almost all children in the United States are infected with rotavirus before their fifth birthday. Children are most likely to get rotavirus disease between November and May, depending on the part of the country in which they live, and can become infected by being around other children who have rotavirus diarrhea. Infants should be given the first dose of this vaccine between six and 14 weeks of age.

Rubella virus vaccine live is used to prevent rubella. Rubella virus causes rash, mild fever, and arthritis (mostly in women). If a woman gets rubella while she is pregnant, she could have a miscarriage, or her baby could be born with serious birth defects. Rubella is spread from person to person through the air. Rubella vaccine is given to children between one and six years of age, usually as part of the measles, mumps, and rubella virus vaccine.

Smallpox vaccine helps the body develop immunity to smallpox. Smallpox is caused by the variola virus, a virus that emerged in human populations thousands of years ago. It spreads through close contact with infected individuals or contaminated objects, such as bedding or clothing. There is no FDA-approved treatment for smallpox, and the only prevention is vaccination. Routine smallpox vaccination among the American public stopped in 1972 after the disease was eradicated in the United States. Until recently, the U.S. government provided the vaccine only to a few hundred scientists and medical professionals working with smallpox and similar viruses in a research setting. After the events of September 11, 2001, however, the U.S. government took further actions to improve its level of preparedness against terrorism. One of many such measures—designed specifically to prepare for an intentional release of the smallpox virus—included updating and releasing a smallpox response plan. In addition, the U.S. government has enough vaccine to vaccinate every person in the United States in the event of a smallpox emergency.

Varicella virus vaccine live is indicated for vaccination against varicella in individuals 12 months of age and older. Varicella, also called chicken pox, is a common childhood disease that is usually mild but can be serious, especially in young infants and adults. It causes a rash, itching, fever, and fatigue and can lead to severe skin infection, scars, pneumonia, brain damage, or death. The chicken pox virus can be spread from person to person through the air or by contact with fluid from chicken pox blisters. A person who has had chicken pox can develop shingles later on in life (see below).

Yellow fever vaccine is used to prevent yellow fever in persons nine months of age or older traveling to or living in an area that requires yellow fever vaccination or has reports of the virus occurring. Yellow fever is a serious disease caused by the yellow fever virus. It is spread through the bite of an infected mosquito and cannot be spread directly from person to person. It is found in certain parts of Africa and South America. Yellow fever vaccine is given only at approved vaccination centers.

Zoster vaccine live is used to prevent shingles, a painful skin rash, often with blisters, also called herpes zoster, in persons 60 years of age or older.

Shingles is caused by the varicella zoster virus, the same virus that causes chicken pox. Only someone who has had a case of chicken pox can get shingles. The virus stays in the body and can reappear many years later to cause a case of shingles. At least 500,000 people a year in the United States develop shingles.

Toxoids protect against diphtheria, tetanus, and pertussis, with several forms of combined vaccines against these diseases available. Diphtheria and pertussis are spread from person to person. Tetanus enters the body through cuts or wounds. Diphtheria causes a thick covering in the back of the throat and can lead to breathing problems, paralysis, heart failure, and even death. Tetanus (lockjaw) causes painful tightening of the muscles, usually all over the body, and can lead to "locking" of the jaw so the victim cannot open the mouth or swallow. Tetanus leads to death in about two out of 10 cases. Pertussis (whooping cough) causes coughing spells so bad that it is hard for infants to eat, drink, or breathe, and these spells can last for weeks. Pertussis can lead to pneumonia, seizures, brain damage, and death.

Tetanus toxoid adsorbed is used to immunize adults and children seven years of age or older against tetanus whenever combined preparations are not indicated. Diphtheria tetanus acellular pertussis vaccine (DTaP) is used for routine immunization of children younger than seven years of age. Diphtheria and tetanus toxoids and acellular pertussis and *Haemophilus* b conjugate vaccine (DTaP-Hib) is used to immunize children 15 to 18 months of age for prevention of invasive disease caused by Hib and diphtheria, tetanus, and pertussis. Diphtheria and tetanus toxoids adsorbed is used to immunize adults against diptheria and tetanus and children seven years of age or older when the physician determines the pertussis vaccine is not to be administered. Diphtheria and tetanus toxoids and acellular pertussis vaccine adsorbed, and hepatitis B (recombinant) and inactivated poliovirus vaccine combined is used to prevent diphtheria, tetanus, pertussis, hepatitis B, and polio infections in infants and children under seven years of age.

(*Note:* Because anthrax and smallpox vaccines are not currently routinely administered, they have been left out of the following sections.)

Administration

Vaccines are administered by mouth, by injection, or by nasal spray.

When used to protect against TB, BCG is given as a single percutaneous injection into the skin using a multiple puncture device. When used for bladder cancer, BCG flows into the bladder through a tube or catheter.

Haemophilus b conjugate vaccine and *haemophilus* b conjugate with hepatitis B vaccine are administered in a series of intramuscular injections.

Meningococcal polysaccharide vaccine is administered as a single subcutaneous injection. Meningococcal polysaccharide diphtheria toxoid conjugate vaccine is administered as a single intramuscular injection.

Pneumococcal vaccine polyvalent is administered via subcutaneous or intramuscular injection. Usually one dose is all that is needed. However, under some circumstances, a second dose may be given. A second dose is recommended for those people aged 65 and older who got their first dose when they were under 65 years if five or more years have passed since that dose. A second dose is also recommended at least five years after the first dose was given for people who have a damaged spleen or no spleen; have sickle-cell disease; have HIV infection or acquired immune deficiency syndrome (AIDS); have cancer, leukemia, lymphoma, or multiple myeloma; have kidney failure; have nephrotic syndrome; have had an organ or bone marrow transplant; or are taking medication that lowers immunity (such as chemotherapy or long-term steroids). Children 10 years old and younger may get this second dose three years after the first dose. Those older than 10 years should get it five years after the first dose.

Pneumococcal 7-valent conjugate vaccine is routinely given to infants as a series of four intramuscular injections from age two months to 12 to 15 months old.

Typhoid vaccine live oral Ty21a vaccine is a live, attenuated (weakened) vaccine taken orally via enteric-coated capsules; typhoid Vi polysaccharide vaccine is an inactivated (killed) vaccine administered as an intramuscular injection.

Hepatitis A vaccine inactivated is administered via intramuscular injection. Two doses of the vaccine are needed for lasting protection. These doses should be given at least six to 18 months apart.

Hepatitis B vaccine is usually given as a series of three intramuscular injections.

Hepatitis A inactivated and hepatitis B recombinant vaccine is administered by intramuscular injection. Primary immunization for adults consists of three doses given on a zero-, one-, and six-month schedule. Alternatively, a four-dose schedule, given on days zero, seven, and 21 to 30 followed by a booster dose at month 12 may be used.

Human papillomavirus vaccine is administered by intramuscular injection as three separate doses at the following schedule: zero, two months, six months.

Influenza virus vaccine trivalent inactivated is administered as a single intramuscular injection. Influenza virus vaccine live intranasal is sprayed as a single dose into the nostrils. Protection lasts up to a year for both forms of the vaccine.

JE virus vaccine inactivated is administered via subcutaneous injection. Three doses of vaccine are given over a 30-day period. A booster dose may be needed after two years.

Measles, mumps, and rubella virus live vaccine is administered via subcutaneous injection. Two doses of vaccine are given. The recommended age for primary vaccination is 12 to 15 months. Revaccination is recommended between age four and six or prior to elementary school entry.

The primary series of poliovirus vaccine inactivated vaccine consists of three doses administered intramuscularly or subcutaneously, preferably eight or more weeks apart and usually at ages two, four, and six to 18 months. Under no circumstances should the vaccine be given more frequently than four weeks apart. A booster dose is then administered at four to six years of age.

Rabies vaccine is administered via intramuscular injection. The pre-exposure schedule for rabies vaccination is three doses, with the second dose being given seven days after the initial dose and the third dose being given 21 to 28 days after the initial dose. For laboratory workers and others who may be repeatedly exposed to rabies virus, periodic testing for immunity is recommended, and booster doses should be given as needed. Persons who are exposed and have never been vaccinated against rabies should get five doses of the vaccine—one dose right away and additional doses on days three, seven, 14, and 28. They should also get a shot of rabies immune globulin at the same time as the first dose, which will provide immediate protection. Persons who are exposed and have been previously vaccinated should get two doses of rabies vaccine—one right away and another on day three, with no rabies immune globulin needed.

Rotavirus vaccine is a liquid administered orally. The dosage regimen differs depending on which product is used. Rotarix is administered as two doses, with the first dose given beginning at six weeks of age and the second dose being given at least four weeks later. This dose series should be completed by 24 weeks of age. RotaTeq is administered as three doses, with the first dose given at six to 12 weeks of age and the subsequent doses administered at four- to 10-week intervals. The third dose should not be given after 32 weeks of age. Varicella vaccine is administered via subcutaneous injection to children 12 months to 12 years of age. In these individuals, a second dose may be administered at least three months later. For those individuals 13 years of age and older who have never had chicken pox or received the varicella vaccine, two doses should be administered separated by four to eight weeks.

Yellow fever vaccine is administered via subcutaneous injection at least 10 days before travel. A booster dose can be given every 10 years for those at continuing risk of exposure.

Zoster vaccine is administered via subcutaneous injection as a single dose.

Toxoids are administered via intramuscular injection. Some toxoids are administered in a series. For example, children receive five doses of DTaP vaccine, one dose at each of the following ages: two months, four months, six months, 15 to 18 months, and four to six years. Hib vaccine can be administered any time DTaP vaccine is given. Diphtheria and tetanus toxoids and acellular pertussis adsorbed, inactivated poliovirus vaccine, and *Haemophilus* b conjugate (tetanus toxoid conjugate) vaccine is usually administered as a four-dose series at two, four, and six months of age and between 15 and 18 months of age. Diphtheria and tetanus toxoids and acellular pertussis adsorbed, inactivated poliovirus vaccine is frequently administered as the fifth dose in the DTaP vaccine series and the fourth dose in the inactivated poliovirus vaccine (IPV) series in children four through six years of age.

Cautions and Concerns

Immunodeficient patients or patients under immunosuppressive therapy may not develop the desired protective immune response to vaccines. Live virus vaccines should not be used in these patients, as replication of the viruses used in the vaccines can be enhanced and result in serious adverse reactions. Caution is advised when considering whether to administer live vaccines to individuals with close contacts who are immunocompromised, such as individuals with malignancies or receiving immunosuppressive therapy, because the recent vaccination site contains live virus that can be transmitted to these other individuals.

Vaccines administered via intramuscular injection should be given with caution in persons with bleeding disorders such as hemophilia or thrombocytopenia and in persons on anticoagulant therapy, with steps taken to avoid the risk of hematoma following the injection.

Prior to an injection of any vaccine, all known precautions should be taken to prevent adverse reactions. This includes a review of the patient's history with respect to possible sensitivity to the vaccine or similar vaccines. Health-care providers should question the patient, parent, or guardian about reactions to a previous dose of this product or similar product. Epinephrine injection and other appropriate agents should be available to control immediate allergic reactions. Health-care providers should obtain the previous immunization history of and inquire about the current health status of the vaccinee.

BCG vaccine should not be injected subcutaneously, intradermally, or intravenously. The vaccinated person should avoid contact with all known tuberculous contacts or suspects until the sensitivity to tuberculin is verified (usually within three months). BCG contains live bacteria; use with aseptic technique.

Hib disease may occur in the week after *Haemophilus* b conjugate vaccination or *Haemophilus* b conjugate with hepatitis B vaccination and prior to the onset of the protective effects of the vaccine.

Special care should be taken to avoid injecting meningococcal polysaccharide vaccine intradermally, intramuscularly, or intravenously, as clinical studies have not been done to establish safety and efficacy of the vaccine using these routes of administration.

Caution and appropriate care should be exercised in administering pneumococcal vaccine polyvalent to individuals with severely compromised cardiovascular and/or pulmonary function in whom a systemic reaction would pose a significant risk. Pneumococcal vaccine polyvalent may not be effective in preventing pneumococcal meningitis in patients who have chronic cerebrospinal fluid leakage resulting from congenital lesions, skull fractures, or neurosurgical procedures.

Pneumococcal 7-valent conjugate vaccine is for intramuscular use only and should under no circumstances be administered intravenously. Fever and, rarely, febrile seizure have been reported in children receiving this vaccine. For children at higher risk of seizures than the general population, an antipyretic, such as acetaminophen or ibuprofen, may be administered around the time of vaccination to reduce the possibility of postvaccination fever.

In the case of acute febrile illnesses and acute gastrointestinal illness as well as during and up to three days after treatment with antibiotics, oral typhoid vaccine should not be taken due to possible inhibition of the growth of the vaccine organisms. The capsules must be swallowed whole and not chewed because of the destruction of the organism by gastric acid.

Typhoid Vi polysaccharide vaccine is for intramuscular use only and should not be administered intravenously.

Hepatitis A vaccine inactivated will not prevent hepatitis caused by infectious agents other than HAV.

Because of the long incubation period (approximately 20 to 50 days) for HAV and HBV, it is possible for unrecognized infection to be present at the time the vaccine is given. The vaccine may not prevent hepatitis A or hepatitis B in such individuals.

Caution and appropriate care should be exercised in administering hepatitis B vaccine to individuals with severely compromised cardiopulmonary status or to others in whom a fever or systemic reaction could pose a significant risk.

Human papillomavirus vaccine is not intended to be used for treatment of active genital warts, cervical cancer, or vaginal cancer. This vaccine has not been shown to provide protection against HPV to which a woman has previously been exposed through sexual activity.

Vaccines prepared for a previous influenza season should not be administered to provide protection for the current season. If Guillain-Barre syndrome (GBS) has occurred within six weeks of any prior influenza vaccination, the decision to give influenza virus vaccine live intranasal should be based on careful consid-

eration of the potential benefits and potential risks, such as increased risk of recurrent disease.

The decision to administer JE virus vaccine should balance the risks for exposure to the virus and for developing illness, the availability and acceptability of repellents and other alternative protective measures, and the side effects of vaccination. JE virus vaccine is not a substitute for mosquito precautions.

Because measles, mumps, and rubella vaccines may result in a temporary depression of tuberculin skin sensitivity, if a tuberculin test is to be done, it should be administered either before or simultaneously with the vaccine.

Intramuscular rabies vaccine should be injected into the deltoid muscle. In infants and small children, the mid-lateral aspect of the thigh may be preferable. Never administer rabies vaccine in the gluteal area, as vaccine failure may occur. While the concentration of antibiotics in each dose of rabies vaccine is extremely small, persons with known hypersensitivity to any of these agents could have an allergic reaction.

Rotavirus vaccine will not prevent diarrhea or vomiting caused by other germs. Rotavirus vaccine virus can potentially be transmitted to persons who have contact with the vaccine. The potential risk of transmission of vaccine virus should be weighed against the risk of acquiring and transmitting natural rotavirus. Children who are moderately or severely ill at the time the vaccination is scheduled should probably wait until they recover. This includes children who have diarrhea or vomiting.

The duration of protection from varicella infection after vaccination is unknown. It is not known whether varicella vaccine given immediately after exposure to natural varicella virus will prevent illness.

Vaccination with yellow fever vaccine should be deferred for eight weeks following blood or plasma transfusion.

The duration of protection after vaccination with zoster vaccine is unknown, although in the Shingles Prevention Study, protection from zoster was demonstrated through four years of follow-up. The need for revaccination has not been defined.

There is an increased incidence of local and systemic reactions to booster doses of tetanus toxoid when given to previously immunized persons. Persons who have a history of GBS may be at increased risk of recurrent disease after subsequent doses of tetanus toxoid vaccines.

Warnings

Severe allergic reaction can occur with any vaccine. Prior to administration of any vaccine, all known precautions should be taken to prevent adverse reactions. Anyone who has had a serious allergic reaction to a previous dose of a vaccine should not get another dose.

Immunization should be delayed during the course of an illness with acute high fever. Most vaccines can be administered to persons with minor illnesses such as diarrhea, mild upper-respiratory infection with or without low-grade fever, or other illnesses with low-grade fever (see rotavirus vaccine under *Cautions and Concerns*). Persons with moderate or severe fever should be vaccinated as soon as they have recovered from the acute phase of the illness.

Certain components that might cause allergic reactions (e.g., neomycin, streptomycin, and formaldehyde) are used in the production of many vaccines. Although purification procedures eliminate measurable amounts of these substances, traces may be present, and allergic reactions may occur in persons sensitive to these substances. These vaccines should be avoided in patients with severe allergies to these substances.

Symptoms such as fever of 103° or greater or acute localized inflammation persisting longer than two to three days suggest active BCG infection, and evaluation for serious infectious complication should be considered.

GBS has been reported following administration of meningococcal polysaccharide diphtheria toxoid conjugate vaccine. An evaluation of post-marketing adverse events suggests a potential for an increased risk of GBS following vaccination.

When cancer chemotherapy or other immunosuppressive therapy (e.g., for patients with Hodgkin's disease or those who undergo organ or bone marrow transplantation) is initiated, the timing of pneumococcal vaccine polyvalent vaccination is critical. The interval between vaccination and beginning immunosuppressive therapy should be at least two weeks. Similarly, the vaccine should be given at least two weeks before elective splenectomy.

The use of pneumococcal 7-valent conjugate vaccine does not replace the use of 23-valent pneumococcal polysaccharide vaccine in children at least 24 months of age with sickle-cell disease, asplenia, HIV infection, chronic illness, or who are immunocompromised.

The safety and immunogenicity of typhoid Vi polysaccharide vaccine in children under two years of age has not been established. As with other polysaccharide vaccines, the antibody response may be inadequate in this age group. The decision whether to vaccinate children under two years of age depends upon the risk incurred by the child.

Fainting, at times accompanied by seizures, has been reported following vaccination with human papillomavirus vaccine, sometimes resulting in falling with injury. Observation for 15 minutes after administration is recommended.

Serious allergic reactions to JE vaccine, including swelling of the hands and feet, face, or lips and difficulty breathing, may occur within minutes following vaccination. A possibly related reaction has occurred as late as 17 days after vaccination. Most reactions occur within 10 days of vaccination, with the majority occurring within 48 hours. Vaccinated persons should be observed for 30 minutes after vaccination and warned about the possibility of delayed generalized urticaria (hives). Vaccinated persons should be advised to remain in areas where they have ready access to medical care for 10 days after receiving a dose of JE vaccine. Vaccinated individuals should be instructed to seek medical attention immediately upon onset of any reaction. Persons should not embark on international travel within 10 days of JE vaccine immunization because of the possibility of delayed allergic reactions.

Due caution should be employed in administration of measles virus vaccine live to persons with a history of cerebral injury, individual or family histories of convulsions, or any other condition in which body stress due to fever should be avoided. The physician should be alert to the temperature elevation which may occur following vaccination.

Recently, a significant increase has been noted in "immune complex–like" reactions in persons receiving booster doses of human diploid cell rabies vaccine. The illness, characterized by onset at two to 21 days postbooster, presents with generalized hives and may also include arthralgia, arthritis, angioedema, nausea, vomiting, fever, and malaise. In no case were the illnesses life-threatening. This reaction occurred much less frequently in persons receiving primary immunization.

Anaphylaxis may occur following the use of yellow fever vaccine, even in individuals with no prior history of hypersensitivity to the vaccine components.

Safety and efficacy of zoster vaccine have not been evaluated in individuals on immunosuppressive therapy nor in individuals receiving daily topical or inhaled corticosteroids or low-dose oral corticosteroids. Zoster vaccine live is not a substitute for varicella virus vaccine live and should not be used in children.

A routine tetanus booster should not be given more frequently than every 10 years; however, if someone experiences a deep or puncture wound or a wound contaminated with dirt, an additional booster dose may be given if the last dose was more than five years ago. Persons who experience severe local reactions or temperature greater than 103°F after a previous tetanus injection usually have very high serum tetanus antibody levels and should not be given emergency doses of tetanus toxoid–containing preparation more frequently than every 10 years, even if they have a wound that is neither clean nor minor.

The decision to administer a pertussis-containing vaccine to children with stable central nervous system disorders must be made by the physician on an individual basis, with consideration of all relevant factors and assessment of potential risks and benefits for that individual.

When Not Advised (Contraindications)

Live vaccines should generally not be given to persons who are immunosuppressed (e.g., persons who are HIV-infected) or who are likely to become immunocompromised (e.g., persons who are candidates for organ transplant). (See *Cautions and Concerns*). Live vaccines should not be given during pregnancy.

Haemophilus b conjugate vaccine should not be given to persons who have ever had an allergic reaction to a *Haemophilus* b or a tetanus vaccine or who have received cancer chemotherapy or radiation treatment in the past three months.

Persons previously diagnosed with GBS should not receive meningococcal polysaccharide diphtheria toxoid conjugate vaccine (see *Warnings*).

Hypersensitivity to diphtheria toxoid is a contraindication to the use of pneumococcal 7-valent conjugate vaccine.

Safety of oral typhoid vaccine has not been demonstrated in immunosuppressed patients. These people should not receive the vaccine regardless of benefit.

Hepatitis A vaccine is contraindicated in patients with hypersensitivity to neomycin. Hepatitis B vaccine is contraindicated in patients with hypersensitivity to yeast.

Influenza virus is propagated in eggs for the preparation of influenza virus vaccine. Thus, this vaccine should not be administered to anyone with a history of allergy to chicken eggs, chicken, chicken feathers, or chicken dander. Influenza virus vaccine live intranasal is contraindicated in children and adolescents (two to 17 years of age) receiving aspirin therapy or aspirin-containing therapy because of the association of Reye's syndrome with aspirin and wild-type influenza infection. The nasal influenza vaccine should also not be administered to any individuals with asthma and children under five years of age with recurrent wheezing because of the potential for increased risk of wheezing postvaccination unless the potential benefit outweighs the potential risk.

Measles vaccine and mumps vaccine are produced in chick embryo cell culture. Anyone with a history of anaphylactic, anaphylactoid, or other immediate reactions (e.g., hives, swelling of the mouth and throat, difficulty breathing, hypotension, and shock) to chicken eggs, chicken, chicken feathers, or chicken dander should not be administered these vaccines.

Persons who have experienced anaphylactic reactions to topically or systemically administered neomycin should not receive measles vaccine. Most often, however, neomycin allergy manifests as a skin reaction (contact dermatitis), which is a delayed-type (cell-mediated) immune response rather than anaphylaxis. A history of contact dermatitis to neomycin is not a contraindication to receiving measles vaccine.

JE vaccine is produced in mouse brains and should not be administered to persons with a proven or suspected hypersensitivity to proteins of rodent or neural origin. Hypersensitivity to thimerosal, a mercury derivative, is a contraindication to JE vaccination.

Measles, mumps, and rubella virus vaccine combined should not be given to pregnant females, as the possible effects of the vaccine on fetal development are unknown. If vaccination of postpubertal females is undertaken, pregnancy should be avoided for three months following vaccination.

Mumps virus vaccine is not recommended for infants younger than 12 months because they may retain maternal mumps neutralizing antibodies, which may interfere with the immune response.

Anyone who has ever had a life-threatening allergic reaction to the antibiotics neomycin, streptomycin, or polymyxin B should not get the polio shot (see *Warnings*).

Rotavirus vaccine live oral is contraindicated in infants with a history of uncorrected congenital malformation of the gastrointestinal tract.

Because the yellow fever virus used in the production of yellow fever vaccine is propagated in chicken embryos, this vaccine should not be administered to anyone with a history of acute hypersensitivity to eggs or egg products. Yellow fever vaccination of infants less than nine months of age is contraindicated because of the risk of encephalitis. Immunosuppressed individuals should not be immunized, and travel to yellow fever endemic areas should be postponed or avoided.

Tetanus toxoid should not be administered to anyone with hypersensitivity to thimerosal.

The following events are contraindications to administration of any pertussis-containing vaccine: encephalopathy (e.g., coma, decreased level of consciousness, prolonged seizures) within seven days of administration of a previous dose of a pertussis-containing vaccine that is not attributable to another identifiable cause; and progressive neurologic disorder, including infantile spasms, uncontrolled epilepsy, or progressive encephalopathy. Pertussis vaccine should not be administered to individuals with such conditions until a treatment regimen has been established and the condition has stabilized. In instances when the pertussis vaccine component is contraindicated, diphtheria and tetanus toxoids (DT) vaccine should be administered for the remaining doses in the vaccination schedule.

Side Effects

All injected vaccines may be associated with injection-site reactions, such as itching, pain, redness, swelling, or a small lump. These side effects usually resolve in a few days, although lumps may take weeks or longer to resolve.

Common side effects with BCG vaccine include swollen lymph nodes, fever, blood in the urine, frequent or painful urination, upset stomach, or vomiting.

Common side effects with *Haemophilus* b conjugate vaccine include low fever, mild fussiness or crying, joint pain, body aches, drowsiness, and diarrhea.

Side effects from the meningococcal vaccine are mild and consist principally of drowsiness, irritability, and diarrhea.

Common side effects with pneumococcal 7-valent conjugate vaccine include decreased appetite, vomiting, diarrhea, irritability, drowsiness, fever, and restless sleep.

Common side effects with oral typhoid vaccine include constipation, abdominal cramps, diarrhea, nausea, vomiting, loss of appetite, fever, headache, and skin rash.

Common side effects with injected typhoid vaccine include malaise, headache, fever, and muscle pain.

Hepatitis A vaccine inactivated is generally well tolerated; mild side effects include headache, loss of appetite, and tiredness.

Hepatitis B vaccine recombinant is a very safe vaccine and is well tolerated. The most commonly reported side effects have included irritability, fever, diarrhea, fatigue/weakness, diminished appetite, and rhinitis.

Mild fever is a common side effect with human papillomavirus vaccine.

Common side effects with influenza virus vaccine trivalent inactivated are fever and aches. Common side effects with influenza virus vaccine live intranasal include runny nose, nasal congestion, cough, fever, headache and muscle aches, wheezing, abdominal pain or occasional vomiting or diarrhea, sore throat, chills, and tiredness/weakness.

Common side effects with JE virus vaccine inactivated include swelling (see *Warnings*), fever, headache, malaise, rash, chills, dizziness, muscle pain, nausea, vomiting, and abdominal pain.

Common side effects with measles virus vaccine live include fever, fainting, headache, dizziness, irritability, diarrhea, vomiting, and nausea.

Common side effects with mumps virus vaccine live include mild fever, mildly swollen glands, and diarrhea.

Common side effects with measles, mumps, and rubella virus vaccine live include temporary pain and stiffness in the joints (mostly in teenage or adult women), fever, and mild rash.

Common side effects with measles, mumps, rubella, and varicella virus vaccine live include fever and irritability.

Common side effects with rabies vaccine include headache, nausea, abdominal pain, muscle aches, and dizziness.

Most babies who get rotavirus vaccine do not have any problems with it. Babies may become slightly irritable or have mild, temporary diarrhea or vomiting after receiving a dose of rotavirus vaccine.

Common side effects with rubella virus vaccine live include itching, rash, fever, and sore throat.

Common side effects with varicella virus vaccine live include fever and mild rash for up to a month following vaccination.

Common side effects with yellow fever vaccine include mild headaches, myalgia, and low-grade fevers for five to 10 days.

Headache is a common side effect with zoster vaccine.

Common side effects with tetanus toxoid include redness, warmth, edema, itching, rash, malaise, transient fever, pain, and nausea.

Common side effects with DTaP vaccine include loss of appetite, fever, drowsiness, and irritability.

Interactions

Drugs that suppress the immune system, such as chemotherapy agents or corticosteroids, and drugs to treat tuberculosis may interfere with the development of the immune response of vaccines.

The immune response to a live vaccine may be impaired if administered within 30 days of another live vaccine.

Meningococcal polysaccharide vaccine should not be given at the same time as whole-cell pertussis or whole-cell typhoid vaccines due to combined endotoxin content.

Oral typhoid vaccine should not be administered concurrently with antibiotics or other drugs that are active against salmonella. The vaccine should be administered first, and at least three days should elapse between the final dose of the vaccine and administering such drugs. There are no known interactions of typhoid Vi polysaccharide vaccine with drugs or foods.

Generally, injectable vaccines should not be mixed with any other vaccine in the same syringe or vial except for those already commercially available as combo vaccines. When multiple injectable vaccines are administered at the same time, they should be given at different injection sites.

The safety and immunity of nasal influenza vaccine when administered concurrently with inactivated vaccines have not been determined. Therefore, health-care providers should consider the risks and benefits of concurrent administration of influenza virus vaccine live intranasal with inactivated vaccines.

Administration of immune globulins concurrently with rubella virus vaccine live may interfere with the expected immune response.

It is not known whether varicella vaccine given immediately after exposure to natural varicella virus will prevent illness. Vaccination should be deferred for at least five months following blood or plasma transfusions or administration of immune globulin or varicella zoster immune globulin. Administration of immune globulin products can diminish the antibody response to varicella vaccine. Vaccine recipients should avoid use of salicylates (e.g., aspirin) for six weeks after vaccination with varicella vaccine, as Reye's syndrome has been reported following the use of salicylates during natural varicella infection.

Because clinical trials in infants younger than 15 months of age have indicated that the combination of DTaP vaccine with DTap-HIB vaccine may induce a lower immune response to the *Haemophilus* b vaccine component than DTap-HIB vaccine given separately, this combination should not be used in infants for the first three doses. DTaP vaccine combined with DTap-HIB vaccine should be used only for the booster dose at 15 to 18 months of age.

Sales/Statistics

According to the CDC's National Center for Health Statistics and National Immunization Program, National Immunization Survey, in 2006, 77 percent of children 19 to 35 months of age received the combined vaccination series of four doses of DTaP (diphtheria-tetanus-acellular pertussis) vaccine, three doses of polio vaccine, one dose of MMR (measles-mumps-rubella vaccine), three doses of *Haemophilus* b conjugate vaccine, three doses of hepatitis B vaccine, and one dose of varicella vaccine. Children living below the poverty threshold were less likely than were children living at or above poverty to have received the combined vaccination series (74 percent compared with 78 percent).

For the 2006–07 school year, all states except Nevada submitted reports of vaccination coverage levels for children entering kindergarten for the U.S. Department of Health and Human Services *Healthy People 2010* initiative. Among the reporting states, coverage ranged from 32 states with at least 95 percent coverage for varicella vaccine to 35 states with at least 95 percent coverage for hepatitis B vaccine; 35 states reported at least 95 percent coverage for MMR, and 13 of the reporting states did not meet the 95 percent coverage target for one or more of the vaccines.

According to a report from the IMS Institute for Healthcare Informatics (the public reporting arm of IMS Health), vaccines were the 17th largest therapeutic class by spending in the United States in 2010, with $5 billion in sales, up from $3.9 billion in 2006.

Demographics and Cultural Groups

According to 2007 vaccine coverage estimates by the CDC, there were no differences in coverage among any racial or ethnic groups for the complete series of recommended vaccines for children.

Development History

An article on the Smithsonian Institution's Web site notes that it has been recognized for centuries that some diseases never reinfect a person after recovery and that inoculation originated in

India or China some time before 200 B.C. "The concept of immunization, or how to artificially induce the body to resist infection, received a big boost in 1796, when physician Edward Jenner inoculated a young boy in England and successfully prevented him from getting smallpox."

In addition, the article says, "World War II accelerated vaccine development. Fear of a repetition of the 1918–19 world epidemic of influenza focused urgent attention on all viral diseases, while commercial production of antibiotics taught researchers to grow viruses with less microbe contamination. Also, investigators paid closer attention to vaccine safety and effectiveness through clinical studies before release of a vaccine to the public, especially after the yellow fever vaccine apparently caused hepatitis B in many U.S. soldiers in 1942."

Approvals for some of the current vaccines:

Anthrax vaccine was licensed in 1970.

Meningococcal polysaccharide vaccine has been available since the 1970s, and meningococcal conjugate vaccine was licensed in 2005.

According to Vaccine Information for the Public and Health Professionals, the first hepatitis B vaccine became commercially available in the United States in 1982. In 1986, a hepatitis B vaccine produced by recombinant DNA technology was licensed, and a second recombinant-type hepatitis B vaccine was licensed in 1989.

The first DTaP product was approved in 1991.

JE virus vaccine inactivated was approved on December 10, 1992.

Hepatitis A vaccine inactivated was approved on February 22, 1995 (Havrix) and March 29, 1996 (Vaqta).

Pneumococcal 7-valent conjugate vaccine was approved on February 17, 2000.

Zoster vaccine live was approved on May 26, 2006.

On June 20, 2008 the FDA licensed a combined DTaP, inactivated poliovirus vaccine, and Hib conjugate (tetanus toxoid conjugate) vaccine, DTaP-IPV/Hib (Pentacel).

Future Drugs

Plotkin, writing in *Nature Medicine,* notes that until now, most vaccines have been aimed at infants and children, but adolescents and adults are increasingly being targeted. Among his other noted trends: Combinations of vaccines are becoming more common, and vaccines containing five or more components are used in many parts of the world. New methods of administering vaccines are being developed, such as skin patches, aerosols via inhalation devices, and eating genetically engineered plants. Attempts are being made to develop vaccines to help cure chronic infections as opposed to preventing disease. New vaccines are being developed to defend against bioterrorist attacks such as anthrax, plague, and smallpox.

Due to the complexity of the vaccine-licensing process and the large number of vaccines on the horizon, the American Academy of Pediatrics (AAP) has developed a Web information page to provide current information about the licensing process and AAP recommendations about vaccines being developed: http://aapredbook. aappublications.org/news/vaccstatus.shtml. The page is updated as changes occur.

"History of Vaccines." Smithsonian National Museum of American History. Available online. URL: http://americanhistory.si.edu/polio/virusvaccine/history. htm. Downloaded on January 16, 2009.

Plotkin, Stanley A. "Vaccines: Past, Present and Future." *Nature Medicine* 11, no. 4 Suppl. (April 2005): S5–S11. Available online. URL: http://www. nature.com/nm/journal/v11/n4s/full/nm1209. html.

wiseGEEK. "How Do Vaccines Work?" Available online. URL: http://www.wisegeek.com/ how-do-vaccines-work.htm. Accessed August 4, 2011.

APPENDIXES

APPENDIX I
COMMON RX ABBREVIATIONS

ac   before meals
bid   two times a day
c̄ or o   with
caps   capsules
daw   dispense as written
i   one
ii   two
iii   three
OD   right eye
OS   left eye
OU   both eyes
p̄   after
pc   after meals
po   by mouth
prn   as needed

q   every
q2h   every two hours
q3h   every three hours
q4h   every four hours
qAM   every morning
qd   once a day; every day
qhs or hs   at bedtime
qid   four times a day
s̄ or ø   without
sig   the Latin abbreviation meaning "Let it be labeled"—often appears before the dosing instructions.
tabs   tablets
tid   three times a day

Note: Some doctors may use variations of these symbols.

APPENDIX II
COMMON MEDICATION ERRORS
AND RECOMMENDATIONS

The National Coordinating Council for Medication Error Reporting and Prevention offers the following information and recommendations.

RECOMMENDATIONS TO ENHANCE ACCURACY OF PRESCRIPTION WRITING

Personnel to whom this applies: Prescribers; Nursing or Pharmacy staff (who transcribe verbal prescription orders or rewrite transfer or admission orders when entering or leaving a health care facility); Healthcare administrators/managers.

Technology plays an important role in the delivery of health care. Utilize technology, as appropriate, but evaluate its effectiveness on an ongoing basis. While technology can reduce medication errors and enhance patient safety, it also has the potential to cause new types of unintentional errors. The Council recommends:

1. . . . all prescription documents be legible. Verbal orders should be minimized. [See the Council's Recommendations to Reduce Medication Errors Associated with Verbal Medication Orders and Prescriptions on page 388.]
2. . . . prescription orders include a brief notation of purpose (e.g., for cough), unless considered inappropriate by the prescriber. Notation of purpose can help further assure that the proper medication is dispensed and creates an extra safety check in the process of prescribing and dispensing a medication. The Council does recognize, however, that certain medications and disease states may warrant maintaining confidentiality.
3. . . . all prescription orders be written in the metric system except for therapies that use standard units such as insulin, vitamins, etc. Units should be spelled out rather than writing "U." The change to the use of the metric system from the archaic apothecary and avoirdupois systems will help avoid misinterpretations of these abbreviations and symbols, and miscalculations when converting to metric, which is used in product labeling and package inserts.
4. . . . prescribers include age and, when appropriate, weight of the patient on the prescription or medication order. The most common errors in dosage result in pediatric and geriatric populations. The age (and weight) of a patient can help dispensing healthcare professionals in their double check of the appropriate drug and dose.
5. . . . medication orders include drug name, exact metric weight or concentration, and dosage form. Strength should be expressed in metric amounts and concentration should be specified. Each order for a medication should be complete. The pharmacist should check with the prescriber if any information is missing or questionable.
6. . . . a leading zero always precede a decimal expression of less than one. A terminal or trailing zero should never be used after a decimal. Ten-fold errors in drug strength and dosage have occurred with decimals due to the use of a trailing zero or the absence of a leading zero.

7. . . . prescribers avoid the use of abbreviations including those for drug names (e.g., MOM, HCTZ) and Latin directions for use. The abbreviations in the chart below are found to be particularly dangerous because they have been consistently misunderstood and therefore, should never be used. The Council reviewed the uses for many abbreviations and determined that any attempt at standardization of abbreviations would not adequately address the problems of illegibility and misuse.

Abbreviation	Intended meaning	Common Error
U	Units	Mistaken as a zero or a four (4) resulting in overdose. Also mistaken for *cc* (cubic centimeters) when poorly written.
:g	Micrograms	Mistaken for *mg* (milligrams) resulting in an overdose.
Q.D.	Latin abbreviation for every day	The period after the *Q* has sometimes been mistaken for an *I*, and the drug has been given *QID* (four times daily) rather than daily.
Q.O.D.	Latin abbreviation for every other day	Misinterpreted as *QD* (daily) or *QID* (four times daily). If the *O* is poorly written, it looks like a period or *I*.
SC or SQ	Subcutaneous	Mistaken as *SL* (sublingual) when poorly written.
T I W	Three times a week	Misinterpreted as *three times a day* or *twice a week*.
D/C	Discharge; also discontinue	Patients' medications have been prematurely discontinued when D/C, (intended to mean *discharge*) was misinterpreted as *discontinue*, because it was followed by a list of drugs.
HS	Half strength	Misinterpreted as the Latin abbreviation *HS* (hour of sleep).
cc	Cubic centimeters	Mistaken as *U* (units) when poorly written.
AU, AS, AD	Latin abbreviation for both ears; left ear; right ear	Misinterpreted as the Latin abbreviation *OU* (both eyes); *OS* (left eye); *OD* (right eye)
IU	International Unit	Mistaken as *IV* (intravenous) or *10* (ten)
MS, MSO4, MgSO4	Confused for one another	Can mean morphine sulfate or magnesium sulfate

8. . . . prescribers avoid vague instructions such as "Take as directed" or "Take/Use as needed" as the sole direction for use. Specific directions to the patient are useful to help reinforce proper medication use, particularly if therapy is to be interrupted for a time. Clear directions are a necessity for the dispenser to: (1) check the proper dose for the patient and (2) enable effective patient counseling. In summary, the Council recommends:

Don't Wait . . . Automate!
When In Doubt, Write It Out!
When In Doubt, Check It Out!
Lead, Don't Trail

RECOMMENDATIONS TO ENHANCE ACCURACY OF ADMINISTRATION OF MEDICATIONS

Personnel to whom this applies: Nursing staff involved in administration of medications; other personnel involved in administration of medications (e.g., respiratory therapists, non-licensed personnel who are delegated tasks by a licensed professional, etc); Pharmacy staff; Healthcare administrators/managers.

The Council recommends:

1. . . . any order that is incomplete, illegible, or of any other concern be clarified prior to administration using an established process for resolving questions.
2. . . . as one aspect of the overall medication use system, the following checks be performed immediately prior to medication administration: the right medication, in the right dose, to the right person, by the right route using the right dosage form, at the right time, with the right documentation.
3. . . . organizations/companies provide employees with adequate training regarding medication administration devices and routinely

monitor or verify that users of such devices demonstrate competency regarding the device, its operation, and its limitations.

4. . . . when electronic infusion control devices are employed, only those that prevent free-flow upon removal of the administration set should be used.

5. . . . the use of integrated automated systems (e.g., direct order entry, computerized medication administration record, bar coding) to facilitate review of prescriptions, increase the accuracy of administration, and reduce transcription errors.

6. . . . all persons who administer medications have adequate and/or appropriate access to patient information, as close to the point of use as possible, including medical history, known allergies, diagnoses, list of current medications, and treatment plan, to assess the appropriateness of administering the medication.

7. . . . all persons who administer medications have easily accessible product information as close to the point of use as possible, and are knowledgeable about:
   • indications for use of the medication as well as precautions and contraindications;
   • the expected outcome from its use;
   • potential adverse reactions and interactions with food or other medication;
   • actions to take when adverse reactions or interactions occur;
   • storage requirements

8. . . . health care professionals administer only medications that are properly labeled and that during the administration process, labels be read three times: when reaching for or preparing the medication, immediately prior to administering the medication, and when discarding the container or replacing it into its storage location.

9. . . . at the time of administration, the name, purpose, and effects of the medication be discussed with the patient and/or caregiver, especially upon first time administration and reviewed upon subsequent administrations.

10. . . . ongoing patient monitoring for therapeutic and/or adverse medication effects.

11. . . . the role of the work environment be considered when assessing safety of the drug administration process. Factors such as lighting, temperature control, noise-level, occurrence of distractions (e.g., telephone and personal interruptions, performance of unrelated tasks, etc.) should be examined. Sufficient staffing and other resources must be provided for the given workload. The science of ergonomics should be employed in the design of safe systems.

12. . . . data be collected and analyzed regarding the actual and potential errors of administration for the purpose of continuous quality improvement.

13. . . . both initial and ongoing training of staff, including licensed staff, support staff or non-licensed staff, and relief staff on accepted standards of practice related to accurate medication administration with the ultimate goal of medication error reduction.

14. . . . every organization establish policies and procedures for the medication administration process. This will ensure that all personnel, including licensed staff, support staff or non-licensed staff, and relief staff are informed of expectations related to the medication administration process.

RECOMMENDATIONS TO ENHANCE ACCURACY OF DISPENSING MEDICATIONS

Personnel to whom this applies: Pharmacy staff including pharmacists and pharmacy technicians; Nursing staff that utilize automated dispensing machines/cabinets; Nurse Managers that utilize pharmacy stock after hours; Healthcare administrators/managers.

The Council recommends:

1. . . . prescriptions/orders always be reviewed by a pharmacist prior to dispensing. Any orders that are incomplete, illegible, or of any other concern should be clarified using an established process for resolving questions.

2. . . . patient profiles be current and contain adequate information that allows the pharmacist to assess the appropriateness of a prescription/order.

3. . . . the dispensing area be properly designed to prevent errors. Design should address fatigue-reducing environmental conditions (e.g. adequate lighting, air conditioning, noise level abatement, ergonomic fixtures); minimize distractions (e.g. telephone and personnel interruptions, clutter, unrelated tasks); and provide sufficient staffing and other resources for workload.

4. . . . product inventory be arranged to help differentiate medications from one another. This may include the use of visual discriminators such as signs or markers. This is particularly important when confusion exists between or among strengths, similar looking labels, and names that sound or appear similar.

5. . . . a series of checks be established to assess the accuracy of the dispensing process prior to the medication being provided to the patient. Whenever possible, an independent check by a second individual should be used. Other methods of checking include the use of automation (e.g. bar coding systems), computer systems, and patient profiles.

6. . . . labels be read at least three times (e.g., when selecting the product, when packaging the product, and when returning the product to the shelf).

7. . . . pharmacy staff triple check replenishment of regular medication stock or automated dispensing machines/cabinets (e.g., Pyxis, etc.) to ensure accuracy of product and precision of placement (e.g., when selecting the product, before the product leaves the pharmacy, and prior to placing the product in the automated dispensing machine/cabinet).

8. . . . pharmacists counsel patients at the time of dispensing. Counseling should be viewed as an opportunity to verify the accuracy of dispensing and the patient's understanding of proper medication use. Counseling should include:
   A. Indications for the use of the medication as well as precautions and warnings;

B. Expected outcome from the medication;
   C. Potential adverse reactions and interactions with food or other medications;
   D. Actions to take when adverse reactions or interactions occur;
   E. Storage requirements of the medication.

9. . . . pharmacies collect and analyze data regarding actual and potential errors for the purpose of continuous quality improvement (e.g., provide feedback to local prescribers, provide error information to national reporting programs/databases).

10. . . . both initial and ongoing training of pharmacy staff on accepted standards of practice related to accurate dispensing processes with the ultimate goal of medication error reduction.

11. . . . each pharmacy establish policies and procedures for the medication dispensing process. This will ensure that all personnel, including pharmacists, support staff, and relief staff, are informed of expectations related to the dispensing process.

RECOMMENDATIONS TO REDUCE MEDICATION ERRORS IN NON-HEALTHCARE SETTINGS*

Medications are often stored and administered in a variety of non-healthcare settings. These settings include:

- Elementary and secondary schools
- Child day care centers
- Summer camps
- Adult day service centers (adult day care)
- Group homes for the developmentally disabled (mentally retarded)
- Assisted living/Residential care
- Board and care homes
- Jails (city and county)
- Prisons (state)

---

* Where state licensure laws apply to a setting, follow the implementing regulations and use these recommendations as supplementary guidance, as appropriate.

In all these settings, employees frequently are responsible for handling and administering prescription and over-the-counter medications to clients or residents. Some organizations may employ licensed health professionals to directly manage the medication administration process. However, many of these settings have no licensed health professionals involved.

Without adequate safeguards and supervision, medications present significant risks. Medication errors result if doses of medication are omitted, or if medication is administered to the wrong person, or given in the wrong dose. Controlled medications (e.g. Ritalin, morphine) may be stolen or diverted.

Settings in which these activities are conducted often are licensed by the state in which they are located, but licensure requirements and oversight vary substantially from state to state. States may not address medication responsibilities in their licensure requirements or may not consistently monitor and enforce requirements related to medications.

Anecdotal reports and results of state licensure surveys indicate that medication errors can be a significant problem in these settings. In the absence of licensed health professionals, and without adequate training for personnel involved with medications in these settings, medication errors often go undetected or unreported.

The National Coordinating Council for Medication Error Reporting and Prevention has developed these recommendations as guidance to non-healthcare settings to help ensure protection of clients, residents, and others who must depend on assistance for medication management in these settings. These recommendations apply to non-healthcare settings regardless of whether licensed health professionals are involved in managing medications.

1. Where medications are stored and administered to individuals, written policies and procedures should address the following:
   - Acquisition of medications (e.g., from parents, caregivers, pharmacies)
   - Documentation of medication order from licensed practitioner when applicable
   - Specification of which personnel are allowed access to medications and allowed to administer medications to students, clients or residents
   - Labeling and packaging of medications managed for students, clients or residents
   - Storage of medications, including medications that may require refrigeration
   - Secure storage and accountability of controlled drugs
   - Limitations on the type(s) of medications permissible for use or storage in the organization
   - Administration of medications (including double-checking by another staff person when feasible)
   - Documentation of medication administration
   - Documentation and reporting of medication errors and adverse drug reactions
   - Disposition of medications that are no longer needed or in use

2. Where medications are stored and administered, training should be provided to personnel with responsibilities related to medication management. The training should correspond to the written policies and procedures, and the person's scope of duties associated with medications.

3. Where controlled medications are stored and/or administered, safeguards should be in place to prevent and detect theft and diversion of controlled drugs.

4. Encourage the reporting of medication errors to appropriate state and national medication error reporting programs. These medication error reports may be used to identify significant trends or patterns that can lead to improved quality and safety of health care, and to teach others how to prevent similar errors.

5. When a medication error occurs, evaluate possible causes in order to improve the facility's system for medication management and to prevent future errors.

RECOMMENDATIONS TO REDUCE MEDICATION ERRORS ASSOCIATED WITH VERBAL MEDICATION ORDERS AND PRESCRIPTIONS

Confusion over the similarity of drug names accounts for approximately 25 percent of all reports to the USP Medication Errors Reporting (MER) Program. To reduce confusion pertaining to verbal orders and to further support the Council's mission to minimize medication errors, the following recommendations have been developed.

In these recommendations, verbal orders are prescriptions or medication orders that are communicated as oral, spoken communications between senders and receivers face to face, by telephone, or by other auditory device.

1. Verbal communication of prescription or medication orders should be limited to urgent situations where immediate written or electronic communication is not feasible.
2. Healthcare organizations (community pharmacies, physicians' offices, hospitals, nursing homes, home care agencies, etc.) should establish policies and procedures that:
   - Describe limitations or prohibitions on use of verbal orders
   - Provide a mechanism to ensure validity/authenticity of the prescriber
   - List the elements required for inclusion in a complete verbal order
   - Describe situations in which verbal orders may be used
   - List and define the individuals who may send and receive verbal orders
   - Provide guidelines for clear and effective communication of verbal orders
3. Leaders of healthcare organizations should promote a culture in which it is acceptable, and strongly encouraged, for staff to question prescribers when there are any questions or disagreements about verbal orders. Questions about verbal orders should be resolved prior to the preparation, or dispensing, or administration of the medication.
4. Verbal orders for antineoplastic agents should NOT be permitted under any circumstances. These medications are not administered in emergency or urgent situations, and they have a narrow margin of safety.
5. Elements that should be included in a verbal order include:
   - Name of patient
   - Age and weight of patient, when appropriate
   - Drug name
   - Dosage form (e.g., tablets, capsules, inhalants)
   - Exact strength or concentration
   - Dose, frequency, and route
   - Quantity and/or duration
   - Purpose or indication (unless disclosure is considered inappropriate by the prescriber)
   - Specific instructions for use
   - Name of prescriber, and telephone number when appropriate
   - Name of individual transmitting the order, if different from the prescriber.
6. The content of verbal orders should be clearly communicated:
   - The name of the drug should be confirmed by any of the following:
     - Spelling
     - Providing both the brand and generic names of the medication
     - Providing the indication for use
   - In order to avoid confusion with spoken numbers, a dose such as 50 mg should be dictated as "fifty milligrams . . . five zero milligrams" to distinguish from "fifteen milligrams . . . one five milligrams."
   - Instructions for use should be provided without abbreviations. For example, "1tab tid" should be communicated as "Take/give one tablet three times daily."
7. The entire verbal order should be repeated back to the prescriber, or the individual transmitting the order, using the principles outlined in these recommendations.
8. All verbal orders should be reduced immediately to writing and signed by the individual receiving the order.

9. Verbal orders should be documented in the patient's medical record, reviewed, and countersigned by the prescriber as soon as possible.

APPENDIX III
ONLINE PHARMACEUTICAL DRUG LISTS AND DATABASES

Alternate Drug Information
A–Z Index (formerly PDR Consumer Drug Information)
http://www.drugs.com/pdr/

DailyMed
Drug content and labeling as found in drug package inserts. Search by drug name.
http://dailymed.nlm.nih.gov/dailymed/about.cfm

Davis's Drug Guide
http://www.drugguide.com/ddo/ub

Drug Approval Reports
http://www.accessdata.fda.gov/scripts/cder/drugsatfda/index.cfm?fuseaction =Reports.ReportsMenu

DrugDigest
A noncommercial, evidence-based, consumer health and drug information site
http://www.drugdigest.org/wps/portal/ddigest

Drugs, Supplements, and Herbal Information
http://www.nlm.nih.gov/medlineplus/druginformation.html

Epocrates Drug and Clinical Reference
http://www.epocrates.com/products/online/

Food and Drug Administration
FDA approved drugs with Healthcare Professional, Patient, and Consumer Information Sheets, Medication Guides, and Information Pages.
http://www.fda.gov/cder/drug/DrugSafety/DrugIndex.htm

National Drug Code Directory
http://www.fda.gov/cder/ndc/database/default.htm

Online PDR Resource Center
Nurse's Physicians Desk Reference—Bonus Monographs
http://www.nursespdr.delmar.cengage.com/resources/monographs.aspx

The Orange Book
Lists approved drug products with therapeutic equivalence evaluations
http://www.fda.gov/cder/ob/

Potentially Inappropriate Medications for the Elderly According to the Revised Beers Criteria
http://www.dcri.duke.edu/ccge/curtis/beers.html

Recently Approved Drugs
http://www.centerwatch.com/drug-information/fda-approvals/default.aspx

Recently Approved Drugs/Indications
http://www.pslgroup.com/newdrugs.htm

RxList
Drug index for prescription drugs
http://www.rxlist.com/drugs/alpha_a.htm

RxMed: Prescribing Information
Complete pharmaceutical monographs
http://www.rxmed.com/b.main/b2.pharmaceutical/b2.prescribe.html

Yahoo! Health Drug Guide
http://health.yahoo.com/drugs/a

APPENDIX IV
TOP TEN DANGEROUS DRUG INTERACTIONS IN LONG-TERM CARE

The Multidisciplinary Medication Management Project, established through a joint effort of The American Medical Directors Association and the American Society of Consultant Pharmacists, developed a list of 10 drug interactions that are particularly problematic in long-term care settings. Each of these drug interactions involves medications that are commonly used in long-term care and has the potential to cause significant harm if not managed appropriately.

Medications chosen for the Top Ten list were based on their frequency of use in older adults in the long-term care setting and on the potential for adverse consequences if used together. Due to individual variability, not every older adult who takes these medications together will experience an adverse reaction. However, these combinations have the potential to produce harmful effects.

1. Warfarin—NSAIDs (does not include COX-2 inhibitors)
   Danger: Potential for serious gastrointestinal bleeding
2. Warfarin—Sulfa drugs
   Danger: Increased effects of warfarin, with potential for bleeding
3. Warfarin—Macrolides
   Danger: Increased effects of warfarin, with potential for bleeding
4. Warfarin—Quinolones (specifically, ciprofloxacin, enoxacin, norfloxacin, and ofloxacin)
   Danger: Increased effects of warfarin, with potential for bleeding
5. Warfarin—Phenytoin
   Danger: Increased effects of warfarin and/or phenytoin
6. ACE inhibitors—Potassium supplements
   Danger: Elevated serum potassium
7. ACE inhibitors—Spironolactone
   Danger: Elevated serum potassium levels
8. Digoxin—Amiodarone
   Danger: Digoxin toxicity
9. Digoxin—Verapamil
   Danger: Digoxin toxicity
10. Theophylline—Quinolones (especially with ciprofloxacin, enoxacin, and norfloxacin)
    Danger: Theophylline toxicity

Source: Brown, Karen E. "Top Ten Dangerous Drug Interactions in Long-Term Care." Medication Management Project. Available online. URL: http://www.sccg.biz/generalDocuments/Top%20Ten%20Dangerous%20Drug%20Interactions%20in%20Long%5B1%5D%5D.pdf. Accessed July 22, 2011.

APPENDIX V
ABUSABLE PRESCRIPTION DRUGS

(The following information is from The National Institute on Drug Abuse [NIDA], part of the National Institutes of Health [NIH], a component of the U.S. Department of Health and Human Services. Additional information is available on their Web site at http://www.drugabuse.gov.)

Three types of prescription drugs are misused or abused most often:

- Opioids—prescribed for pain relief
- CNS depressants—barbiturates and benzodiazepines prescribed for anxiety or sleep problems (often referred to as sedatives or tranquilizers)
- Stimulants—prescribed for attention-deficit hyperactivity disorder (ADHD), the sleep disorder narcolepsy, or obesity

For the sake of regulation, controlled substances are classified into five groups or "schedules" based on:

- whether they have an accepted medical use
- their relative potential for abuse
- the degree of dependence that may be caused by abuse of the drug

Schedule I and II drugs have a high potential for abuse. They require greater storage security and have a quota on manufacturing, among other restrictions. Schedule I drugs are available for research only and have no approved medical use. Schedule II drugs are available only by prescription (unrefillable) and require a form for ordering. Schedule III and IV drugs are available by prescription, may have five refills in six months, and may be ordered orally. Most Schedule V drugs are available over the counter.

Examples of Abusable Prescription Drugs (Schedule I drugs not included)

Opioids and Morphine Derivatives—Intoxication effects: pain relief, euphoria, drowsiness. *Potential health consequences:* respiratory depression and arrest, nausea, confusion, constipation, sedation, unconsciousness, coma, tolerance, addiction

1. **codeine**—*Commercial names:* Empirin with Codeine, Fiorinal with Codeine, Robitussin A-C, Tylenol with Codeine. *Street names:* Captain Cody, Cody, schoolboy; (with glutethimide) doors & fours, loads, pancakes and syrup. *Schedules:* II, III, IV. *How administered:* injected, swallowed. *Notes:* less analgesia, sedation, and respiratory depression than morphine
2. **fentanyl**—*Commercial names:* Actiq, Duragesic, Sublimaze. *Street names:* Apache, China girl, China white, dance fever, friend, goodfella, jackpot, murder 8, TNT, Tango and Cash. *Schedule:* II. *How administered:* injected, smoked, snorted
3. **morphine**—*Commercial names:* Roxanol, Duramorph. *Street names:* M, Miss Emma, monkey, white stuff. *Schedules:* II, III. *How administered:* injected, swallowed, smoked
4. **opium**—*Commercial names:* laudanum, paregoric. *Street names:* big O, black stuff, block, gum, hop. *Schedules:* II, III, V. *How administered:* swallowed, smoked

5. **oxycodone**—*Commercial names:* Tylox, Oxy-Contin, Percodan, Percocet. *Street names:* oxy 80s, oxycotton, oxycet, O.C., killer, hillbilly heroin, percs. *Schedule:* II. *How administered:* swallowed, snorted, injected

6. **hydrocodone**—*Commercial name:* Vicodin. *Street names:* vike, Watson-387. *Schedule:* II. *How administered:* swallowed

7. **meperidine, hydromorphone, propoxyphene**—*Commercial names:* Demerol, meperidine hydrochloride, Dilaudid, Lortab, Lorcet; Darvon, Darvocet. *Street names:* demmies, pain killer, juice, dillies. *Schedules:* II, III, IV. *How administered:* swallowed, injected, suppositories, chewed, crushed, snorted

Depressants—*Intoxication effects:* reduced pain and anxiety, feeling of well-being, lowered inhibitions, slowed pulse and breathing, lowered blood pressure, poor concentration. *Potential health consequences:* confusion, fatigue; impaired coordination, memory, judgment; respiratory depression and arrest, addiction

1. **barbiturates**—*Commercial names:* Amytal, Nembutal, Seconal, Phenobarbital. *Street names:* barbs, reds, red birds, phennies, tooies, yellows, yellow jackets. *Schedules:* II, III, V. *How administered:* injected, swallowed. *Additional intoxication effects:* sedation, drowsiness. *Additional potential health consequences:* depression, unusual excitement, fever, irritability, poor judgment, slurred speech, dizziness

2. **benzodiazepines (other than flunitrazepam)**—*Commercial names:* Ativan, Halcion, Librium, Valium, Xanax. *Street names:* candy, downers, sleeping pills, tranks. *Schedule:* IV. *How administered:* swallowed. *Additional intoxication effects:* sedation, drowsiness. *Additional intoxication effect:* dizziness

3. **flunitrazepam**—*Commercial name:* Rohypnol. *Street names:* forget-me pill, Mexican Valium, R2, Roche, roofies, roofinol, rope, rophies. *Schedule:* IV. *How administered:* swallowed, snorted. *Additional intoxication effects:* visual and gastrointestinal disturbances, urinary retention, memory loss for the time under the drug's effects. *Notes:* associated with sexual assaults

Stimulants—*Intoxication effects:* increased heart rate, blood pressure, metabolism; feelings of exhilaration, energy, increased mental alertness. *Potential health consequences:* rapid or irregular heart beat; reduced appetite, weight loss, heart failure

1. **amphetamines**—*Commercial names:* Biphetamine, Dexedrine. *Street names:* bennies, black beauties, crosses, hearts, LA turnaround, speed, truck drivers, uppers. *Schedule:* II. *How administered:* injected, swallowed, smoked, snorted. *Additional intoxication effects:* rapid breathing; hallucinations. *Additional potential health consequences:* tremor, loss of coordination; irritability, anxiousness, restlessness, delirium, panic, paranoia, impulsive behavior, aggressiveness, tolerance, addiction

2. **cocaine**—*Commercial name:* Cocaine hydrochloride. *Street names:* blow, bump, C, candy, Charlie, coke, crack, flake, rock, snow, toot. *Schedule:* II. *How administered:* injected, smoked, snorted. *Additional potential health consequences:* increased temperature/chest pain, respiratory failure, nausea, abdominal pain, strokes, seizures, headaches, malnutrition, panic attacks

3. **methamphetamine**—*Commercial name:* Desoxyn. *Street names:* chalk, crank, crystal, fire, glass, go fast, ice, meth, speed. *Schedule:* II. *How administered:* injected, swallowed, smoked, snorted. *Additional intoxication effects:* aggression, violence, psychotic behavior. *Additional potential health consequences:* aggression, violence, psychotic behavior/memory loss, cardiac and neurological damage; impaired memory and learning, tolerance, addiction

4. **methylphenidate**—*Commercial name:* Ritalin. *Street names:* JIF, MPH, R-ball, Skippy, the smart drug, vitamin R. *Schedule:* II. *How administered:* injected, swallowed, snorted. *Additional intoxication effects:* increase or decrease in blood

pressure, psychotic episodes. *Additional potential health consequences:* digestive problems, loss of appetite, weight loss

Other compounds

1. **anabolic   steroids**—*Commercial   names:* Anadrol, Oxandrin, Durabolin, Depo-Testosterone, Equipoise. *Street names:* roids, juice. *Schedule:* III. *How administered:* injected, swallowed, applied to skin. *Intoxication effects:* None. *Potential health consequences:* hypertension, blood clotting and cholesterol changes, liver cysts and cancer, kidney cancer, hostility and aggression, acne; in adolescents, prema-ture stoppage of growth; in males, prostate cancer, reduced sperm production, shrunken testicles, breast enlargement; in females, menstrual irregularities, development of beard and other masculine characteristics

2. **Dextromethorphan (DXM)**—*Commercial names:* Found in some cough and cold medications. *Street names:* Robotripping, Robo, Triple C. *Schedule:* not scheduled. *How administered:* swallowed. *Intoxication effects:* none. *Potential health consequences:* dissociative effects, distorted visual perceptions to complete dissociative effects. At high doses, delirium, depression, respiratory depression and arrest

APPENDIX VI
PRESCRIPTION DRUG ASSISTANCE PROGRAMS

The high cost of many drugs, especially those to treat long-term diseases such as cancer, HIV, and autoimmune disorders make it impossible for many people to purchase the drugs they need. Numerous prescription drug assistance programs exist to help the poor, the uninsured, and the underinsured.

FDA Consumer magazine noted in 2005 that two main types of assistance are available from pharmaceutical companies. Several companies offer programs that allow consumers to take a discount drug card to the pharmacy to get a discount on the price of prescription drugs. In addition, most major pharmaceutical companies offer patient assistance programs (PAPs), which provide free or low-cost medicines to people in need.

Access to Benefits Coalition
http://www.accesstobenefits.org

AIDS Drug Assistance Program (ADAP)
www.kff.org/hivaids/upload/1584_10.pdf

GSK patient assistance programs
http://www.gskforyou.com/

The HealthWell Foundation is a 501(c)(3) non-profit, charitable organization that helps individuals afford prescription medications they are taking for specific illnesses.
http://www.healthwellfoundation.org

Help With Prescription Drug Costs for Medicare beneficiaries
http://www.ssa.gov/prescriptionhelp

Medicare Access for Patients Rx
http://www.maprx.info/

National Council on Aging
Find and enroll in federal, state, local, and private programs that help pay for prescription drugs
http://www.benefitscheckup.org

NeedyMeds lists information about state programs, discount drug cards, federal poverty guidelines, and patient assistance programs and includes copies of the forms.
http://www.needymeds.com

The Partnership for Prescription Assistance (PPA)
A resource for patient-assistance programs, run by the Pharmaceutical Research and Manufacturers of America. The PPA also will help potential recipients sign up for Medicare Part D coverage.
http://www.pparx.org also http://www.helpingpatients.org
(888) 4PPA-NOW (477-2669).
The PPA has dedicated a Web site to make it easier for patients to learn about help available for children
http://kids.pparx.org/

RxAssist offers a directory of Patient Assistance Programs. Search by drug name, company name, or assistance program. Sponsored by AstraZeneca.
http://www.rxassist.org

State Pharmaceutical Assistance Programs
(includes subsidies and discounts for seniors, disabled, uninsured, and others)
http://www.ncsl.org/programs/health/drugaid.htm

Together Rx Access Program
http://www.togetherrxaccess.com/

APPENDIX VII
PHARMACEUTICAL COMPANIES

Abbott Laboratories
100 Abbott Park Road
Abbott Park, IL 60064
(847) 937-6100
(847) 937-1511 (fax)
http://www.abbott.com

Allergan, Inc.
P.O. Box 19534
Irvine, CA 92623
(714) 246-4500
(714) 246-4971 (fax)
http://www.allergan.com

Amgen, Inc.
One Amgen Center Drive
Thousand Oaks, CA 91320
(805) 447-1000
(805) 447-1010 (fax)
http://www.amgen.com

Amylin Pharmaceuticals, Inc.
9360 Towne Centre Drive
San Diego, CA 92121
(858) 552-2200
(858) 552-2212 fax
http://www.amylin.com

Astellas Pharma Inc.
Three Parkway North
Deerfield, IL 60015
(847) 317-8212
(847) 317-5983 (fax)
http://www.astellas.com

AstraZeneca LP
1800 Concord Pike
P.O. Box 15437
Wilmington, DE 19850

(302) 886-3000
(302) 886-1889 (fax)
http://www.astrazeneca.com

Baxter Healthcare Corp.
One Baxter Parkway
Deerfield, IL 60015
(847) 948-2000
(847) 948-3642 (fax)
http://www.baxter.com

Bayer HealthCare Pharmaceuticals
400 Morgan Lane
West Haven, CT 06516
(203) 812-2000
(203) 812-5300 (fax)
http://www.bayerus.com

Boehringer Ingelheim Pharmaceuticals, Inc.
900 Ridgebury Road
Ridgefield, CT 06877
(203) 798-9988
(203) 791-6234 (fax)
http://www.boehringer-ingelheim.com

Bristol-Myers Squibb Company
345 Park Avenue
New York, NY 10154
(212) 546-4000
(212) 546-4094 (fax)
http://www.bms.com

Celgene Corporation
86 Morris Avenue
Summit, NJ 07901
(908) 673-9000
(908) 673-9001 (fax)
http://www.celgene.com

Daiichi Sankyo, Inc.
Two Hilton Court
Parsippany, NJ 07054
(973) 359-2600
(973) 359-2645 (fax)
http://www.sankyopharma.com

Eisai, Inc.
Glenpointe Centre West
500 Frank W. Burr Boulevard
Teaneck, NJ 07666
(201) 692-1100
(201) 692-1804 (fax)
http://www.eisai.co.jp/index-e.html

EMD Serono
One Technology Place
Rockland, MA 02370
(781) 982-9000
(781) 982-9478 (fax)
http://www.seronousa.com

Endo Pharmaceuticals, Inc.
100 Endo Boulevard
Chadds Ford, PA 19317
(610) 558-9800
http://www.endo.com

Genzyme Corporation
500 Kendall Square
Cambridge, MA 02139
(617) 252-7500
(617) 252-7600 (fax)
http://www.genzyme.com

GlaxoSmithKline
Five Moore Drive
P.O. Box 13398
Research Triangle Park, NC 27709
(919) 483-2100
(919) 483-6002 (fax)
http://www.gsk.com

Hoffmann-La Roche, Inc.
340 Kingsland Street
Nutley, NJ 07110
(973) 235-5000
http://www.rocheusa.com

Johnson & Johnson
One Johnson & Johnson Plaza
New Brunswick, NJ 08933
(732) 524-0400
(732) 214-0332 (fax)
http://www.jnj.com

Eli Lilly and Company
Lilly Corporate Center
Indianapolis, IN 46285
(317) 276-2000
(317) 276-9707 (fax)
http://www.lilly.com

Lundbeck, Inc.
Four Parkway North
Deerfield, IL 60015
(847) 282-1000
(847) 282-1001 (fax)
http://www.lundbeckinc.com

Merck & Co., Inc.
One Merck Drive
P.O. Box 100
Whitehouse Station, NJ 08889
(908) 423-1000
(908) 423-1160 (fax)
http://www.merck.com

Millennium Pharmaceuticals, Inc.
40 Landsdowne Street
Cambridge, MA 02139
(617) 679-7000
(617) 621-0264 (fax)
http://www.millennium.com

Novartis Corporation Pharmaceuticals
1 Health Plaza
East Hanover, NJ 07936
(973) 781-8300
(973) 781-8265 (fax)
http://www.novartis.com

Otsuka America, Inc.
1 Embarcerdo Center
San Francisco, CA 94113
(240) 683-3049
(301) 721-7049 (fax)
http://www.otsuka.com

Pfizer, Inc
235 East 42nd Street
New York, NY 10017
(212) 573-2323
(212) 573-7851 (fax)
http://www.pfizer.com

Purdue Pharma L.P.
One Stamford Forum
Stamford, CT 06901
(203) 588-8000
(203) 588-8850 (fax)
http://www.purduepharma.com

Sanofi-aventis U.S.
300 Somerset Corporate Boulevard
Bridgewater, NJ 08807

(908) 243-6000
(908) 243-6483 (fax)
http://www.sanofi-aventis.us

Sigma-Tau Pharmaceuticals, Inc.
9841 Washingtonian Boulevard, Suite 500
Gaithersburg, MD 20878
(301) 948-1041
(301) 948-1862 (fax)
http://www.sigmatau.com

Takeda Pharmaceuticals North America, Inc.
1 Takeda Parkway
Deerfield, IL 60015
(224) 554-6500
http://www.takedapharm.com

APPENDIX VIII
STATE BOARDS OF PHARMACY

Alabama State Board of Pharmacy
10 Inverness Center, Suite 110
Birmingham, AL 35242
(205) 981-2280
http://www.albop.com

Alaska Board of Pharmacy
P.O. Box 110806
Juneau, AK 99811-0806
(907) 465-2589
http://www.commerce.state.ak.us/occ/ppha.htm

Arizona State Board of Pharmacy
1700 W Washington, Suite 250
Phoenix, AZ 85007
(602) 771-2727
http://www.azpharmacy.gov

Arkansas State Board of Pharmacy
101 E Capitol, Suite 218
Little Rock, AR 72201
(501) 682-0190
http://www.arkansas.gov/asbp

California State Board of Pharmacy
1625 N Market Boulevard, Suite N-219
Sacramento, CA 95834
(916) 574-7900
http://www.pharmacy.ca.gov

Colorado State Board of Pharmacy
1560 Broadway, Suite 1300
Denver, CO 80202-5146
(303) 894-7800
http://www.dora.state.co.us/pharmacy/

Connecticut Commission of Pharmacy
State Office Building
165 Capitol Avenue, Room 147
Hartford, CT 06106
(860) 713-6070
http://www.ct.gov/dcp/site/default.asp

Delaware State Board of Pharmacy
Division of Professional Regulation
Cannon Building
861 Silver Lake Boulevard, Suite 203
Dover, DE 19904
(302) 744-4526
http://www.dpr.delaware.gov

District of Columbia Pharmaceutical Division
717 14th Street NW, 6th Floor
Washington, DC 20005
(202) 724-4900
http://www.dchealth.dc.gov/

Florida Board of Pharmacy
4052 Bald Cypress Way, Bin C04
Tallahassee, FL 32399-3254
(850) 245-4292
http://www.doh.state.fl.us/mqa/pharmacy/

Georgia State Board of Pharmacy
Professional Licensing Boards
237 Coliseum Drive
Macon, GA 31217
(478) 207-2440
http://www.sos.state.ga.us/plb/pharmacy/

Guam Board of Examiners for Pharmacy
123 Chalan Kareta Vietnam Veterans Highway
Mangilao, GU 96923
(671) 735-7406
http://dphss.guam.gov/about/licensing.htm

Hawaii State Board of Pharmacy
P.O. Box 3469
Honolulu, HI 96801
(808) 586-2694
http://www.hawaii.gov/dcca/areas/pvl/boards/
  pharmacy/

Idaho State Board of Pharmacy
3380 Americana Terrace, Suite 320
Boise, ID 83706
(208) 334-2356
http://bop.accessidaho.org/

Illinois State Board of Pharmacy
Department of Professional Regulation
320 W Washington Street, 3rd Floor
Springfield, IL 62786
(217) 782-8556
http://www.idfpr.com

Indiana Board of Pharmacy
402 W Washington Street, Room W072
Indianapolis, IN 46204
(317) 234-2067
http://www.in.gov/pla/pharmacy.htm

Iowa Board of Pharmacy
400 SW 8th Street, Suite E
Des Moines, IA 50309-4688
(515) 281-5944
http://www.state.ia.us/ibpe

Kansas State Board of Pharmacy
Landon State Office Building, 900 SW Jackson,
  Room 560
Topeka, KS 66612
(785) 296-4056
http://www.kansas.gov/pharmacy/

Kentucky Board of Pharmacy
2624 Research Park Drive, Suite 302
Lexington, KY 40511
(859) 246-2820
http://pharmacy.ky.gov/

Louisiana Board of Pharmacy
5615 Corporate Boulevard, Suite 8E
Baton Rouge, LA 70808
(225) 925-6496
http://www.labp.com

Maine Board of Pharmacy
Department of Professional and Financial
  Regulation
35 State House Station
Augusta, ME 04333
(207) 624-8603
http://maine.gov/pfr/professionallicensing/
  professions/pharmacy/index.htm

Maryland Board of Pharmacy
4201 Patterson Avenue
Baltimore, MD 21215
(410) 764-4755
http://www.mdbop.org/

**Massachusetts Board of Registration in
  Pharmacy**
239 Causeway Street, 2nd Floor, Suite 200
Boston, MA 02114
(617) 973-0950
http://www.mass.gov/reg/boards/ph

Michigan Board of Pharmacy
611 W Ottawa, 1st Floor
P.O. Box 30670
Lansing, MI 48909
(517) 335-0918
http://www.michigan.gov/healthlicense

Minnesota Board of Pharmacy
2829 University Avenue SE, Suite 530
Minneapolis, MN 55414
(651) 201-2825
http://www.phcybrd.state.mn.us

Mississippi Board of Pharmacy
204 Key Drive, Suite D
Madison, MS 39110
(601) 605-5388
http://www.mbp.state.ms.us

Missouri Board of Pharmacy
P.O. Box 625
Jefferson City, MO 65102
(573) 751-0091
http://www.pr.mo.gov/pharmacists.asp

Montana Board of Pharmacy
301 South Park, 4th Floor

P.O. Box 200513
Helena, MT 59620
(406) 841-2371
http://mt.gov/dli/bsd/license/bsd_boards/pha_
    board/board_page.asp

Nebraska Board of Pharmacy
P.O. Box 94986
Lincoln, NE 68509
(402) 471-2118
http://www.hhs.state.ne.us

Nevada State Board of Pharmacy
431 W. Plumb Lane
Reno, NV 89509
(775) 850-1440
http://bop.nv.gov

**State of New Hampshire Board of
    Pharmacy**
57 Regional Drive
Concord, NH 03301
(603) 271-2350
http://www.nh.gov/pharmacy/

New Jersey Board of Pharmacy
P.O. Box 45013
Newark, NJ 07101
(973) 504-6450
http://www.state.nj.us/lps/ca/medical/
    pharmacy.htm

New Mexico Board of Pharmacy
5200 Oakland NE, Suite A
Albuquerque, NM 87113
(505) 222-9830
http://www.rld.state.nm.us/pharmacy/

New York State Board of Pharmacy
89 Washington Avenue, 2nd Floor W
Albany, NY 12234
(518) 474-3817
http://www.op.nysed.gov

North Carolina Board of Pharmacy
P.O. Box 4560
Chapel Hill, NC 27515-4560
(919) 246-1050
http://www.ncbop.org

North Dakota State Board of Pharmacy
P.O. Box 1354
Bismarck, ND 58502
(701) 328-9535
http://www.nodakpharmacy.com

Ohio State Board of Pharmacy
77 S High Street, Room 1702
Columbus, OH 43215-6126
(614) 466-4143
http://www.pharmacy.ohio.gov

Oklahoma State Board of Pharmacy
4545 Lincoln Boulevard, Suite 112
Oklahoma City, OK 73105
(405) 521-3815
http://www.pharmacy.ok.gov

Oregon State Board of Pharmacy
800 NE Oregon Street, Suite 150
Portland, OR 97232
(971) 673-0001
http://www.pharmacy.state.or.us

Pennsylvania State Board of Pharmacy
P.O. Box 2649
Harrisburg, PA 17105
(717) 783-7156
http://www.dos.state.pa.us/pharm

Puerto Rico Board of Pharmacy
Call Box 10200
Santurce, PR 00908
(787) 725-7506
No Web site

Rhode Island Board of Pharmacy
3 Capitol Hill, Room 205
Providence, RI 02908
(401) 222-5960
http://www.health.ri.gov/hsr/professions/
    pharmacy.php

South Carolina Board of Pharmacy
Department of Labor, Licensing,
    and Regulation
Kingstree Building
110 Centerview Drive, Suite 306
Columbia, SC 29210

(803) 896-4700
http://www.llr.state.sc.us/pol/pharmacy

South Dakota State Board of Pharmacy
4305 S Louise Avenue, Suite 104
Sioux Falls, SD 57106
(605) 362-2737
http://doh.sd.gov/boards/pharmacy/

Tennessee Board of Pharmacy
227 French Landing, Suite 300
Nashville, TN 37243
(615) 741-2718
http://health.state.tn.us/Boards/Pharmacy/
    index.shtml

Texas State Board of Pharmacy
333 Guadalupe, Tower 3, Suite 600
Austin, TX 78701
(512) 305-8000
http://www.tsbp.state.tx.us

Utah Board of Pharmacy
Division of Occupational and Professional
    Licensing
P.O. Box 146741
Salt Lake City, UT 84114
(801) 530-6628
http://www.dopl.utah.gov/licensing/pharmacy.
    html

Vermont Board of Pharmacy
Office of Professional Regulation
26 Terrace Street
Montpelier, VT 05609
(802) 828-2373
http://www.vtprofessionals.org/opr1/
    pharmacists/

Virgin Islands Board of Pharmacy
Department of Health
48 Sugar Estate
Saint Thomas, VI 00802
(340) 774-0117
No Web site

Virginia Board of Pharmacy
Perimeter Center
9960 Mayland Drive, Suite 300
Richmond, VA 23233
(804) 367-4456
http://www.dhp.virginia.gov/pharmacy

Washington State Board of Pharmacy
P.O. Box 47863
Olympia, WA 98504
(360) 236-4825
https://fortress.wa.gov/doh/hpqa1/hps4/
    pharmacy/default.htm

West Virginia Board of Pharmacy
232 Capitol Street
Charleston, WV 25301
(304) 558-0558
http://www.wvbop.com

Wisconsin Pharmacy Examining Board
Department of Regulation & Licensing
P.O. Box 8935
Madison, WI 53708
(608) 266-2112
http://drl.wi.gov/boards/phm/index.htm

Wyoming State Board of Pharmacy
1712 Carey Avenue, Suite 200
Cheyenne, WY 82002
(307) 634-9636
http://pharmacyboard.state.wy.us/

APPENDIX IX
PHARMACEUTICAL ASSOCIATIONS AND ORGANIZATIONS

Academy of Managed Care Pharmacy
100 North Pitt Street, Suite 400
Alexandria, VA 22314
(800) 827-2627
(703) 683-8416
http://www.amcp.org

Alliance for the Prudent Use of Antibiotics
75 Kneeland Street
Boston, MA 02111
(617) 636-0966
http://www.tufts.edu/med/apua/

American Association of Colleges of Pharmacy
1727 King Street
Alexandria, VA 22314
(703) 739-2330
http://www.aacp.org

American Association of Pharmaceutical Sales Professionals
2541 IH 35, #176
Round Rock, TX 78664
http://www.pharmaceuticalsales.org

American Association of Pharmaceutical Scientists
2107 Wilson Boulevard, Suite 700
Arlington, VA 22201
(703) 243-2800
http://www.aapspharmaceutica.com

American Association of Pharmacy Technicians
P.O. Box 1447
Greensboro, NC 27402
(877) 368-4771
http://www.pharmacytechnician.com

American Association of Colleges of Pharmacy
1727 King Street
Alexandria, VA 22314
(703) 739-2330
http://www.aacp.org

American College of Apothecaries
P.O. Box 341266
Memphis, TN 38184
(901) 383-8119
http://www.americancollegeofapothecaries.com

American College of Clinical Pharmacy
13000 W. 87th Street Parkway
Lenexa, KS 66215-4530
(913) 492-3311
http://www.accp.com

American Council on Pharmaceutical Education
20 North Clark Street, Suite 2500
Chicago, IL 60602
(312) 664-3575
http://www.acpe-accredit.org

American Institute of the History of Pharmacy
777 Highland Avenue
Madison, WI 53705
(608) 262-5378
http://cms.pharmacy.wisc.edu/aihp

American Pharmacists Association (previously American Pharmaceutical Association)
2215 Constitution Avenue NW
Washington, DC 20037
(202) 628-4410
http://www.pharmacist.com

American Society for Automation in Pharmacy
492 Norristown Road, Suite 160
Blue Bell, PA 19422
(610) 825-7783
http://www.asapnet.org

American Society for Clinical Pharmacology and Therapeutics
528 North Washington Street
Alexandria, VA 22314
(703) 836-5223
http://www.ascpt.org/

American Society for Pharmacology & Experimental Therapeutics
9650 Rockville Pike
Bethesda, MD 20814
(301) 634-7060
http://www.aspet.org

American Society of Consultant Pharmacists
1321 Duke Street
Alexandria, VA 22314
(703) 739-1300
http://www.ascp.com

American Society of Health-System Pharmacists
7272 Wisconsin Avenue
Bethesda, MD 20814
(301) 657-3000
http://www.ashp.org

Association of Natural Medicine Pharmacists
4815 Minneapolis Avenue
Minnetrista, MN 55364
(952) 472-5689
http://www.anmp.org

American Society of Pharmacognosy
3149 Dundee Road, #260
Northbrook, IL 60062
(773) 995-3748
http://www.phcog.org

Board of Pharmaceutical Specialties
1100 15th Street NW, Suite 400
Washington, DC 20005
(202) 429-7591
http://www.bpsweb.org

Center for Medication Use, Policy & Economics
University of Michigan
428 Church Street
Ann Arbor, MI 48109
(734) 764-7312
http://sitemaker.umich.edu/cmupe/cmupe

Commission for Certification in Geriatric Pharmacy
1321 Duke Street, Suite 400
Alexandria, VA 22314
(703) 535-3036
http://www.ccgp.org

Controlled Release Society
3340 Pilot Knob Road
St. Paul, MN 55121
(651) 454-7250
http://www.ccgp.org

Drug, Chemical and Allied Trades Association
One Washington Boulevard, Suite 7
Robbinsville, NJ 08691
(609) 448-1000
http://www.dcat.org

Drug Information Association
800 Enterprise Road, Suite 200
Horsham, PA 19044
(215) 442-6100
http://www.diahome.org

Food and Drug Law Institute
1155 15th Street NW, Suite 800
Washington, DC 20005

(202) 371-1420
http://www.fdli.org

Generic Pharmaceutical Association
2300 Clarendon Boulevard, Suite 400
Arlington, VA 22201
(703) 647-2480
http://www.gphaonline.org

Institute for Safe Medication Practices
200 Lakeside Drive, Suite 200
Horsham, PA 19044-2321
(215) 947-7797
http://www.ismp.org

International Society for Pharmaceutical Engineering
3109 W. Dr. Martin Luther King, Jr. Boulevard, Suite 250
Tampa, FL 33607
(813) 960-2105
http://www.ispe.org

National Association of Boards of Pharmacy
1600 Feehanville Drive
Mount Prospect, IL 60056
(847) 391-4406
http://www.nabp.net

National Association of Chain Drug Stores
413 North Lee Street
P.O. Box 1417-D49
Alexandria, VA 22313
(703) 549-3001
http://www.nacds.org

National Association of Drug Diversion Investigators
1810 York Road #435
Lutherville, MD 21093
http://www.naddi.org

National Association of Pharmaceutical Representatives
2020 Pennsylvania Avenue NW, Suite 5050
Washington, DC 20006
(800) 913-0701
http://www.napsronline.org

National Community Pharmacists Association
100 Daingerfield Road
Alexandria, VA 22314
(703) 683-8200
http://www.ncpanet.org

National Council for Prescription Drug Programs
9240 E Raintree Drive
Scottsdale, AZ 85260
(480) 477-1000
http://www.ncpdp.org

National Pharmaceutical Council
1894 Preston White Drive
Reston, VA 20191-5433
(703) 620-6390
http://www.npcnow.org/Home.aspx

National Pharmacy Technician Association
P.O. Box 683148
Houston, TX 77268
(888) 247-8700
http://www.pharmacytechnician.org

Parenteral Drug Association
Bethesda Towers
4350 East West Highway, Suite 150
Bethesda, MD 20814
(301) 656-5900
http://www.pda.org

Pediatric Pharmacy Advocacy Group
7975 Stage Hills Boulevard, Suite 6
Memphis, TN 38133
(901) 380-3617
http://www.ppag.org

Pharmaceutical Care Management Association
601 Pennsylvania Avenue NW, Suite 740
Washington, DC 20004
(202) 207-3610
http://www.pcmanet.org

Pharmaceutical Research and Manufacturers of America
950 F Street NW

Washington, DC 20004
(202)-835-3400
http://www.phrma.org

Society of Infectious Disease Pharmacists
823 Congress Avenue, Suite 230
Austin, TX 78701
(512) 479-0425
http://www.sidp.org

U.S. Pharmacopeia
12601 Twinbrook Parkway
Rockville, MD 20852
(301) 881-0666
http://www.usp.org

APPENDIX X
DRUG INDUSTRY PUBLICATIONS

American Journal of Health-System Pharmacy
American Society of Health-System Pharmacists
7272 Wisconsin Avenue
Bethesda, MD 20814
http://www.ajhp.org

American Journal of Pharmaceutical Education
American Association of Colleges of Pharmacy
1727 King Street
Alexandria, VA 22314
http://www.ajpe.org

BioPharm International
Advanstar Communications, Inc.
485F U.S. Highway 1 South, Suite 100
Iselin, NJ 08830
http://www.biopharminternational.com

Bioscience Technology
Advantage Business Media
100 Enterprise Drive, Suite 600
Rockaway, NJ 07866
http://www.bioprodmag.com

The Consultant Pharmacist
American Society of Consultant Pharmacists
1321 Duke Street
Alexandria, VA 22314
http://www.ascp.com/articles/
    consultant-pharmacist/nm

Drug Development and Industrial Pharmacy
Taylor & Francis
325 Chestnut Street, # 8
Philadelphia, PA 19106
http://informahealthcare.com/loi/ddi

Drug Discovery & Development
100 Enterprise Drive, Suite 600

Rockaway, NJ 07866
http://www.dddmag.com

Drug Store News
425 Park Avenue
New York, NY 10022
http://www.drugstorenews.com/

Drug Topics
Advanstar Communications, Inc.
24950 Country Club Boulevard, Suite 200
North Olmsted, OH 44070
http://www.drugtopics.com

Formulary
Advanstar Communications, Inc.
24950 Country Club Boulevard, Suite 200
North Olmsted, OH 44070
http://www.formularyjournal.com

Journal of Managed Care Pharmacy
Academy of Managed Care Pharmacy
100 North Pitt Street, Suite 400
Alexandria, VA 22314
http://www.amcp.org/jmcphome.aspx

Journal of Pharmacy Practice
SAGE Publications
2455 Teller Road
Thousand Oaks, CA 91320
http://jpp.sagepub.com/

Pharmaceutical Executive
Advanstar Communications, Inc.
641 Lexington Avenue, 8th Floor
New York, NY 10022
http://www.pharmexec.com

Pharmaceutical Processing
Advantage Business Media
100 Enterprise Drive, Suite 600
Rockaway, NJ 07866
http://www.pharmpro.com

Pharmaceutical Representative
Advanstar Communications, Inc.
641 Lexington Avenue, 8th Floor
New York, NY 10022
http://www.pharmrep.com

Pharmaceutical Technology
Advanstar Communications, Inc.
485 Route One South
Building F, 1st Floor
Iselin, NJ 08830
http://www.pharmtech.com

Pharmacy Times
666 Plainsboro Road, Suite 300
Plainsboro, NJ 08536
http://www.pharmacytimes.com

Rx Times Pharmacy Magazine
200 N Broadway
St. Louis, MO 63102
http://www.rxtimes.com/

U.S. Pharmacist
Jobson Medical Information LLC
160 Chubb Avenue, Suite 306
Lyndhurst, NJ 07071
http://www.uspharmacist.com

APPENDIX XI
GLOSSARY

adjuvant therapy treatment given after the primary treatment to increase the chances of a cure. In cancer treatment, for example, adjuvant therapy may include chemotherapy, radiation therapy, hormone therapy, or biological therapy.

bioavailability the efficiency of a drug in getting into the system; the amount of drug that gets absorbed.

biotherapy treatment with genetically engineered biological materials.

blinding a process used in clinical trials to prevent unintentional bias in the evaluations; it is also referred to as masking. In a single-blind study, one party, either the investigator or participant, is unaware of what medication the participant is taking. In a double-blind study, neither the participating individuals nor the study staff know which participants are receiving the experimental drug and which are receiving a placebo (or another therapy). Double-blind trials are thought to produce more objective results because any expectations of the doctor or the participants about the experimental drug do not affect the outcome. The FDA does not require that a drug study include a placebo group, only that its design be capable of establishing a drug's safety and effectiveness.

cohort study a study in which subjects who presently have a certain condition and/or receive a particular treatment and/or share some other common characteristic are followed over time and compared with another group that is not affected by the condition under investigation.

formulary a list of covered drugs chosen by a health plan or a pharmacy benefit management company's pharmacy and therapeutics (P&T) committee based on effectiveness, safety, and cost considerations.

ex vivo outside of a living organism. Commonly refers to a medical procedure in which an organ, cells, or tissue are taken from a living body for a treatment or procedure and then returned to the living body. Ex vivo cell responses may not be the same as those observed in the more complex in vivo environment.

Gram staining a method of differentiating bacterial species into two large groups (Gram-positive and Gram-negative) based on the chemical and physical properties of their cell walls. Also referred to as Gram's method.

idiopathic a disorder of unknown etiology; no known cause.

incidence a measure of disease that tells the number of newly diagnosed cases during a given time period, usually a year. An incidence rate is the number of new cases of a disease divided by the number of persons at risk for it. If, for example, over the course of one year, five women are diagnosed with breast cancer out of a total female study population of 200 (who do not have breast cancer at the beginning of the study period), then the incidence of breast cancer in this population would be 0.025. (or 2,500 per 100,000 women). Incidence helps determine a person's probability of being diagnosed with a disease during a given period of time. See also **prevalence.**

in vivo occurring in a living body. Animal testing and clinical trials are forms of in vivo research.

in vitro applied to conditions outside the living body, such as in a test tube or other artificial environment.

morbidity   another term for illness. A person can have several comorbidities simultaneously. So, morbidities can range from Alzheimer's disease to cancer to traumatic brain injury. Morbidities are not deaths.

mortality   another term for death. A mortality rate is the number of deaths due to a disease divided by the total population. If there are 25 lung cancer deaths in one year in a population of 30,000, then the mortality rate for that population is 83 per 100,000.

placebo   an inactive pill, liquid, or powder that has no treatment value.

placebo effect   improvement in a patient's condition from a placebo simply because the person thinks he or she is receiving the control drug and so has the expectation that it will be helpful. Research has confirmed that as many as one-third of patients may feel better in response to treatment with placebo. For additional information, see "The Healing Power of Placebos," by Tamar Nordenberg, *FDA Consumer* (January–February 2000). Avail-able online. URL: http://www.fda.gov/fdac/features/2000/100_heal.html. Accessed May 7, 2009.

prevalence   a measure of disease that provides the total number of cases of a given disease existing in a population at any given time. A prevalence rate is the total number of cases of a disease existing in a population divided by the total population. Thus, if a measurement of cancer is taken in a population of 40,000 people and 1,200 were recently diagnosed with cancer and 3,500 are living with cancer, then the prevalence of cancer is 0.118. (or 11,750 per 100,000 persons). Prevalence helps determine a person's likelihood of having a disease. See also **incidence.**

prospective study   investigators follow participants forward in time for weeks, months, or years and record what happens to them, watching for outcomes.

retrospective study   investigators look back at what happened to a group of people in the past, examining exposures to specified risks or protection factors.

APPENDIX XII
PHARMACEUTICAL WEB SITES OF INTEREST

Buying Prescription Medicine Online: A Consumer Safety Guide
http://www.fda.gov/Drugs/ResourcesForYou/ucm080588.htm

ClinicalTrials.gov—Registry of Federally and Privately Supported Clinical Trials
http://www.clinicaltrials.gov

Compare Prescription Drug Prices
http://www.pharmacychecker.com
http://www.pillbot.com
http://www.rxaminer.com/consult/consult_mydrugs.asp

Consumer Education: What You Need to Know to Use Medicine Safely
http://www.fda.gov/Drugs/Emergency
Preparedness/Bioterrorismand
DrugPreparedness/ucm133279.htm

Consumer Reports Best Buy Drugs—Free Guidance for Consumers on Prescription Medicines
http://www.consumerreports.org/health/best-buy-drugs/index.htm

Drug Interactions Checker
http://www.drugs.com/drug_interactions.php

FDA Safety Information and Adverse Event Reporting Program
http://www.fda.gov/medwatch/index.html

National Guideline Clearinghouse Database of Evidence-Based Clinical Practice Guidelines
http://www.guideline.gov

Pharmaceutical & Drug Manufacturers Portal
http://www.pharmaceutical-drug-manufacturers.com

Pharmacy Schools
http://www.uspharmd.com/school/
http://www.pharmacy.org/schools.html

Protecting Yourself: Buying Medicines and Medical Products Online
http://www.fda.gov/ForConsumers/ProtectYourself/default.htm

United States Food and Drug Administration Home Page
http://www.fda.gov

APPENDIX XIII
AUDIOVISUAL MATERIALS

ADDICTION CAUSED BY
MIXING MEDICINES

(VHS or DVD, 19 minutes, unknown date)

Nonaddictive prescription drugs can and often do lead to addiction, and one of the primary dangers of mixing prescription drugs—individually prescribed for specific purposes—is the addictive effect. In this program, an addiction-ologist and a clinical pharmacist explain how mixing medicines can lead to problems, which groupings of drugs are likely to cause problems, and how dangers can be minimized.

ANTIBIOTICS:
THE DOUBLE-EDGED SWORD

(VHS or DVD, 53 minutes, 2003)

Antibiotics initially worked miracles, saving millions of lives. In just decades, many of the wonder drugs are ineffective. How did this happen? This program reports on a battle for survival between humans and microbes, providing a concise history of antibiotics, as well as tracing their decline in efficacy. Their overuse and misuse is examined in medicine, agriculture, and domestic cleaning products. Special attention is given to the world's first case of vancomycin-resistant *Staphylococcus aureus*, or VRSA. Among those who discuss the issue are Dr. Richard Besser, ABC News senior health and medical editor and former director of the Centers for Disease Control's national campaign to reduce antimicrobial resistance, and Dr. Stuart Levy, author of *The Antibiotic Paradox* and founder of the Alliance for the Prudent Use of Antibiotics.

BIOTECHNOLOGY AND YOUR HEALTH:
PHARMACEUTICAL APPLICATIONS

(VHS or DVD, 24 minutes, 2009)

Scientists have come a long, long way since Alexander Fleming's discovery of penicillin, the wonder drug of the 20th century. This program explains the function of infection-fighting antibiotics; vaccinations and insulin, crucial to the prevention of diseases such as smallpox and the management of diabetes; recombinant drugs; treatments involving genetically engineered DNA; and stem cells, those chameleon-like building blocks of the body. Commentary is provided by Drs. James Baker, Brian Athey, and Elliott Hill, of the University of Michigan; Susanne Kleff of MBI International; and Bob Forgey of ProNAi Therapeutics. A Films for the Humanities & Sciences Production.

THE CURE: HEART DISEASE AND
ANTI-CHOLESTEROL DRUGS

(VHS or DVD, 55 minutes, 2005)

Drugs that can cure cardiovascular disease, rather than simply slowing cholesterol buildup, are currently in development. This program examines the history of anti-cholesterol drug production, as well as current biochemical research that might lead to the eradication of heart attacks and strokes. Describing scientific studies of isolated populations—most notably the inhabitants of Limone, Italy, where a genetic mutation has produced a natural cure for arterial plaque accumulation—the video also investigates the extraordinary level of competition that exists among pharmaceutical companies racing to create lifesaving chemical compounds.

CURING CANCER: CLINICAL RESEARCH TRIALS

(VHS or DVD, 28 minutes, 2003)

No drug or medicine has ever been proven safe and effective without a clinical trial. This program demonstrates the vital role of clinical trials in current cancer research, and explains why many medical experts view the clinical trial system as the basis for curing all forms of cancer—or turning it into a manageable disease that patients can live with. Personal testimony from trial participants who have survived lung, breast, and other types of cancer is juxtaposed with the problem of cultural and psychological barriers to participation, providing valuable insight into the sometimes mysterious clinical trial process.

DEATH OF A WONDER DRUG: THE VIOXX RECALL

(VHS or DVD, 44 minutes, 2004)

On September 30, 2004, pharmaceutical giant Merck voluntarily withdrew its popular pain-killer Vioxx after it was linked to increased risks of heart attack and stroke. Was Merck's move driven by genuine concern for patients? Or, given findings from earlier studies, was the recall a self-protective move that came too late? This CNBC investigation takes viewers through the process by which one of Big Pharma's most widely pre-scribed products was tested, approved, and mar-keted—at the expense, many say, of thousands of consumers. Several medical experts provide commentary, in addition to FDA whistle-blower David Graham, who has cited numerous faults in the government's handling of Vioxx testing.

DRUG DANGERS: MEDICAL, LEGAL, AND SOCIAL

(VHS or DVD, 4-part series, 25–30 minutes each part, 2009)

What causes addiction? Is experimenting with drugs just a dangerous gamble or an expressway to the gutter? Can common sense override the urge to rebel and the yearning to fit in? This four-part series reveals the pitfalls of substance abuse in terms of health threats and psychologi-cal problems, as well as the many ways an addict can run afoul of the law and society. Featuring commentary from medical and legal experts and candid testimonials from current and former users, the series shows how easily addiction can occur and explores ways to help those afflicted break their deadly habits. Viewable/printable educational resources are available online.

FIGHTING THE MICROBES: THE HISTORY OF ANTIBIOTICS

(VHS or DVD, 30 minutes, 2006)

The prescription of antibiotics is a medical tightrope walk. The drugs save lives, but because of overuse, may soon usher in a new era of super-germs. This program outlines the discov-eries of bacteria and penicillin and sheds light on the frightening emergence of multi-resistant, often deadly microbes during the last six decades. Presenting interviews with researchers who are deeply involved with the issue, including Tufts University microbiology professor Stuart Levy and Eva Nathanson of the World Health Orga-nization's Stop TB Program, the film examines the implications of antibiotic-enhanced livestock feed and the dangers that staphylococcus poses to hospital patients. Viewer discretion is advised (contains footage of injections, surgeries, and open wounds).

A HISTORY OF ANTIBIOTICS

(VHS or DVD, 47 minutes, 1999)

In this program, experts from the Centers for Disease Control and Prevention, the World Health Organization, and elsewhere use case studies and research findings to discuss key issues in the war against infectious diseases such as pneumococcal meningitis, toxic shock syn-drome, and ulcers. Decades of overuse and mis-use of antibiotics are targeted as key factors in the birth of antibiotic-resistant bacteria and the reemergence of TB, bubonic plague, and other deadly organisms. Factors contributing to the spread of diseases, including crowded day-care facilities and international travel, are also examined, along with the development of the drug Zyvox. Produced by CBS News Productions.

IMPORTING DRUGS: THE CANADIAN CONNECTION

(VHS or DVD, 22 minutes, 2004)

Pharmaceutical prices in the United States are pushing patients to have their prescriptions filled in Canada, where drugs such as Lipitor cost less. Budget-conscious state governments are also eyeing Canadian distributors as a way to manage their prescription plans while making fiscal ends meet. But officially speaking, such transactions are still illegal in the Unite States, and the medicines themselves, traveling outside the domain of the FDA, may not even be safe. In this two-segment program, News-Hour health correspondent Susan Dentzer taps senators, governors, FDA officials, pharmacists, and the CEO of drug manufacturing giant Pfizer to present a balanced view of one of today's most controversial topics.

MULTIPLE MEDS

(VHS or DVD, 24 minutes, 2007)

Confusion over multiple prescriptions and appropriate dosages might seem like a minor nuisance, but it can be dangerous or even fatal. This program explores the challenges that patients often face as they cope with drug interactions. An informative case study features a woman who regularly takes more than 12 medications for various health problems and who, while hospitalized, experienced a drug regimen error that led to cognitive side effects. Guests include Dr. Leslie Brandwin of Erickson Health, who provides essential know-how on properly monitoring drug intake at home and in the hospital, and Anne Burns of the American Pharmacists Association, who discusses the importance of communication between patient, physician, and pharmacist.

NSAID OPTIONS

(VHS or DVD, 28 minutes, 2005)

People who live with chronic pain often face a no-win situation. They usually rely on medications known as NSAIDs or nonsteroidal anti-inflammatory drugs, which, unfortunately, can damage their stomachs and may even threaten their lives. This program details new strategies for helping patients with chronic pain, enabling them to fight it without giving up NSAIDs. Interviews with University of Michigan gastroenterologist James Scheiman and rheumatologist Daniel Clauw shed light on the importance of COX isozymes and the effects of aspirin, ibuprofen, naproxen, and other pain relievers. The use of PPIs, or proton pump inhibitors, is also studied.

PAIN MANAGEMENT: DOCTORS, PATIENTS, AND THE DEA

(VHS or DVD, 22 minutes, 2005)

High-dose pain-management therapy involving narcotics has placed doctors and patients under scrutiny by federal regulators. Is the Drug Enforcement Administration simply cracking down on criminal overprescription and prescription forgery, or is it unfairly targeting doctors for merely doing their jobs, and punishing people with chronic pain? This ABC News program weighs in on the question through interviews with DEA administrator Karen Tandy, a doctor convicted of overprescribing, and a patient serving a 25-year prison sentence for possessing too much pain medication.

PENICILLIN: DISCOVERING THE TRUTH

(VHS or DVD, 51 minutes, 1991)

Although Alexander Fleming is usually credited with the discovery of penicillin in 1928, no penicillin-based antibiotic was actually developed for human use until 1938, through the work of Australian pathologist Howard Florey and German biochemist Ernst Chain. This program puts Fleming's contribution in scientific perspective. Live interviews, journal accounts, and archival footage lead the viewer through the discovery of the drug from a by-product of the tiny fungus *Penicillium notatum*. The roles played by luck, politics, and society both in scientific research and bestowing credit for the discovery are explored. Original BBC broadcast title: *The Mold, the Myth and the Microbe.*

PHARMACOLOGY

(VHS or DVD, 23 minutes, 1989)

Modern medicine owes much of its success to drugs. How do these chemical molecules treat and cure aches and illnesses? This program explains that these substances are usually "copies" of natural substances produced by our own bodies. We witness the invention of a new drug by two researchers working at a major pharmaceutical laboratory. Finally, we are introduced to some promising new weapons against cancer—drugs designed to zero in on cancer cells and destroy them.

PRESCRIPTION FOR TROUBLE

(VHS or DVD, 26 minutes, 2003)

Taking medicine is ingrained in American culture. Is it any surprise, then, that adolescents are abusing prescription and over-the-counter drugs in record numbers? In this program, recovering teenage addicts come clean about which medications they abused, when and why they started, and how their addictions severely damaged their lives, while frontline experts from schools and the medical community—including a substance abuse counselor, a child psychologist, and an adolescent psychiatrist—fill in the blanks about the effects of America's medicine mindset. A Discovery Channel Production.

PRESCRIPTION MEDICATIONS: A PATIENT'S PRIMER

(VHS or DVD, 24 minutes, 2003)

With thousands of prescription drugs on the market, patients, physicians, and pharmacists must work together as never before to ensure that medicines yield their intended effects without exposing those taking them to unnecessary health risks. This overview of prescription medications emphasizes the dangers of interactions between prescription drugs and other prescription drugs, over-the-counter medications, herbal and dietary supplements, and foods and beverages. Patient involvement through sharing information with the health-care team, accepting accountability for compliance with the dosage regimen, and becoming informed of drug side effects is stressed.

REVOLUTIONIZING "CHEMO"

(VHS or DVD, 28 minutes, 2000)

The word conjures fears of debilitation and hair loss, but today's "chemo" treatments are far more endurable than in past decades. This program explores advances in chemotherapy that have transformed dread into relief for many cancer patients. The video shows how chemo medications are administered and how, unlike past regimens, which forced a high number of patients to quit or delay therapy, new drugs have reduced nausea, fatigue, and other side effects. Dr. Lee Schwartzberg of the West Clinic and oncology dietician Debi Kreiman of the Memorial Cancer Institute explain how chemo patients can remain active, eat properly, and maintain an attractive appearance.

APPENDIX XIV
BIBLIOGRAPHY—ARTICLES IN JOURNALS

Altman, R. D., and H. R. Barthel. "Topical Therapies for Osteoarthritis." *Drugs* 71, no. 21 (July 9, 2011): 1,259–1,279.

Astrand, P. "Avoiding Drug-Drug Interactions." *Chemotherapy* 55, no. 4 (May 12, 2009): 215–220.

Bradbury, J. "Beyond Pills and Jabs. Researchers Develop New Ways to Get Drugs to the Right Place at the Right Time." *Lancet* 362, no. 9400 (December 13, 2003): 1,984–1,985.

Calmy, A., B. Hirschel, D. A. Cooper, and A. Carr. "A New Era of Antiretroviral Drug Toxicity." *Antiviral Therapy* 14, no. 2 (2009): 165–179.

Corsonello, A., C. Pedone, F. Lattanzio, M. Lucchetti, S. Garasto, C. Carbone, C. Greco, P. Fabbietti, and R. A. Incalzi. "Regimen Complexity and Medication Nonadherence in Elderly Patients." *Therapeutics and Clinical Risk Management* 5, no. 1 (February 2009): 209–216.

Cullen, G., E. Kelly, and F. E. Murray. "Patients' Knowledge of Adverse Reactions to Current Medications." *British Journal of Clinical Pharmacology* 62, no. 2 (August 2006): 232–236.

Ezziane, Z. "Challenging Issues in Molecular-Targeted Therapy." *Therapeutics and Clinical Risk Management* 5, no. 1 (February 2009): 239–245.

Fleming, W. K. "Pharmacy Management Strategies for Improving Drug Adherence." *Journal of Managed Care Pharmacy* 14, no. 6 Suppl. B (July 2008): 16–20.

Galimberti, D., and E. Scarpini. "Disease-Modifying Treatments for Alzheimer's Disease." *Therapeutic Advances in Neurological Disorders* 4, no. 4 (July 2011): 203–216.

Gjesdal, K. "Non-investigational Antiarrhythmic Drugs: Long-term Use and Limitations." *Expert Opinion on Drug Safety* 8, no. 3 (May 2009): 345–355.

Haaheim, L. R. "Vaccines for an Influenza Pandemic: Scientific and Political Challenges." *Influenza Other Respiratory Viruses* 1, no. 2 (March 2007): 55–60.

Hunt, R. H., A. Lanas, D. O. Stichtenoth, and C. Scarpignato. "Myths and Facts in the Use of Anti-inflammatory Drugs." *Annals of Medicine* 41, no. 6 (2009): 423–437.

Jiang, W., B. Y. Kim, J. T. Rutka, and W. C. Chan. "Advances and Challenges of Nanotechnology-Based Drug Delivery Systems." *Expert Opinion on Drug Delivery* 4, no. 6 (November 2007): 621–633.

Martin, C. M. "Prescription Drug Abuse in the Elderly." *The Consultant Pharmacist* 23, no. 12 (December 2008): 941–942.

Martinez, L. S., and N. Lewis. "The Role of Direct-to-Consumer Advertising in Shaping Public Opinion Surrounding Prescription Drug Use to Treat Depression or Anxiety in Youth." *Journal of Health Communication* 14, no. 3 (April–May 2009): 249–261.

Owen, A. and S. H. Khoo. "Pharmacogenetics of Anti-retroviral Agents." *Current Opinion in HIV and AIDS* 3, no. 3 (May 2008): 288–295.

Palmer, A. M. "Pharmacotherapy for Multiple Sclerosis: Progress and Prospects." *Current Opinion in Investigational Drugs* 10, no. 5 (May 2009): 407–417.

Patrono, C., and B. Rocca. "Nonsteroidal Antiinflammatory Drugs: Past, Present and Future." *Pharmacological Research* 59, no. 5 (May 2009): 285–289.

Pedan, A., J. Lu, and L. T. Varasteh. "Assessment of Drug Consumption Patterns for Medicare Part D Patients." *American Journal of Managed Care* 15, no. 5 (May 2009): 323–327.

Pedersen, C. A., P. J. Schneider, and D. J. Scheckelhoff. "ASHP National Survey of Pharmacy Practice in Hospital Settings: Dispensing and Administration—2008." *American Journal of Health-System Pharmacy* 66, no. 10 (May 2009): 926–946.

Rosen, H., and T. Abribat. "The Rise and Rise of Drug Delivery." *Nature Reviews. Drug Discovery* 4, no. 5 (May 2005): 381–385.

Solomon, M. D., D. P. Goldman, G. F. Joyce, and J. J. Escarce. "Cost Sharing and the Initiation of Drug Therapy for the Chronically Ill." *Archives of Internal Medicine* 169, no. 8 (April 27, 2009): 740–749.

van der Most, P. J., A. M. Dolga, I. M. Nijholt, P. G. Luiten, and U. L. Eisel. "Statins: Mechanisms of Neuroprotection." *Progress in Neurobiology* 88, no. 1 (May 2009): 64–75.

APPENDIX XV
BIBLIOGRAPHY—BOOKS

Angell, Marcia. *The Truth about the Drug Companies.* New York: Random House Trade Paperbacks, 2005.

Campbell, John J. *Understanding Pharma.* 2nd ed. Raleigh, N.C.: Pharmaceutical Institute, 2008.

Critser, Greg. *Generation Rx: How Prescription Drugs Are Altering American Lives, Minds, and Bodies.* Boston: Mariner Books, 2007.

DiPiro, Joseph, Robert L. Talbert, Gary Yee, Gary Matzke, Barbara Wells, and L. Michael Posey. *Pharmacotherapy: A Pathophysiologic Approach.* 8th ed. New York: McGraw-Hill Medical, 2011.

Figg, William D., and Cindy H. Chau. *Get into Pharmacy School: Rx for Success!* 3rd ed. New York: Kaplan Publishing, 2011.

Gallagher, Jason, and Conan MacDougall. *Antibiotics Simplified.* 2nd ed. Sudbury, Mass.: Jones and Bartlett Learning, 2011.

Jackson, Stephen, Paul Jansen, and Arduino Mangoni, eds. *Prescribing for Elderly Patients.* Hoboken, N.J.: John Wiley & Sons, 2009.

Kelly, William N. *Pharmacy: What It Is and How It Works.* 2nd Ed. Boca Raton, Fla.: CRC Press, 2006.

Koda-Kimble, Mary Anne, Lloyd Yee Young, Wayne A. Kradjan, B. Joseph Guglielmo, and Brian K. Alldredge, eds. *Applied Therapeutics: The Clinical Use of Drugs.* 9th Ed. Philadelphia: Lippincott Williams & Wilkins, 2008.

Llenz, Thomas L. *Lifestyle Modifications in Pharmacotherapy.* Philadelphia: Lippincott Williams & Wilkins, 2007.

Linn, William, Marion Wofford, Mary Elizabeth O'Keefe, and L. Michael Posey. *Pharmacotherapy in Primary Care.* New York: McGraw-Hill Medical, 2008.

Madsen, Ulf, Povl Krogsgaard-Larsen, and Kristian Stromgaard. *Textbook of Drug Design and Discovery.* 4th Ed. Boca Raton, Fla.: CRC Press, 2009.

Nahler, Gerhard. *Dictionary of Pharmaceutical Medicine.* 2nd Ed. New York: Springer, 2009.

Orum-Alexander, Gail, and James Minzer. *Pharmacy Technician: Practice and Procedures w/Student CD.* New York: McGraw-Hill Career Education, 2010.

Posey, L. Michael. *Pharmacy: An Introduction to the Profession.* 2nd ed. Washington, D.C.: American Pharmacists Association, 2008.

Rees, Hedley. *Supply Chain Management in the Drug Industry: Delivering Patient Value for Pharmaceuticals and Biologics.* Hoboken, N.J.: John Wiley & Sons, 2011.

Reiss, Barry S., and Gary D. Hall. *Guide to Federal Pharmacy Law.* 7th ed. Boynton Beach, Fla.: Apothecary Press, 2010.

Shargel, Leon, Alan H. Mutnick, Paul F. Souney, and Larry N. Swanson. *Comprehensive Pharmacy Review.* 7th Ed. Philadelphia: Lippincott Williams & Wilkins, 2009.

Thompson, Judith E., and Lawrence Davidow. *A Practical Guide to Contemporary Pharmacy Practice.* 3rd Ed. Philadelphia: Lippincott Williams & Wilkins, 2009

Wells, Barbara, Joseph DiPiro, Terry Schwinghammer, and Cecily DiPiro. *Pharmacotherapy Handbook.* 8th Ed. New York: McGraw-Hill Medical, 2011.

Winter, Michael E. *Basic Clinical Pharmacokinetics.* 5th Ed. Philadelphia: Lippincott Williams & Wilkins, 2009.

INDEX

Note: **Boldface** page numbers indicate extensive treatment of a topic.

A

abacavir 230–234, 238
abacavir/lamivudine 230, 238
abacavir/lamivudine/zidovudine
 230, 238
abatacept 280–291
Abbokinase. *See* urokinase
Abbreviated New Drug Application
 (ANDA) xlvii, lvii–lviii
abbreviations, ambiguous lxviii
abciximab 210–215
Abelcet. *See* amphotericin B, lipid-
 based
Abilify. *See* aripiprazole
Abraxane. *See* paclitaxel
absorption xxii
abuse, drug lxxxiii–lxxxiv
ACAM 2000. *See* smallpox vaccine
acarbose 81, 83, 91
Accelerated Approval lvii
Acclaim (antianginal) 19–20
Accolate. *See* zafirlukast
Accupril. *See* quinapril
acebutolol 128
ACE inhibitors. *See* angiotensin-
 converting enzyme inhibitors
Aceon. *See* perindopril
acetaminophen
 as analgesic 7–14
 as antimigraine agent 140
acetazolamide 64–71
acetohexamide 81, 90
acetylcholine chloride 263–270
acetylcysteine 338–344
achexin 196
Achromycin. *See* tetracycline
acid-suppressives **1–6**
 administration of 2–3
 approved uses of 2
 cautions and concerns with 3

classes of 1–2
companion drugs with 2
contraindications to 3–4
demographics and cultural
 factors 5
development history of 5
interactions of 4
mechanisms of action 2
off-label uses of 2
sales/statistics 4–5
side effects of 4
warnings on 3
Aciphex. *See* rabeprazole
Aclovate. *See* alclometasone
acrivastine 117, 118
acrivastine/pseudoephedrine 118
Actemra. *See* tocilizumab
ACTH. *See* adrenocorticotropin
 hormone
ActHIB. *See Haemophilus* b conjugate
 vaccine
Actiq. *See* fentanyl
Activase. *See* alteplase
Actonel. *See* risedronate
Actoplus Met. *See* pioglitazone plus
 metformin
Actos. *See* pioglitazone
acyclovir 243–250
Adacel. *See* diphtheria and tetanus
 toxoids and acellular pertussis
 vaccine adsorbed
Adalat CC. *See* nifedipine
adalimumab 280–291, 305–313
Adams, Samuel Hopkins xliv
Adderall. *See* dextroamphetamine
 saccharate
Adderall XR. *See*
 dextroamphetamine saccharate
addiction xxv
adefovir dipivoxil 242–250

Adenocard. *See* adenosine
adenosine 28–35
adenosine diphosphate receptor
 antagonists 210
Adipex-P. *See* phentermine
adjuvant therapy 152
ADME (absorption, distribution,
 metabolism, excretion) xxii–xxiii
adrenocorticotropin hormone
 (ACTH) 272–276
Adrucil. *See* fluorouracil
adsorbents, intestinal 92–95
Advair. *See* salmeterol/fluticasone
adverse drug reactions/events lxxii–
 lxxiv
advertising lxv–lxvii
Advicor. *See* lovastatin/niacin
Advil. *See* ibuprofen
Advil Migraine 140
Advisory Committee on
 Investigational Drugs xlvii
Aerobid. *See* flunisolide
Aerospan. *See* flunisolide
Afeditab CR. *See* nifedipine
Afinitor. *See* everolimus
Afluria. *See* influenza virus vaccine
 trivalent inactivated
Afrin Original. *See* oxymetazoline
Aggrastat. *See* tirofiban
Aggrenox. *See* dipyrimadole/aspirin
AIDS 230
Akineton. *See* biperiden
Alavert. *See* loratadine
albaconazole 113
Albert, Adrien 271
Albright, Fuller 228, 358
albuterol 251–254
albuterol/ipratropium 251, 252, 254
alclometasone 272
Aldactone. *See* spironolactone